# Surgical Innovations in Glaucoma

John R. Samples  •  Iqbal Ike K. Ahmed

Editors

# Surgical Innovations in Glaucoma

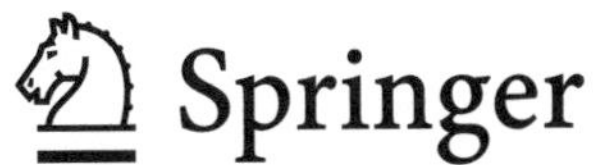 Springer

*Editors*
John R. Samples, MD
Department of Surgery
Rocky Vista University
Parker, CO
USA

Western Glaucoma Foundation
Portland, OR
USA

Cornea Consultants of Colorado
Littleton, CO
USA

The Eye Clinic
Portland, OR
USA

Iqbal Ike K. Ahmed, MD, FRCSC
Department of Ophthalmology
and Vision Sciences
University of Toronto
Toronto, ON
Canada

Videos to this book can be accessed at http://www.springerimages.com/videos/978-1-4614-8347-2

Corrected at 2nd printing 2014

ISBN 978-1-4939-4554-2        ISBN 978-1-4614-8348-9    (eBook)
DOI 10.1007/978-1-4614-8348-9
Springer New York Heidelberg Dordrecht London

# The Wisdom in Putting Clinical Innovation in Glaucoma Surgery Together

Trabeculectomy has been a gold standard for almost 100 years. We believe that many of the emerging technologies can offer significant improvements for our patients. In this volume, we seek to present the most significant new technologies offering promise for glaucoma surgery; some are still investigational, and some are already on the market. These alternatives raise a host of issues which we seek to address throughout the book. We are confident that many of the technologies in this volume will prevail and go on to become mainstream over time. In many instances, these are the first reviews of new devices. Authors have been asked to provide videos, and we provide links to those videos. We will include videos which will really work at the "how to" level for those interested in doing these procedures.

The new approaches described herein use laser, ultrasound, and incisional surgery. In many instances, the new technologies use fibers, stents, or tubes in Schlemm's canal, the suprachoroidal space, or the subconjunctival space. At the outset, we have provided a discussion of anatomy of these spaces, as well as a discussion of the intellectual property issues and regulatory issues pertinent to glaucoma. Regulatory issues for approval of the devices are rapidly changing, and we realize, as we hope the reader will, the limitations of discussing them in a book, which de facto, in this rapidly changing environment, means some elements are subject to going out-of-date.

In the middle of the book, we include a cross section of the therapeutic targets which include the subconjunctival space with improved forms of filtration, Schlemm's canal and its collector channels, the suprachoroidal space, and the ciliary body. These areas are treated with a variety of modalities, each with its own potential pitfalls. A uniform goal for all the procedures is for them to be routine and efficiently performed. Glaucoma is a worldwide problem, and the best and most successful procedures will be those which can succeed with a variety of skill levels in a variety of environments, including third-world settings.

All procedures need to be evaluated while thinking about the risk/reward/effort balance. Risk must always be balanced against the natural history of the disease in glaucoma, as well as the type of glaucoma. Even open-angle glaucoma is really a group of diseases as proven by the genes which have been discovered. Often, glaucoma surgeons get trapped in a rut of doing the most familiar procedure; we need to customize procedures to the life of the patient taking into account expectations, progression, and the surgical risks.

A lot of the things in this book are going to be used outside of their approved use(s) in the USA. Cost and regulatory issues remain concerns with these new procedures. Data needs to constantly be reevaluated keeping in mind our responsibility to do the best that we can for the patient. In some instances, the best available data may suggest "off-label" use which is permitted in the USA when it is clearly in the best interest of the patient. However, going off-label with any drug or device must always be well documented so that the patient and the patient's family have a clear understanding of the reasons for going off-label. As of our December 2013 publication date, off-label use can be discussed in the context of continuing medical education lectures but not in promotional discussions of products. The legal landscape of off-label discussions may be changing with the current finding (subject to reversal) in a federal court that off-label discussions may be constitutionally protected free speech in the USA. Transparency through candid and accurate discussions with patients of potential surgical procedures is an important part of the implementation of these new devices.

These new techniques throw into question long-standing assumptions which – in light of new technologies – need to be challenged. We have both often taught our children to question authority (often, but not always, with good results). Phacoemulsification and the development of the posterior chamber lens are good examples. These hallmark developments in ophthalmology were not well received at inception. It was only with time that they were accepted, particularly by the ophthalmic academic community. Don't forget that phacoemulsification was initially perceived to be almost impossibly difficult to do. Yet, today, it is practically the standard of care and complications are rare. So it will be with some of the procedures outlined in this book.

We thank Rebekah Amos and Daniel Dominguez for their help in assembling this book. We thank all of the chapter authors, some of whom had to put up with all sorts of questions and harassment; they were very kind to put up with us. We thank our families for putting up with us (for JRS that means Griff, Wes, Laura, Andrew, and Lily, and for IKA that means Ruby, Yusuf, Aadam, and Issa).

This book is not comprehensive. At the time we are writing this, we are aware of a number of very new endeavors to surgically treat glaucoma that are not yet ready to be discussed in a volume such as this. Some will undoubtedly find their way "onto the radar" in the very near future.

We thank you who have purchased this book. We are both extremely interested in your feedback on this volume and hope that when you see us at glaucoma meetings you won't hesitate to visit with us about what we could have done better or worse so that we can improve in the future.

Portland, OR, USA                                                    John R. Samples, MD
Toronto, ON, Canada                                       Iqbal Ike K. Ahmed, MD, FRCSC

# Contents

**Part IV    Internal Outflow Enhancement**



**Part V    External Outflow Enhancement**



**Part VI    Suprchoroidal Outflow Devices**



**Part VII    Cataract Surgery**



**Part VIII    Future Developments**

# Contributors

**Iqbal Ike K. Ahmed, MD, FRCSC** Department of Ophthalmology and Vision Sciences, University of Toronto, Toronto, ON, Canada

**Florent Aptel, MD, PhD** Department of Ophthalmology, University Hospital of Grenoble, Grenoble, France

**Michael S. Berlin, MD, MS** Glaucoma Institute of Beverly Hills, Jules Stein Eye Institute, UCLA, Los Angeles, CA, USA

**Toby Yiu Bong Chan, MD, FRCSC** Division of Ophthalmology, Department of Surgery, McMaster University, Waterloo Regional Campus, Kitchener, ON, Canada

**Nathalie J.M. Collignon, MD, PhD** Division of Neuro-Ophthalmology and Glaucoma, Department of Ophthalmology, University Hospital of Liège, Liège, Belgium

**E. Randy Craven, MD** Division of Glaucoma, Department of Ophthalmology, Wilmer Eye Institute at Johns Hopkins University, King Khaled Eye Specialist Hospital, Baltimore, MD, USA

**Philippe Denis, MD, PhD** Department of Ophthalmology, University Hospital of Lyon, Hôpital de la Croix-Rousse, Lyon, France

**Giorgio Dorin** Clinical Applications Development, IRIDEX Corporation, Mountain View, CA, USA

**Rich A. Eiferman, MD, FACS** Department of Ophthalmology, University of Louisville, Louisville, KY, USA

**Antonio Fea, MD, PhD** Clinica Oculistica-Universita' di Torino, Ospedale Oftalmico, Torino, Italy

**Ronald Leigh Fellman, MD** Department of Ophthalmology, Glaucoma Associates of Texas, Eye Institute of Texas, Dallas, TX, USA

Department of Ophthalmology, University of Texas Southwestern Medical Center, Dallas, TX, USA

**Andrew Francis, MD** Department of Ophthalmology and Visual Sciences, University of Illinois at Chicago, Chicago, IL, USA

**Jeffrey Freedman, MBBCh, FRCS (Edin), FCS (SA)** Department of Ophthalmology, SUNY, Downstate University Hospital, Brooklyn, NY, USA

**Ulrich Giers, MD** Augen-klinik OWL, Detmold, Germany

**Ivan Goldberg, AM, MBBS, FRANZCO, FRACS** Department of Ophthalmology, Sydney Eye Hospital, Sydney, NSW, Australia

**Haiyan Gong, MD, PhD** Department of Ophthalmology, Boston University School of Medicine, Boston, MA, USA

**Judy F. Gordon, DVM** ClinReg Consulting Services, Inc., Laguna Beach, CA, USA

**Veva De Groot, MD, PhD** Department of Ophthalmology, University Hospital Antwerp, Edegem, Belgium

**Algis Grybauskas** Department of Ophthalmology and Visual Sciences, University of Illinois at Chicago, Chicago, IL, USA

**David Haffner** Vice President, Product Development, Glaukos Corp., Laguna Hills, CA, USA

**Richard A. Hill, MD** Orange County Glaucoma Inc., Santa Anna, CA, USA

**Christopher Horvath, PhD** AqueSys, Inc, Aliso Viejo, CA, USA

**Guofu Huang, MD, PhD** Department of Ophthalmology, University of California, San Francisco, CA, USA

State Key Laboratory of Ophthalmology, Zhongshan Ophthalmic Center, Sun Yat-sen University, Guangzhou, China

**Tsontcho Ianchulev, MD, MPH** Department of Ophthalmology, University of California, San Francisco (UCSF), San Francisco, CA, USA

**Parul Ichhpujani, MS, MD** Glaucoma Service, Department of Ophthalmology, Level III, Block D, Government Medical College and Hospital, Chandigarh, India

**Jeffrey A. Kammer, MD** Department of Ophthalmology and Visual Sciences, Vanderbilt Eye Institute, Vanderbilt University Medical Center, Nashville, TN, USA

**Kevin Kaplowitz, MD** Department of Ophthalmology, Health Sciences Center, Stony Brook University, Stony Brook, NY, USA

**Toshimitsu Kasuga, MD** Department of Ophthalmology, University of California, San Francisco, CA, USA

Department of Ophthalmology, Juntendo University School of Medicine, Tokyo, Japan

**Edward Kim, BA** Glaucoma Institute of Beverly Hills, Los Angeles, CA, USA

**Paul A. Knepper, MD, PhD** Department of Ophthalmology and Visual Sciences, University of Illinois at Chicago, Chicago, IL, USA

Department of Ophthalmology, Northwestern University Medical School, Chicago, IL, USA

**Robert L. Kramm, MD, MSE** ClinReg Consulting Services, Inc., Ft. Lauderdale, FL, USA

**Paulius V. Kuprys** Department of Ophthalmology and Visual Sciences, University of Illinois at Chicago, Chicago, IL, USA

**Gabrielle LaHatte** Formerly a Staff Attorney with Tarolli, Sundheim, Covell & Tummino, LLP, Cleveland, OH, USA

**Graham A. Lee, MBBS (Qld), MD, FRANZCO** Department of Ophthalmology, City Eye Center, University of Queensland, Brisbane, QLD, Australia

**Shan C. Lin, MD** Department of Ophthalmology, University of California, San Francisco, CA, USA

**Nils A. Loewen, MD, PhD** Department of Ophthalmology, University of Pittsburgh School of Medicine, Pittsburgh, PA, USA

**Steven L. Mansberger, MD, MPH** Devers Eye Institute at Legacy Health, Portland, OR, USA

**Andrew J. Marshall, PhD** Healionics Corporation, Seattle, WA, USA

**Lindsay A. McGrath, MBBS** Department of Ophthalmology, City Eye Center, University of Queensland, Brisbane, QLD, Australia

**Shlomo Melamed, MD** The Sam Rothberg Glaucoma Center, Goldschleger Eye Institute, Sheba Medical Center, Tel Aviv University, Tel Hashomer, Ramat Gan, Israel

**Marlene R. Moster, MD** Anne and William Goldberg Glaucoma Service, Wills Eye Institute, Jefferson Medical College, Philadelphia, PA, USA

**Peter A. Netland, MD, PhD** Department of Ophthalmology, University of Virginia School of Medicine, Charlottesville, VA, USA

**Sayeh Pourjavan, MD, PhD** Department of Ophthalmology, Cliniques Universitaires St. Luc, UCL, Brussels, Belgium

**Cecile J. Roy, PhD** iSTAR Medical SA, Isnes, Belgium

**John R. Samples, MD** Department of Surgery, Rocky Vista University, Parker, CO, USA

Western Glaucoma Foundation, Portland, OR, USA

Cornea Consultants of Colorado, Littleton, CO, USA

The Eye Clinic, Portland, OR, USA

**J. Wesley Samples** Formerly an Intellectual Property Litigation Associate with Klarquist Sparkman, LLP, Portland, OR, USA

**Donald Schwartz, MD, OD, MPA, MOpt** Department of Ophthalmology, Long Beach EyeCare Associates, Long Beach, CA, USA

**Shakeel Shareef, MD** Flaum Eye Institute, University of Rochester Medical Center, School of Medicine and Dentistry, Rochester, NY, USA

**Alon Skaat, MD** New York Eye & Ear Infirmary, New York, NY, USA

The Sam Rothberg Glaucoma Center, Goldschleger Eye Institute, Sheba Medical Center, Tel Aviv University, Tel Hashomer, Ramat Gan, Israel

**Kevin Skuran** Department of Ophthalmology and Visual Sciences, University of Illinois, Chicago, IL, USA

**Diamond Y. Tam, MD** Department of Ophthalmology, University of Toronto, Toronto, ON, Canada

**Marc Töteberg-Harms, MD** Department of Ophthalmology, University Hospital Zurich, Zurich, Switzerland

**Vanessa I. Vera, MD** Unidad Oftalmologica De Caracas, Caracas, Venezuela

**Lilit Voskanyan, MD, PhD** Glaucoma, S.V. Malayan Eye Center, Yerevan, Arabkir, Armenia

**Iris Vuong** Glaucoma Institute of Beverly Hills, Los Angeles, CA, USA

# Part I

# Considerations in Device Development

# Schlemm's Canal and Collector Channels as Therapeutic Targets

Haiyan Gong and Andrew Francis

## Introduction

Intraocular pressure (IOP) is maintained within a normal range from a dynamic balance between aqueous humor formation and drainage. Dysfunctional aqueous drainage results in elevated IOP, which is a causative risk factor for the development and progression of primary open-angle glaucoma (POAG) [1]. An understanding of how to lower IOP using microinvasive glaucoma surgery (MIGS) begins with an understanding of the normal anatomy of the structures related to the drainage of aqueous humor and changes in POAG. The major drainage structures for aqueous humor are the conventional or trabecular outflow pathway, which is comprised of the uveal and corneoscleral portions of the trabecular meshwork, the juxtacanalicular connective tissue, Schlemm's canal, the collector channels, and the aqueous veins. Aqueous humor drains from the anterior chamber through progressively smaller channels of the trabecular meshwork into a circumferentially-oriented channel called Schlemm's canal. From this canal, circuitous channels weave toward the surface of the sclera, ultimately joining the episcleral vasculature which drains into the venous system. Flow through this system is driven by a bulk-flow pressure gradient, and active transport is not involved as neither metabolic poisons nor temperature affects this system to any significant degree [2, 3]. 10–20 % of total aqueous outflow has been reported to leave the normal eye via the uveoscleral

pathway [4, 5] which has become a primary target for medical intervention in glaucoma. However, this chapter will only focus on the conventional trabecular outflow pathway.

## Normal Anatomy of Aqueous Outflow Pathway

### Trabecular Meshwork

The trabecular meshwork (TM) is a triangular-shaped band of tissue encircling the anterior chamber angle (Figs. 1.1 and 1.2). The apex of the triangle is attached to the terminal edge of Descemet's membrane of the cornea which is termed Schwalbe's line. From this point of origin, the TM expands as it bridges the iridocorneal angle and ends posteriorly by blending with the stroma of the iris, ciliary body, and scleral spur. The scleral spur projects like a shelf onto the base of this triangle and also serves as a point of insertion for the longitudinal bundle of the ciliary muscle. The length of the TM from Schwalbe's line to the scleral spur is $694.9 \pm 109$ μm in men and $713.2 \pm 107$ μm in women by histological assessment [8]. Using optical coherence tomography (OCT), the mean length of the TM was found to be $466.9 \pm 60.7$ μm in vivo [9]. An imaginary line drawn from Schwalbe's line to the tip of the scleral spur separates the TM into two major parts. The portions of the TM external to the imaginary line include the corneoscleral meshwork, the juxtacanalicular tissue, and Schlemm's canal. The portion of the TM closer to the anterior chamber internal to this imaginary line is termed the uveal meshwork because it extends from Schwalbe's line to the stromas of the ciliary body and iris (Figs. 1.1 and 1.2). Uveal meshwork is readily viewed gonioscopically.

It is important to understand the relationship of the anterior chamber angle structures as viewed from at least two perspectives—the view obtained from meridional sections and the view obtained gonioscopically. These two views are compared in Figs. 1.3 and 1.4. Figure 1.3 shows a macrophotograph of the angle in a meridional view, while Fig. 1.4 depicts an en


H. Gong, MD, PhD (✉)
Department of Ophthalmology, Boston University School of Medicine, 72 East Concord Street, L-905, Boston, MA 02118, USA
e-mail: hgong@bu.edu

A. Francis, MD
Department of Ophthalmology and Visual Sciences, University of Illinois at Chicago, 1855 West Polk St, Chicago, IL 60612, USA
e-mail: afranc1@uic.edu



J.R. Samples, I.I.K. Ahmed (eds.), *Surgical Innovations in Glaucoma*,
DOI 10.1007/978-1-4614-8348-9_1, © Springer Science+Business Media New York 2014

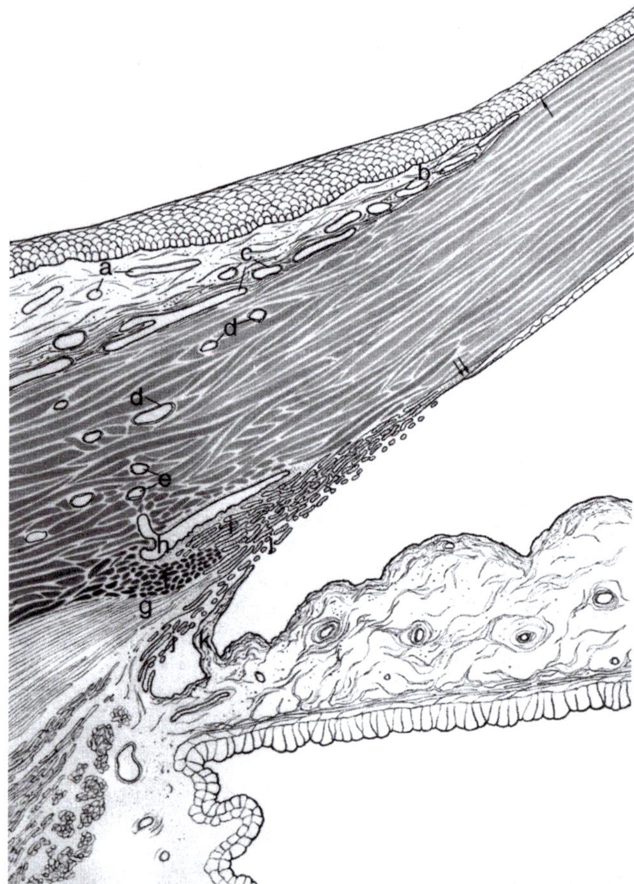

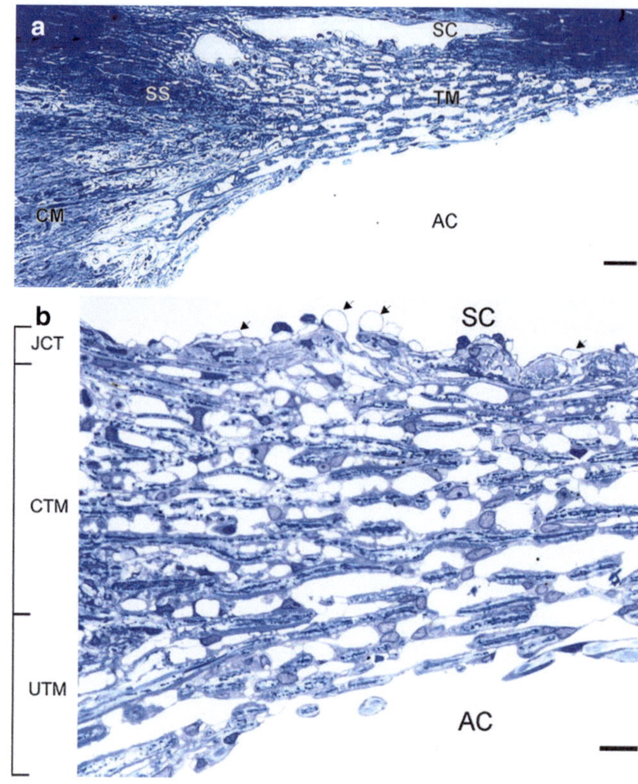


**Fig. 1.1** Drawing of the limbus to illustrate structures evident by microscopic examination. (**a**) Conjunctival vessels, (**b**) corneal arcades, (**c**) episcleral vessels, (**d**) intrascleral plexus, (**e**) deep scleral plexus, (**f**) scleral spur, (**g**) longitudinal bundle of the ciliary muscle, (**h**) canal of Schlemm, (**i**) trabecular meshwork, (**j**) ciliary body band, (**k**) iris process. *Single arrow* represents the terminus of Bowman's membrane and *double arrow* represents the terminus of Descemet's membrane, also known as Schwalbe's line (Modified from Hogan et al. [6])

**Fig. 1.2** Light micrograph of a meridional section of the trabecular meshwork. (**a**) Light micrograph of the anterior chamber angle is shown. Schlemm's canal (*SC*) appears in the plane of section with two lumens that are separated by a septum. The ciliary muscle (*CM*), scleral spur (*SS*), and trabecular meshwork (*TM*) are labeled. (**b**) The trabecular meshwork is shown. From proximal to distal, the uveal trabecular meshwork (*UTM*), the corneoscleral trabecular meshwork (*CTM*), and the juxtacanalicular tissue (*JCT*) are labeled. Giant vacuoles in the inner-wall endothelium of SC are also present (*arrows*). The anterior chamber (*AC*) and Schlemm's canal (*SC*) are also labeled. Magnification bars: 20 mm (**a**), 5 mm (**b**) (Modified from Tamm [7])

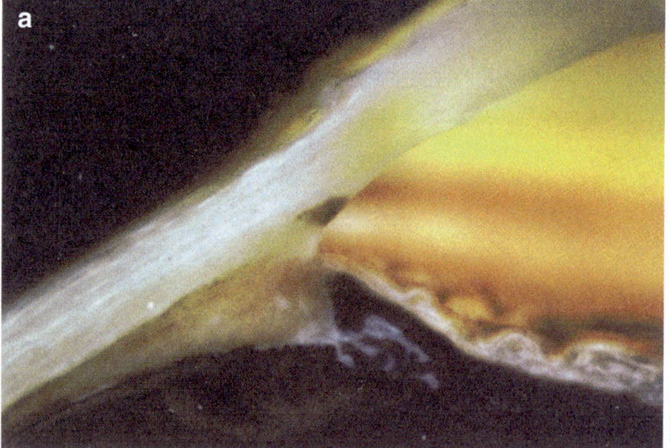


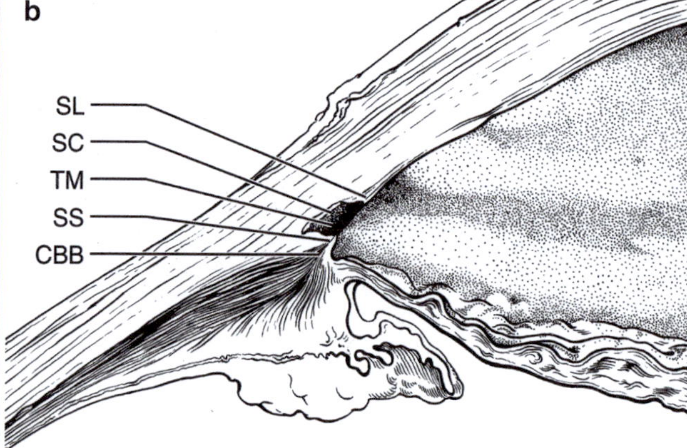


**Fig. 1.3** Macroscopic photograph (**a**) and corresponding sketch (**b**) identifying structures visible in a meridional section of the normal anterior chamber angle. The anterior chamber is artificially deepened because of posterior sagging of the iris following removal of the crystalline lens. The heavily pigmented region corresponds to the posterior or "filtering" meshwork. *SL* Schwalbe's line, *SC* Schlemm's canal, *TM* trabecular meshwork, *SS* scleral spur, *CBB* ciliary body band (From Freddo [10])

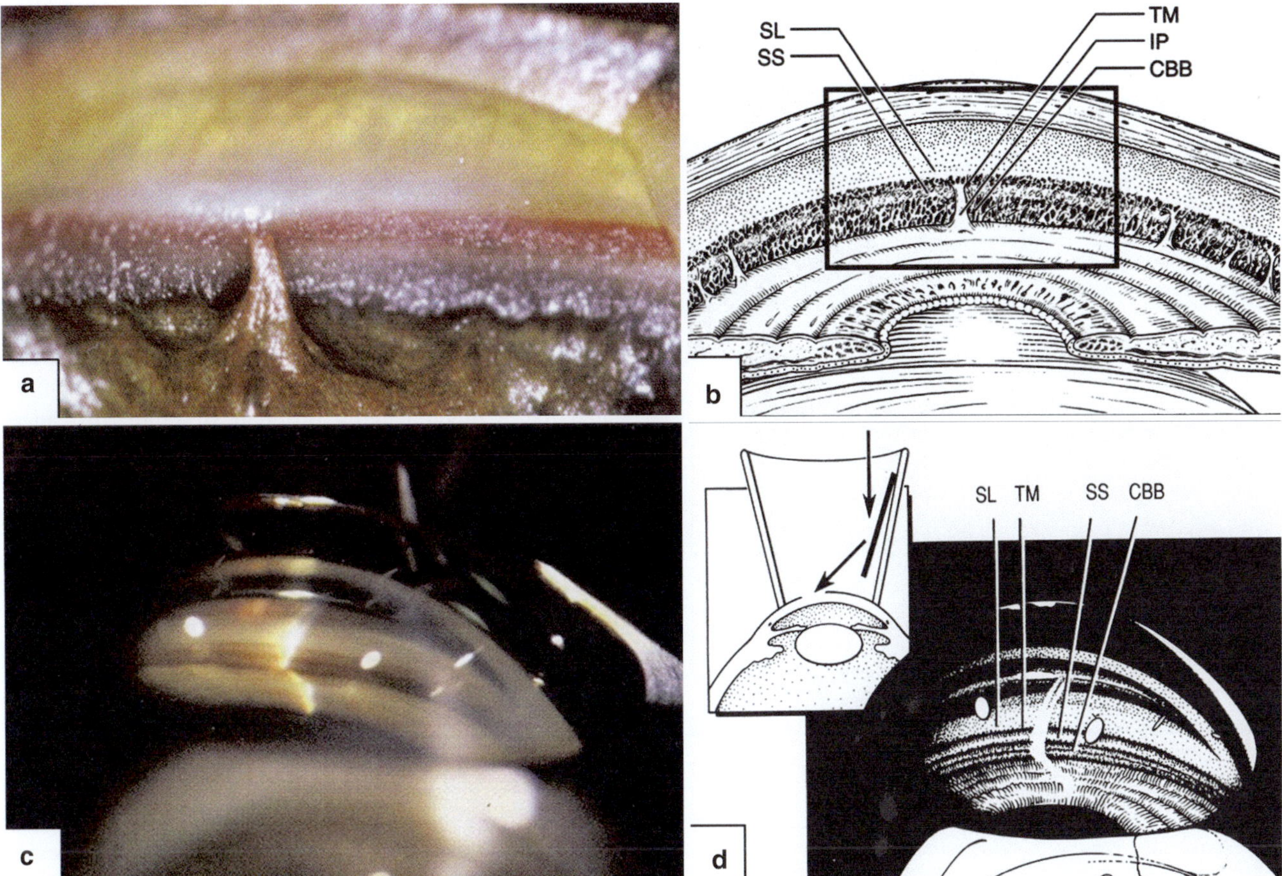

**Fig. 1.4** The anterior chamber angle viewed with both microscopy and gonioscopy. (**a**) Macroscopic photograph of angle structures as seen from the gonioscopic perspective. Schlemm's canal is filled with blood in this specimen, demonstrating its relationship to the other angle structures. An iris process, a normal anatomical variant, is also shown. (**b**) A corresponding sketch of A (*black box*) showing the angle structures from superior to inferior: Schwalbe's line (*SL*), trabecular meshwork (*TM*), scleral spur (*SS*), iris process (*IP*), and ciliary body band (*CBB*). (**c**) Goniophotograph of a normal open angle and corresponding sketch (**d**) representing a view analogous to that in image (**a**) and (**b**). Five alternating dark and light bands are evident in the angle. The termination of Descemet's membrane (Schwalbe's line, *SL*) is the most anterior dark band seen followed by the light band corresponding to the anterior or "nonfiltering" trabecular meshwork (*TM*). The next dark band corresponds to the posterior or "filtering" meshwork, followed by the light band corresponding to the scleral spur (*SS*). The final dark band, just above the peripheral iris, corresponds to the ciliary body band (*CBB*) (From Freddo [10])

face view of the anterior chamber angle in a monkey eye. The light reflection from Schwalbe's line and the TM below it overlying the blood-filled Schlemm's canal can be clearly seen. Below Schlemm's canal, the lighter coloration from the scleral spur is evident, and finally, below the scleral spur, the very dark coloration given by the pigment in the ciliary body stroma is seen. This lowest "layer" of the meshwork, seen from the gonioscopic perspective, is referred to as the ciliary body band (Fig. 1.4a, b). For comparison, these same structures are depicted in a goniophotograph of a normal open angle in Fig. 1.4c, d. A series of alternating dark and light bands is evident corresponding to the areas shown in Fig. 1.5. The uppermost dark band is Schwalbe's line, which is commonly decorated with various amounts of pigment even in the normal eye. The lighter line below represents the anterior or "nonfiltering" meshwork. This portion of the meshwork is not adjacent to Schlemm's canal and no aqueous humor drains in this region. Therefore, aqueous outflow in this portion of the meshwork is small and the amount of pigment phagocytosed by the trabecular cells in this region is low and results in minimal pigmentation. Below this lighter line is a darker line corresponding to the posterior or "filtering" meshwork. This is the portion of the meshwork that leads most directly to Schlemm's canal. Here, both the flow and phagocytosed pigment are greater resulting in a darker appearance on gonioscopy (Fig. 1.6). Below this dark line is another lighter line corresponding to the scleral spur. Finally, just below this, the lowest dark line corresponds to the ciliary body band [12, 13].

## The Uveal and Corneoscleral Meshwork

The uveal and corneoscleral meshwork are composed of a series of trabecular lamella or beams that delimit a system of

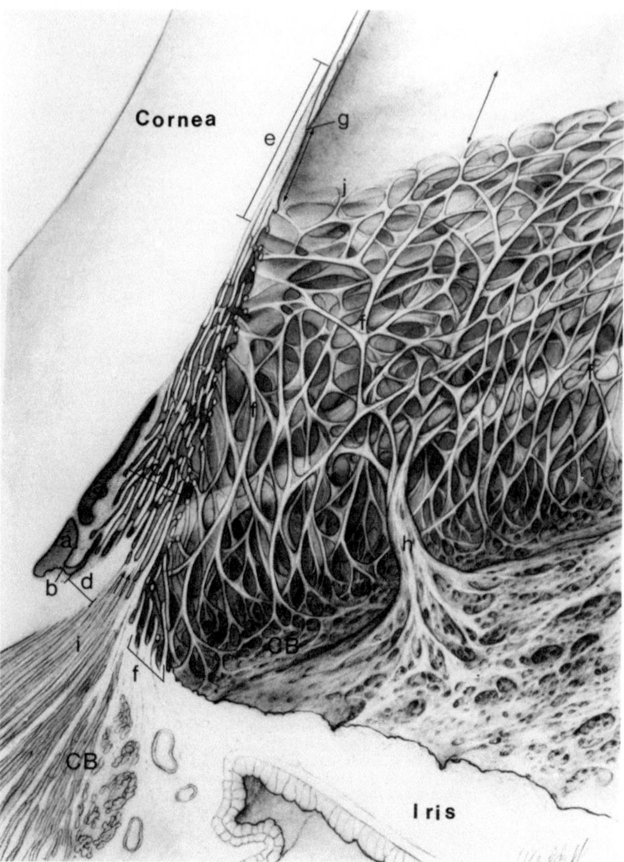



**Fig. 1.5** Drawing of the aqueous outflow pathway and adjacent tissues. (**a**) Schlemm's canal; (**b**) internal collector channel opening into the posterior part of Schlemm's canal; (**c**) corneoscleral beams; (**d**) scleral spur (**e**) limbus; (**f**) uveal beams; (**g**) Schwalbe's line, or the terminus of Descemet's membrane; (**h**) iris process extending from the root of the iris to merge with the uveal meshwork; (**i**) longitudinal ciliary muscle attached to the scleral spur, but with a portion joining the corneoscleral meshwork; (**j**) corneal endothelium continuous with the deep limbus. *Double-headed arrows* represent a transition zone that begins near Schwalbe's line and ends to where the uveal meshwork joins the deep limbus (Modified from Hogan et al. [6])

debris. A progressive age-related loss of trabecular cells has been reported in normal eyes, and compared to normal subjects, additional cell loss was reported in the TM of POAG eyes [18, 20, 21]. Fusion of trabecular beams observed in POAG eyes may result from adhesions between denuded portions of adjacent trabecular beams.

## The Juxtacanalicular Region

The portion of the trabecular meshwork between the outermost corneoscleral beam and the inner wall of Schlemm's canal has a fundamentally different structure. Instead of connective tissue beams confined within endothelial wrappings, the juxtacanalicular (JCT) region is an open connective tissue matrix in which fibroblast-like cells which lack a basal lamina are located. The cells in the JCT form long processes by which they attach to each other, to an extracellular matrix, and to the inner-wall endothelial cells of Schlemm's canal (Fig. 1.8a). In addition, studies have documented that tendons from the longitudinal bundle of the ciliary muscle extend into the meshwork, culminating in a system of elastic fibers that connect to the inner wall of Schlemm's canal which has been termed the cribriform plexus (Fig. 1.9a, b) [23, 24]. The majority of the resistance to aqueous outflow is believed to reside in the JCT region and the inner wall of Schlemm's canal [25], but the actual source of this resistance has remained elusive. The balance between extracellular matrix (ECM) synthesis and degradation plays an important role in the regulation of aqueous outflow resistance and IOP [26]. Abnormal accumulations of ECM in the JCT region have been reported in both primary and secondary open-angle glaucoma [27–30] including POAG patients with no medical treatment [27]. Thus, this accumulation of ECM appears to be a early pathophysiologic event in POAG.

aqueous flow channels (Figs. 1.2 and 1.5). The corneoscleral and outer uveal trabecular beams are flattened, perforated sheets that are oriented circumferentially parallel to the surface of the limbus. The inner 1–2 layers of uveal sheets closest to the anterior chamber, however, have a round, cord-like profile and are oriented in a radial, netlike fashion enclosing large open spaces for aqueous outflow. The spaces become progressively smaller from the uveal to the corneoscleral meshwork (Fig. 1.2). Ultrastructurally, the uveal and corneoscleral beams consist of a central connective tissue core that is enveloped in a continuous wrapping of thin endothelial cells and a subcellular basal lamina (Fig. 1.7). Trabecular cells are phagocytic [15] and capable of removing endogenous [16, 17] and exogenous [18, 19] particles to keep the trabecular outflow channels free of potentially obstructive

## Schlemm's Canal

Schlemm's canal (SC) is a continuous channel oriented circumferentially deep within the internal scleral sulcus. Its lumen is in direct continuity with the venous system of the eye. Despite this connection, blood is not usually seen in the canal unless IOP falls below the episcleral venous pressure or when the limbal vessels are compressed as occurs with the use of a flanged gonioscope. When cut in cross section, the canal has an elliptical appearance with its major length varying from $264 \pm 55$ μm by histological assessments [31] to $347.2 \pm 42.3$ μm as measured with OCT [9]. In frontal section, the mean width of SC (the distance between the inner and outer wall of the canal) is between 13 and 29 μm in human eyes (Gong et al., unpublished data, 2013).

**Fig. 1.6** Light micrograph of trabecular meshwork demonstrating phagocytosis of melanin by trabecular endothelial cells in posterior trabecular meshwork. Note the abrupt reduction in the amount of pigmentation in the anterior meshwork beyond the anterior edge of Schlemm's canal (line). This difference in pigmentation is evident clinically viewed by gonioscopy (see Fig. 1.4) (With permission from Freddo et al. [11], Chapter 191)

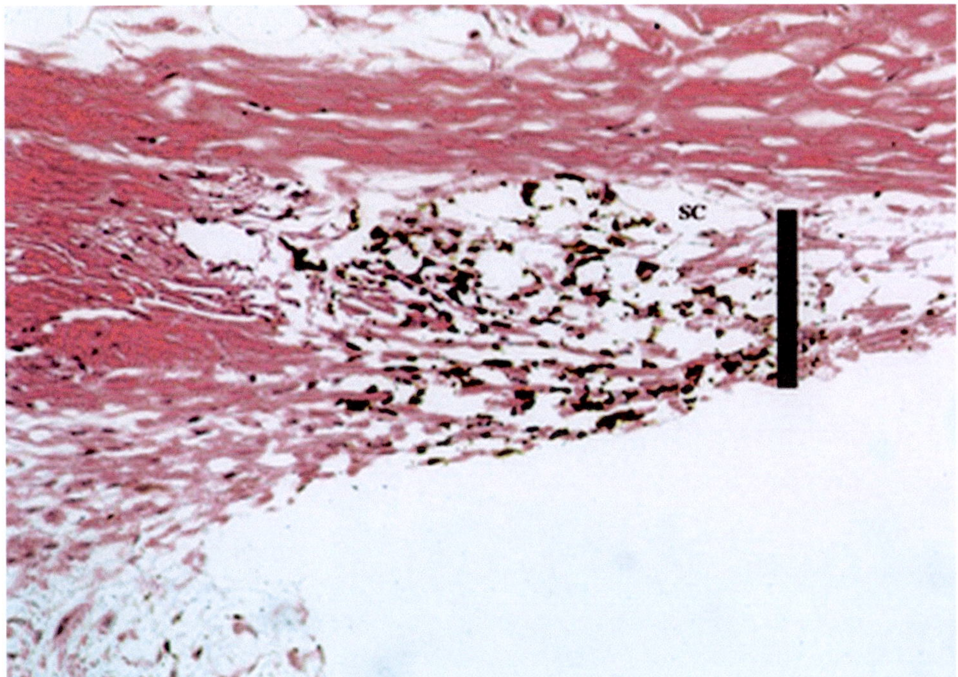


**Fig. 1.7** Transmission electron micrograph showing a cross section of a trabecular beam. The trabecular beam is covered by a single layer of trabecular endothelial cells (*TEC*) that rest on the basal lamina (*BL*) which surrounds a central connective tissue core. *C* collagen, *EL* elastic fiber, *SM* sheath material of elastic fiber, *ITS* intertrabecular spaces (Modified with permission from Gong et al. [14])

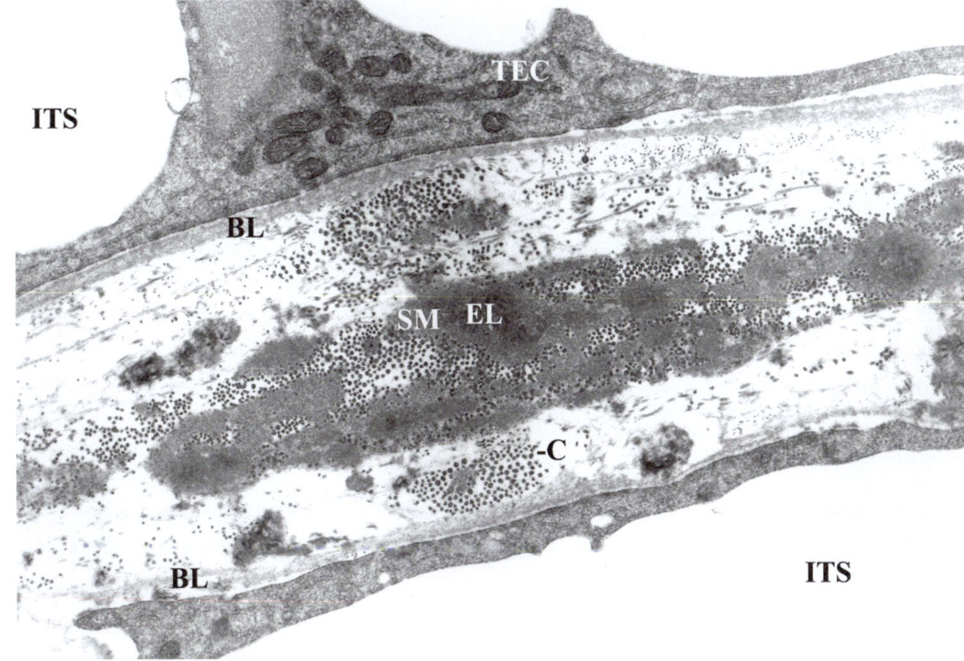


The canal usually appears slit-like (Fig. 1.2a) and at several points around the circumference of the eye is divided into two parallel channels that rejoin one another after a short distance. The endothelial lining of SC is composed of a single layer of cells that rest on a discontinuous basal lamina. Tight junctions between adjacent endothelial cells are present (Fig. 1.8) [32]. One side of the canal directly abuts the sclera which is termed the outer wall of SC. The opposite side is connected to the JCT region of the meshwork and is

termed the inner wall of SC. Aqueous humor must traverse the continuous endothelial lining of Schlemm's canal from the JCT to enter its lumen. Exactly how aqueous humor traverses the endothelium of SC remains one of the enigmatic problems of ocular anatomy and physiology. A characteristic aspect of the inner-wall endothelium of SC is the formation of cellular outpouchings that are termed giant vacuoles (Figs. 1.10 and 1.11). The giant vacuoles form when aqueous humor pushes against the basal side of the inner-wall

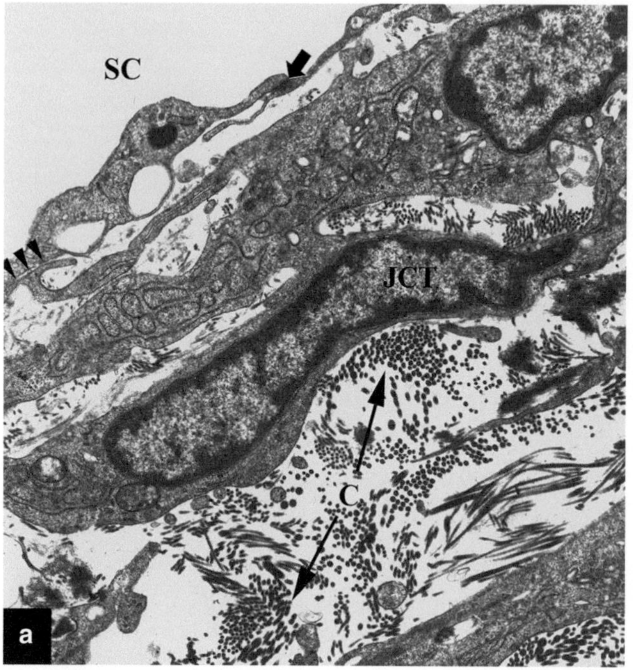

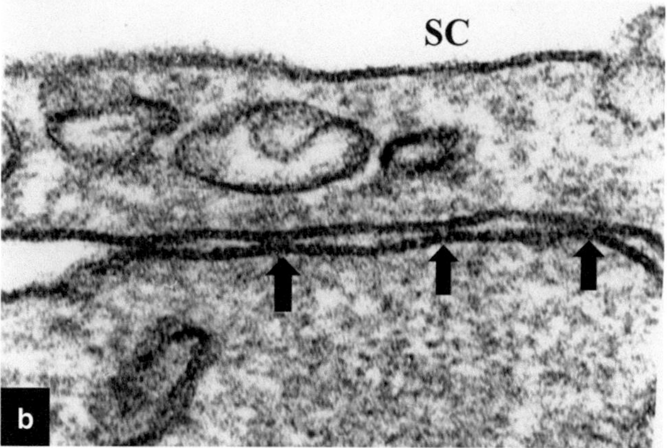

**Fig. 1.8** (**a**) Transmission electron micrograph demonstrating the appearance of the connective tissue matrix and cells in the juxtacanalicular region (*JCT*). The matrix is composed of collagen (*C*) and elastin and the cells are devoid of a basal lamina. The JCT cells extend mushroom-like cell processes (*arrowheads*) that attach to endothelial cells (*E*) of the inner wall of Schlemm's canal (*SC*). (**b**) The tight junction between SC endothelial cells appears as fusion points between plasma membranes of two adjacent cells (*arrows*) (From Gong et al. [22])

endothelium [35]. These vacuoles appear to be pressure-dependent and are not found unless the inner wall is fixed under conditions of active flow [36]. Aqueous humor is believed to traverse the inner wall of Schlemm's canal through small openings or pores (Fig. 1.10) [37]. There are two types of pores that are termed intracellular and paracellular pores (Fig. 1.11) [38]. Intercellular pores (I pores) are often associated with giant vacuoles with a size between 0.1 and 0.2 μm [39]. Paracellular pores are located at the border between two adjacent endothelial cells (B pores) with similar size [38] (Fig. 1.11). Pores are reported to be responsible for

about 10 % of total outflow resistance in normal eyes [39]; however, glaucomatous eyes exhibit fewer pores compared to normal eyes [33, 40] suggesting that endothelial cells lining SC lose their ability to produce pores which may contribute to increased outflow resistance in eyes with POAG. Increasing IOP leads to progressive collapse of the canal [35, 41]. As SC collapses, the outflow resistance increases and the IOP rises [42, 43]. The dimensions of SC in eyes with POAG were reported to be significantly smaller than in the normal eye. This reduction in the dimensions of SC may account for nearly half of the decrease in outflow facility observed in POAG eyes [31].

## The Ciliary Muscle and Trabecular Outflow

Attached to the posterior surface of the scleral spur are tendons of the longitudinal bundle of the ciliary muscle which are continuous with the ECM of the TM [44]. Contraction of these longitudinal muscles pulls the scleral spur posteriorly and separates the layers of the corneoscleral meshwork attached to the anterior surface of this structure. This appears to facilitate aqueous drainage and is the basis for the use of miotics in increasing aqueous outflow to reduce IOP in glaucoma. Surgical disinsertion of the ciliary muscle has been shown to eliminate the outflow-enhancing effects of pilocarpine [45]. In addition, the elastic fibers of the scleral spur are continuous with the elastic fibers in the trabecular beams and the cribriform plexus in the JCT [23] (Fig. 1.9) and extend to the basal lamina of the inner-wall endothelial cells of SC [24]. These tendons are thought to put tension on the inner wall of SC, resisting the pressure-related collapse of SC when pressure is elevated [46].

## Flow Pathways Beyond Schlemm's Canal

### Collector Channels

Aqueous flow into Schlemm's canal is not evenly distributed throughout the inner wall but occurs preferentially in certain areas. Drainage of aqueous humor preferentially occurs near collector channels (CCs) in the human eye [47]. Twice as many giant vacuoles have been shown to be present near regions with CCs indicating that aqueous flow across the inner wall is sensitive to downstream pressure [48]. Studies using fluorescent beads also show increased levels of beads in pigmented trabecular meshwork adjacent to CCs suggesting preferential flow pathways are present near CCs [47].

Histological studies of the human eye have shown that between the ages of 25 and 30, CCs are randomly distributed around the eye with a higher distribution on the inferior-nasal side than on the temporal side of the eye [49, 50]. This has been confirmed by studies using 3-dimensional micro-CT [51]

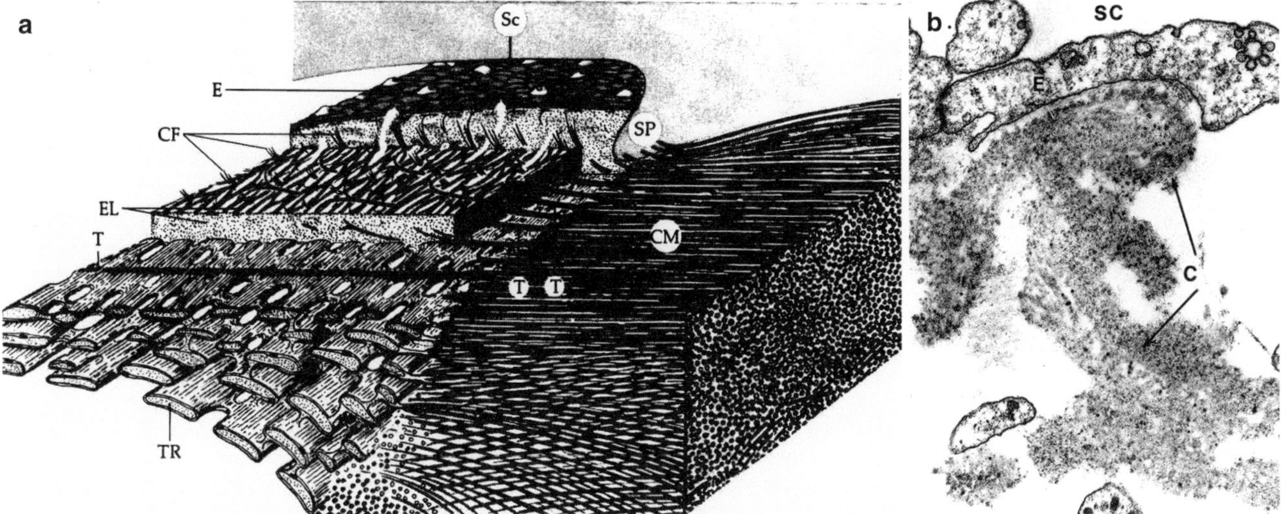



**Fig. 1.9** (a) Anterior ciliary muscle tendons (*T*) and their connections with the trabecular meshwork are shown. Tendons from the longitudinal bundle of the ciliary muscle (*CM*) extend to the scleral spur (*SP*), into the outermost corneoscleral trabeculae, and finally into the juxtacanalicular region contributing to the cribriform plexus. Connecting fibrils (*CF*) extend from the plexus toward the endothelial cells (*E*) lining the inner wall of Schlemm's canal (*SC*). (b) Immunoelectron micrograph shows a single connecting fibril (c) attaching to the endothelium (E) of the inner wall of Schlemm's canal (*SC*). Scattered small black dots represent colloidal gold staining for elastin, confirming that these connecting fibrils contain this protein (Image **a** reproduced with permission from Rohen [23]; Image **b** reproduced with permission from Gong et al. [24])

**Fig. 1.10** Scanning electron micrograph of the luminal surface of the inner wall of Schlemm's canal. Numerous bulging giant vacuoles are seen on the luminal surface of the inner wall of Schlemm's canal. Several pores are evident (*arrowheads*) and are shown at higher magnification in the inset (Modified from Allingham et al. [33] and from Gong et al. [22])

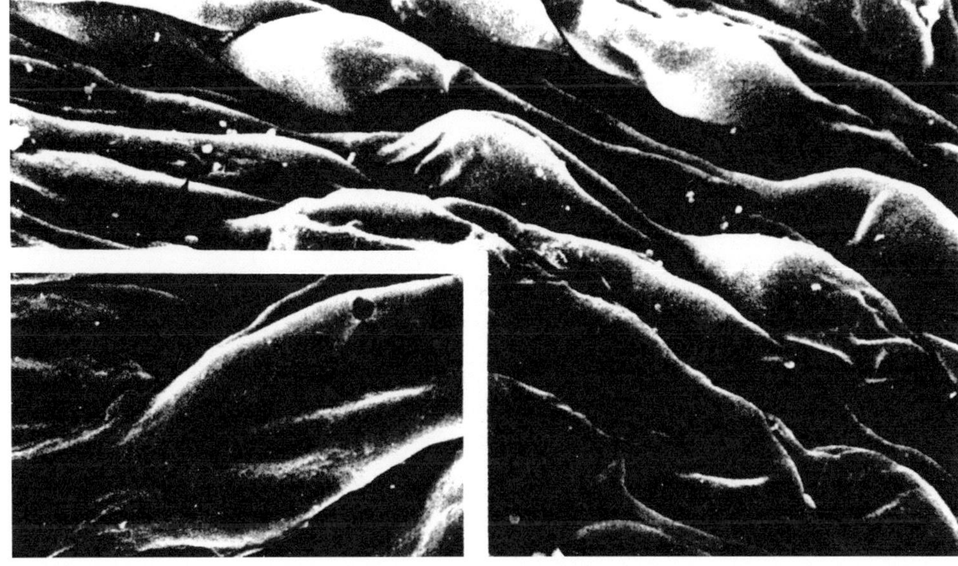

(Fig. 1.12). There is great variability in the orifice size of collector channels with a range between 5 and 50 μm to as high as 70 μm depending on the study design [49–51].

From the CCs, aqueous humor passes through a tortuous system of passages termed the deep, midlimbal, and superficial intrascleral venous plexus that lead in turn to episcleral veins (Fig. 1.13) [6]. The intrascleral venous plexus is composed of a series of small, interconnected venules 10–50 μm in diameter with many interconnecting branch points forming a dense vascular network. The venous plexus is drained posteriorly by several larger veins forming a series of radial arcades. These vessels are 50–100 μm in diameter and progressively converge into larger vessels moving posteriorly away from the image margin and SC. These vessels eventually converge with larger episcleral veins. Visualization of these vessels using optical coherence tomography (OCT) [52, 53], fluorescent microsphere tracer studies [53], and 3D micro-CT [51] has been reported.

The major source of aqueous humor outflow resistance is believed to lie in the JCT and inner-wall endothelium of SC. Structures distal to this including the collector channels, intrascleral venous plexus, and aqueous veins are assumed to

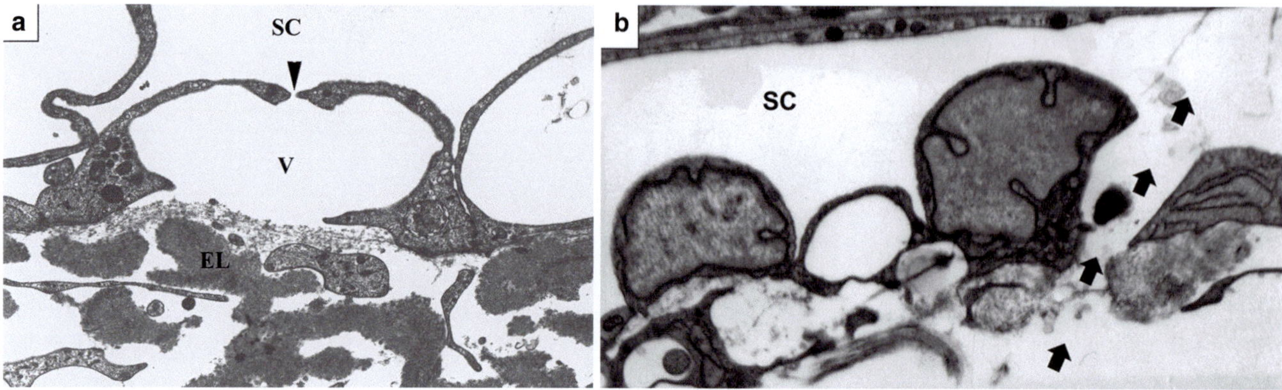



**Fig. 1.11** Transmission electron micrograph of two types of pores I and B in the inner wall of Schlemm's canal. (**a**) The juxtacanalicular tissue region with elastic fibers (*EL*) and the basement membrane (*BM*) of the inner-wall endothelium of Schlemm's canal (*SC*) with giant vacuole (*V*) and an intracellular pore leading into SC (*arrowhead*) are shown. Aqueous humor is believed to traverse the inner wall of Schlemm's canal (*SC*) through small openings or pores. There are two types of pores that are termed intracellular and paracellular pores. Intercellular pores (I pores) are often associated with giant vacuoles with a size between 0.1 and 0.2 μm. (**b**) Paracellular pores (B pores) are located at the border between two adjacent endothelial cells with similar size (Image **a** from Gong et al. [14]; Image **b** from Ye et al. [34])

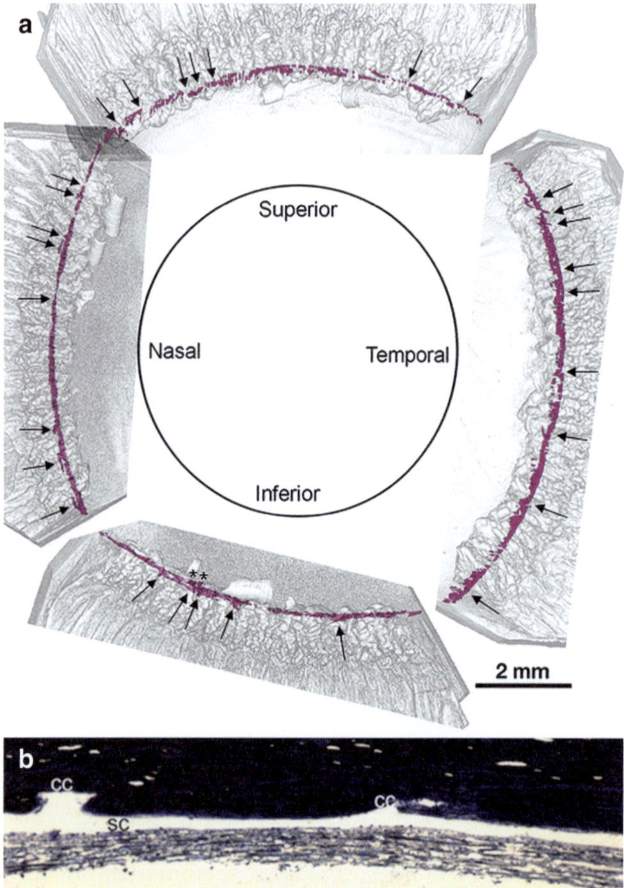



**Fig. 1.12** Distribution of collector channels in the normal eye. (**a**) Up to 30 collector channels can be found in the normal eye with an uneven distribution around Schlemm's canal. The majority are found in the inferior-nasal quadrant followed by the superotemporal quadrant. (**b**) A light micrograph of a frontal section showing the trabecular meshwork (*TM*), Schlemm's canal (*SC*), and collector channel (*CC*) ostia in the normal human eye (Image **a** from Hann et al. [51]; Image **b** provided by Haiyan Gong, MD, PhD)

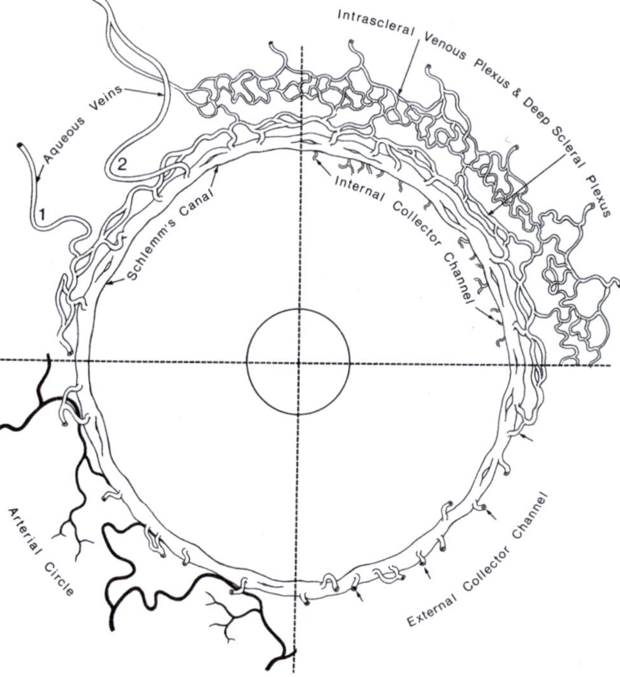



**Fig. 1.13** Diagram representing the distal portion of the aqueous outflow pathways from Schlemm's canal. External collector channels (*lower right*), deep and intrascleral plexi (*upper right*), aqueous veins (*1* and *2*) (*upper left*), and arterial circle (*lower left*) (From Hogan et al. [6])

contribute less to outflow resistance [54–56]. Early studies reported that 75 % of aqueous outflow resistance was localized to the TM and SC with 25 % occurring from the structures distal to SC [57]. A study has reported that smooth muscle actin was found near the CC ostia regions [58], whether these vessels are capable of contraction and thus contribute to regulating aqueous outflow is still unknown. Studies have shown that

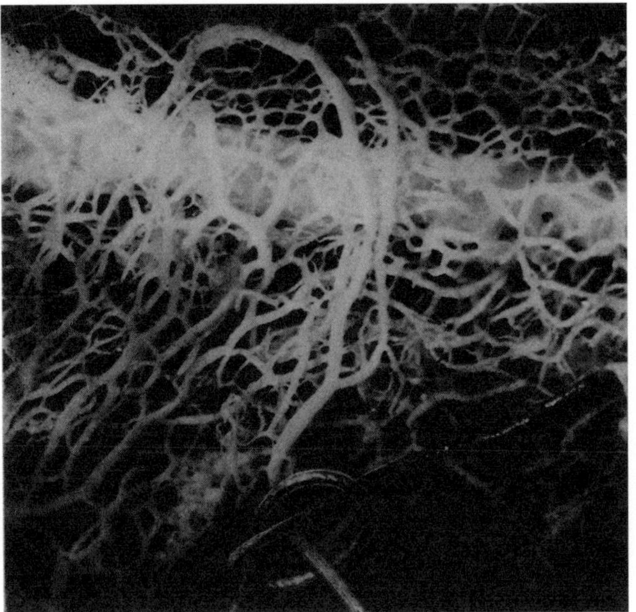

**Fig. 1.14** Aqueous veins. Neoprene cast of Schlemm's canal and limbal vessels after enucleation showing sector containing marked aqueous vein. The tantalum wire loop around the aqueous vein is still visualized in situ (Image adapted from Norman [65]; with permission from BMJ Publishing Group Ltd.)

aqueous and blood. Direct observation of these changes is a reliable method to gauge the efficacy of medical and surgical treatments aimed at reducing IOP in glaucoma [66].

AVs vary in their position, size, and anatomical arrangements. On slit-lamp examination, two to three AVs are typically visible with up to a maximum of six occasionally seen [67]. AVs have unequal distribution and are present most abundantly in the inferior-nasal quadrants with the remainder in the inferior-temporal quadrants [67]. Their size varies from 20 to 100 µm with an average of 50 µm [67–69]. Histologically, AVs are indistinguishable from conjunctival and episcleral veins.

A dynamic equilibrium exists in AVs based on current understanding of pulsatile flow driving aqueous outflow (Fig. 1.15) [71–73]. Pulsatile flow occurs from an oscillatory compressive force provided by the cardiac pulse and blinking, inlet channels from the JCT and the inner-wall endothelium to SC, and outlet channels via CCs and aqueous veins. Glaucoma patients show a decrease in pulsatile flow compared to normal subjects [74, 75]. The reduction of pulsatile flow in glaucoma patients can be accounted for by physiologic changes in the elasticity of the TM. The TM must be deformable to dynamic pressure and volume changes in inflow and outflow for normal aqueous outflow to occur from the anterior chamber to SC [62].

following complete trabeculotomy, 49 % of outflow resistance is eliminated at a perfusion pressure at 7 mmHg (corresponding to the normal IOP in enucleated human eyes with no episcleral venous pressure) [59] and 71 % of outflow resistance was eliminated at a perfusion pressure at 25 mmHg [60]. This suggests that pressure-dependent changes in outflow resistance are present in the TM and SC with additional resistance distal to SC likely. An additional study reported that 35 % of outflow resistance was eliminated after a 1-clock-hour ablation of the tissue from the outer wall of SC and distal by using the excimer laser at a perfusion pressure at 10 mmHg [61]. These studies indicate that a portion (one third to half) of the outflow resistance lies distal to the inner wall of SC.

## Aqueous Veins

The human eye contains a small number of unique vessels termed aqueous veins (of Ascher) which are of great importance to normal aqueous outflow. Aqueous veins (AVs) have a lumen in direct communication with collector channels and in turn communicate directly with episcleral veins that return blood to the general circulation [62]. Thus, AVs can bypass the deep and intrascleral venous plexus and connect directly to episcleral veins [63, 64] (Fig. 1.14). AVs contain clear aqueous at their origins, but anastomose with episcleral vessels that contain blood. Transitional zones are often identified in AVs on the conjunctival surface as a large vessel with a clear central lumen bordered on either side by dark blood. With changes in IOP, these transitional zones vary in their composition of

## Aqueous Outflow Patterns

### Aqueous Outflow Is Not Uniform (Segmental) in Normal Eyes

Aqueous humor outflow has been reported to be nonuniform or "segmental" circumferentially as observed from the distribution of pigment in the trabecular meshwork [47] and tracer perfused into the anterior chamber [41, 76–78]. At any given time, only a fraction of the outflow pathways are actively involved in aqueous humor drainage (Fig. 1.16). This active area is termed the effective filtration area (EFA). Segmental outflow has been reported in mouse [79], porcine [80], bovine [41, 77], monkey [78], and human eyes [47, 80, 81]. A greater concentration tracer was observed in the trabecular meshwork adjacent to CC ostia where more pigment was also observed in human eyes (Fig. 1.17), suggesting that preferential flow pathways are present and pigment may serve as a useful internal marker to identify the area with active flow.

### Reduction of Aqueous Outflow Area with Increasing IOP and in POAG

EFA [measured by length: percentage effective filtration length = (length of the inner wall exhibiting tracer labeling/total length of inner wall) × 100 %] was found to be reduced with

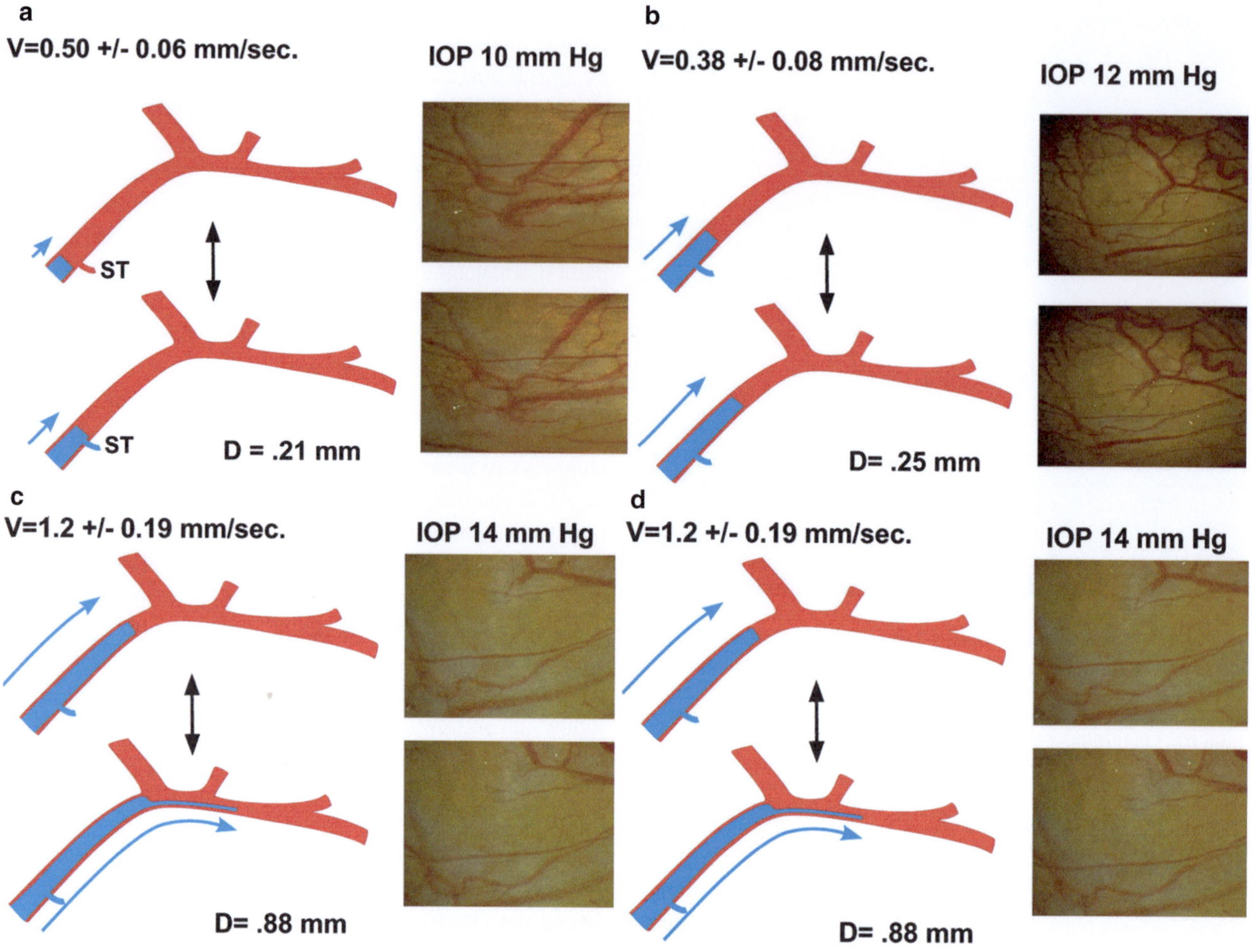

**Fig. 1.15** Pulsatile flow changes in the normal eye. Illustration of characteristic pulsatile flow changes caused by increasing IOP or addition of medications. Still frames and illustrations derived from video images of a 59-year-old male subject. (**a**) Baseline IOP: velocity (*V*) is low and aqueous pulse wave travel (*D*) with each stroke is small. A standing transverse interface of aqueous and blood oscillates resulting in systolic discharge of aqueous into a small venous tributary (*ST*). (**b**) Slightly increased IOP: the oscillatory aqueous fluid wave travels an increased distance. (**c**) Highest IOP: increased velocity and travel of the aqueous fluid wave. At each systole, a lamina of clear aqueous discharges into an episcleral vein. (**d**) Decreasing IOP: velocity and travel of the fluid wave increase further. Continuous oscillating laminar flow is present in a more distal episcleral vein. Two hours after drinking water, IOP was again 10 mmHg and stroke volume returned to appearance seen in image (a) (Image with permission from Johnstone et al. [70], Fig. 7.2)

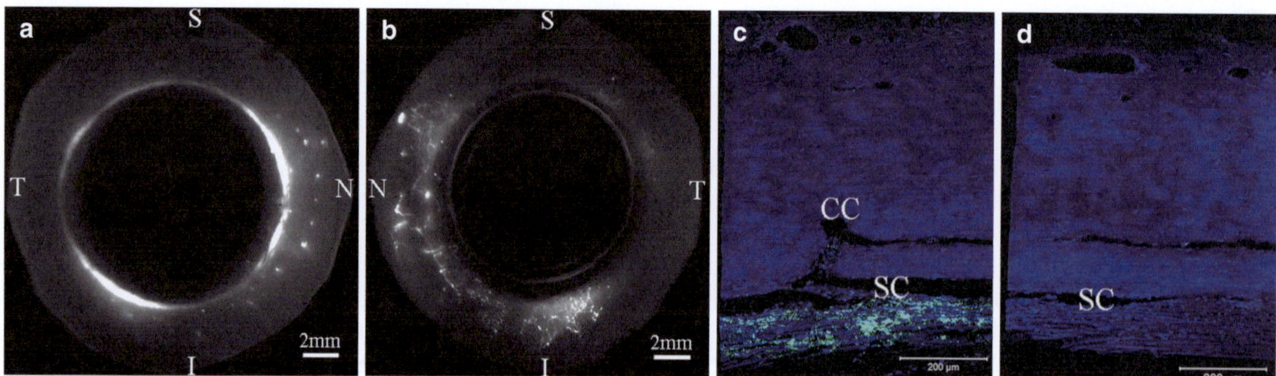



**Fig. 1.16** Segmental aqueous flow pattern in normal human eyes. (**a**) Posterior view of the tracer distribution in the trabecular meshwork (*TM*) in a global imaging. Segmental tracer distribution is seen. (**b**) Segmental tracer distribution is seen in the scleral veins in the anterior view of a global imaging. (**c**) A confocal microscopic image showing tracer distribution in the trabecular meshwork is segmental, and more tracer (green) is near collector channel (*CC*) ostia region. (**d**) A confocal microscopic image showing no tracer was seen in this region of the TM. *S* superior, *N* nasal, *I* inferior, *T* temporal (Images are provided by Haiyan Gong, MD, PhD)

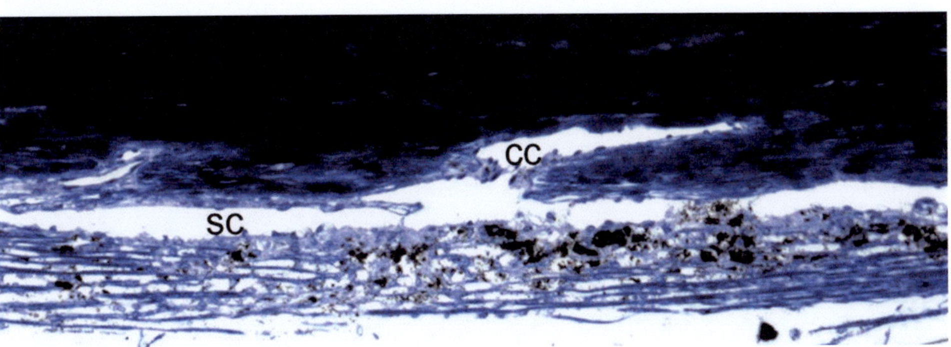

**Fig. 1.17** Pigmentation near collector channel ostia. Light micrograph of trabecular meshwork demonstrates phagocytosis of melanin by trabecular endothelial cells. More pigmentation is observation in the trabecular meshwork near the collector channel (*CC*) ostia than away from these regions (Image is provided by Haiyan Gong, MD, PhD)

acute elevation of IOP in bovine eyes. A greater concentration of tracer was observed near CC ostia with acute elevation of IOP. Outflow patterns in the JCT and inner wall transitioned from less segmental (more uniform) patterns at normal IOP (7 mmHg in enucleated eyes) to an increased segmental pattern at higher IOP (15–45 mmHg) (Fig. 1.18) [41]. This decrease in EFA is associated with decreased outflow facility and is reversible when pressure is reduced from a high to a normal level [82]. A decrease in EFA was also reported in chronic elevation of IOP in the laser-induced monkey glaucoma model [83]. In this study, reduced tracer was found in areas of the trabecular meshwork that had received laser injury including the CC ostia region. Active outflow was found to be shifted away from areas with laser injury to areas without (Fig. 1.19). Significant reduction of EFA was also reported in POAG eyes compared to normal eyes in a tracer study [84]. Additionally, an inverse correlation between EFA and IOP was recently documented in an ocular hypotensive mouse model [79]. Collectively, these results suggest that the EFA is a valuable method of measuring outflow resistance and the effects of changes in IOP in humans and a number of different species.

## Morphological Changes Responsible for Reduced Outflow Area

### Increasing Extracellular Matrix in the JCT

An increase in the amount of extracellular matrix (ECM) or "plaque material" in the JCT has been reported in the eyes of patients with POAG with and without medical treatment [27, 29]. This increase is associated with increasing severity of optic nerve damage in POAG [85]. In laser-induced glaucoma monkey models, increased ECM in the JCT occurs in response to the severity of laser damage observed in areas of the trabecular meshwork. This has been shown to result in a reduction in the active outflow area. This reduction contributes to a decrease in outflow facility and corresponding elevation of IOP [83]. More continuous and thicker basement membranes observed along the inner wall of SC and increased ECM in the JCT may account for the reduction of active outflow areas and outflow facility in POAG [84].

## Collapse of SC and Herniations of the TM into CC Ostia

In an acute IOP elevation study in bovine eyes, morphological changes responsible for reduced outflow area include a progressive collapse of the aqueous plexus (equivalent to Schlemm's canal in human eyes) and increasing numbers of herniations into CC ostia (Fig. 1.20) [41]. These morphological changes were associated with decreases in effective outflow area and outflow facility; however, they were reversible when IOP was returned to a normal level [82]. A progressive collapse of SC and an increasing number of tissue herniations into CC ostia following an acute elevation of IOP were also found to be associated with a decrease in outflow facility in normal human eyes. These changes were reversible when IOP was decreased from high to normal levels (Fig. 1.21) [86]. This data suggests that collapse of SC and increasing numbers of herniations into CC ostia may be important factors contributing to the decrease in outflow facility following acute IOP elevation.

A study compared the light microscopic images in frontal sections between normal autopsy eyes and those with primary open-angle glaucoma (POAG). The collapse of SC and the herniations into the CC ostia were found to be common among eyes with POAG (61 %) even when the eye was fixed at zero pressure (Fig. 1.22) [87]. The longer the IOP remains high, the less pliable the changes in the trabecular meshwork tissue seem to become. The disturbing implication of these findings is that normally reversible morphological changes after an acute elevation in IOP (Fig. 1.21) may become permanent in cases of POAG. Occluded collector channel ostia may explain the variable success of surgical procedures intended to restore outflow into the episcleral venous system via the canal.

## Blockage of Collector Channels by Clinical Observation in POAG

Blockages of CC ostia were also reported in black South African patients with POAG in both retrospective [88] and prospective studies [89]. In the retrospective study, clinical data was analyzed including the video records of surgical procedures for 19 untreated black South African POAG

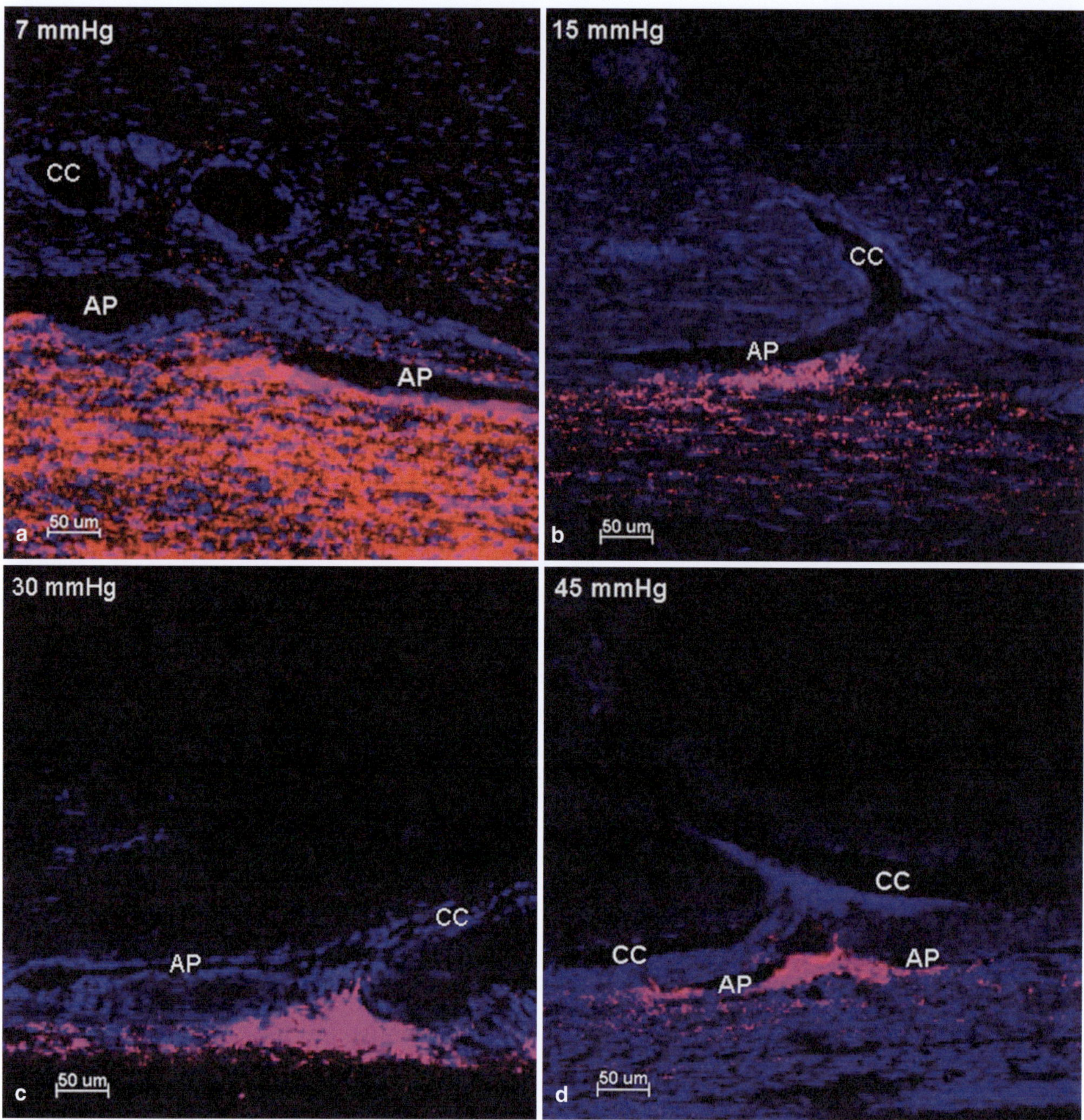

**Fig. 1.18** Confocal microscopy of fluorescent microspheres perfused at 4 different IOPs. (**a**) At 7 mmHg, a uniform distribution of microspheres (*red*) was seen along the inner wall of the aqueous plexus (*AP*). In contrast, at pressures of 15 mmHg (**b**), 30 mmHg (**c**), and 45 mmHg (**d**), there was a segmental pattern of microsphere distribution with a greater concentration of microspheres in the trabecular meshwork near the collector channel (*CC*) ostia. This concentrated distribution was visually more dramatic at 45 mmHg than at 15 mmHg. Scale bar = 50 μm (Image with permission from Battista et al. [41])

patients (24 eyes) undergoing canaloplasty. Preoperative paracentesis was followed by provocative gonioscopy to elicit and grade patterns of inducible blood reflux into SC. After exposing SC, a flexible microcatheter was inserted into SC circumferentially and fluorescein was injected into SC in each quadrant to evaluate the fluorescent outflow patterns from SC into the episcleral veins. Quadrants exhibiting fluorescein egress were counted and analyzed. Three patterns of blood reflux were observed (Fig. 1.23): "good reflux" (blood observed along the entire circumference of SC, $N=9$), "patchy" reflux (attenuated blood reflux observed, $N=6$), and no reflux (no observable blood in SC, $N=9$). Fifteen eyes (patchy + no blood reflux, 60.8 %) demonstrated some degree of blockage for blood reflux into the

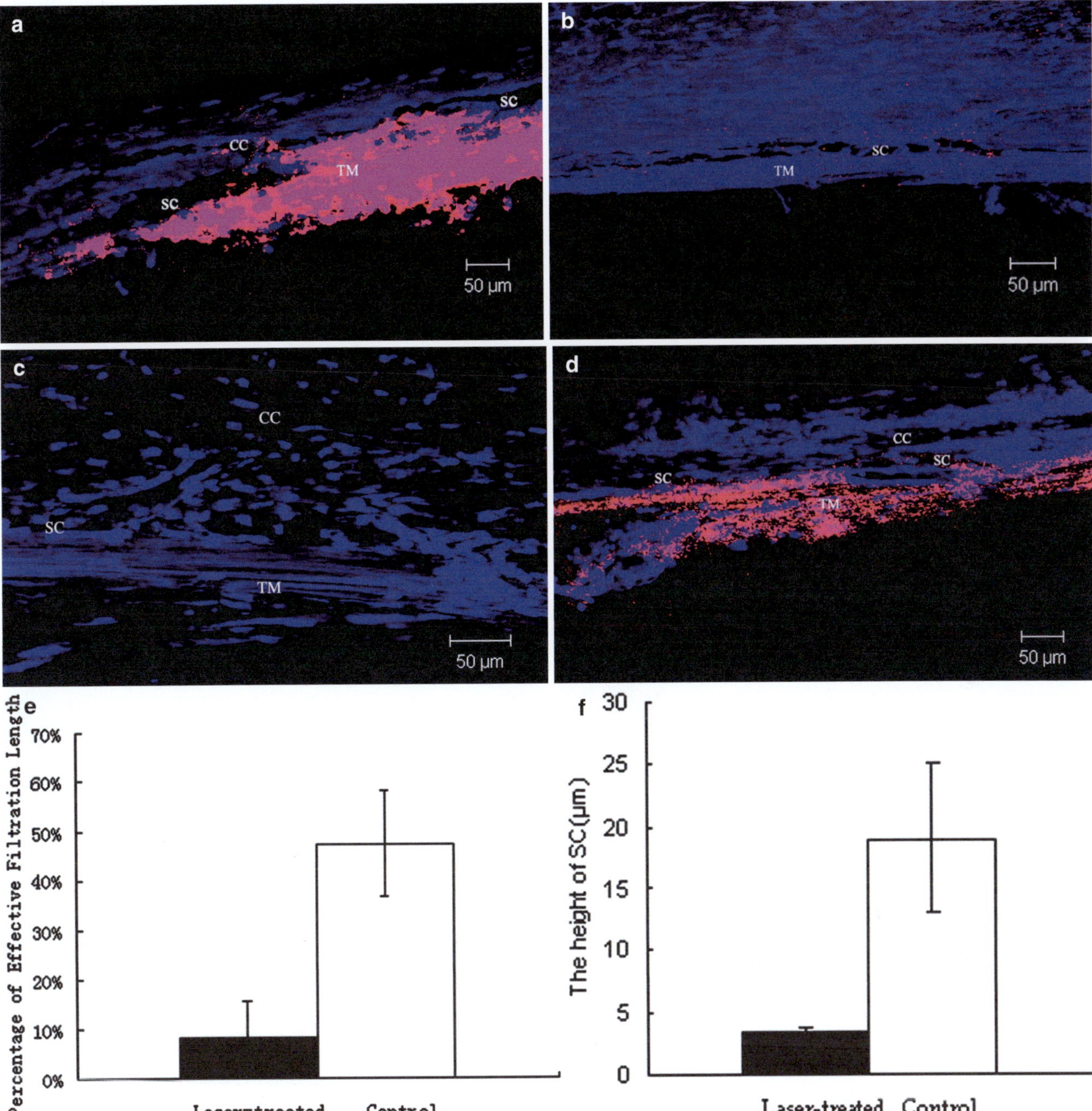


**Fig. 1.19** Comparison of effective filtration length and width of SC in control and laser-induced glaucoma eyes. (**a**) In control eyes, Schlemm's canal (*SC*) was open and segmental distribution of microspheres (*pink*) was found with a greater concentration in the trabecular meshwork (*TM*) near the collector channel (*CC*) ostia. (**b**) In the lasered region of laser-treated eyes, SC was collapsed and fewer or no microspheres were found in most areas of the TM. (**c**) In the lasered region of laser-treated eyes, no microspheres were found in the CC ostia region. (**d**) In the non-lasered region of laser-treated eyes, a large amount of microspheres (*pink*) were seen near CC ostia. (**e**) The average percent effective filtration length (PEFL = L/TL) in control eyes (47.47 ± 10.79 %) was 6-fold larger than in laser-treated eyes (8.40 ± 4.81 %, $p = 0.013$). (**f**) The mean distance between the inner and outer wall of SC of control eyes (18.99 ± 6.03 μm) was 5-fold greater than laser-treated eyes (3.47 ± 0.33 μm, $p = 0.01$). (Modified from Zhang et al. [83])

SC from episcleral veins. In the "good reflux" group, fluorescein egress into episcleral veins was seen in more than three quadrants (3.67 ± 0.5, mean ± SD) of the eyes. In the "patchy reflux" group, fluorescein egress into episcleral veins was seen in more than two quadrants (2.67 ± 1.21), while in the "no reflux" group, fluorescein egress into episcleral veins was decreased to less than one quadrant or between 1 and 2 quadrants (0.89 ± 0.93). Significant differences were found between the patients with "good" reflux vs. no reflux ($p = 4 \times 10^{-6}$) and between "patchy" blood

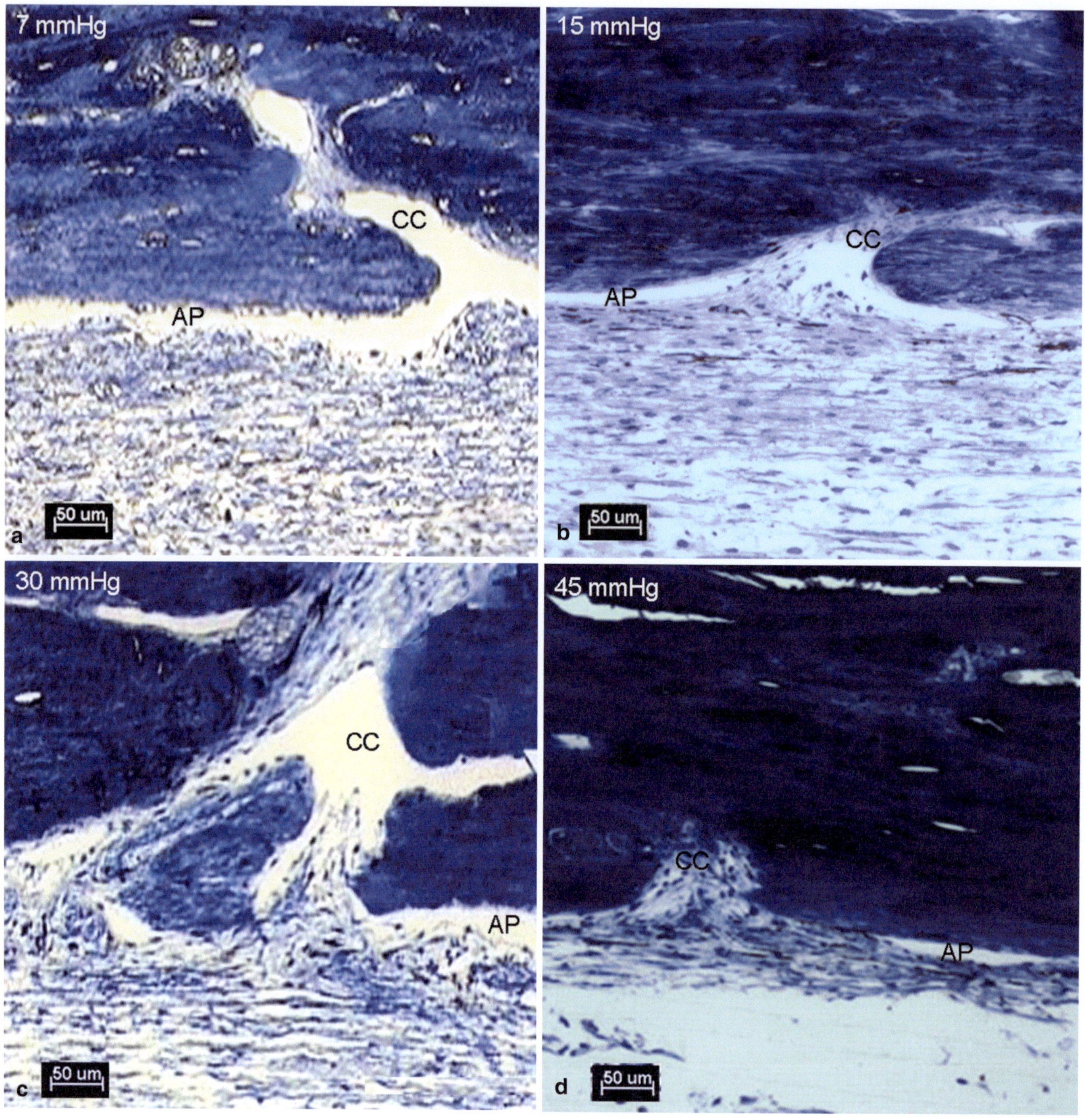


**Fig. 1.20** Light microscopy of the aqueous plexus and collector channels at four different IOPs. At 7 mmHg (**a**), the aqueous plexus (*AP*) is more open compared to the tissue perfused at higher pressures. At 15 mmHg (**b**), the inner wall and juxtacanalicular tissue (*JCT*) were partially herniated into the collector channel (*CC*) ostia. At 30 mmHg (**c**) and 45 mmHg (**d**), the aqueous plexus was collapsed adjacent to the CC ostia. At higher IOP, there is a more dramatic herniation of the inner wall and JCT into the CC ostia. Scale bar = 50 μm (Image with permission from Battista et al. [41])

reflux vs. no blood reflux ($p = 0.01$). No significant difference was found between "good" vs. "patchy" reflux groups ($p = 0.1$). This study suggests that attenuated and interrupted blood reflux into SC from CCs is consistent with decreased numbers of quadrants exhibiting fluorescein egress into episcleral veins via CCs and that blockage of CC ostia exists in vivo. Whether the cause of these blockages is the irreversible herniations into CC ostia observed histologically warrants further study. Since occluded CC ostia affect success of surgical procedures intended to restore outflow into the episcleral venous system via SC, observing the reflux of blood from the collector system into the canal could serve as an indication of a patent system in that region.

**Fig. 1.21** Light microscopy images of the collector channel ostia of normal human eyes after an acute elevation in IOP. (**a**) When the eye was continually perfused at 45 mmHg, Schlemm's canal (*SC*) was collapsed, and the trabecular meshwork was herniated into the collector channel (*CC*) ostium compared with the eyes perfused at lower pressures. (**b**) When the eye was first perfused at 45 mmHg and then the IOP was reduced to 7 mmHg, the herniation into the CC ostia seen at 45 mmHg in image A was reversed; only deformation of the trabecular meshwork was seen facing the CC ostium region. SC was wider in this eye than in the one perfused continually at 45 mmHg. (**c**) When the eye was continually perfused at 7 mmHg, SC was open, and no herniations were visible (Image provided by Haiyan Gong, MD, PhD)

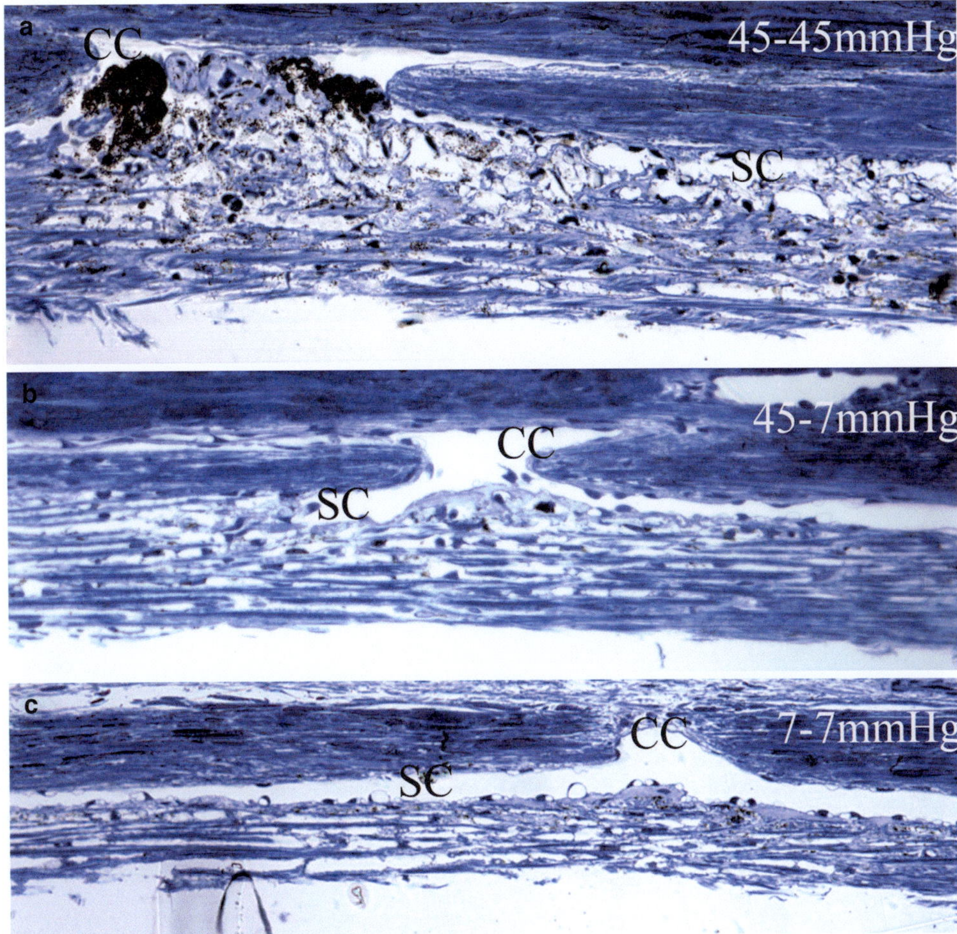


**Fig. 1.22** Light microscopic comparison between the POAG and normal ostia regions. (**a**) A micrograph of a normal eye. Schlemm's canal (*SC*) was open and the herniation was not observed in the collector channel (*CC*) ostia region. (**b**) In comparison, an eye with primary open-angle glaucoma demonstrated a collapse of SC adjacent to both sides of CC ostium with focal adhesions between the inner wall and outer wall. In addition, herniations of the inner wall and JCT into CC ostia were also observed. Scale bar = 25 μm (Images are provided by Haiyan Gong, MD, PhD)

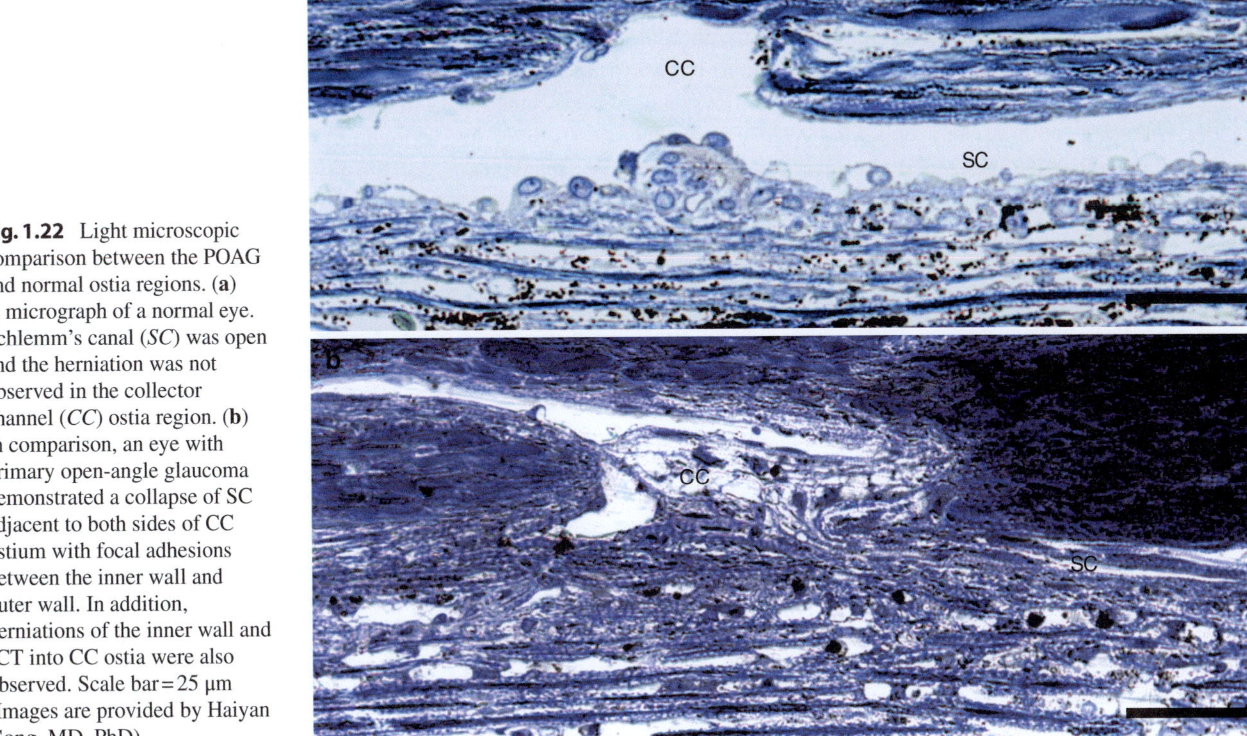

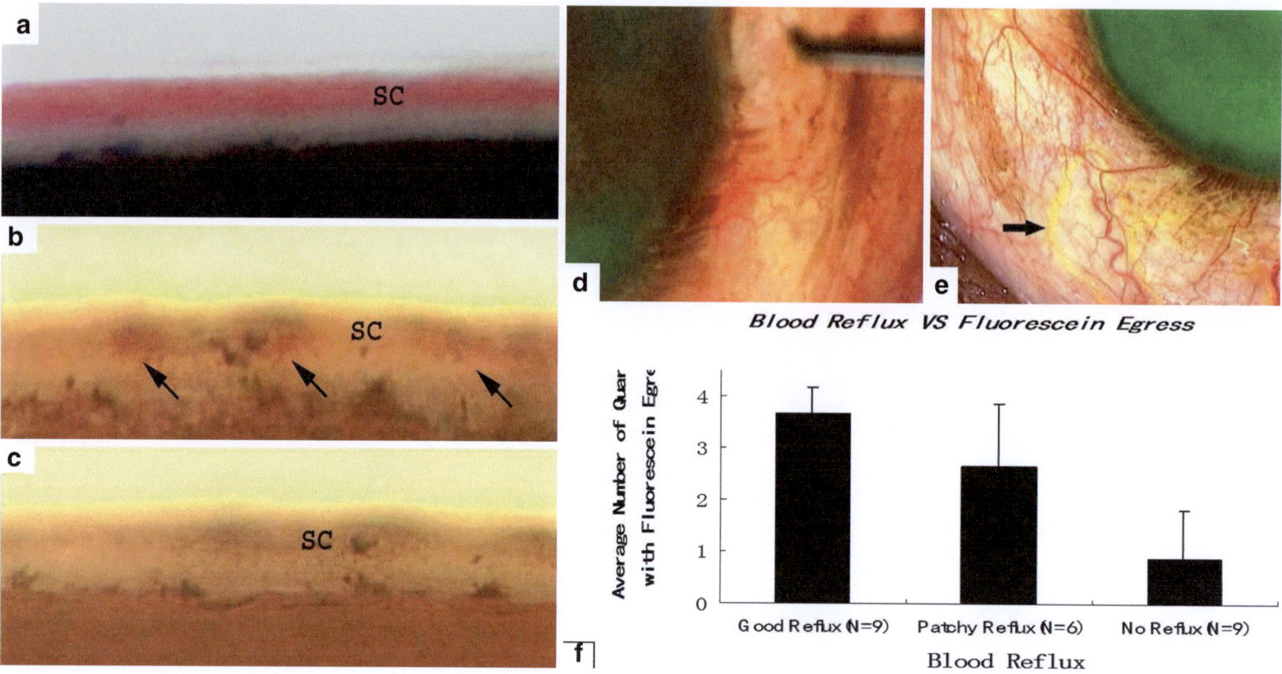



**Fig. 1.23** Evaluation of blockage of collector channel by blood reflux into Schlemm's canal and fluorescein egress pattern in the episcleral veins. (**a–c**) Gonioscopic view of blood into Schlemm's canal after preoperative paracentesis of the anterior chamber. (**a**) Schlemm's canal (*SC*) uniformly filled with blood indicates patent SC and collector channels (*CC*). (**b**) Patchy or irregular filling of SC indicates a partially collapsed SC. Blood is only detectable near the CC ostia (*arrows*). (**c**) No refluxed blood indicating a collapsed SC or blocked CCs. (**d–f**) Analysis of 4 quadrants of each eye with episcleral veins exhibiting fluorescein egress. (**d**) No filling of the episcleral veins. (**e**) Filling of the episcleral veins after injection of fluorescein dye into SC. (**f**) The average number of quadrants exhibiting fluorescein egress is consistent with blood reflux patterns in images (**a–c**) (Images are provided by Robert Stegmann, MD (**a–e**), Data was analyzed by Jinyin Zhu, MD (**f**))

## Increase Aqueous Outflow Area by Medical and Surgical Treatment

An increase in outflow facility by a Rho kinase inhibitor, Y27632, was reported associated with an increase in EFA [77, 78]. A new glaucoma device, trabecular micro-bypass (iStent, Glaukos, Laguna Hills, CA), increases outflow facility by directing outflow into episcleral veins from SC bypassing the trabecular meshwork. However, since the iStent is so small (1 mm length, 120 μm inlet), success of surgery is dependent on the circumferential location (i.e., whether the implant is placed near the larger CC ostia). An increase in outflow facility is associated with implanting more than one iStent [90, 91]. Newer devices undergoing clinical trials would also benefit from preoperative knowledge of CC ostia location. One such device is the Hydrus™ Microstent (Ivantis, CA), a novel intracanalicular scaffold that increases outflow facility by directing flow into more episcleral veins bypassing the trabecular meshwork and scaffolding SC. In one study, the Hydrus Aqueous Implant significantly increased outflow facility by increasing the total area involved in aqueous humor outflow. More scleral veins were accessed by the intracanalicular scaffold via multiple collector channels compared to controls or two iStent Implants [92].

## Evaluation of the Anterior Chamber Angle with Optical Coherence Tomography

### Introduction

Optical coherence tomography (OCT) is a noninvasive, noncontact method of imaging ocular structures in vivo (Fig. 1.24) [94]. Early time-domain (TD-OCT) devices provided cross-sectional images of the retina, nerve fiber layer, and optic nerve head (400-Hz, A-scan rate, Stratus OCT; Carl Zeiss Meditec, Dublin, California) and of the ocular anterior segment (2 kHz, A-scan rate, Visante; Carl Zeiss Meditec) but were limited by slow scan speeds, high signal-to-noise ratios, and motion artifacts. Newer spectral-domain (SD-OCT) and swept-source (SS-OCT) devices with software improvements are capable of distinguishing components of the conventional aqueous outflow pathway including the iridocorneal angle, trabecular meshwork, Schlemm's canal, and the scleral venous plexus (Fig. 1.25). Advances using phase-sensitive OCT devices (PhS-OCT) have even shown pulse-dependent movements in the trabecular meshwork and optic nerve head ex vivo (Fig. 1.26) [95, 96], which provides support to the current theory that proposes glaucoma is a result of resistance to pulsatile aqueous flow by trabecular tissue inelasticity [66].

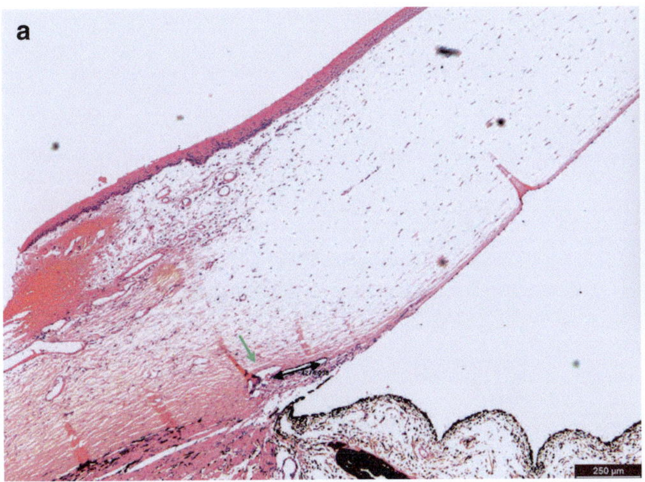
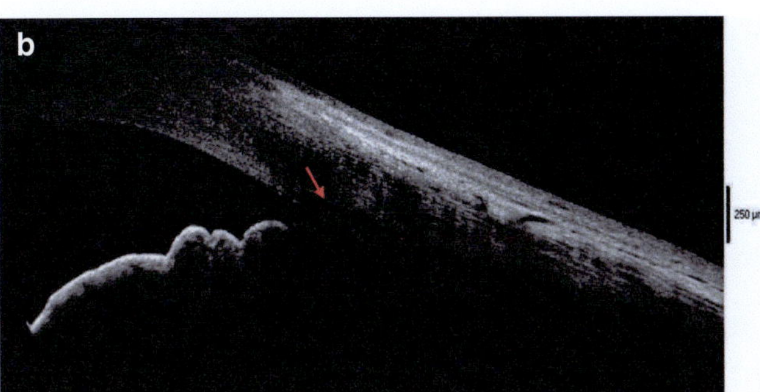

**Fig. 1.24** Anterior segment anatomy as seen with histology and optical coherence tomography (OCT). (**a**) Hematoxylin and eosin (H&E)-stained corneal specimen compared with (**b**) anterior segment optical coherence tomography (OCT) image. Schlemm's canal diameter is clearly visible in the H&E section (*black arrow*) with a collector channel visible nearby (*green arrow*). OCT is also able to identify Schlemm's canal with similar detail (*red arrow*) (With permission from Hong et al. [93])

OCT functions by analyzing interference patterns. Light from a broadband light source is divided into a reference and a sample beam. Light waves that are backscattered from optical structures interfere with the reference beam and a depth and density profile is created [97, 98]. Older time-domain (TD-OCT) systems such as the Stratus OCT (Carl Zeiss Meditec, Inc., Dublin, CA) were limited to 400 A-scans per second with an axial resolution of 8–10 μm in tissue and a high propensity for motion artifact. Newer systems are capable of more than 400,000 A-scans per second and 3-dimensional imaging of ocular structures in vivo [99, 100].

## Identification of Anatomical Structures

An ongoing area of research is noninvasive OCT imaging of the conventional aqueous outflow pathway, including the trabecular meshwork, Schlemm's canal, collector channels, and venous outflow plexus with the goal to optimize surgical treatment of glaucoma. High-definition identification of the anterior chamber angle, the scleral spur, Schwalbe's line, and the anatomical boundaries of the trabecular meshwork has been achieved with excellent reproducibility of angle measurements [100, 101]. Detailed evaluation of the trabecular meshwork, Schlemm's canal, and collector channels is more difficult due to the close association of several different tissues at varying anatomical depths; however, progress continues to be made in identifying several important characteristics of the aqueous outflow structures in vivo.

Allingham et al. first suggested a correlation between decreased Schlemm's canal area in glaucomatous eyes and outflow facility [31]. This was first confirmed using a commercially available spectral-domain (SD-OCT) system [52] and later in a larger cohort where a significant correlation between increasing mean IOP and decreasing Schlemm's canal area in patients with and without POAG was shown [93]. The mechanisms for this relationship is believed to be associated with a reduction in pulsatile flow in glaucomatous eyes where increased resistance to flow occurs by an increase in stiffness of the trabecular meshwork [66]. Actual evidence of this has been provided by newer phase-sensitive (PhS-OCT) OCT systems that have quantitatively visualized trabecular meshwork movement in synch with pulse-induced IOP ex vivo [95].

## Potential Surgical Applications

A number of microinvasive glaucoma surgical devices are FDA approved for the treatment of glaucoma. All function by bypassing the source of aqueous outflow resistance to improve outflow facility by using normal trabecular outflow pathway. The ability for OCT to visualize dynamic movements of the aqueous outflow anatomy in real time may be useful in preoperative planning to optimize placement of microsurgical devices in areas near the collector channels with normal function (Fig. 1.27). This would increase therapeutic efficiency and contribute to better surgical outcomes.

Currently, three microinvasive glaucoma devices are FDA approved for treatment of glaucoma with many more undergoing clinical trials. The iStent trabecular micro-bypass is a heparin-coated, microsurgical shunt placed into Schlemm's canal during cataract surgery that creates a patent bypass of the trabecular meshwork between the anterior chamber and

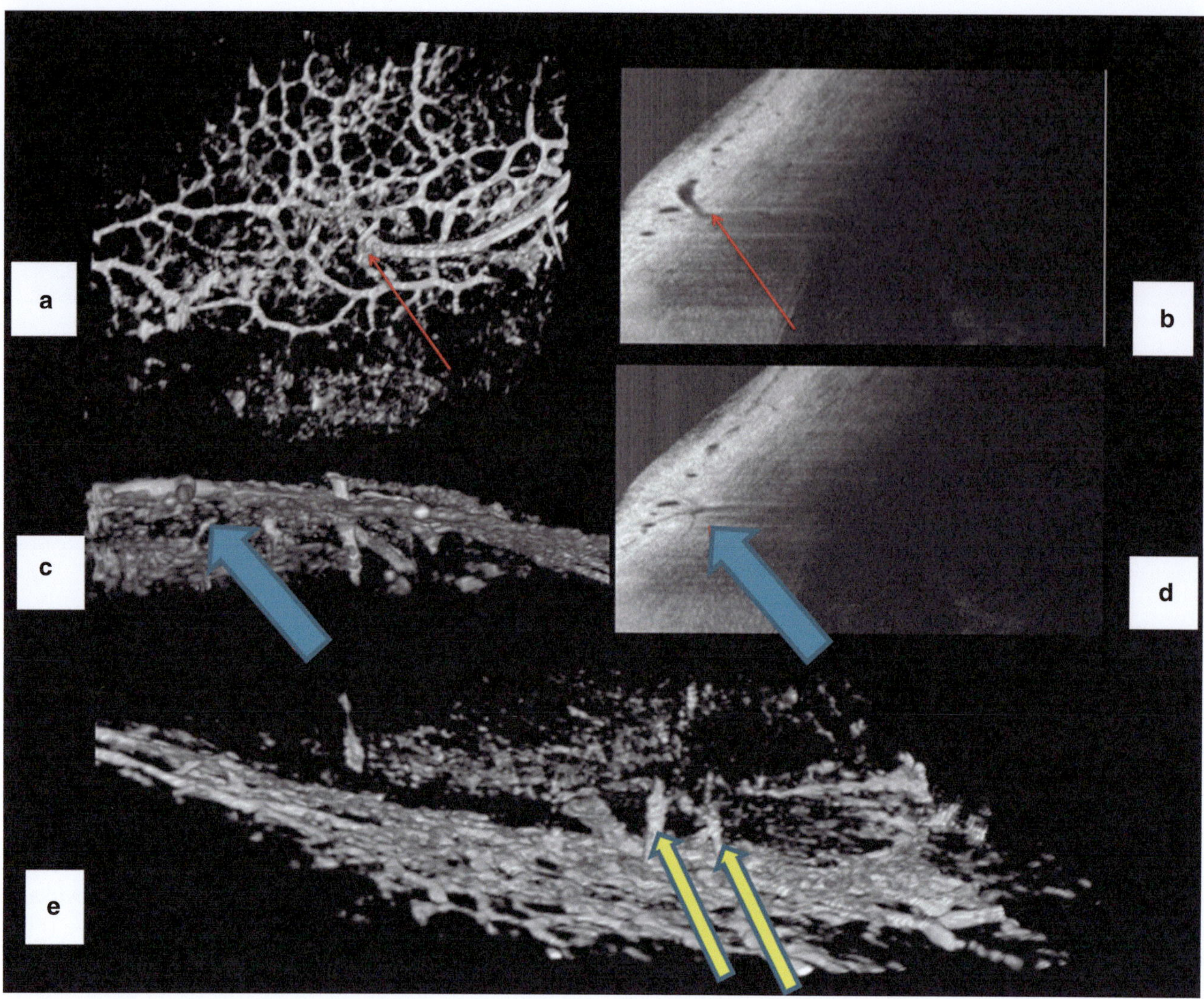

**Fig. 1.25** OCT image of the superficial venous plexus in enucleated human eye. The superficial venous plexus is composed of a series of small interconnected venules between 25 and 100 μm in diameter with many interconnecting branch points forming a dense vascular hexagonal meshwork (**a**). *Red arrows* indicate a vessel seen on the virtual casting (**a**) and its corresponding location in B-scan (**b**). *Blue arrows* indicate a suspected aqueous vein (**c**) descending from the superficial intrascleral venous plexus to the midlimbal intrascleral venous plexus and its corresponding location in B-scan (**d**). *Yellow arrows* indicate two suspected aqueous veins seen in this 180° rotated virtual casting image (**e**) (With permission from Francis et al. [53])

Schlemm's canal. In a prospective, randomized, multicenter, 12-month US study, 68 % of patients who received iStent achieved ≥20 % IOP reduction without medication while sustaining target IOPs of ≤21 mmHg vs. only 48 % of those who underwent cataract surgery alone ($p = .003$) [102]. The device is implanted via the anterior chamber through the trabecular meshwork in the inferior-nasal quadrant, where the greatest number of collector channels is believed to reside,

**Fig. 1.27** Pulse-induced movements in the trabecular meshwork visualized with optical coherence tomography (OCT). Ex vivo pulse-induced movement in the trabecular meshwork (*TM*) and Schlemm's canal (*SC*) in nonhuman primate eye at 8 mmHg mean IOP. Representative cross-sectional images of tissue velocity in the corneoscleral limbus: (**a**) *red* corresponds to TM movement into SC during systole; (**b**) *blue* corresponds to TM movement away from SC during diastole; (**c**) and (**d**) depth-dependent velocity profiles along the *vertical dashed lines* in (**a**) and (**b**), respectively; (**e**) and (**f**) corresponding OCT microstructural images from (**a**) and (**b**). (**g**) Enlarged view of the area marked by the dashed *yellow square* in (**e**). The closed *white curve* in (**g**) depicts the boundary of the SC. (**h**) Schematic of the SC endothelial attachment to the underlying trabecular lamellae. The *bold arrows* in (**h**) indicate tissue responses to deforming forces induced by IOP transients. The *horizontal lines* are used to mark approximately the position of TM, facilitating comparison between figures given (With permission from Li et al. [95])

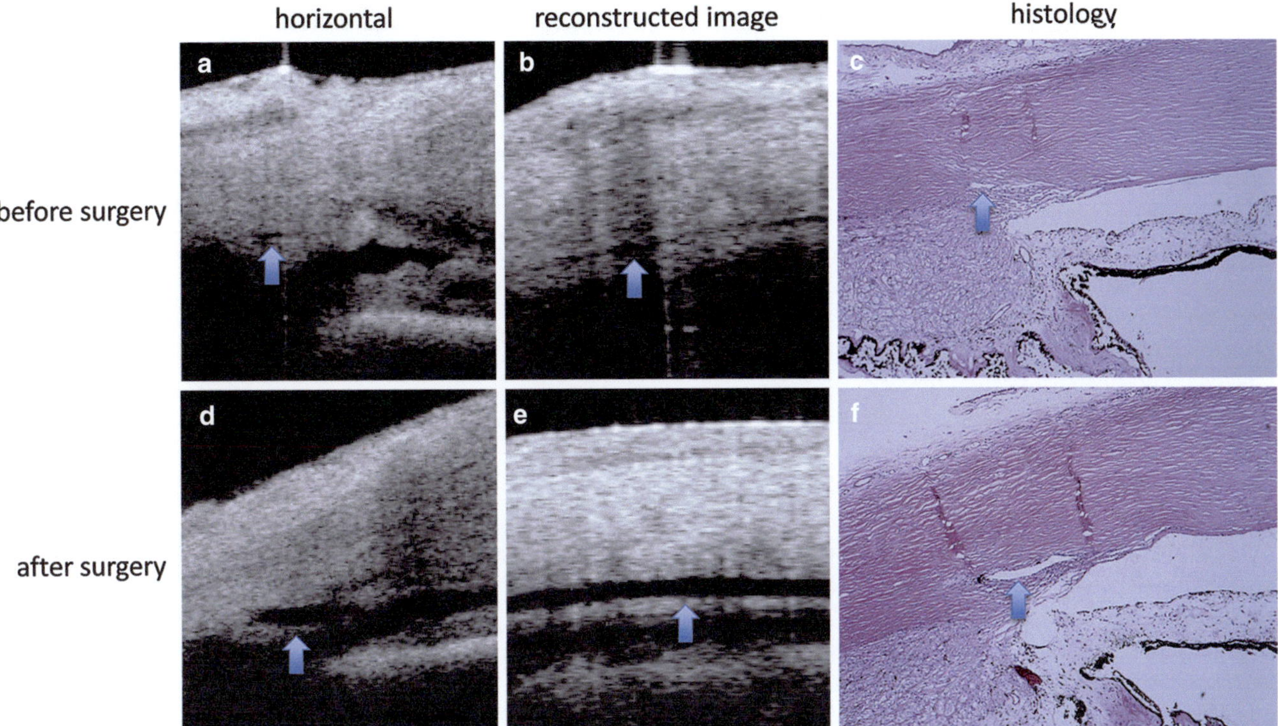


**Fig. 1.26** Assessment of surgical outcome before and after with optical coherence tomography (OCT). A postsurgical change in angle structures in human enucleated eyes is shown before (**a–c**) and after (**d–f**) pseudo viscocanalostomy was performed. A thin lucent space (**a**, **b**; *arrow*) confirmed to be Schlemm's canal on histology (**c**) was visualized. After surgical manipulation, this thin space (**d**, **e**; *arrow*) was enlarged. Histological sections supported the conclusion that this thin black space is SC (*arrows*, **c**, **f**) (Image with permission from Usui et al. [9])

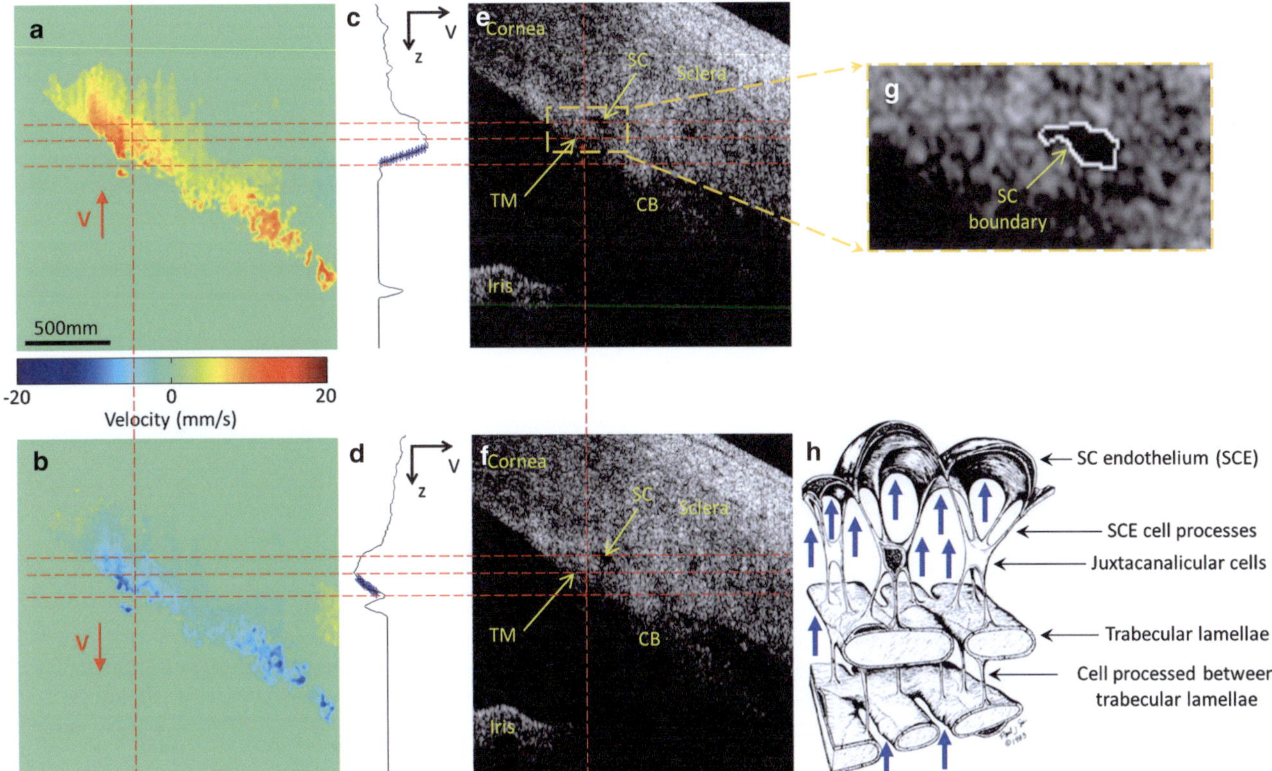

into Schlemm's canal. Advances in intraoperative OCT units may soon offer better visualization of collector channel anatomy than high magnification with a gonioprism alone.

The trabectome is an FDA-approved device for minimally invasive surgical treatment of glaucoma. The trabectome is an alternative to trabeculectomy and does not require the creation of an external filtering bleb. Instead, access to Schlemm's canal is provided by ablating a 60–120° strip of trabecular meshwork using a focused electrosurgical pulse from the anterior chamber. Studies have shown this surgery is an effective method of reducing IOP both alone and combined with phacoemulsification surgery [103].

Canaloplasty is an FDA-approved procedure for the treatment of open-angle glaucoma. The procedure involves circumferential viscodilation and tensioning of the inner wall of Schlemm's canal to treat open-angle glaucoma. To perform a canaloplasty, an incision is made into the eye to gain access to Schlemm's canal and a microcatheter is placed that will circumnavigate the canal around the limbus. The purpose is to enlarge Schlemm's canal and all associated collector channels through the injection of a viscoelastic substance. By opening the canal, the pressure inside the eye is reduced. Long-term follow-up studies show that canaloplasty leads to a significant and sustained reduction in both IOP and the number of glaucoma medications required for glaucoma control in adult patients with open-angle glaucoma with an excellent short- and long-term postoperative safety profile [104].

With continued development of OCT technology, including OCT units now available in handheld form and advanced intraoperative OCT units, analysis of ocular anatomy may optimize placement of minimally invasive surgical devices in areas near the collector channels with normal function. Other anterior segment surgeries may also benefit from precise localization of areas of outflow for trabeculectomy and bleb creation and anatomical changes in the chamber angle following peripheral iridotomies and goniotomy. Real-time, intraoperative feedback on structural changes following anterior segment procedures may soon become standard of care with new OCT technologies [105].

## Summary

This chapter reviewed the basic anatomy of the trabecular outflow pathway and the structural changes observed in experimentally induced elevation of IOP and in eyes with POAG. The structural changes in the outflow pathway that may be related to the reduction of active outflow area and thus increasing outflow resistance were also discussed. Using medical and surgical strategies to restore reduced active flow area in the eyes with POAG to a normal level lowers IOP. With further development of OCT, it is possible that, in the future, some of the structural changes, which currently are only able to be assessed histologically, could be evaluated by OCT before and after medical or surgical treatments in POAG patients.

**Acknowledgements** The original work reported in this chapter was supported in part by NIH/EY018712, EY022634, the American Health Assistance Foundation (now called BrightFocus Foundation), and the Massachusetts Lions Eye Research Fund.

## References

1. The Advanced Glaucoma Intervention Study (AGIS): 7. The relationship between control of intraocular pressure and visual field deterioration. The AGIS Investigators. Am J Ophthalmol. 2000; 130(4):429–40.
2. Barany E. In vitro studies of the resistance to flow through the angle of the anterior chamber. Acta Soc Med Ups. 1954;59:260–76.
3. VanBuskirk EM, Grant WM. Influence of temperature and the question of involvement of cellular metabolism in aqueous outflow. Am J Ophthalmol. 1974;77(4):565–72.
4. Bill A, Phillips CI. Uveoscleral drainage of aqueous humour in human eyes. Exp Eye Res. 1971;12(3):275–81.
5. Pederson JE, Gaasterland DE, MacLellan HM. Uveoscleral aqueous outflow in the rhesus monkey: importance of uveal reabsorption. Invest Ophthalmol Vis Sci. 1977;16(11):1008–7.
6. Hogan M, Alvarado J, Weddell J. Histology of the human eye. Philadelphia: WB Saunders Co; 1971.
7. Tamm ER. The trabecular meshwork outflow pathways: structural and functional aspects. Exp Eye Res. 2009;88(4):648–55.
8. Kasuga T, Chen YC, Bloomer MM, Hirabayashi KE, Hiratsuka Y, Murakami A, et al. Trabecular meshwork length in men and women by histological assessment. Curr Eye Res. 2013;38(1): 75–9.
9. Usui T, Tomidokoro A, Mishima K, Mataki N, Mayama C, Honda N, et al. Identification of Schlemm's canal and its surrounding tissues by anterior segment Fourier domain optical coherence tomography. Invest Ophthalmol Vis Sci. 2011;52(9):6934–9.
10. Freddo T. Ocular anatomy and physiology related to aqueous production and outflow. In: Fingeret M, Lewis T, editors. Primary care of the glaucomas. 2nd ed. New York: McGraw -Hill; 2001.
11. Freddo TF, Civan M, Gong H. Chapter 191: Aqueous humor and the dynamics of its flow: mechanisms and routes of aqueous humor drainage. In: Albert DM, Jakobiec F, editors. Principles and practice of ophthalmology. 3rd ed. Philadelphia: Saunders/Elsevier; 2008.
12. Freddo T. Primary care of the glaucomas. 2nd ed. New York: McGraw Hill Professional; 2001.
13. Freddo T, Gong H, Civan M. Duane's clinical ophthalmology. Philadelphia: Lippincott, Williams & Wilkins; 2011.
14. Gong H, et al. A new view of the human trabecular meshwork using quick-freeze, deep-etch electron microscopy. Exp Eye Res. 2002;75:347–58.
15. Rohen JW, van der Zypen E. The phagocytic activity of the trabecular meshwork endothelium. Albrecht Von Graefes Arch Klin Exp Ophthalmol. 1968;175:143–60.
16. Richardson TM, Hutchinson BT, Grant WM. The outflow tract in pigmentary glaucoma: a light and electron microscopic study. Arch Ophthalmol. 1977;95(6):1015–25.
17. Epstein DL, Freddo TF, Anderson PJ, Patterson MM, Bassett-Chu S. Experimental obstruction to aqueous outflow by pigment particles in living monkeys. Invest Ophthalmol Vis Sci. 1986;27(3):387–95.
18. Grierson I, Howes RC. Age-related depletion of the cell population in the human trabecular meshwork. Eye (Lond). 1987;1(Pt 2): 204–10.

19. Buller C, Johnson DH, Tschumper RC. Human trabecular mesh-work phagocytosis. Observations in an organ culture system. Invest Ophthalmol Vis Sci. 1990;31(10):2156–63.

20. Alvarado J, Murphy C, Polansky J, Juster R. Age-related changes in trabecular meshwork cellularity. Invest Ophthalmol Vis Sci. 1981;21(5):714–27.

21. Alvarado J, Murphy C, Juster R. Trabecular meshwork cellularity in primary open-angle glaucoma and nonglaucomatous normals. Ophthalmology. 1984;91(6):564–79.

22. Gong H, Tripathi RC, Tripathi BJ. Morphology of the aqueous out-flow pathway. Microsc Res Tech. 1996;33:336–67.

23. Rohen JW. Why is intraocular pressure elevated in chronic simple glaucoma? Anatomical considerations. Ophthalmology. 1983;90(7):758–65.

24. Gong HY, Trinkaus-Randall V, Freddo TF. Ultrastructural immuno-cytochemical localization of elastin in normal human trabecular meshwork. Curr Eye Res. 1989;8(10):1071–82.

25. Mäepea O, Bill A. Pressures in the juxtacanalicular tissue and Schlemm's canal in monkeys. Exp Eye Res. 1992;54(6):879–83.

26. Keller KE, Aga M, Bradley JM, Kelley MJ, Acott TS. Extracellular matrix turnover and outflow resistance. Exp Eye Res. 2009;88(4):676–82.

27. Rohen JW, Lütjen-Drecoll E, Flügel C, Meyer M, Grierson I. Ultrastructure of the trabecular meshwork in untreated cases of pri-mary open-angle glaucoma (POAG). Exp Eye Res. 1993;56(6):683–92.

28. Rohen JW, Linnér E, Witmer R. Electron microscopic studies on the trabecular meshwork in two cases of corticosteroid-glaucoma. Exp Eye Res. 1973;17(1):19–31.

29. Lütjen-Drecoll E, Shimizu T, Rohrbach M, Rohen JW. Quantitative analysis of 'plaque material' between ciliary muscle tips in normal- and glaucomatous eyes. Exp Eye Res. 1986;42(5):457–65.

30. Johnson D, Gottanka J, Flügel C, Hoffmann F, Futa R, Lütjen-Drecoll E. Ultrastructural changes in the trabecular meshwork of human eyes treated with corticosteroids. Arch Ophthalmol. 1997;115(3):375–83.

31. Allingham RR, de Kater AW, Ethier CR. Schlemm's canal and pri-mary open angle glaucoma: correlation between Schlemm's canal dimensions and outflow facility. Exp Eye Res. 1996;62(1):101–9.

32. Bhatt K, Gong H, Freddo TF. Freeze-fracture studies of interendo-thelial junctions in the angle of the human eye. Invest Ophthalmol Vis Sci. 1995;36(7):1379–89.

33. Allingham RR, de Kater AW, Ethier CR, Anderson PJ, Hertzmark E, Epstein DL. The relationship between pore density and outflow facility in human eyes. Invest Ophthalmol Vis Sci. 1992;33(5):1661–9.

34. Ye W, Gong H, Sit A, Johnson M, Freddo TF. Immersion fixation vs. fixation under flow: a study of changes in the structure of inter-endothelial junctions of Schlemm's canal in normal human eyes. Invest Ophthalmol Vis Sci. 1995;36(suppl):S729.

35. Johnstone M, Grant W. Microsurgery of Schlemm's canal and the human aqueous outflow system. Am J Ophthalmol. 1973;76:906–17.

36. Ten Hulzen RD, Johnson DH. Effect of fixation pressure on juxta-canalicular tissue and Schlemm's canal. Invest Ophthalmol Vis Sci. 1996;37(1):114–24.

37. Tripathi R, Tripathi B. Functional anatomy of the anterior chamber of the angle. In: Duane TD, Jaeger EA, editors. Biomedical founda-tions of ophthalmology. Philadelphia: Harper & Row; 1982.

38. Ethier CR, Coloma FM, Sit AJ, Johnson M. Two pore types in the inner-wall endothelium of Schlemm's canal. Invest Ophthalmol Vis Sci. 1998;39(11):2041–8.

39. Bill A, Svedbergh B. Scanning electron microscopic studies of the trabecular meshwork and the canal of Schlemm–an attempt to localize the main resistance to outflow of aqueous humor in man. Acta Ophthalmol (Copenh). 1972;50(3):295–320.

40. Johnson M, Chan D, Read AT, Christensen C, Sit A, Ethier CR. The pore density in the inner wall endothelium of Schlemm's canal of glaucomatous eyes. Invest Ophthalmol Vis Sci. 2002;43(9):2950–5.

41. Battista SA, Lu Z, Hofmann S, Freddo T, Overby DR, Gong H. Reduction of the available area for aqueous humor outflow and increase in meshwork herniations into collector channels following acute IOP elevation in bovine eyes. Invest Ophthalmol Vis Sci. 2008;49(12):5346–52.

42. Moses RA. Circumferential flow in Schlemm's canal. Am J Ophthalmol. 1979;88(3 Pt 2):585–91.

43. Van Buskirk EM. Anatomic correlates of changing aqueous outflow facility in excised human eyes. Invest Ophthalmol Vis Sci. 1982;22(5):625–32.

44. Rohen JW, Lütjen E, Bárány E. The relation between the ciliary mus-cle and the trabecular meshwork and its importance for the effect of miotics on aqueous outflow resistance. A study in two contrasting monkey species, Macaca irus and Cercopithecus aethiops. Albrecht Von Graefes Arch Klin Exp Ophthalmol. 1967;172(1):23–47.

45. Kaufman PL, Bárány EH. Residual pilocarpine effects on outflow facility after ciliary muscle disinsertion in the cynomolgus monkey. Invest Ophthalmol. 1976;15(7):558–61.

46. Johnson M, Erickson K. Mechanisms and routes of aqueous humor drainage. In: Albert DM, Jakobiec FA, editors. Principles and practice of ophthalmology. Philadelphia: WB Saunders Co; 2000. p. 2577.

47. Hann CR, Fautsch MP. Preferential fluid flow in the human trabecu-lar meshwork near collector channels. Invest Ophthalmol Vis Sci. 2009;50(4):1692–7.

48. Parc CE, Johnson DH, Brilakis HS. Giant vacuoles are found pref-erentially near collector channels. Invest Ophthalmol Vis Sci. 2000;41(10):2984–90.

49. Dvorak-Theobald G. Further studies on the canal of Schlemm; its anastomoses and anatomic relations. Am J Ophthalmol. 1955;39(4 Pt 2):65–89.

50. Rohen JW, Rentsch FJ. Morphology of Schlemm's canal and related vessels in the human eye. Albrecht Von Graefes Arch Klin Exp Ophthalmol. 1968;176(4):309–29.

51. Hann CR, Bentley MD, Vercnocke A, Ritman EL, Fautsch MP. Imaging the aqueous humor outflow pathway in human eyes by three-dimensional micro-computed tomography (3D micro-CT). Exp Eye Res. 2011;92(2):104–11.

52. Kagemann L, Wollstein G, Ishikawa H, Bilonick RA, Brennen PM, Folio LS, et al. Identification and assessment of Schlemm's canal by spectral-domain optical coherence tomography. Invest Ophthalmol Vis Sci. 2010;51(8):4054–9.

53. Francis AW, Kagemann L, Wollstein G, Ishikawa H, Folz S, Overby DR, et al. Morphometric analysis of aqueous humor outflow struc-tures with spectral-domain optical coherence tomography. Invest Ophthalmol Vis Sci. 2012;53(9):5198–207.

54. Lutjen-Drecoll E, Rohen JW. Morphology of aqueous outflow path-ways in normal and glaucomatous eyes. In: Ritch R, Shields MB, Krupin T, editors. The glaucomas. St. Louis: Mosby; 1989.

55. Lütgen-Drecoll E, Rohen J. Morphology of aqueous outflow path-ways in normal and glaucomatous eyes. In: Ritch R, Shields MB, Krupin T, editors. The glaucomas. St. Louis: Mosby; 1989.

56. Johnson M. What controls aqueous humour outflow resistance? Exp Eye Res. 2006;82(4):545–57.

57. Grant WM. Further studies on facility of flow through the trabecular meshwork. AMA Arch Ophthalmol. 1958;60(4 Part 1):523–33.

58. de Kater AW, Spurr-Michaud SJ, Gipson IK. Localization of smooth muscle myosin-containing cells in the aqueous outflow pathway. Invest Ophthalmol Vis Sci. 1990;31(2):347–53.

59. Rosenquist R, Epstein D, Melamed S, Johnson M, Grant WM. Outflow resistance of enucleated human eyes at two different perfu-sion pressures and different extents of trabeculotomy. Curr Eye Res. 1989;8(12):1233–40.

60. Grant WM. Experimental aqueous perfusion in enucleated human eyes. 1963;69:783–801.
61. Schuman JS, Chang W, Wang N, de Kater AW, Allingham RR. Excimer laser effects on outflow facility and outflow pathway morphology. Invest Ophthalmol Vis Sci. 1999;40(8):1676–80.
62. Schacknow PN, Samples JR. The glaucoma book: a practical, evidence-based approach to patient care. 1st ed. Medford: Springer-Verlag New York, LLC; 2010.
63. Ascher KW. Aqueous veins. Am J Ophthalmol. 1942;25:31–8.
64. Ascher KW. Physiologic importance of the visible elimination of intraocular fluid. Am J Ophthalmol. 1942;25:1174–209.
65. Norman A. Anatomical study of Schlemm's canal and aqueous veins by means of neoprene casts: part II. aqueous veins (continued). Br J Ophthalmol. 1952;36:265–7.
66. Johnstone MA. The aqueous outflow system as a mechanical pump: evidence from examination of tissue and aqueous movement in human and non-human primates. J Glaucoma. 2004;13(5): 421–38.
67. DeVries S. De Zichtbare Afvoer Van Het Kamerwater. 1st ed. Amsterdam: Drukkerij Kinsbergen; 1947.
68. Goldmann H. Weitere Mitteilung über den Abfluss des Kammer wassers beim Menschen. Ophthalmologica. 1946;112(6):344–9.
69. Stepanik J. Measuring velocity of flow in aqueous veins. Am J Ophthalmol. 1954;37:918–22.
70. Johnstone M, et al. The glaucoma book, aqueous veins and open angle glaucoma. New York: Springer; 2010. p. 67.
71. LaBarbera M, Vogel S. The design of fluid transport systems in organisms. Am Sci. 1982;70:54–60.
72. LaBarbera M. Principles of design of fluid transport systems in zoology. Science. 1990;249(4972):992–1000.
73. Zamir M, Ritman E. The physics of pulsatile flow. New York: Springer; 2000.
74. Kleinert H. The visible flow of aqueous humor in the epibulbar veins. II. The pulsating blood vessels of the aqueous humor. Albrecht Von Graefes Arch Ophthalmol. 1952;152(6):587–608.
75. Kleinert H. The compensation maximum: a new glaucoma sign in aqueous veins. Arch Ophthalmol. 1951;46:618.
76. Camp JJ, Hann CR, Johnson DH, Tarara JE, Robb RA. Three-dimensional reconstruction of aqueous channels in human trabecular meshwork using light microscopy and confocal microscopy. Scanning. 1997;19(4):258–63.
77. Lu Z, Overby DR, Scott PA, Freddo TF, Gong H. The mechanism of increasing outflow facility by rho-kinase inhibition with Y-27632 in bovine eyes. Exp Eye Res. 2008;86(2):271–81.
78. Lu Z, Zhang Y, Freddo TF, Gong H. Similar hydrodynamic and morphological changes in the aqueous humor outflow pathway after washout and Y27632 treatment in monkey eyes. Exp Eye Res. 2011;93(4):397–404.
79. Swaminathan SS, Oh DJ, Kang MH, Ren R, Jin R, Gong H, et al. Secreted protein acidic and rich in cysteine (SPARC)-null mice exhibit more uniform outflow. Invest Ophthalmol Vis Sci. 2013;54(3):2035–47.
80. Keller KE, Bradley JM, Vranka JA, Acott TS. Segmental versican expression in the trabecular meshwork and involvement in outflow facility. Invest Ophthalmol Vis Sci. 2011;52(8):5049–57.
81. Yang C-Y, Liu Y, Gong H. Effects of Y27632 on aqueous humor outflow facility with changes in hydrodynamic pattern and morphology in human eyes. Invest Ophthalmol Vis Sci. 2013;54: 5859–70.
82. Zhu JY, Ye W, Wang T, Gong HY. Reversible changes in aqueous outflow facility, hydrodynamics, and morphology following acute intraocular pressure variation in bovine eyes. Chin Med J (Engl). 2013;126(8):1451–7.
83. Zhang Y, Toris CB, Liu Y, Ye W, Gong H. Morphological and hydrodynamic correlates in monkey eyes with laser induced glaucoma. Exp Eye Res. 2009;89(5):748–56.
84. Cha E, Jin R, Gong H. The relationship between morphological changes and reduction of active areas of aqueous outflow in eyes with primary open angle glaucoma. Invest Ophthalmol Vis Sci. 2013;54:2291.
85. Gottanka J, Johnson DH, Martus P, Lütjen-Drecoll E. Severity of optic nerve damage in eyes with POAG is correlated with changes in the trabecular meshwork. J Glaucoma. 1997;6(2):123–32.
86. Zhu J, Gong H. Morphological changes contributing to decreased outflow facility following acute IOP elevation in normal human eyes. Invest Ophthalmol Vis Sci. 2008;49:1639.
87. Gong H, Freddo TF, Zhang Y. New morphological findings in primary open-angle glaucoma. Invest Ophthalmol Vis Sci. 2007;48:2079.
88. Gong H, Huang R, Zhu J, Stegmann R. Blockages of collector channel ostia exist in patients with Primary Open Angle Glaucoma (POAG). In: American Glaucoma Society 19th annual meeting, San Diego, CA, March 5–8, 2009.
89. Grieshaber MC, Pienaar A, Olivier J, Stegmann R. Clinical evaluation of the aqueous outflow system in primary open-angle glaucoma for canaloplasty. Invest Ophthalmol Vis Sci. 2010;51(3): 1498–504.
90. Bahler CK, Smedley GT, Zhou J, Johnson DH. Trabecular bypass stents decrease intraocular pressure in cultured human anterior segments. Am J Ophthalmol. 2004;138(6):988–94.
91. Bahler CK, Hann CR, Fjield T, Haffner D, Heitzmann H, Fautsch MP. Second-generation trabecular meshwork bypass stent (iStent inject) increases outflow facility in cultured human anterior segments. Am J Ophthalmol. 2012;153(6):1206–13.
92. Gong H, Cha E, Gorantla V, Gulati V, Fan S, Steiner C, et al. Characterization of aqueous humor outflow through novel glaucoma devices – a tracer study. Invest Ophthalmol Vis Sci. 2012;53:3743.
93. Hong J, Xu J, Wei A, Wen W, Chen J, Yu X, et al. Spectral-domain optical coherence tomographic assessment of Schlemm's canal in Chinese subjects with primary open-angle glaucoma. Ophthalmology. 2013;120(4):709–15.
94. Huang D, Swanson EA, Lin CP, Schuman JS, Stinson WG, Chang W, et al. Optical coherence tomography. Science. 1991;254(5035): 1178–81.
95. Li P, Reif R, Zhi Z, Martin E, Shen TT, Johnstone M, et al. Phase-sensitive optical coherence tomography characterization of pulse-induced trabecular meshwork displacement in ex vivo nonhuman primate eyes. J Biomed Opt. 2012;17(7):076026.
96. An L, Chao J, Johnstone M, Wang RK. Noninvasive imaging of pulsatile movements of the optic nerve head in normal human subjects using phase-sensitive spectral domain optical coherence tomography. Opt Lett. 2013;38(9):1512–4.
97. Adhi M, Duker JS. Optical coherence tomography – current and future applications. Curr Opin Ophthalmol. 2013;24(3): 213–21.
98. Sull AC, Vuong LN, Price LL, Srinivasan VJ, Gorczynska I, Fujimoto JG, et al. Comparison of spectral/Fourier domain optical coherence tomography instruments for assessment of normal macular thickness. Retina. 2010;30(2):235–45.
99. Potsaid B, Baumann B, Huang D, Barry S, Cable AE, Schuman JS, et al. Ultrahigh speed 1050nm swept source/Fourier domain OCT retinal and anterior segment imaging at 100,000 to 400,000 axial scans per second. Opt Express. 2010;18(19):20029–48.
100. Liu S, Yu M, Ye C, Lam DS, Leung CK. Anterior chamber angle imaging with swept-source optical coherence tomography: an investigation on variability of angle measurement. Invest Ophthalmol Vis Sci. 2011;52(12):8598–603.
101. Tun TA, Baskaran M, Zheng C, Sakata LM, Perera SA, Chan AS, et al. Assessment of trabecular meshwork width using swept source optical coherence tomography. Graefes Arch Clin Exp Ophthalmol. 2013;251(6):1587–92.

102. Samuelson TW, Katz LJ, Wells JM, Duh YJ, Giamporcaro JE, US iStent Study Group. Randomized evaluation of the trabecular micro-bypass stent with phacoemulsification in patients with glaucoma and cataract. Ophthalmology. 2011;118(3):459–67.

103. Minckler D, Mosaed S, Dustin L, Ms BF, Group TS. Trabectome (trabeculectomy-internal approach): additional experience and extended follow-up. Trans Am Ophthalmol Soc. 2008;106:149–59; discussion 59–60.

104. Lewis RA, von Wolff K, Tetz M, Koerber N, Kearney JR, Shingleton BJ, et al. Canaloplasty: Three-year results of circumferential viscodilation and tensioning of Schlemm canal using a microcatheter to treat open-angle glaucoma. J Cataract Refract Surg. 2011;37(4):682–90.

105. Folio LS, Wollstein G, Schuman JS. Optical coherence tomography: future trends for imaging in glaucoma. Optom Vis Sci. 2012;89(5):E554–62.

# Intraoperative Assessment of the Conventional Collector Outflow System as Therapeutic Target

Ronald Leigh Fellman

## Introduction

Microinvasive glaucoma surgery (MIGS) for primary open-angle glaucoma is on the rise largely because of enhanced safety, rapid recovery, and the desire to lower IOP with bleb-less glaucoma surgery. Importantly, most of these MIGS may be performed in conjunction with phacoemulsification, meeting an increasing need for aging patients with conjoint cataract and uncontrolled open-angle glaucoma.

In addition, the indications for microinvasive modern-day canal surgery are expanding to include patients with mild to moderate glaucoma that may not require subnormal IOP. Currently available innovations in adult canal surgery include canaloplasty, trabectome, microcatheter trabeculotomy, and iStent with many promising devices on the horizon. The concept of improving flow into the patient's natural drainage system instead of abandoning it with a filter is a major shift in thinking for glaucoma surgeons and their patients.

Most surgeons understand that a bleb is an excellent readily visible outcome marker for filtration surgery. However, at this time, we are limited in correlating the outcome of canal procedures with a readily visible marker seen at slit lamp exam because of the inability to visualize aqueous flow in the collector system. An outcome marker is currently not possible with canal surgery because we do not have a canalogram or an easy method to assess the health or patency of the entire length of the collector system. Gonioscopy remains our only method of seeing the proximal anatomy of the conventional outflow system. From a physiologic viewpoint, we have no method of measuring aqueous flow in the veins, only observing

flow in aqueous veins, especially the aqueous veins of Ascher. Unfortunately, this is a lost art. Experimentally, we are able to visualize the collectors in perfused cadaver eyes [1] with sophisticated imaging systems and the historical methods of observation [2], inks, and neoprene casts [3, 4] to define the anatomy of the collectors. This chapter reviews the current methods of assessing the intraoperative patency of the conventional outflow system and adds a new observation that might help us better understand the anatomy and healing of the distal collector outflow system.

## Scope of the Problem

Canal surgeons are rapidly becoming students of outflow anatomy of the episcleral venous outflow system. Most of the literature on this subject is decades old because once filtration surgery became popular, there was not much of a need to further explore this subject because aqueous was diverted into a bleb and the condition of the collectors was irrelevant. However, the distal outflow system must be functional for canal procedures to work, a very difficult dilemma because we have no way to know if the distal outflow system is functional.

At this time, the preoperative assessment of the canal system is mainly limited to gonioscopy. Even with high-frequency ultrasound and optical coherence tomography (OCT), it is difficult to consistently see Schlemm's canal and there is limited detail of the downstream collector system.

The anatomy of the angle is critical to understand, especially finding the scleral spur which divides conventional from nonconventional outflow. Without this landmark, it is difficult to comprehend angle anatomy and correlate postoperative findings with intraocular pressure (IOP), and no imaging device consistently identifies the scleral spur.

Another part of the puzzle is our difficulty measuring episcleral venous pressure, which may have a major impact on success of canal surgery; again, this is essentially unrelated to the outcome of a filter. An undetected elevated episcleral

R.L. Fellman, MD
Department of Ophthalmology, Glaucoma Associates of Texas,
Eye Institute of Texas, Ste 300, 10740 North Central Expy,
Dallas, TX 75231, USA

Department of Ophthalmology, University of Texas
Southwestern Medical Center, Dallas, TX, USA
e-mail: rfellman@glaucomaassociates.com, rfellman@aol.com

J.R. Samples, I.I.K. Ahmed (eds.), *Surgical Innovations in Glaucoma*,
DOI 10.1007/978-1-4614-8348-9_2, © Springer Science+Business Media New York 2014

## Aqueous Humor Outflow in the Normal Eye

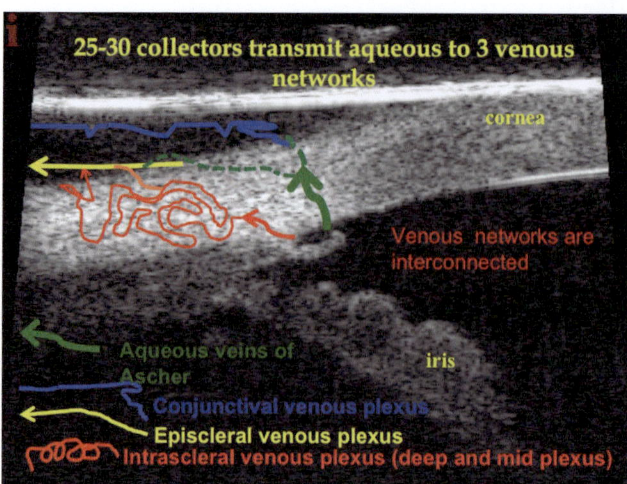


**Fig. 2.2** Aqueous collectors and venous networks. How does aqueous reach the distal collectors from the anterior chamber? There are approximately 25–35 collector channels that drain aqueous from Schlemm's canal into three venous networks: the intrascleral plexus (deep and mid), the episcleral plexus, and the conjunctival plexus. The approximately 30 collectors are comprised of mainly smaller collectors that drain into the deep plexus, then drain into the mid scleral plexus, and then into the episcleral venous plexus. There is a small group of larger veins (8 of the 30) that largely bypass the reticulated intrascleral plexus and drain directly into the episcleral and/or conjunctival networks. These are known as the veins of Ascher and may be seen during slit lamp examination (see reference [3])

**Fig. 2.1** Aqueous outflow. Aqueous exits the eye through either trabecular or uveoscleral channels. Trabecular outflow, seen in red, is also termed pressure-dependent outflow and handles most of the flow of aqueous, estimated to be approximately 75 %. Uveoscleral, or nonpressure-dependent, outflow is nontrabecular and comprises flow through the uveoscleral tissues

venous pressure (EVP), may cause failure of a canal procedure due to an abnormally high venous pressure. At this time, we do not have a rapid reliable way to measure EVP in a routine clinical setting.

## Tracing Trabecular Outflow

The conventional outflow system consists of the trabecular meshwork, juxtacanalicular tissue, Schlemm's canal, and the distal venous collector system (Fig. 2.1). For purposes of this chapter, we will concentrate on Schlemm's canal and the distal collector system. Gonioscopy allows for a view of the proximal conventional collector system such as inspection for peripheral anterior synechiae (PAS), blood, or excessive fibrous tissue that may block the anterior portion of the collector system. However, we are unable to see the collector system as it exits the posterior wall of Schlemm's canal and its pathway through the deep and mid scleral plexus, which together comprise the intrascleral plexus (Fig. 2.2). However, we are able to see the episcleral veins and larger episcleral and conjunctival veins of Ascher. Thus, we are able to see the very beginning of the conventional outflow system with a gonioprism and the termination of the system as it spills into episcleral and conjunctival veins, but nothing in the deep and mid scleral plexus or the collectors as they exit the canal. If an angle procedure such as a trabectome fails but gonioscopy reveals no PAS and a nice trabecular opening, why did the procedure fail? Where is the point of obstruction that caused the failure, closure of the collector channels as they leave Schlemm's canal, an atrophic intrascleral plexus that did not allow the aqueous to get to the episcleral veins or elevated episcleral venous pressure that we are unable to measure?

If we were able to view the distal collector system at the time of surgery, it might give us a clue as to the point of obstruction. At this time, we do not have a routine reliable way to assess the collectors intraoperatively or preoperatively or postoperatively. No doubt, this will change as technology progresses and supplies us with a functional map of the distal outflow system.

## Mapping the Conventional Aqueous Collector System

Ashton's Doyne's memorial lecture revealed groundbreaking work on the canal of Schlemm and outlet channels [5]. His neoprene cast worked and confirmed an irregular number of collector channels, 17–35 in number, that vary considerably in size. Immediately after leaving the canal, the smaller collectors form a deep scleral plexus located just external to the canal. The aqueous is then transmitted to the mid-scleral plexus, together with the deep scleral plexus, forming the intrascleral venous plexus. This drains into the episcleral venous plexus. In addition, Ascher described larger collector vessels that span from Schlemm's canal directly to the episcleral veins and/or the conjunctival plexus and largely bypass the intrascleral plexus. Thus, the aqueous exits Schlemm's canal through approximately 30 collectors passing into three venous systems: the intrascleral, episcleral, and conjunctival networks. Six to eight of the larger collectors comprise the veins of Ascher, which may be seen at the slit lamp. Ascher described the aqueous veins in his landmark 1942 article and defined them as biomicroscopically visible pathways of blood-vessel-like appearance containing a clear colorless fluid or diluted blood and intercalated between Schlemm's canal and conjunctival and subconjunctival veins.

Schlemm's canal is an endothelial-lined circular tube that transmits aqueous from the trabecular meshwork to the distal collector outflow system. It is approximately 36 mm in circumference, 300 μm wide (meridional), and 25 μm in height with the majority of the roughly 30 collector channels located mainly nasally and then inferiorly. This location is quite fortunate for canal surgeons from an accessibility issue. The majority of the collector channels are small, around 20–40 μm, but up to eight of these vessels may be considerably larger and connect directly to the canal (Ascher's veins) and avoid the plexus by communicating directly with either an episcleral or conjunctival vein.

## Assessment of the Conventional Outflow System

### Preoperative Assessment of the Conventional Collector System

It is difficult to study the collector outflow system in vivo, much less a diseased one or an outflow path that has been altered due to canal surgery. From a historical viewpoint, the first in vivo assessment of the collector system was truly the identification of blood in the canal of Schlemm. Investigators eventually discovered that blood could reflux into the canal by applying episcleral pressure with a flanged gonioprism or suction gonioprism. This raised EVP and reversed the pressure gradient causing the blood to reflux. In retrospect, this was an evaluation of the collector system between the canal and some of the distal collectors. The other way to reverse the pressure gradient is to artificially lower IOP below the EVP, and blood will collect in Schlemm's canal in normal eyes and probably less so in glaucomatous eyes. This information in conjunction with Ascher's studies of aqueous veins helped establish the path of aqueous once it left the canal of Schlemm. Therefore, preoperative gonioscopic maneuvers to cause blood to reflux into Schlemm's canal may help predict that there is a communication from the distal to more proximal collectors, but the gonioprism induces obvious mechanical and pressure distortion. OCT with special imaging attachments and altered wavelengths are improving the ability to image the collector system. However, a preoperative commercially available imaging method of the collector system is not widely available. It is possible to see Schlemm's canal with ultrasound biomicroscopic devices [6], but the smaller collectors are very difficult to see.

## Intraoperative Assessment of the Aqueous Channels

Canal surgery presents a unique opportunity to evaluate and explore the conventional aqueous outflow system. Why is it that a canaloplasty, trabectome, or iStent procedure fails? If we were able to assess the entirety of the channel anatomy at the time of surgery and it appeared to be patent but the procedure failed, it would more likely be due to postoperative scarring in or adjacent to the canal, not the fact that the downstream collector system was atrophic and/or unsalvageable. This is imperative to understand in order to advance the field of canal surgery and make pathophysiologic correlations. Gonioscopy or endoscopy is still a key method of visualizing the trabecular meshwork and canal of Schlemm intraoperatively for these structures are large enough to appreciate, but what is happening in the downstream aqueous channels is difficult to ascertain. Typically, we are unable to appreciate if the downstream aqueous channels are intact or totally atrophic from years of glaucomatous downstream collector atrophy from lack of aqueous flow. The other possibility is that the glaucomatous process not only involves the proximal trabecular meshwork but also, in some patients, involves the mid or distal system of collectors. Of course, this might vary depending on the genetic makeup of the individual with primary open-angle glaucoma (POAG).

When viscocanalostomy was introduced, it was not uncommon to see laminar flow into adjacent collectors and episcleral veins while injecting balanced salt solution (BSS) into the orifice of the canal. This phenomenon was also observed during canaloplasty (Fig. 2.3). This exciting observation verified the correct location of the canal and demonstrated flow through the collectors. Intraoperatively, some investigators have infused dye into the anterior chamber adjacent to an iStent with identification of various episcleral collector structures, but we await further published reports on this technique. Grieshaber [7] and colleagues published the intraoperative evaluation of aqueous channels during canaloplasty. They evaluated blood reflux into Schlemm's canal and fluorescein tracer channelography during canaloplasty. The blood reflux in the canal of Schlemm was observed after acutely lowering IOP by paracentesis. They found that excellent blood reflux into Schlemm's canal was associated with a lower preoperative IOP and poor to no reflux was associated with a high preoperative IOP. The tracer was injected directly into the canal through the iTrack microcatheter during canaloplasty (iScience Interventional, Menlo Park, CA). The investigators observed egress of dye through the episcleral venous plexus and graded the dispersion of dye. A broader

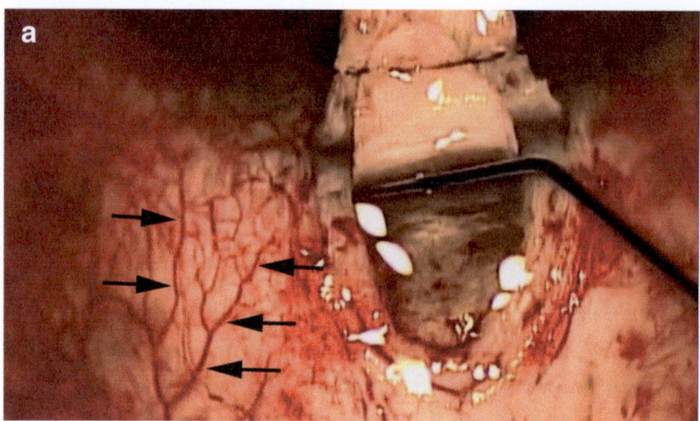
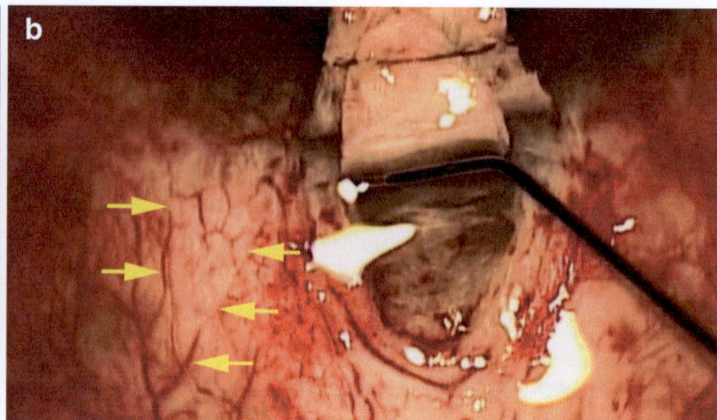

**Fig. 2.3** Episcleral venous laminar flow during canaloplasty. (**a**) Appearance of episcleral veins adjacent to canaloplasty dissection immediately before injection of balanced salt solution (BSS) into Schlemm's canal. Visualize the veins denoted by the *black arrows* and the plexus of veins between the groupings. Theoretically, if the cannula is in the canal and there is a nearby collector, there should be flow of BSS into the adjacent episcleral veins. (**b**) Appearance of episcleral veins immediately after injection of BSS into Schlemm's canal. There is a marked washout of blood from the veins by BSS. The *yellow arrows* are in the same position as the *black arrows* in (**a**). Note the marked decrease of blood in the plexus between the *yellow grouping of arrows*. This is evidence of flow from Schlemm's canal into adjacent collectors. Theoretically, this is anatomic evidence of patency of the collector system

dispersal of dye into the aqueous channels was associated with a lower postoperative IOP. The authors felt that provocative gonioscopy and channelography may reflect the function of the outflow pathway and correlate with canaloplasty outcome. This intuitively makes sense because a higher preoperative IOP is more likely associated with collapse of the canal of Schlemm along with distal compromise of the collectors.

## Episcleral Venous Fluid Wave: A New Intraoperative Method of Assessing Aqueous Outflow

Another recently described method of intraoperative assessment of aqueous channels was described as a wave of BSS coursing through episcleral and conjunctival vessels during the irrigation and aspiration phase of a combined phacotrabectome procedure. The investigators hypothesized that the trabeculotomy created by the trabectome might remove enough resistance in order to allow BSS to surge through an exposed collector and flow down the collector system during irrigation and aspiration associated with phacoemulsification. The trabectome procedure is performed first followed by the phacoemulsification with intraocular lens. After the viscoelastic is removed, the wave may be elicited. The technique of the episcleral venous fluid wave (EFW) [8] is performed by the following maneuvers: (1) start at foot position zero during I and A, whereby the IOP drops to near zero which reverses the pressure gradient allowing reflux of blood into the anterior chamber, and then (2) proceed to foot position two (with bottle height raised) allowing a surge of BSS into the anterior chamber and out the distal collectors associated with the cleaved trabeculotomy site. This was observed in every combined case, in varying degrees, and is associated with the final IOP, as observed by Grieshaber during canaloplasty. The EFW is easy to elicit and likely indicates anatomic patency of the distal aqueous channels. If there is no downstream flow during the propagation of the wave, it is likely that the distal collector system is severely atrophic or the episcleral venous pressure is high. One major problem is the inability to measure episcleral venous pressure in a reliable way, and we await the accuracy and practicality of this measurement.

## Types of Episcleral Venous Waves

During wave propagation, several types of EFWs were noticed. One of the most striking waves was down a large conjunctival vein (Fig. 2.4). It appears that conjunctival vessels are a likely source of the egress of aqueous, a fact that is poorly appreciated, but well described by Ascher. Although not commonly appreciated, it appears that a conjunctival peritomy may adversely affect outflow by destroying egress of aqueous through some conjunctival veins. Another type of common EFW was seen in the larger episcleral veins (Fig. 2.5). This is certainly expected considering our understanding of outflow. The third type of EFW was a marked blanching in the episcleral venous plexus which typically covers several clock hours (Fig. 2.5). There were various combinations of these waves and blanches, some eyes having all three forms (Fig. 2.6). The authors are currently studying the correlation of phacotrabectome outcome with the intraoperative EFW patterns. The videos also are an excellent way to better understand the EFW phenomena.

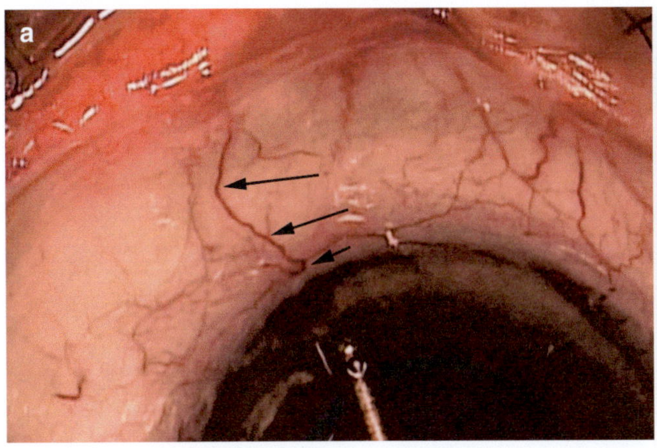
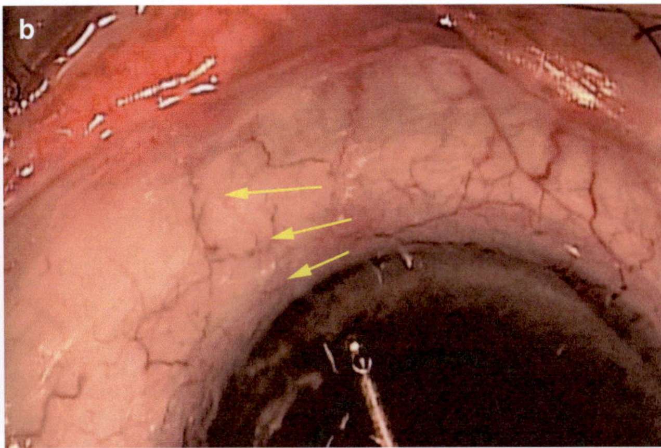

**Fig. 2.4** Episcleral venous fluid wave: conjunctival. (**a**) Irrigation and aspiration phase during phacotrabectome, foot position zero. The *black arrows* denote a conjunctival vein adjacent to the trabectome area. Reflux of blood into the anterior chamber from the area of the vein occurs with foot position zero that causes a reversal of pressure gradient from the episcleral veins to the anterior chamber. (**b**) Irrigation and aspiration phase during phacotrabectome, foot position two. The sudden influx of BSS into the anterior chamber forces aqueous to surge into Schlemm's canal and into a venous collector, now absent (*yellow arrows*), adjacent to the trabectome site nearby conjunctival vein causing it to disappear, *yellow arrows*. It appears that this is likely to be an aqueous vein of Ascher, one of the major collectors coming from the canal. After returning to foot position zero, the vein refills as the pressure gradient reverses and blood refluxes into the anterior chamber as in figure (**a**)

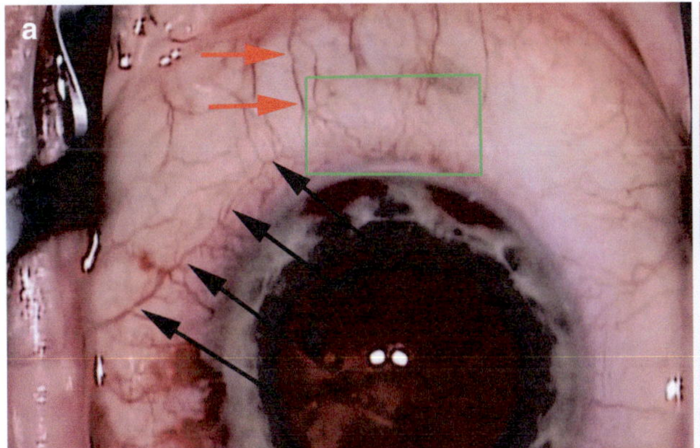
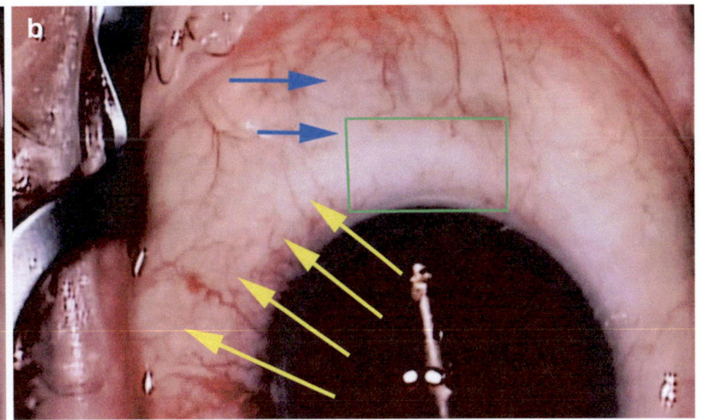

**Fig. 2.5** Episcleral venous fluid wave: episcleral vein and episcleral venous plexus. (**a**) Irrigation and aspiration phase during phacotrabectome, foot position zero. The *black arrows* denote a long episcleral vein and the *red arrows* a shorter episcleral vein. The *green box* reveals the reticulated pattern of veins in the episcleral venous plexus. The blood in the anterior chamber represents the reflux of blood seen with low IOP during foot position zero. (**b**) Irrigation and aspiration phase during phacotrabectome, foot position two. The surge of BSS during transition to foot position two allows a rapid filling of the anterior chamber along with BSS flowing into the cleaved open collectors. The *yellow arrows* represent where the long episcleral vein was located; it is invisible due to total flow of clear BSS. And a similar phenomena for the *blue arrows* representing where the *red arrows* were in figure (**a**). The *green box* demonstrates a significant flush of BSS into the episcleral plexus blanching the entire area exemplified in the box. Thus, this case demonstrates prominent episcleral veins and significant blanching of the tissues from flow into the episcleral plexus

As glaucoma surgery shifts more and more to minimally invasive canal procedures, there is a need to image the delicate collector vessels that must convey aqueous in order for these procedures to lower IOP. This is especially important for patients with mild to moderate glaucomatous disease that might be candidates for minimally invasive glaucoma procedures. These patients may turn out to be optimal candidates especially if they have only had glaucoma for a few years before their natural distal collectors undergo potential atrophy. The ability to image the conventional collector system preoperatively would point the way for surgeons to either enhance the patient's present collectors or abandon them and pursue, for example, uveoscleral outflow or filtration procedures. In addition, the ability to image the collector system would explain the outcomes of canaloplasty, trabectome, trabeculotomy, and iStent procedures, especially when gonioscopy reveals that the angle, device, or trabecular cleft are open.

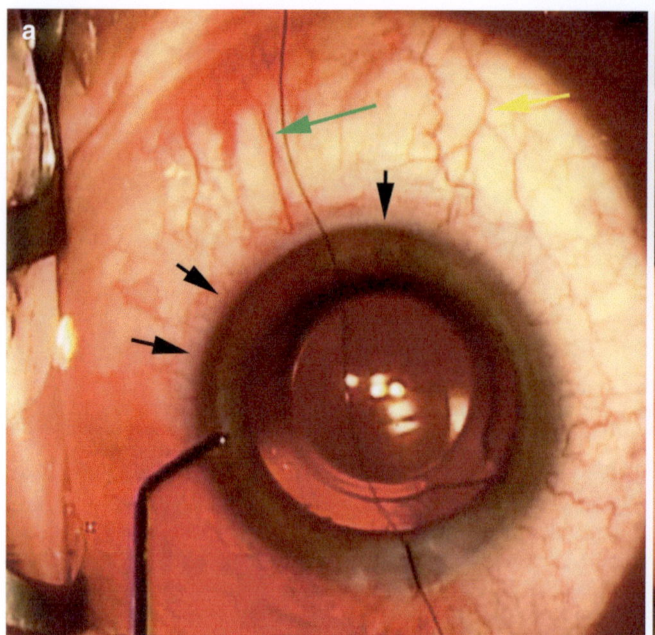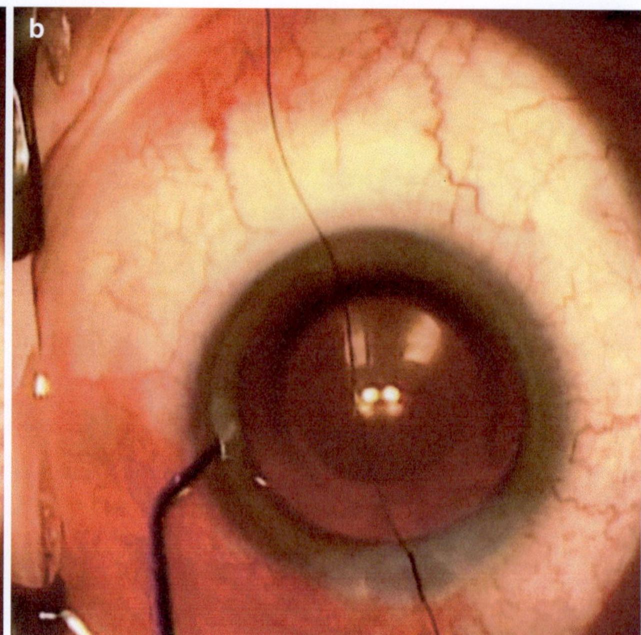

**Fig. 2.6** Episcleral venous fluid wave: episcleral plexus and vein and conjunctival vein. (**a**) Irrigation and aspiration phase during phacotrabectome, foot position zero. The *black arrows* point to the episcleral venous plexus, the *green arrow* to a prominent conjunctival vein, and the *yellow arrow* to an episcleral vein. All three of these venous outflow channels are easily seen. (**b**) Irrigation and aspiration phase during phacotrabectome, foot position two. All three of the venous outflow channels demonstrate a considerable flow of BSS during injection of BSS through a cannula. The only vessels that remain that are easily seen are the anterior ciliary arteries

## References

1. Kagemann L, Wollstein G, Ishikawa H, Sigal IA, Folio LS, Xu J, et al. 3D visualization of aqueous humor outflow structures in-situ in humans. Exp Eye Res. 2011;93:308–15.
2. Ascher KW. The aqueous veins. I. Physiologic importance of the visible elimination of intraocular fluid. Am J Ophthalmol. 1942;25:1174–209.
3. Ashton N. Anatomical study of Schlemm's canal and aqueous veins by means of neoprene casts. Part I aqueous veins. Br J Ophthalmol. 1951;35:291.
4. Ashton N. Anatomic study of Schlemm's canal and aqueous veins by means of neoprene casts. Part II. Aqueous veins (continued). Br J Ophthalmol. 1951;36:265–7.
5. Ashton N. The exit pathway of the aqueous. Doyne Memorial Lecture. Trans Ophthalmol Soc UK. 1960;80:397–421.
6. Irshad FA, Marfield MS, Zurakowski D, Ayyala RS. Variation in Schlemm's canal diameter and location by ultrasound biomicroscopy. Ophthalmology. 2010;117(5):916–20.
7. Grieshaber MC, Pienaar A, Olivier J, Stegmann R. Clinical evaluation of the aqueous outflow system in primary open-angle glaucoma for canaloplasty. Invest Ophthalmol Vis Sci. 2010;51:1498–504.
8. Fellman RL, Grover DS. Episcleral venous fluid wave: intraoperative evidence for patency of the conventional outflow system. J Glaucoma. 2012. doi:10.1097/IJG.0b013e31827a06d8.

# Suprachoroidal Space as a Therapeutic Target

Tsontcho Ianchulev

## Background: The Uveal Tract and the Suprachoroidal Space

The uveal tract, or vascular layer of the eye, comprises the ciliary body, iris, and choroid [1]. Aqueous humor (AH) produced by the ciliary body, or more specifically the ciliary processes in the pars plicata segment [2], can exit the eye through either the trabecular meshwork, moving into the Schlemm's canal and then into the intrascleral and episcleral venous plexus (the primary, so-called conventional pathway, which has been well characterized and is the more typical target of surgical interventions for glaucoma) or through the less studied uveoscleral route (the "unconventional pathway").

A non-trabecular route of AH outflow, identified as the uveoscleral route based initially on radioactive tracer experiments in cynomolgus monkeys, was first described by Anders Bill in the mid-1960s [3, 4]. The uveoscleral pathway of AH outflow has been subsequently demonstrated in humans as well as several other species (including cats, dogs, rabbits). In monkey eyes, 35–60 % of total AH outflow can be attributed to the unconventional (non-trabecular) pathway, whereas that fraction is much smaller in cats and rabbits [5]. Estimates of the total amount of AH outflow that can be attributed to the uveoscleral pathway in humans have varied widely, which is unsurprising considering the difficulty in its measurement (discussed below). Bill and Phillips [6] estimated that approximately 20 % of total AH outflow is via this route, whereas Toris et al. [7] estimated about 54 % in younger healthy adults.

No epithelial barrier exists between the anterior chamber and the clefts between the ciliary muscle bundles [8], so AH flows with little resistance from the anterior chamber through the face of the ciliary body and iris root to the interstitial tissue of the ciliary muscle, then into the suprachoroidal space (SCS) [8, 9]. Anatomically, the SCS is a potential space, a transitional zone between the external surface of the choroid and the internal surface of the sclera. Physiologically, it acts as an isoporous membrane and a molecular sieve which allows size-restricted passage of proteins as evidenced by distribution analyses of serum proteins of different molecular weights in suprachoroidal fluid in humans [10]. Molecular sieving rather than simple diffusing seems to be the physiologic mechanism at play, which becomes increasingly evident when the filtration rate is accelerated in the setting of elevated episcleral venous pressure.

From the SCS the AH enters scleral blood vessels or the choriocapillaris, or transits through scleral pores into episcleral tissue [2, 4, 11–13]. Transscleral drainage occurs through perivascular spaces and through veins communicating with the intrascleral venous plexus [8, 13, 14]. Potential transscleral flow has been estimated to be 4.3 µL/min [15]. The scleral and choroidal vessels carry the AH to the ocular orbit, where, external to the eye, AH enters the systemic circulation via lymphatic vessels [9].

Subtle morphological changes in the uveoscleral pathway occur as the eye ages. The spaces between the ciliary muscle bundles are reduced as the amount of connective tissue is increased, especially in the reticular segment of the ciliary muscle (facing the anterior chamber). By age 60, connective tissue has increased by more than 50 % in that area [16].

## Physiology

The physiology of the trabecular route and uveoscleral route of AH outflow differs in many respects [8, 9]. One key difference is that outflow through the trabecular route is nearly linear in its dependence on IOP (and a greater IOP than episcleral venous pressure [17]), whereas uveoscleral outflow is relatively insensitive to IOP—"relatively" because it is affected by extremely low or very high IOP [12, 18–20] and

T. Ianchulev, MD, MPH
Department of Ophthalmology, University of California,
San Francisco (UCSF), 707 Oregon Ave,
San Francisco, CA 94402, USA
e-mail: sianchulev@transcendmedical.com

J.R. Samples, I.I.K. Ahmed (eds.), *Surgical Innovations in Glaucoma*,
DOI 10.1007/978-1-4614-8348-9_3, © Springer Science+Business Media New York 2014

becomes more intraocular pressure (IOP) dependent when surgically manipulated using cyclodialysis [19].

Uveoscleral outflow is mostly driven by the hydrostatic pressure difference between the anterior chamber (higher) and the SCS (a few mmHg lower) [21]. Emi et al. measured the hydrostatic pressure in the SCS in cynomolgus monkey eyes under various IOP levels between 5 and 60 mmHg using two techniques and determined that a change in IOP produced a corresponding change in the pressure in the anterior SCS (i.e., the supraciliary space), but that at higher IOPs the pressure difference between the anterior chamber and the posterior SCS was increased. During spontaneous measurement, the hydrostatic pressure was significantly lower in the supraciliary space compared with the anterior chamber but higher in the supraciliary space compared with the posterior SCS. This pressure gradient is created and maintained by colloid osmotic absorption by the choroidal vessels and, to some degree, by the outflow of fluid across the sclera and emissaria. Uveoscleral outflow has been described as analogous to lymphatic drainage of tissue fluids in other organs, since the fluid may be drawn osmotically into the veins and may mix with tissue fluid from the ciliary muscle, ciliary processes, and choroid [2, 18].

Another key difference between the physiology of the conventional and unconventional outflow pathways is the factors affecting outflow resistance. Whereas the main resistance in the trabecular pathway is flow facility through Schlemm's canal, the main resistance to uveoscleral outflow appears to be within the ciliary muscle (the scleral and choroidal tissues provide little resistance). This theory is supported by several lines of evidence. A decrease in uveoscleral outflow with age that is consistent with the age-related morphological changes in the ciliary muscle is noted above. Decreased production of AH with aging balances this ciliary muscle change, so that IOP in the healthy aging eye is maintained [7]. Another line of evidence is the observation that in monkeys the degree of uveoscleral flow is affected by the degree of pharmacologically induced ciliary muscle contraction [22]. The trabecular and uveoscleral pathways respond differently to the various pharmacological interventions used to manipulate IOP, which is consistent with their differing effects on the ciliary muscle. Contraction of the ciliary muscle (e.g., induced by muscarinic agents like pilocarpine) moves it into an anterior and inward direction, which spreads the trabecular meshwork and dilates Schlemm's canal—thereby actually decreasing resistance in the conventional pathway; however, the opposite occurs when the ciliary muscle is relaxed (e.g., by adrenergic agonists and prostaglandins) [23, 24].

A hindrance to a more complete understanding of the physiology of the uveoscleral outflow pathway and therefore to the development of therapeutic interventions to increase its functionality when the trabecular pathway is compromised is the difficulty in measuring uveoscleral outflow alluded to above. Measurement of uveoscleral outflow in humans is by necessity indirect, and its accuracy is problematic because of variability inherent in the measurement of contributing parameters [2, 18]. Three measurement techniques have been described [18]:

- Use of tracers to determine where and to what extent the tracers accumulate in the uveoscleral pathway [6, 20, 25–27]
- Use of tracers to determine their concentration in the general circulation following a perfusion through the uveoscleral pathway [12]
- Measurements of parameters that are more easily assessed (total outflow resistance, AH inflow rate, IOP, and episcleral venous pressure) and using these to calculate uveoscleral outflow based on several assumptions (discussed below)

Theoretically, calculations can be made using an expanded Goldman equation that takes into account the rate of AH formation ($F$), the IOP ($P_i$), the episcleral venous pressure ($P_e$), and the tonographic facility of trabecular outflow ($C$): $F = (P_i - P_e) \times C + U$, where $U$ symbolizes the uveoscleral outflow, or alternatively $P_i = P_e + (F - U)/C$. As noted by Alm and Nilsson in their excellent review of uveoscleral outflow [8], there are several potential sources of imprecision in these calculations. First, there can be large errors in measurement of each of the individual parameters used in the equation and especially for episcleral venous pressure and outflow facility through the trabecular meshwork. Second, the various parameters are measured under very different conditions (e.g., IOP is measured instantly, AH flow is averaged over several hours, and clinical tonography artificially increases IOP). In studies in normal human eyes, estimates of $U$ calculated from the Goldman equation based on measurement of the other parameters have ranged from 0.80 µL/min (representing 36 % of $F$) [28] to 1.52 µL/min (representing 54 % of $F$) [7] in young adults. In older adults (age $\geq$60 years) with normal eyes, estimates of $U$ have ranged from 0.14 to 1.09 µL/min, representing 12–46 % of $F$ [7, 29–31]. In human eyes with ocular hypertension, estimated $U$ has ranged from 0.12 to 1.24 µL/min, representing 5–40 % of $F$ [30–35]. In human eyes with exfoliation syndrome with or without ocular hypertension, $U$ was estimated at 0.11 µL/min, representing 5 % of $F$ [31]. The assumption that uveoscleral flow is pressure independent can also lead to significant error in measurement, particularly given the pressure dependence of other parameters in the equation used [18].

## Targeted Drug Delivery via the Uveoscleral Pathway

The ocular distribution of fluid injected into the anterior SCS was investigated by Seiler et al. [26] using ex vivo eyes from pigs and dogs. Ultrasound tracking of the distribution of injected contrast medium revealed that the fluid flowed from the injection site to the opposite ventral anterior SCS and to the posterior SCS, arriving at these locations at a mean time of just under 8 s. In 10 of the 12 eyes injected, contrast medium reached the posterior pole. It was also demonstrated that the SCS is capable of dose-dependent expansion to accommodate injected fluids of various volumes up to 250 µL. Although a modest, dose-dependent, transient rise in IOP was also observed, these results support injection into the anterior SCS as a potentially effective procedure for delivering drugs to the back of the eye, including the macula, and treating posterior segment diseases. The feasibility of this method of drug delivery had been suggested previously by Einmahl et al. in 2002 [36], who used a solid, olive-tipped cannula for suprachoroidal injections of poly(ortho ester), a polymer they were evaluating for the development of sustained drug delivery systems, in rabbit eyes in vivo. The injected biomaterial was confirmed to have reached the posterior pole and remained present in the SCS in animals sacrificed at 3 weeks postinjection.

A modest, transient elevation of IOP with injection into the SCS such as was reported by Seiler et al. was actually hypothesized to be a potential advantage in delivering drugs to the posterior segment via microneedle injection by another team of investigators [37]. Patel et al. reasoned that such elevation would increase the firmness of the scleral surface, thereby allowing a deeper penetration of the microneedle into the sclera and increasing the rate of infusion success. Their hypothesis was supported in a study of SCS delivery of nanoparticle and microparticle suspensions to the posterior segment in rabbit, pig, and human ex vivo eyes. At IOP of 36 mmHg, but not at IOP of 18 mmHg, particles were sometimes successfully delivered at the lowest infusion pressure (300 kPa) or shortest microneedle length (700 µm), and a 100 % delivery success was achieved using 900 and 1,000 µm microneedles. In another study, in which the microneedle SCS delivery method was directly compared with intravitreal delivery of fluorescein, fluorescently tagged dextrans (40 and 250 kDa), bevacizumab, and polymeric particles (20 nm and 10 µm diameter) in vivo in rabbits, Patel et al. demonstrated that the SCS route achieved a 10-fold higher concentration of the injected material in the back of the eye than in the anterior tissues, whereas there was no significant posterior versus anterior segment selectivity with intravitreal injection [38]. Half-lives of the particles injected into the SCS depended on size: those with molecular weight of 0.3–250 kDA had a half-life from 1.2 to 7.9 h, but particles ranging from 20 nm to 10 µm had not cleared the eye after a period of months and were still detected primarily in the SCS and choroid.

Evidence obtained using a flexible fiber-optic microcannula for injection of drugs into the SCS in pigs suggests that this route may prove to be more practical for the delivery of small molecules than for larger biological molecules [39], presumably because of the collagen matrix of the scleral tissue [40]. In a 2006 study, Olsen et al. had demonstrated in a porcine model that microcannulation of the SCS delivered a small molecule, triamcinolone in a sustained-release matrix, to the macula for at least 120 days [41]. In their 2011 study, Olsen et al. compared the pharmacokinetics and tissue response to the macromolecule bevacizumab when injected via the typical intravitreal route versus the SCS route. Bevacizumab had a more sustained pharmacological profile when delivered intravitreally and achieved more direct distribution to the inner retina tissues than when delivered via the SCS route. The investigators concluded that sustained-release formulations should be considered for optimizing delivery of larger biological molecules using the SCS pathway.

Pilot studies of suprachoroidal drug delivery of triamcinolone and/or bevacizumab using a microcatheter have been performed in patients with advanced macular disease and/or who have not responded to conventional therapies (see Augustin et al. for a brief review of these studies [42]). Pathologies treated in these studies included choroidal neovascularization secondary to exudative age-related macular degeneration and retinal vein occlusion or diffuse diabetic macular edema accompanied by subfoveal hard exudates. These small studies have provided encouraging results, including some increase in residual vision and significant reduction of macular edema, without surgical complications or unmanageable postoperative adverse events.

If larger prospective clinical trials support the promising results obtained in the animal models and human pilot studies, it is expected that the delivery of drugs via the SCS would offer several advantages over the conventional drug delivery methods used to target the back of the eye. As noted by Patel et al. [37], the four characteristics desirable for effective drug delivery to the posterior segment include the following: (1) that the procedure be minimally invasive and safe; (2) the procedure should effectively target the desired tissues, with limited exposure to the drug in other ocular regions; (3) sustained drug exposure should be possible, so that repetition of the procedure is minimized and better therapeutic control is achieved; and (4) the procedure should be sufficiently simple so that it can be performed at a routine office visit. Delivery of drugs via the uveoscleral route has the potential to meet all of these criteria. Moreover, a recent study in a rabbit model demonstrated that the SCS can be utilized for virally vectored gene delivery— potentially a less invasive and safer method than currently used procedures for gene delivery in eyes with hereditary pathologies such as Leber's congenital amaurosis [43].

## Role of the Uveoscleral Outflow Pathway in Glaucoma and IOP Control

The clinical significance and physiologic role of AH outflow via the uveoscleral route is not yet clear, either in normal eyes or in those with glaucoma [8, 44].

In beagle dogs, one of the few nonhuman species that spontaneously develops glaucoma, radiotracer studies showed that advanced glaucoma reduced uveoscleral flow to 3 % of total outflow, compared with 15 % in nonglaucomatous eyes [45]. In cynomolgus monkeys with laser-induced glaucoma, fluorophotometry showed that uveoscleral flow was increased compared with control eyes, but this increase was insufficient to prevent a rise in IOP caused by a 63 % reduction in outflow facility in the trabecular pathway [46].

Toris et al. investigated AH dynamics in the presence of ocular hypertension (OH) by comparing IOP, aqueous flow, uveoscleral outflow, episcleral venous pressure, fluorophotometric outflow facility, anterior chamber volume, and corneal thickness in two age-matched groups, one with normal IOP and one with elevated IOP not due to glaucoma [30]. Compared with the normal group, the group with OH exhibited statistically significantly higher mean IOP ($21.4\pm0.6$ with OH vs. $14.9\pm0.3$ mmHg in normal) accompanied by both significantly reduced outflow facility ($0.17\pm0.01$ vs. $0.27\pm0.002$ μL/min/mmHg) and uveoscleral outflow ($0.66\pm0.11$ $1.09\pm0.11$ μL/min). Noting elevated rates of uveoscleral outflow in a small study of patients with advanced POAG characterized by uncontrolled IOP on maximally tolerated medical therapy and high resistance in the trabecular meshwork [47], Toris and Camras [44] hypothesize that in the initial stages of glaucoma, both trabecular outflow facility and uveoscleral outflow may be subnormal, but with glaucoma disease progression and increasing trabecular meshwork resistance, there may be redirection of AH into the uveoscleral pathway, where flow is far less IOP dependent. This may be an oversimplified model which highlights our lack of advanced physiologic understanding of uveoscleral outflow and the need for additional basic research.

## Pharmacotherapies Targeting Uveoscleral Outflow for Reducing IOP

One of the most effective pharmacotherapies for glaucoma, the prostaglandin analogs, lowers IOP primarily by increasing uveoscleral outflow. Prostaglandins (PGs), as well as PG analogs and prodrugs, have become widely used in pharmacotherapy for reducing glaucoma-related IOP elevation, although the mechanism(s) contributing to this effect has not yet been fully characterized.

PGs, locally acting hormones (autocoids) with potent proinflammatory effects, are synthesized and secreted throughout the body, including in the trabecular meshwork and other ocular tissues [48]. An inflammatory effect of PGs on ocular tissues, accompanied by an elevation of IOP, was well documented [49, 50] before the potential clinical utility of PGs in lowering IOP was discovered. One of the earliest observations suggesting PGs might be useful as ocular hypotensive

agents came from an in vivo rabbit study [51], which demonstrated that although topical application of 25–200 μg of PG initially raised IOP, it was followed by a prolonged (15–20 h) ocular hypotony of up to 7 mmHg compared to control values. The same study demonstrated that topical application of a very low dose (5 μg) of $PGF_2\alpha$, which was insufficient to cause the initial rise in IOP, was nonetheless effective in reducing IOP by up to 7 mmHg for $\geq12$ h. Thus, the hypotensive phase was not a compensatory response to an initial hypertensive phase and suggested that PGs or their analogs could be useful in treating ocular hypertension.

It is generally accepted that the primary mechanism of action of PGs in lowering IOP is an increase in uveoscleral outflow [48, 52, 53], with minimal effect on trabecular outflow, episcleral venous pressure, or aqueous humor formation [48, 54]. However, there is evidence that at least one of the four PG analogs available commercially for the treatment of glaucoma, unoprostone, does increase trabecular outflow facility [35]. Evidence suggesting that PGs increase the pressure sensitivity of uveoscleral outflow has been inconsistent [44].

Several different PG receptors are located in the ciliary muscle, with FP and EP2 receptors predominating [53]. A cascade of effects following exposure to $PGF_2\alpha$ has been shown in cultured human ciliary muscle: intracellular cAMP is increased [55], leading to activation of nuclear regulatory proteins such as c-Fos and c-Jun, followed by increased biosynthesis and secretion of matrix metalloproteinases (MMPs) [56, 57]. Increased MMP expression in tissues typically results in increased turnover and remodeling of extracellular matrix (ECM) [48, 58]. The action of MMPs on ciliary muscle appears to be an alteration of the collagens I, III, and IV, such that the ECM is reduced and the permeability increased, and the spacing of ciliary muscle fibers is widened; consequently, the hydraulic resistance to uveoscleral outflow is decreased [54, 59, 60]. Because different MMPs differ in their ability to cleave at specific sites within ECM components, activation of several MMPs may be involved in the remodeling of ECM [61].

Other hypothesized mechanisms of PG enhancement of uveoscleral outflow include ciliary muscle relaxation, changes in ciliary muscle cell shape due to changes in actin and vinculin localization within the cells, cytoskeletal alteration, and /or compaction of the ECM within the tissues of the uveoscleral pathway [48, 54]. Monkey and human evidence suggests that PG-induced changes in sclera are also important in increasing uveoscleral outflow [54, 62–64].

As a class, PGs have proved to be effective and practical as first-line treatment of glaucoma [1]. As experiments revealed more about the mechanisms by which PG lowered IOP, investigators began chemically modifying parent natural PG to optimize topical delivery to intraocular PG receptors (e.g., by increasing the lipophilicity of the agents, allowing greater corneal penetration) and to enhance the

**Table 3.1** Commercially available prostaglandin analog drugs for treatment of glaucoma

| Generic name | Brand name in the USA | Manufacturer |
| --- | --- | --- |
| Unoprostone | Rescula | CIBA Vision Ophthalmics, Bulach, Switzerland (also generically manufactured by other companies) |
| Latanoprost | Xalatan | Pfizer Inc., New York, NY (also generically manufactured by other companies) |
| Travoprost | Travatan | Alcon Inc., Ft Worth, TX |
| Bimatoprost | Lumigan | Allergan Inc., Irvine, CA |

specificity for certain PG receptors [53]. A recent systematic review of glaucoma therapies by the AHRQ (USA) indicated that PG drugs are more effective than dorzolamide (a carbonic anhydrase inhibitor), brimonidine (an alpha-adrenergic agonist), and timolol (a beta-adrenergic blocker) in lowering IOP [65]. An additional positive feature of PG drugs topically applied to the eye is the near absence of any systemic side effects. The small amount of PG that enters the systemic circulation with the use of these drugs is minimal compared with the amount of endogenous PG normally released from virtually all body tissues [66].

Currently, four drugs with IOP-lowering effects mediated by PG activity are marketed (Table 3.1) for treatment of open-angle glaucoma. The first such commercially available PG analog (PGA) was isopropyl unoprostone, launched in Japan in 1994. In 2000, the US FDA approved unoprostone (Rescula) for the treatment of OAG and ocular hypertension but restricted its use to only those patients who were intolerant of or unresponsive to other IOP-lowering drugs. Rescula labeling indicated a lowering of IOP by about 3–4 mmHg throughout the day and is considered the least efficacious of the four drugs. Its lower clinical efficacy compared to later PGAs marketed may be due to its greater activation of certain tissue inhibitors of MMPs in ciliary body smooth muscle cells [67]. Unoprostone also performed less well than timolol in two head-to-head comparative studies [68, 69]. The three PGAs most commonly used to treat COAG are latanoprost, launched in the USA in 1996, and travoprost and bimatoprost, both launched in the USA in 2001 [70]. All three of these drugs are approved for first-line treatment of OAG and ocular hypertension, effectively lower IOP both during the day and during the night (24-h IOP reduction), and have similar efficacy overall, although some studies have reported a greater effect on IOP with bimatoprost [65, 70]. Latanoprost, travoprost, and bimatoprost have also been investigated for treatment of closed-angle glaucoma, with promising results [71]. All three drugs have shown efficacy as monotherapy but are frequently combined with other glaucoma medications such as timolol.

Latanoprost is an ester prodrug of $PGF_{2}\alpha$ [70] that selectively acts as an agonist at prostanoid FP receptors [72].

After absorption through the cornea, the isopropyl ester prodrug is hydrolyzed to acid form to become biologically active. According to latanoprost labeling, patients with mean baseline IOP of 24–25 mmHg treated for 6 months in multicenter, randomized, controlled trials had IOP reductions of 6–8 mmHg; efficacy was comparable to that of timolol. In studies of the use of latanoprost in pediatric glaucoma, the drug appears safe and effective but less effective than in adults and less effective in children with juvenile-onset OAC than in older children [73, 74].

Travoprost is also an ester prodrug of $PGF_{2}\alpha$ that acts as a selective agonist at prostanoid FP receptors [72], with overall efficacy comparable to that of latanoprost and timolol. There is some suggestion that travoprost may be more effective than latanoprost in lowering IOP in black compared with non-black patients, but the evidence is inconsistent [1].

Bimatoprost is a synthetic amide prodrug of 17-phenyl-PGF2α [54, 75] that mimics the activity of $PGF_{2}\alpha$ ethanolamide (prostamide $F_{2}\alpha$) [72]. Efficacy in some patients resistant to latanoprost suggests its effect on uveoscleral flow involves receptor(s) different from those targeted by pure FP receptor agonists [54]. There is some evidence based on a feline iris model that bimatoprost does have FP agonist activity but may also have one or more other mechanisms of action related to trabecular outflow and an alternative signaling pathway [1, 76, 77].

Adverse effects of the PG drugs for glaucoma are consistent throughout the class [1, 70]. Conjunctival hyperemia has been the most common adverse reaction to these drugs in several studies; product labeling indicates that clinical studies showed a rate of 25–45 % of patients with bimatoprost and 30–50 % with travoprost but only 5–15 % for latanoprost. Other adverse reactions reported include iris pigmentation (irreversible or slowly reversible; likely related to increased melanogenesis), hypertrichosis of eyelashes, and periocular skin pigmentation and less commonly cystoid macular edema, anterior uveitis, *Herpes simplex* keratitis, iris cyst, and infrequent systemic events (e.g., upper respiratory infection) via nasopharyngeal mucosal absorption.

As with other topically administered medications for glaucoma, a barrier to compliance is the difficulty of self-administering eye drops. However, latanoprost, travoprost, and bimatoprost at least have the advantage of requiring only once daily dosing.

## Surgical Interventions Targeting Uveoscleral Outflow

Cyclodialysis, i.e., separation of the ciliary body from scleral spur, allowing free communication between anterior chamber and SCS, was the first surgical intervention for glaucoma that increases AH outflow via the uveoscleral pathway.

Classic transscleral cyclodialysis ab externo was first described by Leopold Heine in 1905. When successfully performed, cyclodialysis reduces IOP not only by enhancing drainage of AH via the SCS and choroid but also by reducing AH production because restriction of blood supply to the ciliary body causes atrophy ("ciliary shutdown") [78, 79]. The ab externo cyclodialysis procedure has been abandoned in clinical practice, however, due to an unacceptably high rate of complications (e.g., severe intra- and postoperative bleeding from the scleral vessels, profound postoperative hypotony), the failure of the cyclodialysis cleft to remain open over time (mainly due to scarring), and the advent of trabecular filtration surgery.

In cyclodialysis ab interno procedures, the integrity of the conjunctiva is spared and space-retaining substances with an extended duration are used in an attempt to keep the cyclodialysis cleft open and prevent scarring [80]. A variety of such space-retaining substances have been investigated, but finding substances that stay in place long enough and prevent scarring has been a challenge. Portney treated five eyes with severe, intractable, secondary angle-closure glaucoma with a cyclodialysis procedure that utilized a T-shaped silicone elastomer implantation [81]. The technique was unsuccessful, largely because of an inflammatory reaction and fibrous scar formation that surrounded the implant and obliterated the cyclodialysis cleft. The use of hylan gel as a space retainer was pioneered by Wirt and Draeger, working with Bill, in the cynomolgus monkey model [82] (cited by Klemm et al. [80]). Subsequently, working with Klemm and Balazs, Wirt and Draeger investigated two modified forms of hylan gel with different molecular weights (8,000 kDa and 25,000 kDA) as space retainers in 12 nonglaucomatous eyes of six owl monkeys that underwent cyclodialysis ab interno [80]. Postoperatively, IOP was effectively reduced from the preoperative level. Histological evaluation of enucleated eyes on postoperative days 140, 155, and 210 revealed no tissue reactions or inflammation, and with one exception the cyclodialysis cleft remained widely open for several months.

Jordan et al. reported cyclodialysis ab interno in a series of 20 patients (28 treated eyes) with intractable glaucoma [79]. The viscoelastic substance Healon (1 % sodium hyaluronate with a viscosity of 300,000 mPas and a molecular weight of 4.0 million daltons) was the space retainer left in the SCS at the end of surgery; the substance is usually resorbed within a few days after surgery. The mean baseline IOP was 34.3 mmHg despite maximum therapy, and a mean of 4.4 previous interventions had been performed. Absolute success was defined as lowering IOP to <21 mmHg without further medication or intervention and qualified success as lowering IOP to <21 mmHg with topical medication or further surgery. The mean follow-up was 122 days. Postoperatively, the mean IOP was 14.6 mmHg. After a mean of 60 days, 21 eyes (75 %) required further surgical intervention due to return of uncontrolled IOP. Qualified success was achieved in four eyes (14.3 %), with mean follow-up of 384 days (range 3–573 days), and absolute success in three eyes (10.7 %), with mean follow-up of 203 days (range 20–322 days). The greatest success was observed in phakic eyes, followed by pseudophakic and aphakic eyes. Patients experienced no postoperative hypotony, localized infection or endophthalmitis, or loss of vision. The authors concluded that although they did not demonstrate the functional efficacy of cyclodialysis ab interno, the procedure was easy to perform and offered atraumatic access to the SCS drainage route with a low rate of side effects. They further suggested that other viscoelastic substances with a higher viscosity and molecular weight or the use of slowly resorbable elastic implants might more effectively prevent closure of the cyclodialysis cleft—ideally, for approximately 3 months so that wound healing is completed.

Several attempts have been made to increase AH drainage through the uveoscleral pathway with novel surgical techniques, abandoning the cyclodialysis approach but further pursuing the use of space-retaining substances or devices to keep the pathway open long term. Some of these approaches are reviewed below.

A method reported by Ozdamar et al. employed implantation of a modified (trimmed for size) Krupin eye valve with a disk (typically used for episcleral fixation) into the SCS to increase uveoscleral outflow [83] in four painful-blind eyes of four patients with neovascular glaucoma complicating diabetic retinopathy ($n=3$) and chronic angle-closure glaucoma ($n=1$). The anterior tube part of the implanted device courses from the anterior chamber through the long scleral tunnel to drain AH into the SCS. The mean preoperative IOP in patients on two antiglaucoma medications was 58.5 mmHg (range 45–65 mmHg). Postoperatively, mean IOP was reduced to 14.2 mmHg at 1 week, 13.5 mmHg at 1 month, 15 mmHg at 3 months, and 17 mmHg (range 12–24 mmHg) at the last follow-up (timing not stated). "Successful control of IOP" (not specifically defined in the report, but ranging from 12 to 19 mmHg) at the last examination was achieved in 3 of 4 patients (i.e., 75 %). Postoperative hypotony occurred in only one patient in whom the procedure caused choroidal detachment; there were no serious cases of postoperative bleeding or infection, and none of the eyes had developed tube erosion or suprachoroidal hemorrhage as of the last follow-up.

Yablonski has reported a novel approach to trabeculectomy that utilizes an internal tube shunt for suprachoroidal drainage [84]. In a pilot study in 23 eyes in 23 patients with OAG, only 3 of whom had a history of incisional glaucoma surgery, a deep sclerectomy was performed under a scleral flap, producing an intrascleral lake. A small silicone tube was then placed between the intrascleral lake and the SCS, with a trabeculectomy stoma and a peripheral iridectomy allowing easy flow of AH into the tube. After a mean follow-up of 324 days, the mean postoperative IOP had dropped to 13.8 mmHg from a preoperative value of 25.4 mmHg, and patients were using a mean of 1.1 medications for IOP control compared with 3.0 preoperatively. The size of the surgically created bleb was substantially smaller in these eyes than in 45 control eyes that underwent conventional trabeculectomy, and postoperative outflow facility was significantly increased only in the control eyes. Eighteen of the 23 eyes required laser lysis of the scleral nylon sutures or postoperative 5-fluorouracil to control IOP. Yablonski attributed the success of this trabeculectomy with internal tube shunt procedure mostly to increased access of the AH to the SCS, where the protein colloid osmotic pressure of uveal blood results in AH absorption.

Other techniques utilizing a silicone tube to shunt AH from the anterior chamber to the SCS have been reported by several other investigative teams [85–87]. Jordan et al. reported their study of an ab externo procedure conducted in 31 eyes of 31 patients with uncontrollable refractory glaucoma (i.e., a mean baseline IOP of 44.3 mmHg despite maximum therapy, including a mean of 3.5 previous surgical interventions) [86]. The silicone tube was fed through the anterior chamber and connected intrasclerally to the SCS via a deep posterior scleral flap. Mean IOP was reduced to 13 mmHg in 70 % of all eyes at 30 weeks after surgery. Success, defined as lowering IOP to <21 mmHg without further medication or intervention, was achieved in 60 % of eyes at 52 weeks postoperatively and in 40 % at 76 weeks. There were no serious complications, no severe postoperative hypotony or suprachoroidal bleeding, and no localized or general inflammation related to the implant. However, anterior chamber lavage was required in two patients because of intracameral bleeding, and dislocated tubes had to be removed from two patients because of corneal endothelial contact. The mean functional survival of the shunt was 56 weeks, with an initial peak of failure after only 4 weeks and a second peak after 1 year. Scarring in the SCS was the rate-limiting factor in long-term success, with connective tissue formation (fibroblast reaction) observed under ultrasound biomicroscopy at the posterior lumen of the tube in failed eyes.

Palamar et al. reported their retrospective study of an ab externo procedure similar to that used by Jordan et al. but using a modified silicone implant with no valve implanted into the SCS [87]. They treated 15 eyes in 14 patients with intractable glaucoma (7 eyes with OAG, 4 with glaucoma secondary to trauma, 4 with juvenile glaucoma) who were receiving two or more antiglaucoma medications and who had undergone at least one prior failed glaucoma surgery. The mean follow-up time was 17.1 months (range 10–28 months). The mean baseline IOP in the 15 eyes was 33 mmHg. A 30 % postoperative decrease in IOP was achieved in 66.7 % of eyes. Functional success, defined as

lowering IOP to ≤21 mmHg both with and without medication at 6 months after surgery, was 93.3 %; total success, defined as lowering IOP to ≤21 mmHg without medication at 6 months after surgery, was 13.3 %. The mean number of antiglaucoma medications dropped from a mean of 3.8 (range 2–5) before surgery to a mean of 2.2 (range 0–4) after surgery. Only minor complications were seen, with the occurrence of shallow choroidal detachment in all eyes considered to be proof of uveoscleral drainage of AH.

Unal et al. also used an ab externo procedure similar to that of Jordan et al. to implant a silicone tube with the anterior end in the anterior chamber and the posterior end in the SCS in 24 glaucomatous eyes in 24 patients unresponsive to maximal medical treatment (including seven with earlier trabeculectomy). The glaucoma diagnoses in these eyes included POAG ($n=5$), neovascular ($n=6$), uveitic ($n=5$), secondary to vitreoretinal surgery with silicone injection ($n=2$), pseudoexfoliative ($n=2$), congenital ($n=2$), traumatic ($n=1$), and juvenile ($n=1$). The mean preoperative IOP was 32.8 mmHg (range 24–50 mmHg). Patients were followed for a mean of 24.4 weeks (range 4–78 weeks) after surgery. Mean postoperative IOPs were significantly reduced from preoperative baseline: 8.5, 12.9, 17.0, 15.3, 18.3, and 15.1 mmHg, respectively, for 1 day, 1 week, and 1, 3, 6, and 12 months after surgery. Failure was defined as a postoperative IOP >21 or <5 mmHg after 3 months, complete success was defined as eyes not failed and not on supplemental medical therapy, and qualified success as eyes not failed with or without supplemental medical therapy. The complete success rate was 95.8 % at 1 week after surgery, 79.2 % at 1 and 3 months, and 63.3 % at 6 and 12 months. Qualified success was achieved in 95.8 % at 1 week and 87.5 % at 1, 3, 6, and 12 months. The success rate was significantly higher in eyes without earlier trabeculectomy. The surgery failed in seven eyes, with three requiring reoperation for glaucoma. Complications included early hypotony in six eyes, fibrin reaction in the anterior chamber in three eyes, and intracameral bleeding in two eyes, with one requiring anterior chamber lavage. No postoperative infection or choroidal or retinal detachment was observed. The authors concluded that their SCS implantation procedure effectively reduced IOP with a lower rate of serious complications than frequently occurs with trabeculectomy and could be a preferred initial surgery—particularly in cases without previous trabeculectomy.

Gold has been used as a biocompatible material for the development of another type of shunt connecting the anterior chamber with the SCS. Based on a design concept developed in 2001 by Gabriel Simon, the SOLX Gold Shunt (GMS; SOLX Ltd, Boston, MA) is a micro-device marketed in Canada and select European countries but not yet approved for use in the USA. This shunt is a nonvalved flat-plate, rectangular (2.3 mm W×5.2 mm L×44 μm thick) drainage device made of 24-karat medical-grade gold. Two plates are welded together, with two rounded projections on the distal end for anchoring the device in the SCS and with a gently curved proximal end that projects into the anterior chamber. A grid of holes in the anterior and posterior ends allows AH to flow into and out of the device, respectively. The device is implanted using an ab externo technique.

The first peer-reviewed publication on the gold shunt [88] reported a pilot study in 38 patients with advanced glaucoma (66 % with primary open-angle glaucoma (POAG)) and uncontrolled IOP, more than half of whom had a history of a failed glaucoma surgery or drainage device. After surgery, patients were followed for a mean of 11.7 months. The mean preoperative IOP in these patients was 27.6 mmHg. Surgical success was defined as IOP <22 and >5 mmHg with or without medication at the last follow-up; complete success was defined as achievement of the same mmHg criteria but without medication. Implantation of the device resulted in a statistically significant mean IOP decrease from baseline of 9 mmHg (mean = 18.2 mmHg), with a surgical success rate of 79 % and a complete success rate of 13.2 %. The most frequent complication was mild to moderate hyphema (eight patients; 21 %), with shunt exposure, synechia formation, and exudative inferior retinal detachment reported in one patient each. The authors concluded that the device and procedure were safe and effective and could be an alternative to trabeculectomy.

A series of publications from Italian investigators have further elucidated the efficacy and safety of the gold micro shunt. In 2010, Mastropasqua et al. [89] reported their in vivo analysis of conjunctival features observed using confocal laser-scanning microscopy following implantation of the gold micro shunt in 14 eyes of 14 patients with uncontrolled POAG who had a history of multiple failed incisional surgeries. After implantation of the gold shunt, eyes were examined at follow-up times ranging from 3 to 20 months (mean = 15.4 months). Based on the degree of IOP control achieved and on evidence of surgical success, the patients were divided into two analysis groups. Group 1 ($n=8$) comprised patients with successful implantation, defined as a 1/3 reduction from their preoperative IOP with or without medications. Group 2 ($n=6$) comprised patients with failed implantations, defined as less than 1/3 reduction in IOP with maximal tolerated medical therapy. The mean postoperative IOP was significantly higher in patients with failed implantations than in those with success (32.3 mmHg vs. 14 mmHg, respectively) despite similar preoperative IOP in the two groups. The main outcome measures were the mean density and area of conjunctival mean microcysts. The results showed that successful gold shunt implantation significantly increased conjunctival microcyst density and surface area at the site of device insertion (five- to sixfold higher in Group 1 than in Group 2). The authors considered this finding to be evidence of AH percolation through the scleral layers and then the conjunctiva, leading them to conclude that uveoscleral outflow of AH is enhanced by this device.

The following year, another publication that included authors from the same team as the 2010 report described evaluation of the gold micro shunt in a 2-year study of 55 eyes of 55 patients with refractory glaucoma despite maximal medical treatment [90]. The patients had previously undergone a mean of 1.9 (range 1–5) surgical interventions for glaucoma. Prior to gold shunt implantation, the patients' mean IOP was 30.8 mmHg (range 22–58 mmHg). At 2 years, 37 eyes (67.3 %) were deemed a qualified success and 3 eyes (5.5 %) a complete success. In eyes that achieved success, mean IOP had dropped from a preoperative mean of 27.6 mmHg to 13.7 ± 2.98 mmHg; the mean number of medications decreased from 2.5 preoperatively to 1.4 ± 0.7 postoperatively. Twenty-one of the 55 patients experienced mild to moderate postoperative adverse events, with mild or moderate hyphema the most common. The authors determined that development of a thin membrane that obstructed the anterior holes of the shunt in 12 patients from the failure group (66.7 % of failures) was the most important factor contributing to lack of efficacy.

In 2012, an investigative team including authors from the previous two publications coming out of Italy [91] reported histological features of failed GMS implantations in an interventional case series study of 5 eyes in 5 patients who had received the gold micro shunt for refractory POAG. When the shunts were removed, 4 of 5 were found to have been correctly placed into the anterior chamber and SCS, so mislocation did not appear to be the main issue responsible for the poor efficacy. Examination of the failed shunts revealed connective tissue filling all the inner spaces of the device, creating a thick fibrotic capsule surrounding both ends of the shunt that impeded AH flow through the shunt.

The gold micro shunt, although composed of a biologically inert material, has some of the same problems with fibrotic obstruction as the silicone shunts used to improve uveoscleral outflow. However, an advantage is the ability of the surgeon to successively open the device after implant by applying a laser to the fenestrations in its anterior chamber component, allowing in vivo postoperative adjustment of the outflow [92]. Because the shunt is not resorbable, a disadvantage compared with the silicone shunts is the presence of a permanent implant in the AC and SCS, with risk of erosion or exposure of the device.

Another novel and experimental procedure for improving uveoscleral outflow of AH is ab interno implantation of a fenestrated micro-stent composed of a biocompatible polyamide material—the CyPass Micro-Stent (Transcend Medical, Menlo Park, CA)—into the supraciliary space [93–97]. Because CyPass implantation is ab interno, conjunctiva sparing without surgical trauma to the sclera, it has the additional advantage of minimizing tissue inflammation and subsequent fibrosis. The ab interno surgical approach involves no scleral penetration and also leaves the trabecular meshwork intact. Using a special manual applier, the CyPass Micro-Stent is placed in the supraciliary space below the scleral spur at the iris root, either through a clear corneal incision or through the primary phacoemulsification incision when combined with cataract removal. CyPass stent is approved in the EU and under FDA investigation in the USA.

Ianchulev et al. [93] first reported on 81 glaucomatous (OAG) eyes that underwent cataract surgery (phacoemulsification) followed by CyPass implantation. At 6 months after surgery, the mean IOP had decreased to 16 mmHg from a preoperative mean value of 22.9 mmHg. The procedure was well tolerated, with postoperative complications of shallow anterior chamber and transient hyphema in one patient each. The following year, Craven et al. reported on safety outcomes of 121 eyes that underwent phacoemulsification and CyPass implantation [97]. The adverse events following the procedure were transient hyphema ($n=8$), persistent inflammation ($n=1$), branch retinal vein occlusion ($n=1$), and diabetic macular edema exacerbation ($n=1$).

Encouraging initial results with minimally invasive suprachoroidal stenting as a therapeutic intervention for glaucoma has stimulated further clinical research into the space. A large FDA RCT of more than 500 patients (COMPASS study) is ongoing which will provide definitive evidence on the safety and efficacy of the device. New suprachoroidal stents are also entering clinical investigation with multiple interventional options on the horizon.

# References


1. Allingham RR, Damji KF, Feedman S, Moroi SE, Rhee DJ, editors. Shields textbook of glaucoma. 6th ed. Philadelphia: Lippincott Williams & Wilkins; 2011.
2. Goel M, Picciani RG, Lee RK, Bhattacharya SK. Aqueous humor dynamics: a review. Open Ophthalmol J. 2010;4:52–9.
3. Bill A, Hellsing K. Production and drainage of aqueous humor in the cynomolgus monkey (Macaca irus). Invest Ophthalmol. 1965;4(5):920–6.
4. Bill A. The aqueous humor drainage mechanism in the cynomolgus monkey (Macaca irus) with evidence for unconventional routes. Invest Ophthalmol. 1965;4(5):911–9.
5. Bill A. Uveoscleral drainage of aqueous humor: physiology and pharmacology. Prog Clin Biol Res. 1989;312:417–27.
6. Bill A, Phillips CI. Uveoscleral drainage of aqueous humour in human eyes. Exp Eye Res. 1971;12(3):275–81.
7. Toris CB, Yablonski ME, Wang YL, Camras CB. Aqueous humor dynamics in the aging human eye. Am J Ophthalmol. 1999;127(4):407–12.
8. Alm A, Nilsson SF. Uveoscleral outflow – a review. Exp Eye Res. 2009;88(4):760–8.
9. Nilsson SF. The uveoscleral outflow routes. Eye (Lond). 1997;11(Pt 2): 149–54.
10. Chylack Jr LT, Bellows AR. Molecular sieving in suprachoroidal fluid formation in man. Invest Ophthalmol Vis Sci. 1978;17(5):420–7.
11. Teng CC, Chi HH, Katzin HM. Histology and mechanism of filtering operations. Am J Ophthalmol. 1959;47(1 Part 1):16–33.
12. Pederson JE, Gaasterland DE, MacLellan HM. Uveoscleral aqueous outflow in the rhesus monkey: importance of uveal reabsorption. Invest Ophthalmol Vis Sci. 1977;16(11):1008–17.
13. Krohn J, Bertelsen T. Light microscopy of uveoscleral drainage routes after gelatine injections into the suprachoroidal space. Acta Ophthalmol Scand. 1998;76(5):521–7.
14. Krohn J, Bertelsen T. Corrosion casts of the suprachoroidal space and uveoscleral drainage routes in the human eye. Acta Ophthalmol Scand. 1997;75(1):32–5.
15. Jackson TL, Hussain A, Hodgetts A, Morley AM, Hillenkamp J, Sullivan PM, et al. Human scleral hydraulic conductivity: age-related changes, topographical variation, and potential scleral outflow facility. Invest Ophthalmol Vis Sci. 2006;47(11):4942–6.
16. Tamm S, Tamm E, Rohen JW. Age-related changes of the human ciliary muscle. A quantitative morphometric study. Mech Ageing Dev. 1992;62(2):209–21.
17. Suguro K, Toris CB, Pederson JE. Uveoscleral outflow following cyclodialysis in the monkey eye using a fluorescent tracer. Invest Ophthalmol Vis Sci. 1985;26(6):810–3.
18. Johnson M, Erickson K. Mechanisms and routes of aqueous humor drainage. In: Albert DM, Jakobiec FA, editors. Principles and practice of ophthalmology. Philadelphia: WB Saunders; 2000. p. 2577–95.
19. Toris CB, Pederson JE. Effect of intraocular pressure on uveoscleral outflow following cyclodialysis in the monkey eye. Invest Ophthalmol Vis Sci. 1985;26(12):1745–9.
20. Bill A. Conventional and uveo-scleral drainage of aqueous humour in the cynomolgus monkey (Macaca irus) at normal and high intraocular pressures. Exp Eye Res. 1966;5(1):45–54.
21. Emi K, Pederson JE, Toris CB. Hydrostatic pressure of the suprachoroidal space. Invest Ophthalmol Vis Sci. 1989;30(2):233–8.
22. Bill A. Effects of atropine and pilocarpine on aqueous humour dynamics in cynomolgus monkeys (Macaca irus). Exp Eye Res. 1967;6(2):120–5.
23. Rohen JW, Lutjen E, Barany E. The relation between the ciliary muscle and the trabecular meshwork and its importance for the effect of miotics on aqueous outflow resistance. A study in two contrasting monkey species, Macaca irus and Cercopithecus aethiops. Albrecht Von Graefes Arch Klin Exp Ophthalmol. 1967;172(1):23–47.
24. Barany EH. The mode of action of miotics on outflow resistance. A study of pilocarpine in the vervet monkey Cercopithecus ethiops. Trans Ophthalmol Soc U K. 1966;86:539–78.
25. Gabelt BT, Kaufman PL. Prostaglandin F2 alpha increases uveoscleral outflow in the cynomolgus monkey. Exp Eye Res. 1989;49(3):389–402.
26. Seiler GS, Salmon JH, Mantuo R, Feingold S, Dayton PA, Gilger BC. Effect and distribution of contrast medium after injection into the anterior suprachoroidal space in ex vivo eyes. Invest Ophthalmol Vis Sci. 2011;52(8):5730–6.
27. Bill A. Basic physiology of the drainage of aqueous humor. Exp Eye Res. 1977;25(Suppl):291–304.
28. Townsend DJ, Brubaker RF. Immediate effect of epinephrine on aqueous formation in the normal human eye as measured by fluorophotometry. Invest Ophthalmol Vis Sci. 1980;19(3):256–66.
29. Toris CB, Camras CB, Yablonski ME. Effects of PhXA41, a new prostaglandin F($2\alpha$) analog, on aqueous humor dynamics in human eyes. Ophthalmology. 1993;100(9):1297–304.
30. Toris CB, Koepsell SA, Yablonski ME, Camras CB. Aqueous humor dynamics in ocular hypertensive patients. J Glaucoma. 2002;11(3):253–8.
31. Johnson TV, Fan S, Camras CB, Toris CB. Aqueous humor dynamics in exfoliation syndrome. Arch Ophthalmol. 2008;126(7): 914–20.
32. Toris CB, Tafoya ME, Camras CB, Yablonski ME. Effects of apraclonidine on aqueous humor dynamics in human eyes. Ophthalmology. 1995;102(3):456–61.
33. Toris CB, Gleason ML, Camras CB, Yablonski ME. Effects of brimonidine on aqueous humor dynamics in human eyes. Arch Ophthalmol. 1995;113(12):1514–7.

34. Toris CB, Camras CB, Yablonski ME. Acute versus chronic effects of brimonidine on aqueous humor dynamics in ocular hypertensive patients. Am J Ophthalmol. 1999;128(1):8–14.

35. Toris CB, Zhan G, Camras CB. Increase in outflow facility with unoprostone treatment in ocular hypertensive patients. Arch Ophthalmol. 2004;122(12):1782–7.

36. Einmahl S, Savoldelli M, D'Hermies F, Tabatabay C, Gurny R, Behar-Cohen F. Evaluation of a novel biomaterial in the suprachoroidal space of the rabbit eye. Invest Ophthalmol Vis Sci. 2002; 43(5):1533–9.

37. Patel SR, Lin AS, Edelhauser HF, Prausnitz MR. Suprachoroidal drug delivery to the back of the eye using hollow microneedles. Pharm Res. 2011;28(1):166–76.

38. Patel SR, Berezovsky DE, McCarey BE, Zarnitsyn V, Edelhauser HF, Prausnitz MR. Targeted administration into the suprachoroidal space using a microneedle for drug delivery to the posterior segment of the eye. Invest Ophthalmol Vis Sci. 2012;53(8):4433–41.

39. Olsen TW, Feng X, Wabner K, Csaky K, Pambuccian S, Cameron JD. Pharmacokinetics of pars plana intravitreal injections versus microcannula suprachoroidal injections of bevacizumab in a porcine model. Invest Ophthalmol Vis Sci. 2011;52(7):4749–56.

40. Olsen TW, Edelhauser HF, Lim JI, Geroski DH. Human scleral permeability. Effects of age, cryotherapy, transscleral diode laser, and surgical thinning. Invest Ophthalmol Vis Sci. 1995;36(9): 1893–903.

41. Olsen TW, Feng X, Wabner K, Conston SR, Sierra DH, Folden DV, et al. Cannulation of the suprachoroidal space: a novel drug delivery methodology to the posterior segment. Am J Ophthalmol. 2006;142(5):777–87.

42. Augustin C, Augustin A, Tetz M, Rizzo S. Suprachoroidal drug delivery – a new approach for the treatment of severe macular diseases. Eur Ophthalmic Rev. 2012;6:25–7.

43. Peden MC, Min J, Meyers C, Lukowski Z, Li Q, Boye SL, et al. Ab-externo AAV-mediated gene delivery to the suprachoroidal space using a 250 micron flexible microcatheter. PLoS One. 2011; 6(2):e17140.

44. Toris CB, Camras CB. Aqueous humor dynamics II. Clinical studies. In: Civan MM, editor. The eye's aqueous humor. Waltham, MA: Elsevier Inc; 2008. p. 231–72.

45. Barrie KP, Gum GG, Samuelson DA, Gelatt KN. Quantitation of uveoscleral outflow in normotensive and glaucomatous Beagles by 3H-labeled dextran. Am J Vet Res. 1985;46(1):84–8.

46. Toris CB, Zhan GL, Wang YL, Zhao J, McLaughlin MA, Camras CB, et al. Aqueous humor dynamics in monkeys with laser-induced glaucoma. J Ocul Pharmacol Ther. 2000;16(1):19–27.

47. Yablonski ME, Cook DJ, Gray J. A fluorophotometric study of the effect of argon laser trabeculoplasty on aqueous humor dynamics. Am J Ophthalmol. 1985;99(5):579–82.

48. Weinreb RN, Toris CB, Gabelt BT, Lindsey JD, Kaufman PL. Effects of prostaglandins on the aqueous humor outflow pathways. Surv Ophthalmol. 2002;47 Suppl 1:S53–64.

49. Eakins KE, Whitelocke RA, Bennett A, Martenet AC. Prostaglandin-like activity in ocular inflammation. Br Med J. 1972;3(5824):452–3.

50. Conquet P, Plazonnet B, Le Douarec JC. Arachidonic acid-induced elevation of intraocular pressure and anti-inflammatory agents. Invest Ophthalmol. 1975;14(10):772–5.

51. Camras CB, Bito LZ, Eakins KE. Reduction of intraocular pressure by prostaglandins applied topically to the eyes of conscious rabbits. Invest Ophthalmol Vis Sci. 1977;16(12):1125–34.

52. Lindsey JD, Kashiwagi K, Kashiwagi F, Weinreb RN. Prostaglandin action on ciliary smooth muscle extracellular matrix metabolism: implications for uveoscleral outflow. Surv Ophthalmol. 1997;41 Suppl 2:S53–9.

53. Schachtschabel U, Lindsey JD, Weinreb RN. The mechanism of action of prostaglandins on uveoscleral outflow. Curr Opin Ophthalmol. 2000;11(2):112–5.

54. Toris CB, Gabelt BT, Kaufman PL. Update on the mechanism of action of topical prostaglandins for intraocular pressure reduction. Surv Ophthalmol. 2008;53(Suppl1):S107–20.

55. Zhan GL, Camras CB, Opere C, Tang L, Ohia SE. Effect of prostaglandins on cyclic AMP production in cultured human ciliary muscle cells. J Ocul Pharmacol Ther. 1998;14(1):45–55.

56. Lindsey JD, Kashiwagi K, Boyle D, Kashiwagi F, Firestein GS, Weinreb RN. Prostaglandins increase proMMP-1 and proMMP-3 secretion by human ciliary smooth muscle cells. Curr Eye Res. 1996;15(8):869–75.

57. Weinreb RN, Kashiwagi K, Kashiwagi F, Tsukahara S, Lindsey JD. Prostaglandins increase matrix metalloproteinase release from human ciliary smooth muscle cells. Invest Ophthalmol Vis Sci. 1997;38(13):2772–80.

58. Woessner Jr JF. Matrix metalloproteinases and their inhibitors in connective tissue remodeling. FASEB J. 1991;5(8):2145–54.

59. Lindsey JD, Kashiwagi K, Kashiwagi F, Weinreb RN. Prostaglandins alter extracellular matrix adjacent to human ciliary muscle cells in vitro. Invest Ophthalmol Vis Sci. 1997;38(11):2214–23.

60. Sagara T, Gaton DD, Lindsey JD, Gabelt BT, Kaufman PL, Weinreb RN. Topical prostaglandin F2alpha treatment reduces collagen types I, III, and IV in the monkey uveoscleral outflow pathway. Arch Ophthalmol. 1999;117(6):794–801.

61. Galis ZS, Muszynski M, Sukhova GK, Simon-Morrissey E, Unemori EN, Lark MW, et al. Cytokine-stimulated human vascular smooth muscle cells synthesize a complement of enzymes required for extracellular matrix digestion. Circ Res. 1994;75(1):181–9.

62. Kim JW, Lindsey JD, Wang N, Weinreb RN. Increased human scleral permeability with prostaglandin exposure. Invest Ophthalmol Vis Sci. 2001;42(7):1514–21.

63. Weinreb RN. Enhancement of scleral macromolecular permeability with prostaglandins. Trans Am Ophthalmol Soc. 2001;99:319–43.

64. Weinreb RN, Lindsey JD, Marchenko G, Marchenko N, Angert M, Strongin A. Prostaglandin FP agonists alter metalloproteinase gene expression in sclera. Invest Ophthalmol Vis Sci. 2004;45(12): 4368–77.

65. Boland MV, Ervin AM, Friedman D, Jampel H, Hawkins B, Volenweider D. Treatment for glaucoma: comparative effectiveness. In: (AHRQ) AfHRaQ, editor. Comparative Effectiveness Review No 60 (Prepared by the Johns Hopkins University Evidence-based Practice Center under Contract No HHSA 290-2007-10061-I). Rockville: US Dept of Health and Human Services; 2012.

66. Bito LZ. Prostaglandins and other eicosanoids: their ocular transport, pharmacokinetics, and therapeutic effects. Trans Ophthalmol Soc U K. 1986;105(Pt 2):162–70.

67. Ooi YH, Oh DJ, Rhee DJ. Effect of bimatoprost, latanoprost, and unoprostone on matrix metalloproteinases and their inhibitors in human ciliary body smooth muscle cells. Invest Ophthalmol Vis Sci. 2009;50(11):5259–65.

68. Nordmann JP, Mertz B, Yannoulis NC, Schwenninger C, Kapik B, Shams N. A double-masked randomized comparison of the efficacy and safety of unoprostone with timolol and betaxolol in patients with primary open-angle glaucoma including pseudoexfoliation glaucoma or ocular hypertension. 6 month data. Am J Ophthalmol. 2002;133(1):1–10.

69. Stewart WC, Stewart JA, Kapik BM. The effects of unoprostone isopropyl 0.12% and timolol maleate 0.5% on diurnal intraocular pressure. J Glaucoma. 1998;7(6):388–94.

70. Lee AJ, McCluskey P. Clinical utility and differential effects of prostaglandin analogs in the management of raised intraocular pressure and ocular hypertension. Clin Ophthalmol. 2010;4: 741–64.

71. Cheng JW, Cai JP, Li Y, Wei RL. A meta-analysis of topical prostaglandin analogs in the treatment of chronic angle-closure glaucoma. J Glaucoma. 2009;18(9):652–7.

72. Chen J, Runyan SA, Robinson MR. Novel ocular antihypertensive compounds in clinical trials. Clin Ophthalmol. 2011;5:667–77.

73. Coppens G, Stalmans I, Zeyen T, Casteels I. The safety and efficacy of glaucoma medication in the pediatric population. J Pediatr Ophthalmol Strabismus. 2009;46(1):12–8.

74. Enyedi LB, Freedman SF. Latanoprost for the treatment of pediatric glaucoma. Surv Ophthalmol. 2002;47 Suppl 1:S129–32.

75. Woodward DF, Krauss AH, Chen J, Liang Y, Li C, Protzman CE, et al. Pharmacological characterization of a novel antiglaucoma agent, Bimatoprost (AGN 192024). J Pharmacol Exp Ther. 2003; 305(2):772–85.

76. Woodward DF, Liang Y, Krauss AH. Prostamides (prostaglandin-ethanolamides) and their pharmacology. Br J Pharmacol. 2008; 153(3):410–9.

77. Wan Z, Woodward DF, Cornell CL, Fliri HG, Martos JL, Pettit SN, et al. Bimatoprost, prostamide activity, and conventional drainage. Invest Ophthalmol Vis Sci. 2007;48(9):4107–15.

78. Boke H. History of cyclodialysis. In memory of Leopold Heine 1870–1940. Klin Monbl Augenheilkd. 1990;197(4):340–8.

79. Jordan JF, Dietlein TS, Dinslage S, Luke C, Konen W, Krieglstein GK. Cyclodialysis ab interno as a surgical approach to intractable glaucoma. Graefes Arch Clin Exp Ophthalmol. 2007;245(8): 1071–6.

80. Klemm M, Balazs A, Draeger J, Wiezorrek R. Experimental use of space-retaining substances with extended duration: functional and morphological results. Graefes Arch Clin Exp Ophthalmol. 1995; 233(9):592–7.

81. Portney GL. Silicone elastomer implantation cyclodialysis. A negative report. Arch Ophthalmol. 1973;89(1):10–2.

82. Wirt H, Bill A, Draeger J. Neue aspekte in der operativen behandlung des glaukoms – vergleich viskoelastischer substanzen in der kammerwinkelchirurgie. Fortschr Opththalmol [Suppl]. 1991; 88:234.

83. Ozdamar A, Aras C, Karacorlu M. Suprachoroidal seton implantation in refractory glaucoma: a novel surgical technique. J Glaucoma. 2003;12(4):354–9.

84. Yablonski ME. Trabeculectomy with internal tube shunt: a novel glaucoma surgery. J Glaucoma. 2005;14(2):91–7.

85. Unal M, Kocak Altintas AG, Koklu G, Tuna T. Early results of suprachoroidal drainage tube implantation for the surgical treatment of glaucoma. J Glaucoma. 2011;20(5):307–14.

86. Jordan JF, Engels BF, Dinslage S, Dietlein TS, Ayertey HD, Roters S, et al. A novel approach to suprachoroidal drainage for the surgical treatment of intractable glaucoma. J Glaucoma. 2006;15(3): 200–5.

87. Palamar M, Ates H, Oztas Z, Yusifov E. Suprachoroidal implant surgery in intractable glaucoma. Jpn J Ophthalmol. 2011;55(4): 351–5.

88. Melamed S, Ben Simon GJ, Goldenfeld M, Simon G. Efficacy and safety of gold micro shunt implantation to the supraciliary space in patients with glaucoma: a pilot study. Arch Ophthalmol. 2009; 127(3):264–9.

89. Mastropasqua L, Agnifili L, Ciancaglini M, Nubile M, Carpineto P, Fasanella V, et al. In vivo analysis of conjunctiva in gold micro shunt implantation for glaucoma. Br J Ophthalmol. 2010;94(12): 1592–6.

90. Figus M, Lazzeri S, Fogagnolo P, Iester M, Martinelli P, Nardi M. Supraciliary shunt in refractory glaucoma. Br J Ophthalmol. 2011; 95(11):1537–41.

91. Agnifili L, Costagliola C, Figus M, Iezzi G, Piattelli A, Carpineto P, et al. Histological findings of failed gold micro shunts in primary open-angle glaucoma. Graefes Arch Clin Exp Ophthalmol. 2012; 250(1):143–9.

92. Sharaawy T, Bhartiya S. Surgical management of glaucoma: evolving paradigms. Indian J Ophthalmol. 2011;59(Suppl):S123–30.

93. Ianchulev T, Ahmed K, Hoeh HR, Rau M. Minimally invasive ab interno suprachoroidal device (CyPass) for IOP control in open-angle glaucoma. American Academy of Ophthalmology annual meeting, Chicago, 18–19 Oct 2010.

94. Erb C, Hoeh H, Rau M, Peters S, Nardi M, Ianchulev T. European clinical experience with the CyPass supraciliary micro-stent for IOP lowering. European Society of Cataract and Refractive Surgeons annual meeting, Vienna, 17–22 Sept 2011.

95. Garcia-Feijoo J, Rau M, Ahmed I, Anton A, Grabner G, Ianchulev T. Safety and efficacy of CyPass Micro-Stent as a stand-alone treatment for open-angle glaucoma: Worldwide clinical experience. 2012 Sept 10.

96. Grisanti S, Garcia-Feijoo J, Nardi M, Rapisarda A, Anton A, Craven E, et al. CyPass for the primary treatment of OAG medication-naive patients. European Society of Cataract and Refractive Surgeons annual meeting, Milan, 8–12 Sept 2012.

97. Craven ER, Khatana A, Hoeh H, Rau M, Ianchulev T. Safety of minimally invasive, ab interno suprachoroidal micro-stent for IOP reduction used in combination with phaco cataract surgery. American Academy of Ophthalmology annual meeting, Orlando, FL, 22–25 Oct 2011.

# Ciliary Body as a Therapeutic Target

Jeffrey A. Kammer

## Abbreviations

CPC   Cyclophotocoagulation
IOP    Intraocular pressure

Intraocular pressure (IOP) is a direct reflection of the fine balance between aqueous secretion and outflow. The IOP can be influenced by modifying both of these variables. This can be accomplished by employing medical or surgical intervention to decrease aqueous secretion or increase outflow facility. The ciliary body has become a prime target for both modalities of treatment. In pharmacotherapy, prostaglandin analogs bind to and then activate the FP receptors in the ciliary body smooth muscle, thus increasing uveoscleral outflow. From a surgical perspective, the secretory activity of the ciliary body epithelium can be decreased by ablating a portion of the ciliary body using ultrasonic energy, cyclocryotherapy, diathermy, and thermal lasers. Over the past 20 years, the ciliary body has evolved from being a target of last resort (i.e., cyclocryotherapy) to one that is considered early in the course of the disease (endocyclophotocoagulation).

## Historical Perspective

### Diathermy

The concept of cyclodestruction was introduced by Coppez in 1929 when he reported the successful destruction of ciliary body epithelium in rabbits by heating the sclera overlying the ciliary body [1, 2]. Four years later, Weve was the first to describe the successful use of nonpenetrating diathermy in humans. His technique involved using a blunt-tipped probe that was attached to a cautery device. The heat from this unit was transmitted through the sclera and selectively destroyed sections of the ciliary body [3].

This procedure was modified by Vogt, who favored using the diathermy probe to physically penetrate the sclera. His technique involved placing one or two rows of full-thickness burns 2.5–5 mm from the corneolimbal junction at 180°. Each application lasted 10–20 s and delivered 40–45 mA of electric current [4, 5]. The mechanism of action was postulated to be cell death within the ciliary body and/or a diathermy-induced draining fistula over the pars plana [6, 7].

The results of the early studies were quite encouraging, with documented success rates as high as 78 % [8], albeit with limited follow-up. Cyclodiathermy became the preferred cyclodestructive procedure for years until long-term efficacy concerns dampened the enthusiasm for this technique. Specifically, Berens reported that only 22 % of the treated patients had an IOP under 25 mmHg with or without glaucoma medications at the last follow-up after 7–14 years of observation [9]. The longevity concerns regarding cyclodiathermy were reinforced by a 1970 paper that reported that only 7 % of the patients maintained an IOP less than 25 mmHg for at least 4 months [10].

Given the suboptimal success rates, the relatively high incidence of severe complications, and other viable alternatives, this technique has largely fell out of favor.

### Cyclocryotherapy

As clinicians became increasingly disenchanted with the foibles of cyclodiathermy, several progressive ophthalmologists began looking for alternative methods for cycloablation.

J.A. Kammer, MD
Department of Ophthalmology and Visual Sciences,
Vanderbilt Eye Institute, Vanderbilt University Medical Center,
2311 Pierce Avenue, Nashville, TN 37232, USA
e-mail: jeff.kammer@vanderbilt.edu

**Electronic supplementary material** Supplementary material is available in the online version of this chapter at http://dx.doi.org/10.1007/978-1-4614-8348-9_4. Videos can also be accessed at http://www.springerimages.com/videos/978-1-4614-8347-2

J.R. Samples, I.I.K. Ahmed (eds.), *Surgical Innovations in Glaucoma*,
DOI 10.1007/978-1-4614-8348-9_4, © Springer Science+Business Media New York 2014

The concept of using a freezing source to destroy the ciliary body (cyclocryotherapy) was first reported by Bietti in 1950 [11]. This procedure was considered more predictable with relatively fewer side effects and became the mainstay of cyclodestructive therapy until the advent of lasers.

Indeed, the efficacy of this procedure has been quite impressive. For patients with open-angle glaucoma, there was a 77 and 87 % success rate at the 1 and 3 year follow-up, respectively [12, 13]. Cyclocryotherapy also appears to perform particularly well in patients with glaucoma following penetrating keratoplasty and in aphakic glaucoma—two entities that are historically difficult to treat. Both Bellows and Shields documented that they were able to adequately control the IOP in over 90 % of the patients with aphakic glaucoma after 4 years of follow-up [14, 15]. In patients with glaucoma following corneal transplants, 83 % of the individuals in two separate studies achieved good IOP control following cyclocryotherapy treatment [16, 17]. Unfortunately, patients with neovascular glaucoma met with mixed results. While reports of successful IOP control ranged from 30 to 64 %, the rate of complete visual loss (no light perception) was 46 % [12, 13, 15].

The technique for performing cyclocryotherapy has evolved over time to provide maximum efficacy while minimizing complications. Experimental evidence supports 4 fundamental factors in the success of this procedure: probe size, temperature and duration of the freeze, probe placement, and number of applications. There has been no greater debate than the optimal size of the cryoprobe tip. While studies clearly demonstrate a strong relationship between probe size and IOP lowering, there is also compelling evidence of an increased risk of hypotony and phthisis with a larger cryoprobe. Most practitioners have adopted the 2.5-mm probe tip since it covers the 2-mm pars plicata width and seems to provide the most favorable risk-benefit ratio [18–21].

There has also been extensive research into the optimal freezing technique. Animal studies suggest a probe temperature range between −60 and −80 C for a clinically meaningful drop in IOP [22–24]. Other reports indicate a minimal freeze time of 60 s, with longer times increasing the rates of phthisis [18, 25]. Based on this information, consensus suggests achieving a probe temperature of −60 to −80 C and leaving it in place for 60 s. Some diminution of effect occurs due to the insulating properties of the tissue along with circulatory factors [26]. These effects can be minimized by applying scleral pressure during probe application [27].

The location of the probe placement and the number of treatment applications also impact the ultimate success of cyclocryotherapy. Ideally, the cryoprobe should be positioned with maximal proximity to the ciliary processes. Based upon experimental determination of average ciliary processes position, Prost recommended probe placement 1.0 mm from the limbus for the inferior, temporal, and nasal quadrants and 1.5 mm from the limbus in the superior quadrant [18]. Confirmation of plana plicata position using transillumination is advisable, particularly in patients with atypical axial lengths. The probe placement is vital since the success rate increases considerably with accurate positioning. In fact, one study demonstrated an 85 % success rate when the probe was placed within 1.5 mm of the corneolimbal junction compared to 30 % success in another study using otherwise similar parameters [12, 28].

The number of treatment applications is equally important but highly controversial. A feline study demonstrated a graded IOP-lowering response proportional to the extent of treatment [29]. While aggressive (360°) treatment produces a significant drop in IOP, it is also associated with a proportionately higher rate of complications, including phthisis bulbi, hypotony, and anterior segment ischemia [30, 31]. These devastating complications can be significantly reduced by decreasing the extent of treatment to 180°. Even in neovascular glaucoma, the rate of hypotony can be reduced to 0–18 % and the incidence of phthisis bulbi reduced to 0–10 % [12, 14, 19, 32–34]. Most clinicians modulate the number of cryolesions based upon the type and severity of the glaucoma. Since many surgeons err on the side of undertreatment to minimize the risk of complications, augmenting therapy in the previously untreated regions is commonplace. Bellows and associates have cautioned to wait a month before re-treatment since it can take 2–4 weeks before the full extent of treatment is realized [35].

## Current Therapeutic Options

## Transscleral Cyclophotocoagulation

### Nd:YAG Transscleral Cyclophotocoagulation

Light energy was first employed as a cyclodestructive medium in 1961 when Weekers and colleagues used the transscleral xenon arc photocoagulation in rabbit and human eyes [36]. While it produced a deleterious histologic effect, its clinical impact was unimpressive. In 1969, Smith and Stein introduced the concept of using a ruby laser for cyclodestruction [37]. Beckman and Waeltermann published a retrospective review of their 10-year experience with transscleral ruby laser cyclophotocoagulation (CPC). They documented a 62 % success rate in maintaining IOP between 5 and 22 mmHg, with a particularly good response (86 %) in aphakic glaucoma patients. While 17 % of the treated patients experienced chronic hypotony, most of these individuals maintained their baseline vision [38].

In the early 1970s, Beckman and Sugar experimented with neodymium-yttrium aluminum garnet (Nd:YAG) laser as another option for transscleral CPC. This laser had several attributes which distinguished it from the ruby laser. From a practical standpoint, Nd:YAG lasers were relatively more available and cost effective, thus making this laser a more attractive option. The Nd:YAG laser had other advantages which could be theoretically beneficial in practice. Most notably, the longer (1,064 nm) wavelength facilitates scleral penetration with less backscatter compared to lasers with shorter wavelengths [39, 40]. The combined benefits of availability, cost utility, and putative efficacy resulted in the rise of the Nd:YAG at the expense of the ruby laser.

The Nd:YAG laser consists of a medium of neodymium atoms in a crystal of yttrium, aluminum, and garnet [41]. Transscleral cilioablation with the Nd:YAG laser can be employed using two unique protocols. Contact Nd:YAG CPC is performed with a 2.2-mm fiber-optic tip coupled with a probe that is placed directly on the conjunctiva. The laser system (i.e., SLT CL60 {Surgical Laser Technologies, Montgomeryville, PA}) provides direct delivery of Nd:YAG laser energy in a continuous wave mode of 0.1–10 s. The non-contact laser system transmits the laser energy through air from a slit lamp delivery system (Lasag Microruptor II [Meridian, Switzerland]). The noncontact mode uses a pulsed, free-running, thermal mode that focuses intense energy in a small area for a brief period of time, thus causing mechanical photodisruption [7]. The mechanism of action of Nd:YAG cyclophotocoagulation is incompletely understood but appears to be multifactorial in origin. The proposed mechanisms include (1) destruction of the ciliary processes [42–44], (2) increase uveoscleral outflow [45, 46], (3) inflammatory-induced alterations [7], and (4) ischemic destruction of the microvascular elements supporting the ciliary processes [47].

While each physician takes some artistic license when it comes to treatment parameters, there are some general guidelines that most surgeons follow. For noncontact transscleral Nd:YAG CPC, the general recommendation is to use 4–8 J of energy for a 10–20-ms duration and maximum offset. One prospective study that evaluated noncontact Nd:YAG CPC using two different energy levels (4 J vs. 8 J) found a trend towards greater success with more energy [48]. Thirty-two laser applications are evenly spaced for 360 around the limbus, skipping the 3 and 9 o'clock positions so as not to ablate the long posterior ciliary arteries [49]. The laser beam is typically aimed 1.0–1.5 mm posterior to the limbus. This recommendation is based on two studies that demonstrate maximal destruction of the ciliary body and lower IOPs with laser placement 1.0–1.5 mm behind the surgical limbus [50–52]. By comparison, contact transscleral Nd:YAG CPC uses 4–9 W of power for 0.5–0.7 s. This technique also utilizes 32 burns place circumferentially 0.5–1.0 mm behind the limbus [40]. Once again, histopathology studies were used to determine optimal positioning of the laser probe during treatment [53, 54].

While both forms of Nd:YAG CPC employ the same amount of total energy, the contact method utilizes less power due to functional differences between the two techniques. Specifically, contact Nd:YAG CPC allows for a more efficient transfer of energy through the sclera by pushing the probe firmly against the globe, thus optimizing scleral contact per unit area [49, 55]. When the probe indents the sclera, this enhances the overall efficiency of energy transmission. Decreasing the probe size and tailoring the contour of the tip further optimizes contact and efficiency [56]. Together, these two factors result in improved energy transmission and therefore less power consumption in the contact method for CPC.

Both forms of Nd:YAG CPC have been found to be effective at controlling IOP in patients with glaucoma. Noncontact Nd:YAG CPC has a documented success for achieving target IOP in 45–86 % of patients [57–59, 60–62]. In this group of studies, 21–46 % of the patients required one or more re-treatments to achieve the desired IOP range [58, 60]. The contact Nd:YAG CPC group performed equally well with reported success rates ranging from 66 to 71 % and published re-treatment rates from 11 to 57 % [40, 63–65].

Since a significant percentage of patients require more than one laser session to achieve optimal IOP, this is an important concept to consider before committing to a second treatment. It takes approximately 1 month to reach maximum IOP reduction following Nd:YAG CPC, so it is generally recommended that surgeons wait at least this long before considering repeat laser treatment [7].

Several factors have been identified that portend a higher likelihood for success or failure following Nd:YAG CPC. Simmons et al. found that race was a possible distinguishing risk factor when they reported a significantly higher success rate in whites as compared to blacks. The same study did not identify any predictive value when it comes to age, preoperative IOP, and gender [66]. Nd:YAG CPC also seems to be particularly effective in patients with uveitic glaucoma [67] and in eyes with penetrating keratoplasty-related glaucoma [68, 69].

There are several complications that are common to both types of Nd:YAG CPC. Immediately following the procedure, white conjunctival scars are often present. This complication can be minimized in contact Nd:YAG CPC by utilizing a contact lens during treatment [7, 66]. Transient pain is also relatively common but typically resolves within 3 days for most patients [41]. Uveitis is equally common, although highly variable in terms of severity. While most patients demonstrate a mild to moderate anterior chamber inflammatory reaction, there have been reports of severe inflammation with fibrin and hypopyon [7]. Fortunately, this inflammation is responsive to topical steroids.

Other documented anterior segment complications include hyphema, scleral thinning, corneal graft failure, hypotony, and flat anterior chamber [58, 70–72]. Vitreoretinal complications include choroidal detachments, vitreous hemorrhages, cystoid macular edema, and aqueous misdirection [73, 74]. The two most concerning complications include sympathetic ophthalmia and visual loss. Some form of visual degradation occurs in up to 50 % of all cases of Nd:YAG CPC [7]. The underlying cause of this visual loss is difficult to assess but likely multifactorial. The underlying disease certainly plays a role since we know that patients with complex conditions (like neovascular glaucoma) have the highest rate of visual loss following treatment [75]. That being said, up to 50 % of the cases of vision loss are thought to be directly attributable to the laser treatment [7]. While the definitive mechanism of action is incompletely understood, it is thought to be due to macular edema, inflammation, and phototoxicity [7, 75]. Sympathetic ophthalmia is a rare but potentially devastating complication that can occur following Nd:YAG CPC. The relationship was first described by Edward and associates in 1989 when they published a report that provided compelling clinical and histopathological evidence of a relationship between Nd:YAG CPC and sympathetic ophthalmia [76]. Since that time, this relationship has been reaffirmed in several other reports [77, 78]. There are two risk factors that seem to be associated with a higher likelihood of developing this condition: (1) high laser power and (2) previous incisional surgery [49]. Moderating the total energy delivered and careful selection of patients will help minimize the risk for developing sympathetic ophthalmia.

Compared to its predecessors, Nd:YAG CPC appears to be at least as effective, with advantages that include a lower incidence of phthisis bulbi, hypotony, transient IOP spikes, pain, and ocular inflammation [79]. Both techniques for Nd:YAG CPC yield excellent and nearly equivalent success rates. The contact method has been shown to be more energy efficient and also creates a more localized destruction, which theoretically results in less pain and inflammation [40]. While its relatively high rate of vision loss prohibits Nd:YAG CPC from becoming a first-line treatment in most situations, it remains an excellent option for patients with historically recalcitrant conditions, like neovascular and aphakic glaucoma.

## Diode Laser Transscleral Cyclophotocoagulation

The concept of incorporating diode lasers into clinical medicine was initially proposed by Pratesi in 1984 [80]. The semiconductor material in this particular diode laser is composed of gallium-aluminum-arsenide. When the semiconductor is excited by an electrical current, it emits infrared energy with a peak wavelength of 810 nm [80]. The use of diode laser technology as an option for cilioablative therapy was first described in rabbits [81]. Subsequent histopathology studies in both rabbit and human eyes have demonstrated blanching and shrinking of the ciliary processes on gross examination, along with ciliary body necrosis and epithelial cell disruption on microscopic evaluation [82–84].

While the Nd:YAG laser produced reliable results, the potential benefits of the diode laser were too great to overlook. Compared to the Nd:YAG system, the diode laser was

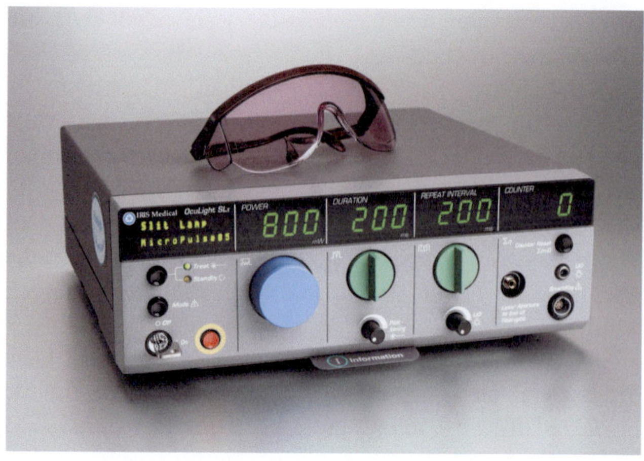

**Fig. 4.1** This is an image of the OcuLight SLx, the most commonly used ophthalmic diode laser in the United States (Image courtesy of Iridex, Mountain View, CA)

more appealing due to its compact size, portability, improved ergonomics, low maintenance costs (i.e., no laser tubes), facile delivery of laser energy, and efficiency at converting electric energy into laser energy [85, 86].

The diode in this light-emitting system produces a combined wavelength of 810 nm compared to the 1,064 nm wavelength emitted by the Nd:YAG laser [87]. The shorter wavelength affords the advantage of greater absorption by the uveal melanin. Thus, for a set amount of energy absorption by uveal melanin, less energy is required using the diode system compared to the Nd:YAG laser [84, 85, 88]. This benefit is tempered by the fact that the longer wavelength emitted by the Nd:YAG laser has significantly better (75 %) scleral transmission compared to the 35 % scleral transmission produced by diode laser. Fortunately, the effective laser transmission can be increased to 70 % by employing a probe that can be used to perform scleral indentation [87, 89]. These attributes have led to the diode laser overtaking the Nd:YAG laser as the preferred method of transscleral CPC.

The commercially available diode units include Microlase (Keeler Instruments, Broomall, PA), DC-300 (Nidek, Inc., Palo Alto, CA), and OcuLight SLX (Iridex, Mountain View, CA). In the OcuLight SLX system (Fig. 4.1), the laser energy is transmitted through a 600-μm diameter quartz fiber with a polished tip that is oriented by a handpiece known as a "G-probe" (Fig. 4.2). The footplate for this probe is curved to match the contour of the sclera and centers the fiber-optic tip 1.2 mm from the corneoscleral limbus. This polished tip protrudes 0.7 mm from the footplate to maximize transmission of laser energy through the sclera. The most commonly used settings start at 2,000 mW for 2,000 ms duration. The traditional teaching recommends increasing the power in standard increments until an audible "pop" (which represents intraocular uveal microexplosions) is heard, at which point the energy is decreased to a power just below the level

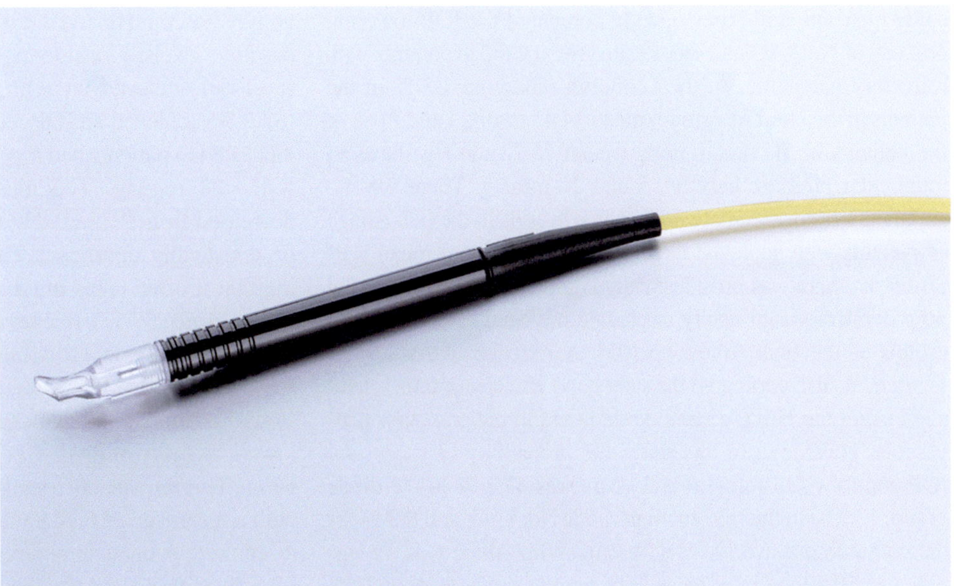

**Fig. 4.2** This is a magnified image of the G-probe, with an excellent view of the curved footplate and the protruding tip (Image courtesy of Iridex, Mountain View, CA)

of the "pop" (Video 4.1). Despite this anecdotal recommendation, Robolleda et al. reported that there were no significant differences in IOP-lowering efficacy between patients in whom the intraoperative "pop" did and did not occur [90]. A new protocol (known as the slow coagulation technique) uses a lower level of power (1,250–1,500 mW) for a longer duration (3,500–4,000 ms) in an effort to maintain efficacy while minimizing postoperative inflammation.

Most surgeons apply six to eight laser spots per quadrant for 360°, with the applications spaced one half probe tip width apart. This strategy produces confluent burns on the ciliary processes in human autopsy eyes [91]. It is highly recommended to avoid the 3 and 9 o'clock meridians so as to minimize trauma to the long posterior ciliary arteries and nerves [89]. It is also advisable to avoid perilimbal regions with excessive scleral or conjunctival pigmentation. Since the shorter wavelength of the diode laser is preferentially absorbed by pigment, laser uptake within pigmented anterior segment tissues can result in partial- or full-thickness ocular surface burns. Applying laser treatment to these highly pigmented regions also reduces energy transmission to the ciliary body, thus reducing efficacy [92].

The efficacy of transscleral diode CPC is directly related to the extent of ciliary body and ciliary process destruction. While the G-probe performs admirably at positioning the laser over the ciliary body in standard eyes, its performance in patients with atypical morphology or axial length (i.e., extreme myopia, congenital glaucoma, or microphthalmos) is deficient. For this reason, many surgeons routinely employ ocular transillumination to facilitate identification of the ciliary body for optimal laser probe placement. This procedure is performed by placing a bright focal light source against the posterior globe, while aiming the light anteriorly. When this is performed in a dark environment, the darker ciliary body will be highlighted against the backdrop of a brighter ruby-colored glow [93, 94].

Historically, the use of transscleral diode CPC in the United States has been relegated to eyes with severe, refractory glaucoma. Its status as a treatment of last resort is due to concerns regarding phthisis, chronic uveitis, pain, and loss of vision. The official recommendations of the American Academy of Ophthalmology Ophthalmic Assessment committee are based on Level III evidence and include [93]:

1. Patients with refractory glaucoma who have failed trabeculectomy or tube shunt procedures
2. Patients with elevated IOP and poor vision
3. Patients with minimal or no visual potential who have eye pain thought to be secondary to the elevated IOP
4. Patients whose ocular surface precludes incisional surgery (i.e., profoundly scarred conjunctiva, ocular cicatricial pemphigoid, thin sclera, history of scleritis)
5. Patients who refuse incisional surgery
6. Patients who are in emergent situations (i.e., neovascular glaucoma)

While this list serves as a useful guideline, the position of transscleral diode CPC in the treatment algorithm is surgeon specific. Ultimately, this decision is based on a careful consideration of the potential risks (i.e., visual loss, hypotony), the potential benefits (i.e., noninvasive procedure), and individualized patient characteristics (i.e., candidate for anesthesia).

Diode CPC has been shown to have both theoretical and practical benefits compared with older forms of cyclodestruction, but widespread adoption required strong clinical data establishing efficacy. The first item that required clarification was comparative efficacy with the other comparable cyclodestructive technique, Nd:YAG CPC. In a prospective, randomized study by Youn et al., they directly compared the IOP-lowering efficacy of Nd:YAG and diode transscleral CPC in patients with refractory glaucoma. At the 12-month follow-up, 83 % of the patients in the Nd:YAG group (mean 14.45 mmHg) and 71 % of the patients in the diode group (mean 15.22 mmHg) have an intraocular pressure between 5 and 20 mmHg. There was no significant difference between the two groups in the percentage of patients who achieved target IOP or in the final mean IOP. Similarly, there was no statistically significant difference in the postoperative visual acuity or change in visual acuity between groups at the final follow-up [95]. A retrospective study by Oguri et al. also compared the safety and efficacy of transscleral CPC using the Nd:YAG and diode lasers in patients with neovascular glaucoma. In this study, the probability of successful IOP control ($\leq$23 mmHg) at 3 years was 47.2 % in the diode group, 13.3 % in the free-running mode Nd:YAG, and 8.8 % for the continuous wave Nd:YAG group. While there was no significant difference in efficacy between the diode laser and the free-running Nd:YAG laser, the diode laser was significantly more effective compared with the Nd:YAG in continuous wave mode. In the Oguri study, there was a significantly high rate of visual loss in all three groups (24 % for the diode group, 56 % for the free-running Nd:YAG, and 44 % for the continuous wave Nd:YAG) [96]. While the rates of visual loss were high, they are similar to other CPC studies that studied patients with neovascular glaucoma [63].

Establishing comparative efficacy was necessary to consider the diode laser as a viable alternative to the Nd:YAG laser for use in transscleral CPC. The next step in validating the diode laser involves documenting long-term IOP control. Kosoko and associates led the way in this endeavor when they designed a prospective, non-comparative study that specifically looked at the long-term efficacy of diode CPC in patients with refractory glaucoma, naïve to previous ciliary ablation. This study followed 27 eyes from 27 patients for 6–28 months, with a mean follow-up of 19 months. These patients were treated with 17–19 applications over 270°, for a total energy of 63.3 J. In this publication, failure was defined as an IOP drop of less than 20 % from baseline and an IOP above 22 mmHg. Based on this definition, the cumulative probability of success in this cohort of patients was 52 % at 2 years [97].

In 2006, Vernon et al. published their own efficacy results that spanned a longer duration of postoperative observation. In this retrospective study, the authors reviewed the results of 42 eyes from 39 patients who underwent diode laser transscleral CPC. These patients were followed for 36–84 months, with a mean duration of 65.7 months. The treatment consisted of 14 burns that were distributed around 270° of the limbus overlying the ciliary body. Each treatment session delivered 56 J of energy. In this study, the mean IOP decreased from a pretreatment level of 31.4±8.8 mmHg to a final value of 15.6±6.3 mmHg. This represents a 50.3 % decrease in the IOP compared with baseline. Treatment failure was defined as

an IOP $\geq$ 22mmHg and a <30% reduction in IOP compared to baseline levels. Considering this criteria, 37 of the 42 eyes (88.1 %) achieved an IOP <22 mmHg, 35 of the 42 eyes (83.3 %) achieved an IOP reduction $\geq$30 %, and 31 out of the 42 (73.8 %) patients had a $\geq$30 % reduction in IOP and a final IOP <22 mmHg. The mean number of glaucoma drops decreased from 2.55±0.83 to 1.71±1.44, which was found to be statistically significant. This study also reinforced the finding that it often takes multiple treatments to achieve optimal success since 59.6 % of eyes required more than one treatment (mean 2.17 sessions) to achieve the desired outcome [98].

While the previous studies focused on efficacy in adults, a study by Autrata and associates considers the long-term IOP-lowering ability of diode CPC in the pediatric glaucoma population. This retrospective study reviewed 69 eyes in 53 children, with a mean age of 6.14±1.29 (range 0.9–15) years. A majority of these patients have already undergone some form of eye surgery, with the average patient having undergone 1.6 previous surgeries. The mean follow-up for these patients was 5.6±2.8 (range 2.2–9.5) years. In this particular study, success was defined as a postoperative IOP of $\leq$21 mmHg, with or without glaucoma medications. In patients who underwent a single treatment session, only 46 % of these patients had an IOP $\leq$21 mmHg at 12 months. With repeat laser procedures, the success rate increased to 79 % at 1 year, 63 % at 2 years, and 48 % at 5 years. The mean final post laser IOP was 20.81±6.38 mmHg after a mean of 2.13±1.47 laser treatment sessions [99]. Pediatric glaucoma patients seem to respond with the same degree of IOP lowering that you would see in an adult glaucoma patient, but the effect has a shorter duration of action. This limitation must be considered in light of its more favorable side effect profile. In pediatric glaucoma patients, diode CPC seems to be particularly useful for patients who are not good candidates for incisional surgery, as a temporizing measure before performing more invasive procedures and as an adjunct to previous tube shunt surgery [100, 101].

The results with diode laser CPC have been good enough that some have considered using it in lieu of a glaucoma drainage device in patients with refractory and neovascular glaucoma. In a study by Malik and associates, they retrospectively compared the use of a double plate Molteno tube shunt to diode CPC in glaucoma patients who failed previous surgery. Twenty-eight eyes in the diode group and 26 eyes in the glaucoma drainage implant group were followed for a mean of 150 (range 21–322) weeks. While the number of patients who achieved an intraocular pressure between 5 and 21 mmHg without adjunctive glaucoma medications strongly favored the Molteno tube shunt group (46 % in the Molteno group to 11 % in the diode laser group), the success rate was comparable in the patients who required postoperative glaucoma medications (81 % in the tube eyes and 64 % in the diode laser eyes) [102]. Yildirim and associates prospectively treated neovascular glaucoma patients with either diode CPC or an Ahmed Glaucoma Valve to compare the long-term safety and efficacy. Of the fifty-eight patients who completed the study, all had at least 2 years of follow-up. The Kaplan-Meier survival analysis demonstrated a 2-year probability of success of 61.18 and 59.26 % for the diode and Ahmed groups, respectively. The two groups also shared a similar rate of postoperative vision loss, with 24 % of the patients in the diode group experiencing a decrease in vision compared with a 27 % rate of vision loss in the Ahmed group [103].

Like all surgical procedures, diode transscleral CPC has its share of potential complications. The most common postoperative issues include visual loss, chronic uveitis, pain, hypotony, and treatment failure [87]. The prevalence of visual loss after diode transscleral CPC has been documented to be 7–31 %, which is lower than that seen in patients following Nd:YAG CPC (30–47 %) and cyclocryotherapy (5–69 %) [49, 57, 86, 87, 89, 97, 104–107]. Similarly, posttreatment discomfort is less pronounced following diode CPC as compared to Nd:YAG CPC and cyclocryotherapy [87, 108]. Other reported complications include phthisis bulbi, malignant glaucoma, anterior segment ischemia, sympathetic ophthalmia, lens subluxation, choroidal effusions, necrotizing scleritis, staphylomas, epiretinal membrane formation, intraocular pressure spikes, and corneal edema [87, 109–115].

## Future Considerations

### New Indications

Historically, cyclodestructive procedures have been reserved for patients with poor vision and refractory glaucoma. This is due to concerns about the high rates of visual loss and phthisis in the cyclocryotherapy literature [116]. A more detailed review of the literature highlights the fact that a majority of the early studies on cyclodestructive procedures targeted patients with refractory glaucomatous conditions, particularly neovascular glaucoma. In fact, a study by Sidoti and associates that evaluated the success rate of Baerveldt tube shunt placement in patients with neovascular glaucoma documented a high complication rate, including a 31 % incidence of complete visual loss (no light perception) and an 11 % incidence of phthisis [117]. This finding highlights the fact that refractory glaucoma conditions are difficult to treat and susceptible to poor outcomes, regardless of the intervention.

The evolution of cilioablative therapy has ushered in the much more refined diode laser procedure. When directly compared against cyclocryotherapy, diode laser cyclophotocoagulation was found to be equally effective at IOP reduction, with a significantly lower rate of profound vision loss (cyclocryotherapy 15.7 %, diode CPC 6.3 %) and phthisis (cyclocryotherapy 5.2 %, diode CPC 3.1 %) [118]. Moreover, as previously discussed, the study by Yildirim and associates documented the equivalent IOP-lowering efficacy of diode CPC and the Ahmed Glaucoma Valve in treating patients with neovascular glaucoma. Similarly, the rate of vision loss was statistically equivalent between the two groups (27 % in the Ahmed valve-treated patients and 24 % in the diode CPC patients). One particularly interesting finding was that this study reported a greater incidence of phthisis bulbi for the Ahmed Glaucoma Valve (6 %) patients as compared to those patients who received diode CPC (0 %) treatment [103].

The excellent results described above have encouraged surgeons to employ diode CPC in early stages of glaucoma and in patients with better vision [119, 120]. In 2001, Egbert and colleagues performed a prospective study of diode laser CPC as the primary surgical treatment in patients with primary open-angle glaucoma. In this study, one eye was treated with diode laser CPC while the fellow eye was treated with glaucoma drops. The IOP decreased in 67 % of the patients, with 48 % achieving a >20 % reduction in IOP compared with baseline eye pressure. There were no reports of phthisis bulbi, hypotony, or sympathetic ophthalmia in patients who were treated with laser. Regarding vision, 76 % (60/79) of the patients had the same or improved visual acuity as compared to baseline. Moreover, the incidence of visual loss was 23 % in both the diode CPC-treated eyes (18/79) and in the medically treated eyes (10/47) [121].

Another study looked at diode CPC as the primary surgical therapy in patients with primary open-angle glaucoma, chronic angle-closure glaucoma, and neovascular glaucoma. The patients in all three groups experienced significant drops in the IOP compared with baseline levels. Specifically, the patients with neovascular glaucoma experienced a 47 % decrease in IOP, the primary open-angle glaucoma patients achieved a 39 % drop in IOP, and the patients with chronic angle-closure glaucoma were found to have a 29.9 % reduction in eye pressure. There were no patients in any subgroup that experienced phthisis bulbi, prolonged hypotony, or vitreous hemorrhage. Importantly, the mean pre-laser visual acuity did not deteriorate following treatment in the primary open-angle glaucoma or chronic angle-closure glaucoma subgroups with good baseline vision [122].

With mounting evidence supporting the safety and efficacy of diode CPC as a primary treatment, an increasing number of surgeons are considering this procedure earlier in the course of the disease and in patients with better vision. In fact, the United Kingdom National Cyclodiode Laser survey reported that only 12.3 % of the respondents reserved diode CPC for patients with poor (≤6/60) vision [123]. It is likely that increasing familiarity and comfort with diode CPC will lead more surgeons to consider this intervention earlier in the course of the glaucoma treatment paradigm.

## Endoscopic Cyclophotocoagulation

While it is difficult to classify endoscopic cyclophotocoagulation (ECP) as a new technology since it was first described in 1985 and then released as a commercially available unit in the early 1990s, it is reasonable to state that its greater acceptance and position in the therapeutic paradigm are still in evolution [15, 124]. ECP is a cilioablative technique that allows direct photocoagulation of the ciliary processes with endoscopic assistance. The E2 Microprobe Laser and Endoscopy Systems (Endo Optiks, Little Silver, NJ) incorporates a diode laser that emits pulsed continuous wave energy at 810 nm with a 175-W xenon light source, a helium-neon laser aiming beam, and a recordable video camera. The image guide, the light guide, and the laser guide are transmitted via fiber-optic technology to an 18- or 20-gauge probe. The 20-gauge endoscope provides a 70° field of view with a depth of focus from 0.5 to 15 mm. The 18-gauge endoscope affords a larger (110°) field of view with a depth of focus from 1 to 30 mm. While the 20G probe has a smaller diameter and can focus close to the target, the larger probe provides improved resolution and a more panoramic view [125].

Endoscopic cyclophotocoagulation can be performed through limbal, clear cornea, and pars plana approaches. A pars plana entry is favored by vitreoretinal surgeons, who often use this technology in combination with a pars plana vitrectomy. The clear corneal and limbal approaches are preferred by anterior segment surgeons, who can perform this procedure without the need for a vitrectomy.

In a clear cornea/limbal approach, viscoelastic is used to stabilize the anterior chamber and then expand the posterior chamber. This technique facilitates endoprobe access to the ciliary processes. Yu and associates reported that 2 mm was the ideal distance between the probe and target tissue to preserve the intended laser energy settings [126]. The initial power is 0.25–0.3 W, which is titratable up to 1.2 W. The laser should be set on continuous mode so that the surgeon is "painting" the laser across the target tissue (Video 4.2). Successful treatment is manifested as a whitening and contraction of the ciliary processes. Utilization of a curved probe allows treatment for up to 270° from a single incision. Kahook and colleagues found that a two-site treatment allowed for 360° of treatment, which resulted in significantly lower intraocular pressure and less dependence on glaucoma medication compared with a one-site approach [127]. At the end of the case, complete removal of viscoelastic is highly recommended since retained viscoelastic is one of the most common causes of post-ECP IOP elevation [128].

Given that ECP is still in its relative infancy, the specific indications are still evolving. Currently, the most common use of ECP is in combination with phacoemulsification for the treatment of early to moderate glaucoma. Other documented indications for ECP include the following: (1) the treatment of plateau iris syndrome, (2) for patients with refractory glaucoma, (3) to augment the effects of a glaucoma drainage implant, and (4) in patients who are not good candidates for filtration surgery or glaucoma drainage implants.

At the 2006 American Glaucoma Society annual meeting, Berke and associates presented the long-term data for the use of combined cataract surgery with ECP (Phaco/ECP) in the setting of medically controlled glaucoma. With a mean follow-up of 3.2 years (range 5 months–5.5 years), the mean IOP decreased 3.4 mmHg in the Phaco/ECP group as compared to a 0.7 mmHg increase in IOP following the straight cataract extraction. The Phaco/ECP group also experienced a >50 % reduction in medication burden, while there was no significant change in medication load for the patients who underwent cataract surgery alone [129].

Chen and associates evaluated the IOP-lowering efficacy of ECP in a large series of patients with refractory glaucoma of various diagnoses. The eyes in this study received 180–360° of laser treatment to the ciliary processes. The mean baseline IOP was 27.7 mmHg preoperatively, which decreased to 17.0 mmHg at the last follow-up. With the definition of success being an IOP ≤21 mmHg, 94 % of the treatments were successful at year one and 82 % were considered a success after 2 years. There was a mean reduction of one glaucoma medication over the course of the study. No significant complications were noted in this report and <10 % of the patients experienced a ≥ 2 line decrease in Snellen visual acuity [130].

Another compelling question is how ECP compares with traditional glaucoma surgeries (trabeculectomy and glaucoma drainage device) in the treatment of elevated IOP. Gayton and colleagues conducted a randomized prospective study that compared Phaco/ECP with combined phacoemulsification and trabeculectomy. Success was defined as a post-treatment IOP <19 mmHg with no deterioration of the visual field and no increase in optic nerve head cupping. Based upon this criterion, 30 % of the Phaco/ECP eyes achieved the target IOP range without medications and 65 % were successful with adjunctive medications. In the phacoemulsification/trabeculectomy group, 40 % of the patients achieved IOP control without medications, while 52 % of these patients reached the desired IOP range with additional glaucoma medications [131]. Lima et al. prospectively compared patients with refractory glaucoma who were randomized to receive either ECP or an Ahmed drainage implant. All of the patients were pseudophakic, status post at least one previous trabeculectomy with adjunctive antimetabolite, possessed vision better than light perception, and had an IOP ≥35 mmHg (mean 41 mmHg in both groups) on maximal tolerated medical therapy. At 24 months of follow-up, the mean postoperative IOP was 14.73 mmHg in the Ahmed group and 14.07 mmHg among ECP-treated patients. Based on a Kaplan-Meier analysis, this represents a 2-year success rate of 70.6 % for the Ahmed patients and 73.5 % for the

ECP patients. Noteworthy, the Ahmed glaucoma implant-treated patients had a significantly higher rate of complications compared with those patients treated with ECP [132].

Neely and Plager published two studies detailing their experience with ECP in the pediatric population. In the first study, they retrospectively evaluated 6 years of data from 36 eyes of 29 patients with refractory glaucoma who underwent ECP. The mean baseline IOP was 35.06 mmHg and the mean IOP at the final visit was 23.63 mmHg, representing a 30 % decrease in IOP. The cumulative success rate for ECP in pediatric glaucoma patients was 43 %, with 25 % of all patients requiring more than one treatment to achieve the desired efficacy. Aphakic patients had a higher rate of complications, which included 2 retinal detachments, 1 episode of chronic hypotony, and 1 case of profound visual loss [133]. In another related study, Carter et al. performed a retrospective review of 34 eyes from 24 children and young adolescents who were followed for a mean of 44 months after being treated with ECP. The mean IOP decreased from 32.6 to 22.9 mmHg during the follow-up period. In this study, treatment failure was defined as a (1) postoperative IOP >24 mmHg and <15 % IOP lowering, despite the addition of adjunctive medications, or (2) the occurrence of a visually significant complication. Based on these qualifiers, the overall success rate was found to be 53 % [134].

One distinct advantage of ECP is that the treatment is performed with direct visualization of the target tissue. This is particularly useful in situations where the patient has abnormal anatomy (i.e., congenital glaucoma) or media opacities (i.e., corneal opacities). As it relates to the former, Barkana and associates reported successfully treating a congenital glaucoma patient with ECP in the setting of a failed transscleral diode CPC. Endoscopic visualization revealed several misplaced laser burns, representing the ill-fated attempt at transscleral CPC [135]. A study by Al-Haddad and colleagues documented a low incidence of successful IOP reduction (17 %) using ECP in patients with corneal opacities but acknowledged that the procedure still played a limited role in this challenging patient population. They also reported significant benefit of endoscopy alone in the intraocular placement of tube shunts when media opacities precluded good visualization. This study was limited by a low sample size, patients with abnormal anatomy and aqueous dynamics, and difficulty measuring the IOP accurately due to the opacified corneas [136].

While ECP has a favorable side effect profile compared to transscleral CPC, several complications have been reported. The largest series of Phaco/ECP patients reported the following complications: IOP elevation (14 %), fibrinous uveitis (7 %), cystoid macular edema (4 %), and transient hypotony (2 %) [137]. Another large case series that included patients with more advanced glaucoma reported fibrinous exudates (24 %), hyphema (12 %), cystoid macular edema (10 %), ≥2

line visual loss (6 %), and choroidal detachment (4 %) [130]. There are several theoretical, albeit currently unsubstantiated, risks such as endophthalmitis and suprachoroidal hemorrhage that are an inherent to any intraocular procedure. There was one reported case of post-ECP phthisis bulbi that occurred 5 months after treatment [138].

## Micropulse Transscleral Diode Laser Cyclophotocoagulation

A new form of transscleral diode laser CPC has been developed that utilizes micropulse technology to denature the target tissue while minimizing collateral tissue damage. The diode laser emits a series of short (microsecond), repetitive bursts of energy. This active phase of the treatment algorithm is referred to as "on" time and confines the thermal effect to the absorbing tissue, with minimal diffusion of heat to the adjacent structures. The cooling period ("off" time) is proportionately longer than the pulse time, thus allowing the thermal relaxation of tissue and a return to baseline temperature [139, 140] (Fig. 4.3).

Micropulse diode laser technology has been successfully used for the treatment of several retinal diseases, including diabetic retinopathy and maculopathy. This same technology is now being evaluated for safety and efficacy as a method for CPC. Based on its mechanism of action, the expectation is that micropulse diode laser CPC will achieve IOP-lowering efficacy that rivals traditional diode CPC, without the associated pain and inflammation.

In 2002, the results of a pilot study were published that documented a mean baseline IOP of 44 mmHg that decreased to 28 mmHg at week 1 and 36 mmHg at week 3. At the end of the first week, 75 % of the patients achieved ≥20 % decrease in IOP, while 63 % of the patients experienced a ≥30 % drop in IOP compared to baseline. These results demonstrate a significant short-term reduction in IOP that tends to regress over time [141]. In 2010, Tan and associates published the results from a prospective interventional case series that evaluated 40 eyes from 38 consecutive patients with refractory glaucoma who were treated with micropulse diode CPC using a redesigned G-probe. The mean baseline IOP was 40.1 mmHg and the patients were followed for an average of 17.3 (range 12–118) months. The mean IOP dropped to 24.6 mmHg at the final follow-up, with 35 % (14/40) requiring a second laser treatment. The mean number of glaucoma medications was reduced from 2.1 before treatment to 1.3 at the final visit. Importantly, only 31.6 % reported any pain during the procedure and none of the patients described the discomfort as moderate or severe. Regarding complications, all of the patients experienced mild inflammation and hyperemia. Fortunately, there were no reports of hypotony and no patients experienced a loss in visual acuity [142].

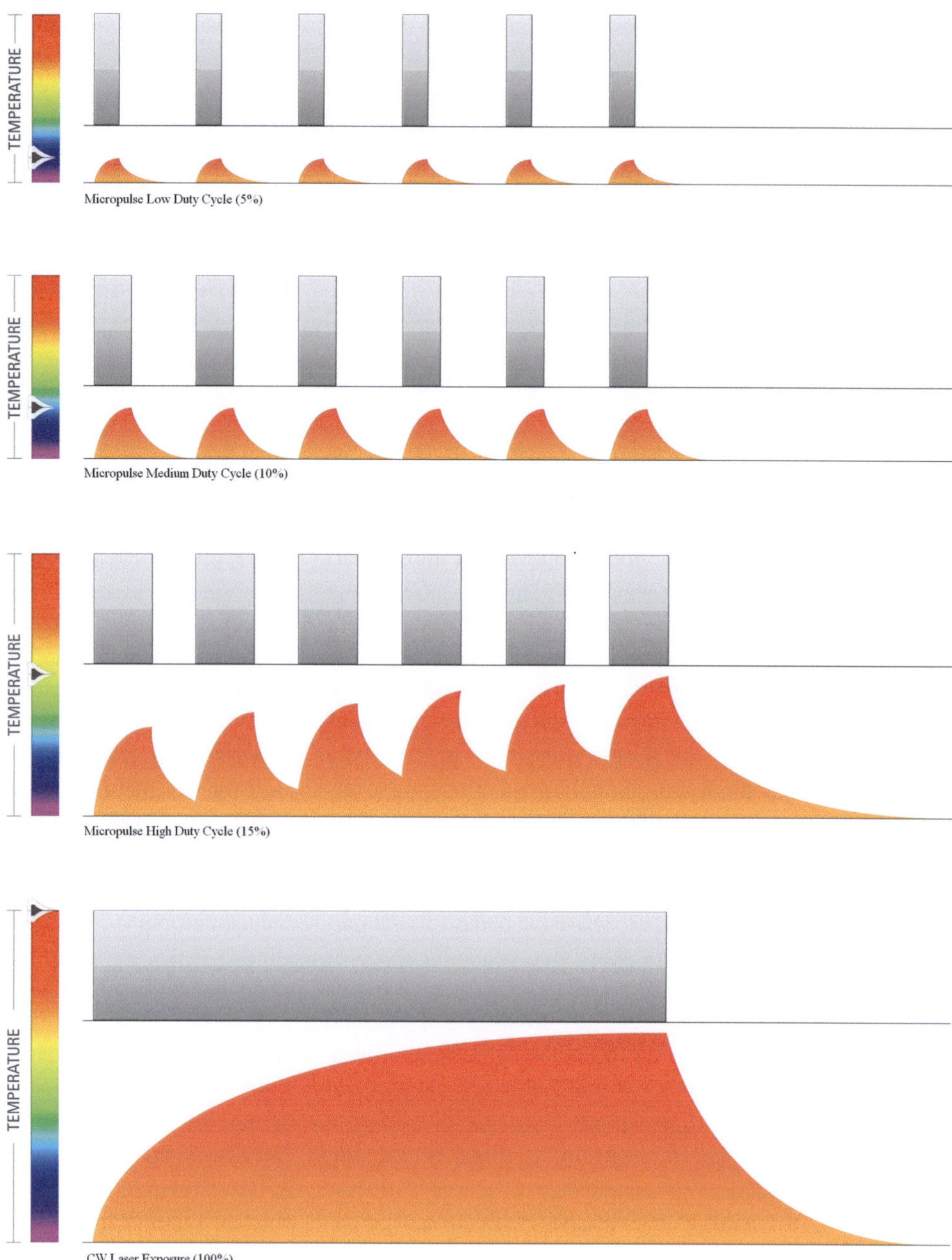



**Fig. 4.3** This is an artistic rendering of micropulse laser delivery. These images demonstrate how continuous wave energy is separated into a series of repetitive microsecond pulses. The pictures provides a graphical representation of the fact that the duration of the laser pulse ("ON") time can be adjusted to deliver adequate energy to the target tissue while minimizing thermal spread (Image courtesy of Iridex, Mountain View, CA)

Indeed, the micropulse diode transscleral CPC appears to be a promising new technology that provides stellar IOP control with a favorable side effect profile. Further testing with longer follow-up is required to have a better sense of where this fits in our treatment algorithm.

## Ultrasound-Mediated Cyclomodification

While effective, traditional cyclodestructive procedures are nonspecific interventions that coagulate the surrounding tissue along with the ciliary body and ciliary processes. This indiscriminate tissue damage results in the feared complications, including hypotony, phthisis, and pain.

These issues have prompted research into other tissue-specific and less destructive alternatives. This effort culminated in the introduction of high-intensity focused ultrasound (HIFU) for the treatment of glaucoma. In 1991, Silverman and colleagues published the results from a multicenter clinical trial, where 880 eyes of patients with refractory glaucoma were treated with HIFU. In this study, successful treatment was defined as an IOP between 6 and 22 mmHg. Given this qualifier, the authors reported a 6-month success rate of 48.7 % with one treatment and

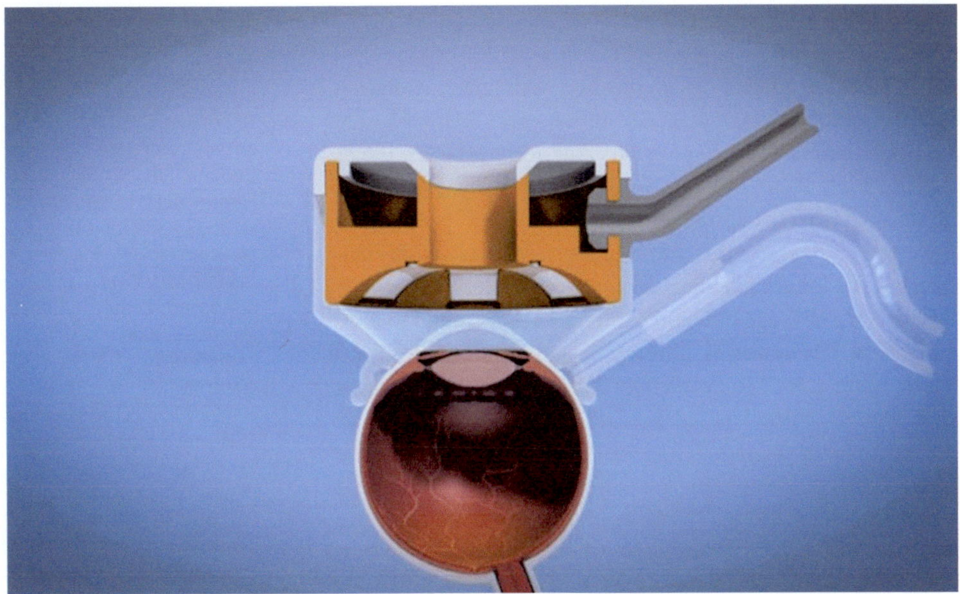

**Fig. 4.4** This is a representation of the HIFU handpiece as it sits on the human eye (Image courtesy of EyeTechCare, Rillieux-la-Pape, France)

79.3 % when re-treatment was allowed. The common complications in this study included mild iritis, scleral thinning, and phthisis (1.1 %) [143]. Unfortunately, the commercial unit was obtrusive and the process was cumbersome, thus leading to the demise of this device (Fig. 4.4) [144].

Improved technology (particularly miniaturized annual transducers) has facilitated the redesign of the HIFU unit into a compact, user-friendly device. The first commercially available HIFU unit is called EyeOP1 (EyeTechCare, Rillieux-la-Pape, France) and consists of a command module and a disposable circular therapy probe. The command module is a computerized system with a touch screen that allows input and adjustment of the setting parameters. The computer controls the two essential components of the system: (1) the generator that delivers the necessary power to the piezoelectric transducers and (2) the pressure reduction system, which modulates the amount of suction applied by the probe. The therapeutic device also consists of two vital parts: (1) the positioning cone, which centers the device on the eye and fixates it in proper position, and (2) the treatment probe, which actually creates the ultrasonic beam [144].

The concept underlying this device is called ultrasound circular cyclocoagulation (UC$^3$). It involves the simultaneous treatment of the entire ciliary body through the use of a circular treatment probe that releases a titratable dose of ultrasonic energy. By incorporating six separate microtransducers, the probe is able to form six distinct ultrasonic beams that treat the circumference of the eye at the required depth in a procedure that takes approximately 1 min [144, 145].

The first clinical pilot study on the EyeOP1 was completed in March 2011. In this prospective, non-comparative study, 12 eyes of patients with refractory glaucoma were treated with the EyeOP1 device. The patients were randomized into groups receiving either three- or four-second duration of ultrasound exposure per shot. In the former group, the IOP decreased from a mean preoperative value of 35.6 to 27.49 mmHg at the 6-month follow-up visit. The IOP in the latter group decreased from a 40.5 mmHg baseline value to 23.4 mmHg at the 6-month follow-up. The complications included three cases of superficial punctate epitheliopathy and one report of a central ulcer. There were no reports of chronic pain, hypotony, or phthisis bulbi in either group [145].

Another IOP-lowering ultrasonic device is being developed by visionary ophthalmologist Donald Schwartz, M.D. This instrument emits a low frequency ultrasonic energy to the targeted perilimbal region that ultimately results in an increased outflow facility. This effect is mediated by two presumptive mechanisms: (1) by initiating an integrin response that leads to a cytokine cascade, culminating in the activation of enzymes, macrophages, and heat shock proteins, and (2) by dislodging debris from the trabecular meshwork.

This procedure is performed by placing an ultrasound probe circumferentially around the limbus at all twelve clock hours. According to Dr. Schwartz, the focused ultrasonic energy (20,000–100,000 Hz) generates a high enough temperature within the trabecular meshwork to stimulate the cytokine cascade without causing tissue destruction. He cites non-published rabbit histopathology studies to support his contention that the IOP-lowering effect is not mediated through ciliary body destruction. Instead, he proposes that the mechanism of action is similar to laser trabeculoplasty, where cytokine activation leads to increased outflow facility. Clinical studies are currently underway to evaluate the short- and long-term safety and efficacy of this exciting new technology [146–147].

## Summary

Over the past 100 years, there has been a dramatic evolution in the technology that is used for cilioablation. Cyclodiathermy was effective but long-term efficacy issues and its high incidence of severe complications led to its demise. Cyclocryotherapy afforded a more predictable IOP-lowering response, but it also had a prohibitively high incidence of vision threatening complications. Diode laser CPC ushered in a new age of ciliodestruction. It was found to have equivalent IOP-lowering efficacy to its predecessors with a much more tolerable side effect profile. This encouraging risk-benefit profile has led to a dramatic expansion in the indications for implementing cilioablative therapy in the treatment of glaucoma. In fact, there has been a shift towards using transscleral diode CPC in patients with much better vision. That trend started in Europe and has now gained some degree of acceptance in the United States. While early utilization of transscleral diode CPC is just starting to catch on, there has been greater acceptance of endoscopic diode CPC for the treatment of early stages of glaucoma. This acceptance is due to good efficacy and minimal side effects and because it can be easily used as an adjunct to cataract surgery. Diode technology continues to evolve and has resulted in micropulse diode CPC. Early results suggest similar IOP-lowering efficacy as traditional diode CPC with less trauma to the surrounding tissue. The ciliary body is also being considered as a target for the similarly benign high-intensity focused ultrasound treatment. This technology is a hybrid between cilioablation and selective laser trabeculoplasty, with early results that produce excitement for the future.

## References

1. Coppez L. Au sujet des applications chirurgicales de la diathermie enophthalmologie. Bull Soc Belge Ophthalmol. 1929;58:56–7.
2. Coppez L. La technique de la diathermie en ophthalmologie. Bull Soc Belge Ophthalmol. 1927;55:91–2.
3. Weve H. Die zyklodiatermie das corpus ciliare bei glaukom. Zentralbl Ophthalmol. 1933;29:562–9.
4. Vogt A. Cyclodiathermy puncture in cases of glaucoma. Br J Ophthalmol. 1940;24:288–97.
5. Vogt A. Versuche zur intraokularen druckherabsetzung mittelst diatermiescha digung des corpus ciliare (Zyklodipatermiestichelung). Klin Monatsbl Augenheilkd. 1936;97:672–7.
6. Edmonds C, De Roeth Jr A, Howard GM. Histopathologic changes following cryosurgery and diathermy of the rabbit ciliary body. Am J Ophthalmol. 1970;69:65–72.
7. Allingham RR, Damji KF, Freedman S, Moroi SE, Shafranov G, Shields MB, editors. Shields' Textbook of Glaucoma. 5th ed. Philadelphia: Lippincott Williams & Wilkins; 2005.
8. Albaugh CH, Dunphy EB. Cyclodiathermy. Arch Ophthalmol. 1942;27:543–57.
9. Berens C. Glaucoma surgery: an evaluation of cycloelectrolysis and cyclodiathermy. Arch Ophthalmol. 1955;54:548–62.
10. Walton DS, Grant WM. Penetrating cyclodiathermy for filtration. Arch Ophthalmol. 1970;83:47–8.
11. Bietti G. Surgical intervention on the ciliary body: new trends for the relief of glaucoma. J Am Med Assoc. 1950;142(12):889–97.
12. Bellows AR, Grant WM. Cyclocryotherapy in advanced inadequately controlled glaucoma. Am J Ophthalmol. 1973;75:679–84.
13. Bellows AR. Cyclocryotherapy for glaucoma. Int Ophthalmol Clin. 1981;21(1):99–111.
14. Bellows AR, Grant WM. Cyclocryotherapy of chronic open angle glaucoma in aphakic eyes. Am J Ophthalmol. 1978;85:615–21.
15. Shields MB. Cyclodestructive surgery for glaucoma: past, present and future. Trans Am Ophthalmol Soc. 1985;83:285–303.
16. West CE, Wood TO, Kaufman HE. Cyclocryotherapy for glaucoma pre or post penetrating keratoplasty. Am J Ophthalmol. 1973;76:485.
17. Binder PS, Abel R, Kaufman HE. Cyclocryotherapy for glaucoma after penetrating keratoplasty. Am J Ophthalmol. 1975;79:489–92.
18. Prost M. Cyclocryotherapy for glaucoma: evaluation of techniques. Surv Ophthalmol. 1983;28:93–100.
19. Faulborn J, Birnbaum F. Zyklokryotherapie hamorrhagischer glaukome: langzeitbeobachtungen und histologische befunde. Klin Monbl Augenheilkd. 1977;170:651–6.
20. Krupin T, Mitchell KB, Becker B. Cyclocryotherapy in neovascular glaucoma. Am J Ophthalmol. 1978;86:24–6.
21. McLean JM, Lincoff HA. Cryosurgery of the ciliary body. Trans Am Ophthalmol Soc. 1964;62:385–407.
22. Demols E, Brihaye-VanGeertruden M. Cyclocryoapplication. Ophthalmologica. 1975;171:332–45.
23. Lincoff H, Cavero R, Nadel A, McLean JM. Cryosurgery of the ciliary body. Arch Ophthalmol. 1968;79:196–204.
24. Paterson CA, Paterson EF. Experimental cryosurgery. Arch Ophthalmol. 1971;86:425–31.
25. De Roeth A. Cryosurgery for glaucoma. Int Ophthalmol Clin. 1967;7(2):351–67.
26. Quigley HA. Histological and physiological studies of cyclocryotherapy in primate and human eyes. Am J Ophthalmol. 1976;82: 722–32.
27. Brihaye M, Oosterhuis JA. Experimental cryoapplication with variations in the pressure exerted on the sclera. Trans Ophthalmol Soc U K. 1972;92:860.
28. Wesley RD, Kielar RA. Cyclocryotherapy in treatment of glaucoma. Glaucoma. 1980;3:533–8.
29. Higginbotham EJ, Lee DA, Bartels SP, Richardson T, Miller M. Effects of cyclocryotherapy on aqueous humor dynamics in cats. Arch Ophthalmol. 1988;106:396–403.
30. Boniuk M. Cryotherapy in neovascular glaucoma. Trans Am Acad Ophthalmol Otolaryngol. 1974;78:337–43.
31. Brindley G, Shields MB. Values and limitations of cyclocryotherapy. Graefes Arch Clin Exp Ophthalmol. 1986;224:545–8.
32. Palmeris G, Moschos M, Chimonidou E, Velissaropoulos P. Einige bemer kungen zur anwendung der zyklokryopexie in der behandlung der verchiedenen glaukomfarnen. Klin Monbl Augenheilkd. 1976;169:439–41.
33. Caprioli J, Strang SL, Spaeth GL, Poryzees EH. Cyclocryotherapy in the treatment of advanced glaucoma. Ophthalmology. 1985;92: 947–54.
34. De Roeth A. Cryosurgery for the treatment of advanced chronic simple glaucoma. Am J Ophthalmol. 1968;66:1034–41.
35. Bellows AR. Cyclocryotherapy. In: Chandler P, Grant WM, editors. Glaucoma. Philadelphia: Lea and Febiger; 1979. p. 311–5.
36. Weekers R, Lavergne G, Watillon M, Gilson M, Legros AM. Effects of photocoagulation of ciliary body upon ocular tension. Am J Ophthalmol. 1961;52:156–63.
37. Smith RS, Stein MN. Ocular hazards of transscleral laser radiation: II. Intraocular injury produced by ruby and neodymium lasers. Am J Ophthalmol. 1969;67:100–10.

38. Beckman H, Waeltermann J. Transscleral ruby laser cyclophotocoagulation. Am J Ophthalmol. 1984;98:788–95.

39. Fankhauser F, van der Zypen E, Kwasniewska S, Rol P, England C. Transscleral cyclophotocoagulation using a neodymium:YAG laser. Ophthalmic Surg. 1986;17:94–100.

40. Schuman JS, Puliafito CA. Laser cyclophotocoagulation. Int Ophthalmol Clin. 1990;30(2):111–9.

41. Gandham SB, Katz LJ. Cyclodestructive procedures. In: Gross RL, editor. Clinical glaucoma management: critical signs in diagnosis and therapy. Philadelphia: W.B. Saunders Company; 2001.

42. England C, Van der Zypen E, Fankhauser F, Kwasniewska A. A comparison of optical methods use for transscleral cyclophotocoagulation in rabbit eyes produced with the Nd:YAG laser: a morphological, physical and clinical analysis. Lasers Light Ophthalmol. 1988;2:87–102.

43. Krasnov MM, Naumidi LP, Federov AA. Morphological research on the ciliary body in contact transscleral laser cyclocoagulation of human and rabbit eyes. Vestn Oftalmol. 1988;04:11–3.

44. Wilensky JT, Welch D, Mirolovich M. Transscleral cyclocoagulation using a neodymium:YAG laser. Ophthalmic Surg. 1985;16:95–8.

45. Schubert HD, Agarwala A, Arbizo V. Changes in aqueous outflow after in vitro neodymium-aluminum-garnet laser cyclophotocoagulation. Invest Ophthalmol Vis Sci. 1990;31:1834–8.

46. Schmidt KG, Vhuytan KG, Camras CB, Zhan G, Podos SM. The role of prostaglandins and uveoscleral outflow in the reduction of intraocular pressure after contact transscleral Nd:YAG laser cyclophotocoagulation. Invest Ophthalmol Vis Sci Abstr Issue. 1992;33:1269.

47. Van der Zypen E, England C, Fankhauser S. The effect of transscleral laser cyclophotocoagulation on rabbit ciliary body vascularization. Graefes Arch Clin Exp Ophthalmol. 1989;227:172–9.

48. Shields MB, Wilkerson MH, Echelman DA. A comparison of two energy levels for noncontact transscleral neodymium-YAG cyclophotocoagulation. Arch Ophthalmol. 1993;111:484–7.

49. Mastrobattista JM, Luntz M. Ciliary body ablation: where are we and how did we get here? Surv Ophthalmol. 1996;41(3):193–213.

50. Crymes BM, Gross RL. The influence of laser lesion placement in neodymium:YAG cyclophotocoagulation (abstract). Invest Ophthalmol Vis Sci. 1989;30(Suppl):353–4.

51. Schubert HD. Noncontact and contact pars plana transscleral neodymium:YAG laser cyclophotocoagulation in postmortem eyes. Ophthalmology. 1989;96:1471–5.

52. Hampton C, Shields MB. Transscleral neodymium-YAG cyclophotocoagulation. A histologic study of human autopsy eyes. Arch Ophthalmol. 1988;106:1121–3.

53. Allingham RR, de Kater AW, Bellows AR, Hsu J. Probe placement and power levels in contact transscleral neodymium:YAG cyclophotocoagulation. Arch Ophthalmol. 1990;108:738–42.

54. Fiore PM, Latina MA. A technique for precise placement of laser applications in transscleral Nd:YAG cyclophotocoagulation. Am J Ophthalmol. 1989;107:292–3.

55. Stolzenburg S, Muller-Stolzenburg N, Krresse S, Muller GJ. Contact cyclophotocoagulation with the continuous wave Nd:YAG laser with quartz fiber. Optimizing coagulation parameters. Ophthalmologe. 1992;89:210–7.

56. Fankhauser F, Kwasniewska S, Van der Zypen E. Cyclodestructive procedures. Clinical and morphological aspects: A review. Ophthalmologica. 2004;218:77–95.

57. Hampton C, Shields MB, Miller KN, Blasin M. Evaluation of a protocol for transscleral neodymium:YAG cyclophotocoagulation in one hundred consecutive patients. Ophthalmology. 1990;97:910–7.

58. Devenyi RG, Trope GE, Hunter WH, Badeeb O. Neodymium-YAG transscleral cyclophotocoagulation in human eyes. Ophthalmology. 1987;94:1519–22.

59. Trope GE, Ma S. Mid term effects of neodymium:YAG thermal cyclophotocoagulation in glaucoma. Ophthalmology. 1990;97:73–5.

60. Klapper RM, Wandel T, Donnenfeld E, Perry HD. Transscleral neodymium:YAG thermal cyclophotocoagulation in refractory glaucoma. A preliminary report. Ophthalmology. 1988;95:719–22.

61. Balazsi G. Noncontact thermal mode Nd:YAG laser transscleral cyclocoagulation in the treatment of glaucoma. Ophthalmology. 1991;98:18581863.

62. Wright MM, Grajewski AL, Feuer WJ. Nd:YAG cyclophotocoagulation: outcome of treatment for uncontrolled glaucoma. Ophthalmic Surg. 1991;22:279–83.

63. Schuman JS, Bellows AR, Shingleton BJ, Latina MA, Allingham RR, Belcher CD, Pulifito CA. Contact transscleral Nd:YAG laser cyclophotocoagulation. Midterm results. Ophthalmology. 1992;99:1089–94; discussion 1095.

64. Schuman JS, Puliafito CA, Allingham RR, Belcher CD, Bellows AR, Latina MA, Shingleton BJ. Contact transscleral Nd:YAG laser cyclophotocoagulation. Ophthalmology. 1990;97:571–80.

65. Brancato R, Giovanni L, Trabbuchi G, Pietroni C. Contact transscleral cyclophotocoagulation with Nd: YAG laser in uncontrolled glaucoma. Ophthalmic Surg. 1989;20:547–51.

66. Simmons RB, Shields MB, Blasini M, Wilkerson M, Stern RA. Transscleral Nd:YAG laser cyclophotocoagulation with a contact lens. Am J Ophthalmol. 1991;112:671–7.

67. Zaidman GW, Wandel T. Transscleral YAG laser photocoagulation for uncontrolled glaucoma in corneal patients. Cornea. 1988;7:112–4.

68. Thofts RA, Gordon JM, Dohlman CH. Glaucoma following keratoplasty. Trans Am Acad Ophthalmol Otolaryngol. 1974;78:352–64.

69. Threlkeld AB, Shields MB. Non-contact transscleral Nd:YAG cyclophotocoagulation for glaucoma after penetrating keratoplasty. Am J Ophthalmol. 1995;120:569–76.

70. Maus M, Katz LJ. Choroidal detachment, flat anterior chamber, and hypotony as complications of neodymium:YAG laser cyclophotocoagulation. Ophthalmology. 1990;97:69–72.

71. Fiore PM, Melamed S, Krug JH. Focal scleral thinning after transscleral Nd:YAG cyclophotocoagulation. Ophthalmic Surg. 1989;20:215–6.

72. Cyrlin MN, Beckman H, Czedik C. Nd:YAG laser transscleral cyclocoagulation treatment for severe glaucoma. Invest Ophthalmol Vis Sci Suppl. 1985;26:157.

73. Wand M, Schuman JS, Puliafito CA. Malignant glaucoma after contact transscleral Nd:YAG cyclophotocoagulation. J Glaucoma. 1993;2:110–1.

74. Hardten DR, Brown JD. Malignant glaucoma after Nd:YAG cyclophotocoagulation. Am J Ophthalmol. 1991;111:245–7.

75. Shields MB, Shields SE. Noncontact transscleral Nd:YAG cyclophotocoagulation: a long-term follow up of 500 patients. Trans Am Ophthalmol Soc. 1994;92:271–87.

76. Edward DP, Brown SVL, Higginbotham E, Jennings T, Tessler HH, Tso MO. Sympathetic ophthalmia following Nd:YAG cyclotherapy. Ophthalmic Surg. 1989;20:544–6.

77. Kalenak JW, Pardinson JM, Kass MA, Kolker AE. Transscleral neodymium:YAG laser cyclocoagulation for uncontrolled glaucoma. Ophthalmic Surg. 1990;21:346–51.

78. Lam S, Tessler HH, Lam BI, Wilensky JT. High incidence of sympathetic ophthalmia after contact and non-contact neodymium:Yag cyclotherapy. Ophthalmology. 1992;99:1818–22.

79. Suzudi Y, Araie M, Yumita A, Yamamoto T. Transscleral Nd:YAG laser cyclophotocoagulation versus cyclocryotherapy. Graefes Arch Clin Exp Ophthalmol. 1991;229(1):33–6.

80. Pratesi R. Diode lasers in photomedicine. J Quantum Electron. 1984;20:1432–9.

81. Peyman GA, Naguid KS, Gaasterland D. Transscleral application of a semiconductor diode laser. Lasers Surg Med. 1990;10:569–75.

82. Hennis HL, Assia E, Stewart WC, Legler UF, Apple DJ. Transscleral cyclophotocoagulation using a semiconductor diode laser in cadaver eyes. Ophthalmic Surg. 1991;22:274–8.

83. Assia E, Hennis HL, Stewart WC, Legler UF, Carlson AN, Apple DJ. A comparison of neodymium:yttrium aluminum garnet and diode laser transscleral cyclophotocoagulation and cyclocryotherapy. Invest Ophthalmol Vis Sci. 1991;32:2774–8.

84. Schuman JS, Jacobson JJ, Puliafito CA, Noecker RJ, Reidy WT. Experimental use of semiconductor diode laser in contact transscleral cyclophotocoagulation in rabbits. Arch Ophthalmol. 1990;108:1152–7.

85. Hennis HL, Stewart WC. Semiconductor diode laser transscleral cyclophotocoagulation in patients with glaucoma. Am J Ophthalmol. 1992;113:81–5.

86. Gaasterland DE, Pollack IP. Initial experience with a new method of laser transscleral cyclophotocoagulation for ciliary ablation in severe glaucoma. Trans Am Ophthalmol Soc. 1992;90:225–43.

87. Chen TC, Pasquale LR, Walton DS, Grosskreutz CL. Diode laser transscleral cyclophotocoagulation. Int Ophthalmol Clin. 1999;39(1):169–76.

88. Gupta N, Weinreb RN. Diode laser transscleral cyclophotocoagulation. J Glaucoma. 1997;6:426–9.

89. Brancato R, Carassa R, Bettin P, Fiori M, Trabucchi G. Contact transscleral cyclophotocoagulation with diode laser in refractory glaucoma. Eur J Ophthalmol. 1995;5(1):32–9.

90. Rebolleda G, Munoz F, Murube J. Audible pops during cyclodiode procedures. J Glauocoma. 1999;8(3):177–83.

91. Monsour M, Albrecht K, Gaasterland D. Contact semiconductor diode laser transscleral cyclophotocoagulation in human autopsy eyes. Invest Ophthalmol Vis Sci. 1991;32:860.

92. Jampel HD, Wells AP, Gupta N. Cyclodestruction. In: Weinreb R, Crowston J, editors. Glaucoma surgery: open angle glaucoma, Consensus series 2. The Netherlands: Kugler Publications; 2005. p. 122–5.

93. Pastor SA, Sing K, Lee DA, Juzych MS, Lin SC, Netland PA, Nguyen NT. Cyclophotocoagulation: a report by the American Academy of Ophthalmology. Ophthalmology. 2001;108(11):2130–8.

94. Sharkey J, Murray T. Identification of the ora serrata and ciliary body by transillumination in eyes undergoing transscleral fixation of posterior chamber intraocular lenses (letter). Ophthalmic Surg. 1994;25:479–80.

95. Youn J, Cox TA, Herndon LW, Allingham RR, Shields MB. A clinical comparison of transscleral cyclophotocoagulation with Neodymium:YAG and semiconductor diode lasers. Am J Ophthalmol. 1998;126:640–7.

96. Oguri A, Takahashi E, Tomita G, Yamamoto T, Jikihara S, Kitazawa Y. Transscleral cyclophotocoagulation with the diode laser for neovascular glaucoma. Ophthalmic Surg Lasers. 1998;29:722–7.

97. Kosoko O, Gaasterland DE, Pollack IP, Enger CL. Long term outcome of initial ciliary ablation with contact diode laser transscleral cyclophotocoagulation for severe glaucoma. The diode laser ciliary ablation study group. Ophthalmology. 1996;103(8):1294–302.

98. Vernon SA, Koppens JM, Menon GJ, Negi AK. Diode laser cycloablation in adult glaucoma: long-term results of a standard protocol and review of current literature. Clin Experiment Ophthalmol. 2006;34:411–20.

99. Utrata R, Rehurek J. Long-term results of transscleral cyclophotocoagulation in refractory pediatric glaucoma patients. Ophthalmologica. 2003;217(6):393–400.

100. Kirwan JF, Shah P, Khaw PT. Diode laser cyclophotocoagulation: role in the management of refractory pediatric glaucoma. Ophthalmology. 2002;109(2):316–23.

101. Sood S, Beck AD. Cyclophotocoagulation versus sequential tube shunt as a secondary intervention following primary tube shunt failure in pediatric glaucoma. J AAPOS. 2009;13(4):379–83.

102. Malik R, Ellingham RB, Suleman H, Morgan WH. Refractory glaucoma – tube or diode? Clin Exp Ophthalmol. 2006;34:771–7.

103. Yildirim N, Yalvac IS, Sahin A, Ozer A, Bozca T. A comparative study between diode laser cyclophotocoagulation and the Ahmed glaucoma valve implant in neovascular glaucoma – A long term follow-up. J Glaucoma. 2009;18(3):192–6.

104. Bloom PA, Tsai JC, Sharma K, Miller MH, Rice NS, Hitchings RA, Khaw PT. Trans-scleral diode laser cyclophotocoagulation in the treatment of advanced refractory glaucoma. Ophthalmology. 1997;104:1508–20.

105. Hawkins TA, Stewart WC. One year results of semiconductor transscleral cyclophotocoagulation in patients with glaucoma. Arch Ophthalmol. 1993;111:488–91.

106. Shah P, Lee GA, Kirwan JK, Bunce C, Bloom PA, Ficker LA, Khaw PT. Cyclodiode photocoagulation for refractory glaucoma after penetrating keratoplasty. Ophthalmology. 2001;108:1986–91.

107. Delgado MF, Dickens CJ, Iwach AG, Novack GD, Nychka DS, Wong PC, Nguyen N. Long-term results of noncontact neodymium:yttrium-aluminum-garnet cyclophotocoagulation in neovascular glaucoma. Ophthalmology. 2003;110(5):895–9.

108. Stinson WG, Sherwood MB. Cyclodestructive procedures for advanced glaucoma: an update. In: Jay B, Kirkness CM, editors. Recent advances in ophthalmology. New York: Churchill Livingstone; 1995. p. 91–103.

109. Kumar N, Chang A, Beaumont P. Sympathetic ophthalmia following ciliary body laser cyclophotocoagulation for rubeotic glaucoma. Clin Experiment Ophthalmol. 2004;32:196–8.

110. Ganesh SK, Rishi K. Necrotizing scleritis following diode laser trans-scleral cyclophotocoagulation. Indian J Ophthalmol. 2006;54(3):199–200.

111. Prata TS, Lima VC, Pinto LM, Costa EF, Melo LA. Diode laser transscleral cyclophotocoagulation – induced staphyloma following trabeculectomy with mitomycin c. Ophthalmic Surg Lasers Imaging. 2008;39(4):343–5.

112. Wagenfeld L, Klemm M, Feuerberg F, Zeitz O. Incidence of vitreoretinal complications following cyclophotocoagulation. Graefes Arch Clin Exp Ophthalmol. 2009;247:1565–6.

113. Contreras I, Noval S, Gonzalez J, Rebolleda G, Munoz-Negrete FJ. IOP spikes following contact transscleral diode laser cyclophotocoagulation. Arch Soc Esp Oftalmol. 2004;79(3):105–9.

114. Kumar H, Gupta S, Agarwal A. Corneal edema following diode laser cyclophotocoagulation in an eye with secondary glaucoma. Indian J Ophthalmol. 2008;56(4):317–8.

115. Quagliano F, Fontana L, Parente G, Tassinari G. Choroidal effusion after diode laser cyclophotocoagulation in Sturge-Weber syndrome. J AAPOS. 2008;12(5):526–7.

116. Benson MT, Nelson ME. Cyclocryotherapy: a review of cases over a 10-year period. Br J Ophthalmol. 1990;74:103–5.

117. Sidoti PA, Dunphy TR, Baerveldt G, LaBree L, Minckler DS, Lee PP, Heuer DK. Experience with the baerveldt glaucoma implant in treating neovascular glaucoma. Ophthalmology. 1995;102:1107–18.

118. Goldenberg-Cohen N, Bahar I, Ostashinski M, Lusky M, Weinberger D, Gaton D. Cyclocryotherapy versus transscleral diode laser cyclophotocoagulation for uncontrolled intraocular pressure. Ophthalmic Surg Lasers Imaging. 2005;36(4):272–9.

119. Wilensky JT, Kammer J. Long-term visual outcome of transscleral laser cyclotherapy in eyes with ambulatory vision. Ophthalmology. 2004;111(7):1389–92.

120. Kramp K, Vick HP, Guthoff R. Transscleral diode laser contact cyclophotocoagulation in the treatment of different glaucomas,

also as primary surgery. Graefes Arch Clin Exp Ophthalmol. 2002;240:698–703.

121. Egbert PR, Fiadoyor S, Budenz DL, Dadzie P, Byrd S. Diode laser transscleral cyclophotocoagulation as a primary surgical treatment for primary open-angle glaucoma. Arch Ophthalmol. 2001;119: 345–50.

122. Ansari E, Gandhewar J. Long-term efficacy and visual acuity following transscleral diode laser photocoagulation in cases of refractory and non-refractory glaucoma. Eye. 2007;21:936–40.

123. Agarwal P, Dulku S, Nolan W, Song V. The UK National Cyclodiode Survey. Eye. 2011;25(2):166–73.

124. Shields MB. Intraocular cyclophotocoagulation. Trans Ophthalmol Soc UK. 1986;105:237–41.

125. Uram M. Endoscopic cyclophotocoagulation in glaucoma management. Curr Opin Ophthalmol. 1995;6(2):19–29.

126. Yu JY, Kahook MY, Lathrop KL, Noecker RJ. The effect of probe placement and type of viscoelastic material on endoscopic cyclophotocoagulation laser energy transmission. Ophthalmic Surg Lasers Imaging. 2008;39(2):133–6.

127. Kahook MY, Lathrop KL, Noecker RJ. One-site versus two-site endoscopic cyclophotocoagulation. J Glaucoma. 2007;16(6):527–30.

128. Nocker RJ, Kahook MY, Berke SJ, Nichamin LD, Weston JM, Mackool R, Tyson F, Lima F, Kleinfeldt N. Uncontrolled intraocular pressure after endoscopic cyclophotocoagulation – comment. J Glaucoma. 2008;17(3):250–1.

129. Berke SJ, Sturm RT, Caronia RM et al. Phacoemulsification combined with endoscopic cyclophotocoagulation (ECP) in the management of cataract and medically controlled glaucoma: a large, long term study. Presented at the AGS annual meeting, Charleston, Mar 2006.

130. Chen J, Cohn RA, Lin SC, Cortes AE, Alvarado JA. Endoscopic photocoagulation of the ciliary body for treatment of refractory glaucomas. Am J Ophthalmol. 1997;124(6):787–96.

131. Gayton JL, Van Der Karr M, Sanders V. Combined cataract and glaucoma surgery: trabeculectomy versus endoscopic laser cycloablation. J Cataract Refract Surg. 1999;25(9):1214–9.

132. Lima FE, Magacho L, Carvalho DM, Susanna R, Avila MP. A prospective, comparative study between endoscopic cyclophotocoagulation and the Ahmed drainage implant in refractory glaucoma. J Glaucoma. 2004;13(3):233–7.

133. Neely DE, Plager DA. Endocyclophotocoagulation for management of difficult pediatric glaucomas. J AAPOS. 2001;5(4):221–9.

134. Carter BC, Plager DA, Neely DE, Sprunger DT, Sondhi N, Roberts GJ. Endoscopic diode laser cyclophotocoagulation in the management of aphakic and pseudophakic glaucoma in children. J AAPOS. 2007;11(1):34–40.

135. Barkana Y, Morad Y, Ben-nun J. Endoscopic photocoagulation of the ciliary body after repeated failure of trans-scleral diode-laser cyclophotocoagulation. Am J Ophthalmol. 2002;133(3): 405–7.

136. Al-Haddad CE, Freedman SF. Endoscopic laser cyclophotocoagulation in pediatric glaucoma with corneal opacities. J AAPOS. 2007;11(1):23–8.

137. Lima FE, Carvalho DM, Avila MP. Phacoemulsification and endoscopic cyclophotocoagulation as primary surgical procedure in coexisting cataract and glaucoma (in Portuguese). Arq Bras Oftalmol. 2010;73:419–22.

138. Ahmad S, Wallace DJ, Herndon LW. Phthisis after endoscopic cyclophotocoagulation. Ophthalmic Surg Lasers Imaging. 2008; 39(5):407–8.

139. Fea AM, Dorin G. Laser treatment of glaucoma: evolution of laser trabeculoplasty techniques. Tech Ophthalmol. 2008;6(2):45–52.

140. Kammer JA. Laser trabeculoplasty: treatment with a diode laser appears to lower IOP while minimizing complications. Glaucoma Today. 2012;10(2):18–28.

141. Ho CL. Micropulse diode transscleral cyclophotocoagulation. Asian J Ophthalmol. 2002;3(3,4) 2001 supplement.

142. Tan AM, Chockalingam M, Aquino MC, Lim ZI, See JL, Chew PT. Micropulse transscleral diode laser cyclophotocoagulation in the treatment of refractory glaucoma. Clin Exp Ophthalmol. 2010;38:266–72.

143. Silverman RH, Vogelsang B, Rondeau MJ, Coleman DJ. Therapeutic ultrasound for the treatment of glaucoma. Am J Ophthalmol. 1991;111(3):327–37.

144. Cato S. Ultrasound circular cyclo-coagulation – innovation in glaucoma with high intensive focused ultrasound. Eur Ophthalmic Rev. 2011;5(2):1–76.

145. Aptel F, Charrel T, Lafon C, et al. Miniaturized high-intensity focused ultrasound device in patients with glaucoma: a clinical pilot study. Invest Ophthalmol Vis Sci. 2011;52(12):8747–53.

146. Schwartz DN. Ultrasonic treatment of glaucoma. U.S. Pat. 0152626A1, 17 Jun 2010.

147. Schwartz DN. Ultrasonic treatment of glaucoma. U.S. Pat. 7909781B2, 22 Mar 2011.

# Clinical Trials for IOP-Lowering Devices to Support an FDA Premarket Submission

Judy F. Gordon and Robert L. Kramm

## The US Food and Drug Administration's Regulation of Medical Devices

The jurisdiction of the US Food and Drug Administration (FDA) encompasses human and animal drugs; therapeutic agents of biological origin; most food products (other than meat and poultry); tobacco products; radiation-emitting products for consumer, medical, and occupational use; cosmetics; animal feed; and medical devices.

Although it was not known by its present name until 1930, the FDA's modern regulatory functions began with the passage of the 1906 Pure Food and Drugs Act which prohibited interstate commerce in adulterated and misbranded food and drugs. It was not until passage in 1938 of the Food, Drug, and Cosmetic Act that medical devices were placed under FDA control; however, this legislation did not require premarket approval for devices. The 1976 Medical Device Amendments, following a public health disaster in which thousands of women were injured by an intrauterine device, provided for three classes of medical devices, each requiring a different level of regulatory scrutiny. This classification scheme depends on the intended use of the device and is based on risk.

Ophthalmic examples of class II devices include most vitrectomy and phacoemulsification instruments, tonometers, slit lamp microscopes, glaucoma lasers, and implantable glaucoma devices for the "refractory" patient population. Ophthalmic examples of class III devices include intraocular lenses, excimer lasers, endotamponades, viscoelastics, and implantable glaucoma devices for the "non-refractory" patient population.

J.F. Gordon, DVM (✉)
ClinReg Consulting Services, Inc., 733 Bolsana Drive, Laguna Beach, CA 92651, USA
e-mail: judy@clinregconsulting.com

R.L. Kramm, MD, MSE
ClinReg Consulting Services, Inc., 1281 South Ocean Drive, Ft. Lauderdale, FL 33316, USA
e-mail: rlkfda@gmail.com

A 510(k) is a premarket submission made to the FDA to demonstrate that the device to be marketed is at least as safe and effective, that is, substantially equivalent, to a legally marketed device (21 CFR 807.92(a)(3)) that is not subject to PMA. Premarket approval (PMA) is the FDA process of scientific and regulatory review to evaluate the safety and effectiveness of class III medical devices. Class III devices are those that support or sustain human life, are of substantial importance in preventing impairment of human health, or present a potential, unreasonable risk of illness or injury.

## History of IOP-Lowering Devices at the FDA

Depending on the nature of the technology, the indications for use, and the claims being made by the company marketing the device, non-implantable devices (i.e., surgical instruments and tools) used to lower IOP may be class I (exempt from a 510(k) submission), class II requiring FDA clearance, or class III requiring FDA approval via a PMA prior to marketing in the United States. For example, the FDA cleared the Trabectome as a class II device via the 510(k) pathway in 2006 for the general claim of "removal, destruction and coagulation of tissue." The iTrack (iScience Interventional) ophthalmic microcannula received 510(k) marketing clearance from the FDA in 2004 for the general purpose of "fluid infusion and aspiration, as well as illumination, during surgery." Subsequently, in 2008 the iScience Microcatheter was specifically cleared for "catheterization and viscodilation of Schlemm's canal to reduce intraocular pressure in adult patients with open-angle glaucoma." Furthermore, in 2004, the FDA cleared the Endo Optiks E2 MicroProbe for endoscopic cyclophotocoagulation (ECP) in patients who have failed conventional topical and systemic medical therapy, previous laser photocoagulation, trabeculectomy, or cyclocryotherapy. The clinical evidence, if any, on which these 510(k) clearances of manual instruments were based is not readily apparent in the FDA database of marketing decision summaries [1].

J.R. Samples, I.I.K. Ahmed (eds.), *Surgical Innovations in Glaucoma*,
DOI 10.1007/978-1-4614-8348-9_5, © Springer Science+Business Media New York 2014

Lasers used for IOP reduction historically have been treated by the FDA as class II devices and were cleared under the general ophthalmic laser regulation, 21 CFR 886.4390[1] under product codes HQF and LQJ; however, claims for specific therapeutic procedures (e.g., trabeculoplasty and iridotomy) can be found in the labeling. The clinical evidence, if any, on which these laser 510(k) clearances were based is not readily apparent in the FDA database of marketing decision summaries.

Like the non-implantable examples listed above, implantable aqueous shunts intended to reduce intraocular pressure (IOP) "refractory" glaucoma[2] patients are usually treated by the FDA as class II consistent with 21 CFR 886.3920 (under product code KYF). What constitutes failure of "medical and conventional surgical treatment" has not been clearly defined and standardized neither by the academic community nor by the FDA. In 1998, the FDA issued a guidance document which describes preclinical and clinical testing requirements for the regulation of class II aqueous shunts through the submission of premarket notifications [510(k)s] [2]. The first generation Ahmed (New World Medical), Baerveldt (Advanced Medical Optics), Krupin (Eagle Vision), and Molteno (Molteno Ophthalmic) aqueous shunts received marketing clearance from the FDA between 1989 and 1993; modified Ahmed and Molteno devices were subsequently cleared in 2006. The Ex-PRESS™ Mini Glaucoma Shunt received 510(k) marketing clearance in 2002 [3].

The FDA considers aqueous shunts intended to reduce intraocular pressure in "non-refractory" eyes which have not failed conventional medical and surgical treatment to be higher risk and as such are regulated as class III devices under product code OGO. An increasing number of companies are pursuing FDA approval of their devices for this patient population. The AquaFlow™ Collagen Glaucoma Drainage Device received PMA approval from the FDA in 2001 for the maintenance of subscleral space following nonpenetrating deep sclerectomy in patients with open-angle glaucoma where intraocular pressure remains uncontrolled while on maximally tolerated medical therapy [4]. The Glaukos iStent® Trabecular Bypass Stent Model GTS100 was PMA approved in 2012 for use in conjunction with cataract surgery for the reduction of intraocular pressure in adult patients with mild to moderate open-angle glaucoma who receiving treatment with ocular hypotensive medication [5].

In addition to aqueous shunts intended for the "non-refractory" glaucoma population, an implantable device intended for the refractory population could be considered class III if there is no legally marketed predicate device that can serve as the basis of a substantial equivalence comparison in a 510(k) notification.

## "Valid Scientific Evidence"

The FDA evaluates medical devices using information provided by the sponsor of the submission. This information typically consists of a technical description and "valid scientific evidence". Among the types of evidence that may be required, when appropriate, to determine that there is reasonable assurance that a device is safe and effective are investigations using animal models, nonclinical investigations including in vitro studies, and investigations involving human subjects. Among the types of nonclinical information evaluated by the FDA review team for an implantable shunt are its mechanical, material, dimensional, and flow characteristics. For lasers intended to lower IOP, the nonclinical aspects of the FDA review may involve an optical radiation safety evaluation and testing in an animal model.

For all class III devices and some class II devices, clinical performance data are required to be included in the premarket regulatory marketing submissions. All clinical evaluations of investigational IOP-lowering devices in the United States, unless exempt or nonsignificant risk [6], must have an approved investigational device exemption (IDE) before the study is initiated.

Clinical data provided in support of any FDA marketing application, including a 510(k) when those data are relevant to a substantial equivalence determination, should also fit the definition of "valid scientific evidence". According to the federal regulation 21 CFR 860.7(c)(2) [7], the FDA defines "valid scientific evidence" derived from a clinical study as, "Evidence from well-controlled investigations, partially controlled studies, studies and objective trials without matched controls, well-documented case histories conducted by qualified experts, and reports of significant human experience with a marketed device, from which it can fairly and responsibly be concluded by qualified experts that there is reasonable assurance of the safety and effectiveness of a device under its conditions of use….The valid scientific evidence used to determine the effectiveness of a device shall consist principally of well-controlled investigations." The regulation goes on to define a well-controlled clinical investigation as one with a documented study plan or protocol, well-defined study objectives and study population, a clear description of the study methods, and a comparison of the results of treatment with a pre-specified control (no treatment, placebo, active treatment, or historical control). Finally, a description of the methods of analysis should be included in the protocol.

The regulations permit the FDA to calibrate the level of clinical evidence required according to the characteristics of the device, its conditions of use, the existence and adequacy of warnings and other restrictions, and the extent of experience with its use. The agency can accept evidence from studies that do not meet all the criteria above if the agency deter-

---

[1] AC-powered device intended to coagulate or cut tissue of the eye, orbit, or surrounding skin by a laser beam.

[2] Defined as eyes with "patients with neovascular glaucoma or with glaucoma when medical and conventional surgical treatments have failed".

mines that they are "not reasonably applicable to the device." Therefore, the FDA typically handles non-implanted devices differently than permanently implanted devices, and the evidentiary standards for class II implantable devices are not always the same as those for class III implantable devices.

While all clinical studies performed inside the United States to support a marketing submission must be conducted in accordance with the investigational device exemption (IDE) regulation, the FDA's purview does not extend to clinical studies performed outside the United States. Theoretically, the FDA is willing to accept data from studies conducted solely outside the United States as support for a PMA under the following conditions:

- The rights, safety, and welfare of human subjects have been protected in accordance with 21 CFR 814.15.
- The data are scientifically valid.
- The foreign data are applicable to the US population and medical practice.
- The studies have been performed by clinical investigators of recognized competence.
- The data may be considered valid without the need for an on-site inspection by the FDA, or if the FDA considers such an inspection to be necessary, the FDA can validate the data through an on-site inspection or other appropriate means.

Realistically, however, the applicability of foreign data to the US population may be limited due to the following confounding factors:

- Demographic factors (e.g., race, sex, ethnicity, age, socioeconomic status, or educational status)
- Clinical factors (e.g., prevalence of smoking, diabetes, or obesity; compliance with medical regimen or follow-up; education level or language; and cultural differences)
- Population/system-related factors (e.g., concomitant medication use, differing physician and medical practices, legal factors, or the use of adjunct devices)
- Protocol-related factors (e.g., inclusion and exclusion criteria, procedural characteristics, or the test materials being used)

In a PMA, applicability of foreign data to the US population and medical practice can be demonstrated by showing baseline homogeneity and outcome comparability and adjusting for differences in important covariates if observed.

## Clinical Study Design for Implantable Glaucoma Devices

Though the recommendations were not limited to studies intended to support an FDA submission, a 2011 Ophthalmic Technology Assessment from the American Academy of Ophthalmology entitled, "Novel Glaucoma Procedures" [8] concluded that "Randomized trials are needed to determine the efficacy of [novel glaucoma] procedures compared with trabeculectomy, with one another, and with phacoemulsification alone (in the case of combined procedures)." The report

also recommended the establishment of "a uniform study design for novel glaucoma procedures so that different studies are more easily compared" including standard inclusion and exclusion criteria, length and retention of follow-up, and definitions of success and failure.

Generally, for all implant device studies intended to support an FDA application, the choice of effectiveness endpoints is dependent on whether the sponsor of the device intends to claim the device is indicated for IOP reduction, for treatment of glaucoma, or for both. Because a marketing claim for stabilization or reversal of glaucomatous optic neuropathy would require a significantly more arduous study design entailing functional (e.g., perimetry) and structural (e.g., retinal nerve fiber layer thickness) endpoints and a longer follow-up period, sponsors typically seek only claims related to the ability of their device to lower IOP.

At the 2008 NEI/FDA CDER Glaucoma Clinical Drug Trial Design and Endpoints Symposium [9], the FDA expressed its willingness to consider additional outcome measures in the approval process for new glaucoma drugs and devices but also indicated that it is the responsibility of the research community to demonstrate that structural measures correlate with clinically relevant functional measures. During the symposium, the FDA encouraged sponsors of glaucoma clinical trials to propose new clinical endpoints and to discuss these with the FDA at a very early phase of research planning.

The level of clinical evidence necessary for clearance of class II implantable shunts has been inconsistent and, as described below, is generally lower than the evidence required for class III shunts. With the 1998 publication of the aforementioned FDA guidance document, the agency described generally applicable requirements for implantable device studies in the "refractory" glaucoma[3] population in order to obtain 510(k) clearance as a class II device. Since that time, the FDA has collaborated within the American National Standards Institute (ANSI) working group to describe the mechanical, physical, and biocompatibility properties, as well as the elements of clinical protocols that are recommended to evaluate the clinical performance of "refractory"[4] as well as

---

[3]Defined in the guidance as eyes "with neovascular glaucoma or with glaucoma when medical and conventional surgical treatments have failed".

[4]Defined in the ANSI standard as "eyes uncontrolled by medical therapy and diagnosed with glaucoma which meet at least one of the following criteria:

1. Failed one or more incisional intraocular glaucoma surgeries (e.g., glaucoma filtering surgery or tube shunt)
2. Failed one or more cilioablative procedures (e.g., cryotherapy, cyclodiode therapy)
3. Have neovascular glaucoma
4. Have any other condition (e.g., conjunctival scarring, uveitis) in which a conventional incisional glaucoma surgery like trabeculectomy would be more likely to fail than for an eye with uncomplicated primary open-angle glaucoma"

"non-refractory"[5] glaucoma devices. The scope of the ANSI standard applies to devices which are implanted in the eye to treat glaucoma by facilitating aqueous outflow but does not apply to implantable glaucoma devices whose effect depends upon metabolic and/or pharmacologic mechanisms.[6]

The clinical protocol should include descriptions of the surgical technique for implantation and considerations for safe explantation of the device and of the use of preoperative, intraoperative, and postoperative medications (anti-infective, anti-inflammatory, IOP lowering, etc.).

The enrollment criteria should specify the type of glaucoma in the study population, e.g., primary open-angle glaucoma and secondary open-angle glaucoma (i.e., pseudo-exfoliation, pigmentary). The visual acuity and the maximum allowable degree of restriction of the visual field of the non-study eye should also be specified. It is recommended that only one eye of each subject should be implanted with the investigational device. If both eyes of a subject qualify for enrollment and only one eye is to be enrolled, then a method by which the eye for enrollment is selected to minimize bias should be specified in the study protocol.

Investigators should consider including the following evaluations in the protocol (not an exhaustive list):
- Best corrected visual acuity
- Tonometry
- Central corneal thickness
- Diurnal IOP measurement
- Motility evaluation
- Gonioscopy
- Lens opacification for phakic eyes
- Slit lamp exam
- Vertical cup/disk ratio assessment
- Dilated fundus exam
- Optic nerve image analysis
- Perimetry
- Specular microscopy
- Patient reported outcomes

In addition to the FDA guidance and ANSI consensus standard, study investigators and sponsors of clinical studies can refer to the 2009 publication from the World Glaucoma Association (WGA) entitled, "Guidelines on Design and Reporting of Glaucoma Surgical Trials" which is endorsed by the American Glaucoma Society [10]. This document is a comprehensive discussion and includes recommendations for the design and conduct of a glaucoma clinical trial irrespective of whether the study is intended to support an FDA regulatory application. Notably this document does not make separate recommendations for "refractory" and "non-refractory" glaucoma populations as is done in the ANSI document described above. Also, this document is not limited to implantable device studies unlike the ANSI document. The following are some the "summary points" from the WGA document:

- The randomized clinical trial is the most valid methodology to determine the safety and efficacy of new glaucoma surgical procedures and to compare their results and complications with those of established glaucoma surgical techniques.
- It is recommended that investigators comply with the CONSORT checklist [11] for reporting randomized clinical trials.
- Though it is understood that non-randomized studies may provide some information regarding outcomes and complications of new glaucoma surgical procedures, however, the non-randomized study design cannot assure the investigation of two comparable groups.
- Investigators should include broad-based study populations to develop widely applicable and generalizable new information about glaucoma surgical care.
- International collaboration of investigators to study new types of glaucoma surgery is supported and encouraged.
- The benefits and risks of any new glaucoma surgical procedure should be compared with those of established and accepted interventions. The participation of concurrent controls rather than previously collected information (historical controls) is strongly encouraged.
- Investigators should consider defining the nature of the glaucoma on the basis of anterior chamber angle anatomy; the structural state of the disease, based on quantitative assessment of the optic nerve or nerve fiber layer or both; and the functional status, as defined with standard automated perimetry.
- The establishment of study endpoints before the initiation of any investigation as critical to the interpretation of the results.
- The importance of determining visual function before and after operative intervention to assess the outcomes of glaucoma surgery is recognized. Use of standard automated perimetry as described in several large randomized clinical trials may facilitate the comparison of results across different studies.
- The surgeon and patient should be masked as to the treatment being performed if this is practical; however, it is recognized that this is not possible for most glaucoma surgical procedures.
- The surgeon who performs the procedure should not evaluate the patient for the purpose of providing information

---

[5]Defined in the ANSI standard as "eyes diagnosed with glaucoma which do not meet any of the criteria for refractory glaucoma and which may have or may not have been treated with medications or laser trabeculoplasty. It includes eyes with glaucoma that are candidates for medical therapy, laser treatment, and glaucoma filtering surgery. Eyes in this category may have undergone uncomplicated cataract surgery, retinal laser, or extraocular muscle surgery."

[6]N.B. The ANSI standard for implantable glaucoma devices has yet to be formally recognized by FDA as of May 2013.

that will be used to judge the success or failure of the procedure.

- The measurement of endpoints by skilled graders who have not been directly involved in patient care is strongly advocated.

## "Refractory Glaucoma" Studies

The types of clinical investigations recommended in the ANSI standard and typically required by FDA for this patient population are a non-comparative study or a comparative study using either an appropriate historical control population or a concurrently studied control population. If the clinical data is intended to serve as a primary means of determining substantial equivalence to a predicate device, the control treatment should be a well-documented glaucoma device, marketed widely for at least the last 5 years and marketed "on-label" for the same indication.

A minimum of 12 months of follow-up from every enrolled subject is recommended; however, any device specific safety and/or effectiveness concerns that might require longer follow-up should be assessed during the protocol development to determine the appropriate study duration. A minimum sample size of 50 investigational device subjects should be evaluable at 12 months; however, enrollment may be hampered by the relatively small number of patients who meet the regulatory definition of "refractory."

## "Non-refractory Glaucoma" Studies

For a PMA application intended to establish reasonable evidence of safety and effectiveness of an implantable device in the "non-refractory" patient population, the FDA recommends a randomized controlled study with an appropriate control group. Depending on the indication and device, the type of control group may vary. With the FDA approval of mitomycin as an adjunct to ab externo glaucoma surgery in 2012, studies of investigational devices are able to utilize conventional trabeculectomy with mitomycin application as a concurrent control group. In comparative studies, the study design should ensure there is sufficient statistical power to address the study's effectiveness endpoints and to support any associated labeling claims which may be requested. The protocol should ensure that a sufficient number of subjects are enrolled to detect clinically relevant and statistically significant differences between study arms in regard to the endpoints.

A minimum of 24 months of follow-up is recommended; however, based on the risk analysis, a shorter or longer study duration may be appropriate. Emergent safety issues identified during the course of the study may also warrant the follow-up period to be extended with adequate informed consent of study subjects.

The sample size should be large enough such that any adverse event (of a given type) that occurs in the population at a rate of 1 % or greater is likely to be observed in the study population. To ensure that there is at least a 95 % probability that at least one adverse event of this type will be detected, it is recommended that safety data from a minimum of 300 subjects be provided in the FDA submission. The sample size should be adequate to allow for 10 % of subjects being lost to follow-up per year; hence, in a study with 24-month endpoints, approximately 375 subjects should be implanted with the investigational device. It is also recommended that no investigator's and no center's total enrollment exceed 25 % of the total number of investigational or control device subjects in the investigation. Because the number of patients who meet the regulatory definition of "non-refractory" glaucoma is relatively large, enrollment for these studies is generally easier than for "refractory" studies.

The FDA recommends that subject enrollment proceed in phases to minimize risks associated with the clinical investigation; however, the extent of prior clinical experience with the device is taken into consideration when the FDA decides whether to require a phased study design. If a phased study is performed in the United States under IDE approval, the data from each phase is evaluated by the FDA and must be found acceptable prior to continuation of the clinical investigation.

## Analysis of Intraocular Pressure Data

There is considerable variability in how the IOP-lowering effect of glaucoma devices is characterized in the medical literature and in FDA studies. The two primary analyses utilized in FDA IDE studies are mean reduction in IOP and proportion of study eyes with a 20 % reduction in IOP. The latter is a responder analysis for which other criteria for failure (e.g., hypotony) are incorporated. Detailed recommendations for standardized IOP analyses can be found in the WGA document and ANSI consensus standard.

Of particular importance in the design and conduct of the study is the confounding influence of IOP-lowering medication used prior to and before implantation and the impact of variability in tonometry measurements on the outcomes. Therefore, the ANSI standard recommends, where feasible, that baseline IOP be established for a randomized clinical study with "washout" of IOP-lowering medications pre- and postoperatively and by averaging the diurnal IOP measurements taken on a single day. If no medication "washout" is utilized, the standard recommends that a baseline IOP be established using methods that reduce the effects of regression to the mean and decrease the variability and confounding resulting from the use of concomitant medications.

Also of importance in designing the protocol is to describe how eyes for which data is missing and for which IOP-lowering procedures (e.g., needling, trabeculectomy, cyclophotocoagulation) are needed postoperatively will be handled in the primary effectiveness analyses. Responder analyses and imputation methods are often used to address the potential for the outcomes to be confounded in these circumstances.

## Post-market Studies

Certain issues that arise during premarket evaluation of a device may be more appropriately addressed through data collection in the post-market period rather than prior to approval or clearance for marketing. Post-market studies are a means by which the FDA collects safety and/or effectiveness data for a 510(k)-cleared or PMA-approved device. One form of post-market study is a post-approval study. A post-approval study is a study that is required as a condition of approval for a PMA. A PMA may actually have more than one post-approval study and may include both clinical and nonclinical studies. In general, a post-approval study is a clinical study intended to collect long-term safety and/or effectiveness data for the approved device or to collect data that shows the device's safety and/or effectiveness in a real-world setting. While a post-approval study cannot be used to answer fundamental safety and effectiveness questions, they serve to complement premarket data.

## References


1. U.S. Food and Drug Administration 510(k) Premarket Notification Database. Available from: http://www.accessdata.fda.gov/scripts/cdrh/cfdocs/cfpmn/pmn.cfm. Updated 3 May 2013.

2. U.S. Food and Drug Administration Guidance for Industry and for FDA Reviewers/Staff: Aqueous Shunts – 510(k) Submissions. Available from: http://www.fda.gov/MedicalDevices/DeviceRegulationandGuidance/GuidanceDocuments/ucm073806.htm. Updated 16 Nov 1998.

3. Ex-Press Miniature Glaucoma Implant, Models R-20, R-30, R-50 STS Versions: Optonol, Ltd. Available from: http://www.accessdata.fda.gov/cdrh_docs/pdf/K012852.pdf. Updated 3 May 2013.

4. STAAR Surgical Company AquaFlow Collagen Glaucoma Drainage Device Model CGDD-20 – P000026. Available from: http://www.accessdata.fda.gov/scripts/cdrh/cfdocs/cftopic/pma/pma.cfm?num=p000026. Updated 27 Aug 2001.

5. Glaukos iStent® Trabecular Micro-Bypass Stent (Models GTS-00R, GTS-100L) and Inserter (GTS-100i) – P080030. Available from: http://www.accessdata.fda.gov/scripts/cdrh/cfdocs/cfTopic/pma/pma.cfm?num=P080030. Updated 16 July 2012.

6. U.S. Department of Health and Human Services Food and Drug Administration. Information Sheet Guidance For IRBs, Clinical Investigators, and Sponsors: significant risk and nonsignificant risk medical device studies. Available from: http://www.fda.gov/downloads/regulatoryinformation/guidances/ucm126418.pdf. Updated Jan 2006.

7. U.S. Food and Drug Administration 21 CFR 860.7 – Code of Federal Regulations Title 21, (Volume 8) Food and Drugs, Chapter 1 – Food and Drug Administration Department of Health and Human Services Subchapter H – Medical Devices – Part 860-Medical Device Classification Procedures- Subpart A- General, Section 860.7 Determination of safety and effectiveness. Available from: http://www.accessdata.fda.gov/scripts/cdrh/cfdocs/cfCFR/CFRSearch.cfm?FR=860.7. Updated 1 Apr 2012.

8. Francis BA, Singh K, Lin SC, Hodapp E, Jampel HD, Samples JR, et al. Novel glaucoma procedures: a report by the American Academy of Ophthalmology. Ophthalmology. 2011;118:1466–80. doi:10.1016/j.ophtha.2011.03.028. PubMed PMID 21724045. Available from http://www.ncbi.nlm.nih.gov/pubmed/21724045.

9. Weinreb RN, Kaufman PL. The glaucoma research community and FDA look to the future: a report from the NEI/FDA CDER Glaucoma Clinical Trial Design and Endpoints Symposium. Invest Ophthalmol Vis Sci. 2009;50(4):1497–505. doi:10.1167/ivos.08-2843.

10. Parrish RK, Minckler DS, Lam D, Pfeifffer N, RojanaPongpun P. Recommended methodology for glaucoma surgical trials. The Hague/Amsterdam/The Netherlands: Kugler Publications; 2008.

11. CONSORT Statement Website. Available from: http://www.consort-statement.org/. Updated 20 Jan 2012.

# Considerations in Patenting New Surgical Devices for Glaucoma: The Changing Patent Law Landscape



J. Wesley Samples and Gabrielle LaHatte

## Disclaimer:

This chapter should not be construed as legal advice or a legal opinion on any specific facts or circumstances. This chapter is not intended to create, and receipt of it does not constitute, an attorney-client relationship. The contents are intended for general informational purposes only, and you are urged to consult your attorney concerning any particular situation or any specific legal questions you may have.

## Introduction

The impetus for physicians to participate in the process that translates clinical and benchtop discoveries to commercializable products has arguably never been greater. Medical innovation increasingly provides physicians with an opportunity to create alternative revenue streams. It can also impact career advancement, as many research universities are beginning to consider whether faculty have any patents or pending patent applications, along with more traditional metrics, such as peer-reviewed publications, when making decisions related to professional advancement. Some innovations have been highly successful, such as Dr. Latina's patent on

selective laser trabeculoplasty.[1] As the pace of medical innovation increases, the strategic importance of physician involvement with intellectual property management and the commercialization process continues to grow. Recent changes to the patent laws in the United States have increased the physician's opportunity to participate in the patent prosecution and the commercialization process.

## Introduction to Commercialization

The origin of university-led biomedical innovation commercialization as we know it today began with the Bayh-Dole Act.[2] Adopted in 1980, the Act permits universities and nonprofit institutions to "elect to retain title" of the federal government's (but not necessarily the inventor's) intellectual property rights arising from federally funded research, provided that affirmative steps are taken to achieve "practical application" of the invention by way of either direct commercialization or licensing.[3] By electing to take title, universities are able to prosecute patents arising from federally funded research at their own expense and reap the financial rewards of any ensuing licensing or commercialization efforts. Today, such university-directed patent prosecution and commercialization efforts are often directed by Technology Transfer Offices ("TTOs").

In general, the Bayh-Dole Act has been regarded as a tremendous success. In the 1970s, before Bayh-Dole, it was estimated that the US government owned over 28,000 patents, only 4 % of which had been developed into products used by the public.[4] Simply put, taxpayers were not realizing

J.W. Samples
Formerly an Intellectual Property Litigation Associate with Klarquist Sparkman, LLP,
Portland, OR, USA

G LaHatte
Formerly a Staff Attorney with Tarolli,
Sundheim, Covell & Tummino, LLP,
Cleveland, OH, USA

[1] *See* US Patent No. 5,549,596 (filed Oct. 20, 1995).

[2] Patent Rights in Inventions Made with Federal Assistance (The Bayh-Dole Act), Pub. L. No. 96–517, 94 Stat. 3019 (1980) (codified at 35 U.S.C. §§ 200–212 (2011)).

[3] *Id.*

[4] Senator Birch Bayh, Statement of Senator Birch Bayh to the National Institutes of Health (March 25, 2004), http://ott.od.nih.gov/policy/meeting/Senator-Birch-Bayh.pdf.

J.R. Samples, I.I.K. Ahmed (eds.), *Surgical Innovations in Glaucoma*,
DOI 10.1007/978-1-4614-8348-9_6, © Springer Science+Business Media New York 2014

the benefits of federally funded research. In contrast, today over 80 universities have each received more than $1 million in running royalty payments from licensed innovations, demonstrating a dramatic upswing in the successful commercialization of federally funded research.[5] Much of this improvement is attributable to the concerted efforts of TTOs. Many important innovations might have failed to make the transition from clinic, operating room, or benchtop discovery to commercial success if it were not for their efforts.

While a university may "elect to retain title" to the government's interest under Bayh-Dole, the employment agreement between university and employee controls the extent to which a university may own an employee's intellectual property.[6] However, determining the extent to which an employment agreement assigns the employer rights to an employee's intellectual property can be complex. The US Supreme Court recently described intellectual property assignment clauses in employment agreements as "technical drafting trap[s] for the unwary."[7] Regardless of the exact language used, it is important for physicians to understand how their employment agreement or employer's intellectual property assignment policy may grant a university rights in any invention developed during the course of the physician's employment. To ensure that an employer does not inadvertently allege ownership of inventions created before employment commences, it may be prudent for a physician to disclose or file patent applications on all preexisting innovations. It may also be wise to consult an attorney.

Additionally, the employment agreement or intellectual property assignment policy may determine what portion of revenue a physician may receive if an invention created during the course of employment is commercialized successfully. Unfortunately, a physician may not have any control over how their invention is commercialized. Recent changes to patent law in the United States have made this issue more poignant than ever before, because inventors are no longer required to actively participate in patent prosecution, as discussed below.

Where an employment agreement or an intellectual property assignment policy controls, it is customary for a TTO to distribute roughly 40 % of net revenue to the inventors. However, this figure varies widely from university to university within the United States. The portion of revenue shared with the physician inventor is often defined as a percentage of net revenue, i.e., revenue earned less the TTO's expenses, including patent prosecution. Patent prosecution expenses

may run into the hundreds of thousands of dollars, depending on a multitude of factors including complexity of the invention and the number of countries where patent protection is sought. In some cases, nothing is distributed to the inventor until all patent prosecution and associated TTO costs have been recouped by the university.

It is worth noting that in some cases the percentage and scheme of revenue sharing may be negotiated, along with other employment terms. For example, an institution may be willing to modify its policy for a well-established physician who has a proven record of successful innovation. However, when negotiating such terms, it is important to remember that the division of revenues should keep the interests of the physician and university substantially parallel, as TTOs can add tremendous value to commercialization outcomes. University administrators often closely scrutinize TTO performance based on metrics such as net revenue generated by all TTO commercialization efforts, as well as the total number of deals completed. Therefore, even if the physician has tremendous leverage, assigning an inadequate portion of revenue to the university may dampen enthusiasm for aggressive commercialization campaigns involving the physician's innovations.

Physicians may find themselves free to pursue their own commercialization efforts in the absence of other obligations, such as might be the case with a physician in private practice. Consultation with an attorney specializing in biomedical commercialization and patent prosecution may be prudent before approaching any potential partners. A physician should carefully consider at least filing a provisional patent application and asking potential partners to sign to nondisclosure agreements before disclosing anything. These and other measures may help protect a physician's intellectual property, even within the context of preliminary and informal commercialization efforts. Given the transition from a first-to-invent to first-to-file patent system, provisional patent applications will arguably become increasingly important to the individual physician approaching industry contacts as part of self-directed commercialization efforts, as discussed below.

## Patent Law Basics

Whether or not patent protection is necessary for the commercialization of any given invention should be evaluated on a case-by-case basis. However, patent applications and issued patents can be powerful tools in the commercialization process.

If the pursuit of patent protection is appropriate, it is prudent to have a handle on the contours of patent law before approaching a TTO or industry partner. It may be particularly useful to roughly understand the legal rights secured by

---

[5]This figure is the total running royalties from all licenses at each of the given universities and therefore includes both federally funded and non-federally funded innovations. Association of University Technology Managers (AUTM) Statistics Access for Tech Transfer (STATT) 2.0.

[6]Bd. of Trs. v. Roche Molecular Sys. (*Stanford*), 131 S. Ct. 2188, 2196 (2011).

[7]*Id.* at 2203 (Breyer, S., dissenting).

an issued patent, what is and is not patentable, what "prior art" is, and what one must do in order to avoid barring the patentability of one's own invention.

The process of obtaining a patent, also known as patent prosecution, begins when a patent application is prepared and filed with the United States Patent and Trademark Office ("USPTO"). After filing an application, a patent examiner will review the application as part of a nuanced process to determine if the application complies with all applicable patent laws. After examination, the patent examiner may allow the application to issue as a patent. However, it is more likely that the examiner will initially reject a portion of the application. In such an event, the applicant may respond to the examiner's rejections and can amend the application in order to put the application in condition for allowance.

In the United States, a patent provides only the right to exclude others from making, using, selling, offering for sale, or importing the patented invention.[8] A patent does not grant the right to practice or use the patented invention. As such, it is possible for an inventor to patent an invention, wherein the rights of other patent holders may limit the actual practice of the invention. For example, if a physician patents a new method for using an already patented surgical apparatus, the physician cannot thereafter make and use the entire apparatus in conjunction with their new method without regard for the preexisting apparatus patent. In such a scenario, the holder of the apparatus patent would be a natural partner with respect to the commercialization of the physician's new method. In fact, the physician's patent may be of little monetary value if the method cannot be practiced without other manufacturer's apparatuses and the singular owner of the patented apparatus is disinterested in partnering with the physician.

To appreciate the potential value of patents, it is helpful to understand why the United States created a patent system in 1790 with the passage of the first Patent Act.[9] The Founding Fathers understood the value of spurring innovation and progress, so they included a provision in the Constitution instructing Congress "[t]o promote the Progress of Science and the useful Arts, by securing for limited Times to … Inventors the exclusive Right to their … Discoveries."[10] Though adverse to the tyranny of monopolies, the Founding Fathers, particularly Thomas Jefferson, believed that "an inventor ought to be allowed a right to the benefit of his invention for some certain time," such that "ingenuity should receive a liberal encouragement."[11] Despite temporarily restricting the public's use of a new invention, this sanctioned monopoly was designed to reward inventors and encourage

commercialization of new technologies while also promoting the disclosure of inventions to the general public.[12] "The patent laws promote this progress by offering a right of exclusion for a limited period as an incentive to inventors to risk often enormous costs in terms of time, research, and development. The productive effort thereby fostered [has] a positive effect on society through the introduction of new products and processes of manufacture into the economy, and the emanations by way of increased employment and better lives for our citizens."[13]

Since then, Congress has occasionally updated the patent system, most recently with the passage of the Leahy-Smith America Invents Act ("AIA") in 2012.[14] However, Congress's authority to promote the useful Arts is tempered with the understanding that Congress may not grant temporary monopolies which "remove existent knowledge from the public domain, or [] restrict free access to materials already available."[15] Thus, Congress has enacted laws to effectuate its goal – laws which define what subject matter is patent eligible and outline the conditions for patentability.[16]

## Patentable Subject Matter

35 U.S.C. § 101 defines the scope of patentable subject matter. Specifically, anyone who "invents or discovers any new and useful process, machine, manufacture, or composition of matter, or any new and useful improvement thereof may obtain a patent."[17] Conversely, a person cannot obtain a patent on "laws of nature, natural phenomena, and abstract ideas."[18] For example, "a new mineral discovered in the earth or a new plant found in the wild is not patentable subject matter. Likewise, Einstein could not [have] patent[ed] his celebrated law that $E = mc^2$; nor could Newton have patented the law of gravity. Such discoveries are 'manifestations of . . . nature, free to all men and reserved exclusively to none.'"[19] These restrictions ensure that the "basic tools of scientific and technological work" remain free and available

---

[8]35 U.S.C. § 154(a) (1)(2011).

[9]Patent Act of 1790, ch. 7, § 1, 1 Stat. 109.

[10]US Const. art I, § 8.

[11]V Writings of Thomas Jefferson, at 75–76 (Washington ed., 1895).

[12]Graham v. John Deere Co., 383 U.S. 1, 9 (1966).

[13]Kewanee Oil Co. v. Bicron Corp., 416 U.S. 470, 480 (1974).

[14]*See* Leahy-Smith America Invents Act (AIA), Pub. L. No. 112–29, 125 Stat. 284 (2011) (codified in scattered sections of 35 U.S.C.); Patent Act of 1952, Pub. L. No. 82–593, § 5, 66 Stat. 792; Patent Act of 1870, ch. 230, 16 Stat. 198; Patent Act of 1836, ch. 357, 5 Stat. 117; Patent Act of 1790, ch. 7, § 1, 1 Stat. 109–112.

[15]*Graham*, 383 U.S. at 6.

[16]*See* 35 U.S.C. §§ 101–103 (2011).

[17]35 U.S.C. § 101.

[18]Diamond v. Diehr, 450 U.S. 175, 185 (1981); Mayo Collaborative Servs v. Prometheus Labs, Inc., 132 S. Ct. 1289, (2012).

[19]Diamond v. Chakrabarty, 447 U.S. 303, 309 (1980) (quoting Funk Brothers Seed Co. v. Kalo Inoculant Co., 333 U.S. 127, 130 (1948)).

to all.[20] However, even though a law of nature or abstract idea by itself is not patentable, "an *application* of a law of nature or mathematical formula to a known structure or process" may be patent eligible.[21]

Historically, this requirement received relatively little attention because it was generally assumed that a patent application was attempting to claim patentable subject matter. However, the Supreme Court recently revisited the issue in *Mayo Collaborative Services v. Prometheus Labs, Inc.*, reminding us that we cannot simply assume a patent meets the requirements of § 101.[22] At issue in the case were patents that claimed a method for optimizing the dosage of thiopurine drugs used in the treatment of immune-mediated gastrointestinal disorders, such as colitis and Crohn's disease.[23] The claims directed physicians to examine levels of certain thiopurine metabolites, namely, 6-thioguanine ("6-TG") and 6-methyl-mercaptopurine ("6-MMP"), to determine if the thiopurine dosage was within the drug's therapeutic range. If the metabolite levels were above a certain number, this indicated that the dosage should be decreased, whereas if the levels were below another value, the dosage should be increased.[24] In finding the claims were directed to unpatentable subject matter, the Supreme Court emphasized that patent protection is only for inventions which apply a law of nature and "one must do more than simply state the law of nature while adding the words 'apply it.'"[25] The Supreme Court found that the patents-in-suit

merely instructed doctors to apply a well-known consequence of thiopurine metabolism in routine, well-understood, or conventional ways previously used by researchers in the field.[26] This case has severe implications for the biotechnology industry, because it has significantly limited the patentability of medical diagnostic methods. For example, this means that a physician cannot patent a diagnostic method that claims the naturally occurring correlation between the severity of glaucoma and a patient's interocular pressure. A physician would have to include additional elements or steps that apply this natural principle in order to have a patent eligible invention. For example, a patentable method of characterizing a disease by measuring levels of a particular protein could be patentable if the method involved detecting the protein with a novel antibody.[27] Alternatively, a method wherein a doctor undertakes a unique and specific treatment plan that applies a well-known law of nature might also be patentable.[28]

## Conditions for Patentability

In addition to claiming patent eligible subject matter, a patentable application must be directed to a novel, useful, and nonobvious invention.[29] Very generally, an invention is considered novel if no one else has previously patented the invention, described it in a printed publication, used the invention publicly, sold the invention, or otherwise made it available to the public.[30] Any reference, such as a printed publication or prior patent, that could be used to demonstrate that an invention lacks novelty is referred to as a "prior art reference." When an examiner rejects a patent application, they will rely upon these references to explain why an application lacks novelty. It is important to note that even prior art created by an inventor themselves may negate novelty and thereby bar patentability. For example, a published journal article authored by an inventor may thereafter bar the inventor from acquiring a patent on the invention that was described in the article. Accordingly, it may be wise to consult a patent attorney before disclosing any inventions in a publication or at a conference, to avoid the inadvertent creation of prior art.

Before the enactment of the AIA, the ability of a third party to submit prior art references to the USPTO for consideration during the prosecution of any given application was

---

[20] Gottschalk v. Benson, 409 U. S. 63, 67 (1972).

[21] *Diehr*, 450 U.S. at 187.

[22] *Mayo Collaborative Servs.*, 132 S. Ct. at 1289 (2012).

[23] *Id* at 1294–95. *See* US Patent No. 6,355,623 col. 20:10–25 ("A method of optimizing therapeutic efficacy for treatment of an immune-mediated gastrointestinal disorder, comprising: (a) administering a drug providing 6-thioguanine to a subject having said immune-mediated gastrointestinal disorder; and (b) determining the level of 6-thioguanine in said subject having said immune-mediated gastrointestinal disorder, wherein the level of 6-thioguanine less than about 230 pmol per $8\times10^8$ red blood cells indicates a need to increase the amount of said drug subsequently administered to said subject and wherein the level of 6-thioguanine greater than about 400 pmol per $8\times10^8$ red blood cells indicates a need to decrease the amount of said drug subsequently administered to said subject."); US Patent No. 6,680,302, col. 20:24–43 ("A method of optimizing therapeutic efficacy for treatment of an immune-mediated gastrointestinal disorder, comprising: (a) administering a drug providing 6-thioguanine to a subject having said immune-mediated gastrointestinal disorder; and (b) determining a level of 6-thioguanine or 6-methyl-mercaptopurine in said subject having said immune-mediated gastrointestinal disorder, wherein a level of 6-thioguanine less than about 230 pmol per $8\times10^8$ red blood cells indicates a need to increase the amount of said drug subsequently administered to said subject and wherein a level of 6-thioguanine greater than about 400 pmol per $8\times10^8$ red blood cells or a level of 6-methyl-mercaptopurine greater than about 7000 pmol per $8\times10^8$ red blood cells indicates a need to decrease the amount of said drug subsequently administered to said subject.").

[24] *Id.* at 1295.

[25] *Id.* at 1294.

[26] *Id.* at 1294, 1299–1300.

[27] *See* 2012 Interim Procedure for Subject Matter Eligibility Analysis of Process Claims Involving Laws of Nature, 3–4, 11–12 (2012).

[28] *Id.* at 10; *see* Classen Immunotherapies, Inc. v. Biogen IDEC, 659 F.3d 1057, 1067–68 (Fed. Cir. 2011).

[29] 35 U.S.C. §§102–103 (2011).

[30] 35 U.S.C. § 102.

limited. A third party could only submit a reference within 2 months from the date the application was published or prior to the USPTO issuing a notice that the application would issue as a patent, whichever was earlier.[31] However, as will be discussed below, the AIA has expanded the ability of individuals not immediately involved with the prosecution of an application to submit relevant publications to the Patent Office for consideration.

Additionally, the AIA has changed the requirements of 35 U.S.C. § 102 by expanding the scope of art that may bar patentability. For example, previously only public use or sales of an invention in the United States would bar an inventor from obtaining a patent.[32] However, now any use by the public or any sales anywhere in the world can bar the acquisition of a patent.[33] These changes will not go into effect until March 16, 2013; therefore, any patent application filed before this date will be evaluated according to the older § 102 requirements.[34] However, there are numerous nuanced exceptions to these general requirements. Thus, it may be advisable to consult with a patent attorney before disclosing any invention to prospective commercialization partners or at any conferences or symposiums, to mitigate the risk that disclosure might inadvertently bar later efforts to obtain patent protection.

In addition to being novel, an invention must also be nonobvious. An invention is considered nonobvious if it was not obvious or apparent to a person having ordinary skill in the art in light of what was known in the field of technology at the time of the invention.[35] Technically a legal fiction, a person of ordinary skill in the art, or a "PHOSITA," is one who can read a patent in a particular field and understand the invention claimed within.[36] To determine whether an invention is obvious, a PHOSITA can consider, for example, a combination of prior art references in the field, references reasonably related to the problem the inventor is attempting to solve, and the PHOSITA's own experiences, in light of their own hypothetical problem-solving skills.[37]

In addition to being novel and nonobvious, a patent must also comply with the disclosure requirements described in 35 U.S.C. § 112. A central tenant of the patent bargain is that the novel invention must be fully disclosed to the public in exchange for the inventor's right to exclude others for a limited

---

[31] 37 C.F.R. § 1.99 (e) (2009). "A submission under this section must be filed within two months from the date of publication of the application (§1.215(a) ) or prior to the mailing of a notice of allowance (§ 1.311 ), whichever is earlier. Any submission under this section not filed within this period is permitted only when the patents or publications could not have been submitted to the Office earlier, and must also be accompanied by the processing fee set forth in § 1.17(i) . A submission by a member of the public to a pending published application that does not comply with the requirements of this section will not be entered."

[32] 35 U.S.C. § 102. The pre-AIA § 102 states "[a] person shall be entitled to a patent unless—(a) the invention was known or used by others in this country, or patented or described in a printed publication in this or a foreign country, before the invention thereof by the applicant for patent, or(b) the invention was patented or described in a printed publication in this or a foreign country or in public use or on sale in this country, more than one year prior to the date of the application for patent in the United States, or (c) he has abandoned the invention, or (d) the invention was first patented or caused to be patented, or was the subject of an inventor's certificate, by the applicant or his legal representatives or assigns in a foreign country prior to the date of the application for patent in this country on an application for patent or inventor's certificate filed more than twelve months before the filing of the application in the United States, or (e) the invention was described in (1) an application for patent, published under section 122 (b), by another filed in the United States before the invention by the applicant for patent or (2) a patent granted on an application for patent by another filed in the United States before the invention by the applicant for patent, except that an international application filed under the treaty defined in section 351 (a) shall have the effects for the purposes of this subsection of an application filed in the United States only if the international application designated the United States and was published under Article 21(2) of such treaty in the English language; or (f) he did not himself invent the subject matter sought to be patented, or (g) (1) during the course of an interference conducted under section 135 or section 291, another inventor involved therein establishes, to the extent permitted in section 104, that before such person's invention thereof the invention was made by such other inventor and not abandoned, suppressed, or concealed, or (2) before such person's invention thereof, the invention was made in this country by another inventor who had not abandoned, suppressed, or concealed it. In determining priority of invention under this subsection, there shall be considered not only the respective dates of conception and reduction to practice of the invention, but also the reasonable diligence of one who was first to conceive and last to reduce to practice, from a time prior to conception by the other."

[33] 35 U.S.C. § 102 (a). The post-AIA §102 states "(a) NOVELTY; PRIOR ART.--A person shall be entitled to a patent unless-- (1) the claimed invention was patented, described in a printed publication, or in public use, on sale, or otherwise available to the public before the effective filing date of the claimed invention; or (2) the claimed invention was described in a patent issued under section 151, or in an application for patent published or deemed published under section 122(b), in which the patent or application, as the case may be, names another inventor and was effectively filed before the effective filing date of the claimed invention."

[34] See Leahy-Smith America Invents Act (AIA), Pub. L. No. 112–29, 125 Stat. 284 (2011) (codified in scattered sections of 35 U.S.C.).

[35] The 35 U.S.C. § 103 was recently updated by the passage of the AIA. This amendment went into effect September 16, 2012. See id.

[36] MPEP § 2141.01 (8th ed. Rev. 9, Aug. 2012); KSR Int'l Co. v. Teleflex Inc., 550 U.S. 398, 417 (2007) (explaining that a PHOSITA is "a person of ordinary creativity, not an automaton"); MPEP § 2144.

[37] MPEP § 2141.03. "Factors that may be considered in determining the level of ordinary skill in the art may include: (A) 'type of problems encountered in the art;' (B) 'prior art solutions to those problems;' (C) 'rapidity with which innovations are made;' (D) 'sophistication of the technology; and' (E) 'educational level of active workers in the field. In a given case, every factor may not be present, and one or more factors may predominate.'" (Citing in re GPAC, 57 F.3d 1573, 1579 (Fed. Cir. 1995); Custom Accessories, Inc. v. Jeffrey-Allan Indus., 807 F.2d 955, 962 (Fed. Cir. 1986); Envtl. Designs, Ltd. v. Union Oil Co., 713 F.2d 693, 696 (Fed. Cir. 1983)).

time.[38] Therefore, this section requires a patent application to contain a written description of the invention, to clearly describe how to use and make the invention such that a PHOSITA could use or make the invention without undue experimentation. The written description must also include the best mode for using the invention, and it must conclude with at least one claim that clearly and precisely claims the subject matter of the present invention.[39] These requirements help to ensure that an inventor only receives a patent covering subject matter which is adequately described in the application.

## Getting a Patent

The path to an issued patent can be lengthy and fraught with complications. There are many different types of patent applications, and determining which application to file depends on several different factors, including the geographic protection sought and the timing of the application. For example, if one wishes to obtain patent protection in several different countries in addition to the United States, it may be best to file a special international patent application, known as a "PCT," instead of filing individual applications in each country. Additionally, if time is of the essence, perhaps due to an inadvertent premature disclosure of the invention at a conference or concerns that someone else may seek patent protection for a similar invention, then filing a provisional patent application may be the best course of action. However, these concerns and others should be discussed with a patent attorney who has a substantial technical background in the relevant field in order to decide how to best proceed at the Patent Office.

*Provisional Patent Applications*: In many cases, filing a provisional application provides the quickest and most affordable route to secure a patent application filing date. Provisional patent applications are unique because they are not examined by the Patent Office and they are not published. This type of application is best viewed as a mere placeholder that preserves a filing date while an inventor decides whether to actively pursue patent protection or while a nonprovisional application is being drafted. A provisional application can be as simple as attaching a special form, known as a "cover sheet," to a manuscript, so long as the manuscript adequately describes the invention and can fully support any claims that may be later added to a nonprovisional application.[40]

A provisional application can be very important because the earliest filing date also determines what references the Patent Office can consider when examining the patent application. For example, if a reference which completely describes an invention was published just 2 days after the earliest filing date of a patent application claiming the invention, then the Patent Office cannot consider the publication because the application was filed first. This concept of priority can have a major impact on patent prosecution. Thus, it is crucial to determine if one has the luxury of taking time to prepare a thorough nonprovisional application or if something needs to be filed as quickly as possible.

However, provisional applications always automatically expire after 12 months and cannot be renewed after expiration.[41] Therefore, a corresponding nonprovisional application must be filed within 1 year. If the provisional application is allowed to expire before the corresponding nonprovisional application is filed, then the earlier filing date of the provisional application will be lost forever.

*Nonprovisional Applications*: If an inventor does decide to pursue patent protection, a nonprovisional application must eventually be filed with the USPTO.[42] In contrast to a provisional application, a nonprovisional must comply with numerous requirements, in addition to those previously discussed, before it can be reviewed by a patent examiner. Specifically, a nonprovisional application must include a specification, which provides a written description of the invention; at least one claim, which defines the boundaries of the invention; drawings if necessary to depict aspects of the invention; an oath from the inventor stating that he is the original inventor; and the necessary filing fees.[43]

*Patent Cooperation Treaty ("PCT") Applications*: As mentioned before, in addition to provisional and nonprovisional applications, an American inventor who is interested in obtaining patent protection abroad can file a PCT application with the USPTO.[44] While patent protection can be obtained by filing an application with a foreign country's patent office directly, a PCT application allows an inventor to file one application that is thereafter forwarded to any of the more than 140 member countries where patent protection is desired.[45] While the application is ultimately individually prosecuted in each country, this mechanism streamlines the filing process if an inventor is interested in patent protection outside the United States. Of course, prosecuting a patent in multiple countries can be very expensive. Therefore, one should carefully consider the cost involved

---

[38] Eldred v. Ashcroft, 537 U.S. 186, 216 (2003).

[39] MPEP § 2164; 35 U.S.C. §112 (2011).

[40] MPEP § 201.11; New Railhead Mfg., L.L.C. v. Vermeer Mfg. Co., 298 F.3d 1290, 1294 (Fed. Cir. 2002) (finding that for a nonprovisional application to be afforded the earlier filing date of the provisional application "the specification of the provisional must 'contain a written description of the invention and the manner and process of making and using it, in such full, clear, concise, and exact terms,' 35 U.S.C. § 112 ¶1, to enable an ordinarily skilled artisan to practice the invention claimed in the nonprovisional application").

[41] 37 C.F.R. § 1.53(c) (2009).

[42] 37 C.F.R. § 1.9.

[43] 35 U.S.C. §§ 111–113, 115. Post-AIA an entity can file a nonprovisional application without the inventor's oath if the inventor is under obligation to assign the invention to the entity. 35 U.S.C. § 115(d).

[44] MPEP §§ 1801–1896 (8th ed. Rev. 9, Aug. 2012).

[45] There are currently 146 contracting countries. *PCT, The International Patent System*, WIPO, http://www.wipo.int/pct/en.

and consult an attorney to determine if seeking patent protection abroad is a wise decision.

## Notable Implications of the AIA

In 2011, Congress passed the AIA, which brought about the most sweeping change to the US patent system since its inception. These changes included (1) a transition from a first-to-invent to a first-to-file system for awarding patent rights, (2) the ability of an assignee of an invention to file and prosecute an application without the input of the inventor, and (3) an expansion of a third party's ability to submit prior art to the USPTO during the examination of other's patent applications.

*Transition to First to File*: The transition to a first-to-file system reflects a fundamental shift in the philosophy of the US patent system. Historically, patent rights in the United States were awarded to whomever was first to conceive of an invention and thereafter exercised reasonable diligence in reducing the invention to practice. As of March 16, 2013, the first applicant to file a patent application will be awarded priority over a later-filed application, regardless of who conceived of the invention first.[46]

As a result of the transition to first-to-file system, it will be necessary to seek patent protection, where appropriate, early and often. Provisional applications provide one possible solution because they require relatively little time and cost to prepare compared to nonprovisional and PCT applications. In a system where patent rights are awarded to whomever gets an application on file first, the focus should be on getting the most thorough and complete disclosure of the application on file as quickly as possible.

Please note that patent applications filed before March 16, 2013, will continue to be prosecuted under the old first-to-invent system.[47]

*Patent Prosecution by the Assignee Without Inventor Involvement*: Generally speaking, a patent can be prosecuted before the USPTO by the inventor, a patent agent, or a registered patent attorney. As of September 16, 2012, an entity who has been assigned the rights to an invention may prosecute a patent on behalf of the inventor, without the inventor's involvement or consent.[48] This allows employers who have been assigned rights in an employee's inventions through an employment agreement to prosecute patents on that employee's inventions without any involvement of the employee.

*Third-Party Submissions*: As mentioned previously, the AIA has greatly expanded the ability of third parties to submit certain prior art references for consideration during patent prosecution. Previously, a party had less than a few months to submit a reference to the USPTO for consideration.[49] Additionally, the party was required to provide the patent applicant a copy of the submission, forcing the submitting party to reveal its interest in narrowing a particular patent application's scope.[50] This notice requirement deterred many third parties from submitting references, in fear of reprisals from industry rivals when later attempting to prosecute their own patents.

With the passage of the AIA, the amount of time allowed for third parties to submit prior art references has been greatly expanded, and third parties are no longer required to inform the patent applicant of its submission. Specifically, a party may file a submission up to 6 months after the publication of a patent application or before the first rejection by an examiner, whichever is later.[51] Acceptable submissions are limited to patents, published patent applications, and printed publications.[52] This expansion of third-party submissions presents a unique opportunity to third parties that wish to limit the scope of a particular patent application. If used effectively, this procedure can help to mitigate overly broad patents. Finding prior art references can be time consuming; however, one can use search tools such as Google Patents and the USPTO's patent database to find patents and patent applications related to particular technologies.[53] Additionally, one can utilize online alert services to monitor the near-real-time publication of patent applications in fields of particular interest.

Ultimately, few individuals are as well positioned as physicians to know which biomedical innovations are within the public domain and which innovations are novel. Thanks to the AIA physicians are now empowered with the ability to help mitigate overreaching patents and to take a more active role in the medical innovation process at large.

---

[46] AIA, Pub. L. No. 112–29, 125 Stat. 284, 285–293 (2011) (codified in scattered sections of 35 U.S.C.).

[47] *Id.*

[48] AIA, 125 Stat. at 293–297.

[49] 37 C.F.R. § 1.99 (2009), MPEP § 1134.01.

[50] *Id.*

[51] 35 U.S.C. § 122 (2011).

[52] *Id.*

[53] *See Patent Search*, Google, https://www.google.com/?tbm=pts; *Search for Patents*, United States Trademark and Patent Office, http://www.uspto.gov/patents/process/search/.

**Part II**

**Laser Technologies**

Giorgio Dorin

## History of Laser Surgery at the Trabecular Meshwork

The 693 nm ruby laser and the 488–514 nm argon laser have been, respectively, the first "pulsed" and first "continuous-wave" (CW) laser sources incorporated in ophthalmic photocoagulator systems. Their availability in the 1970s inspired glaucoma surgeons to use them to perform laser *trabeculotomy ab interno* by directing the laser beam on the trabecular meshwork (TM) through a gonioscopic lens to drill new outflow pathways between the anterior chamber (AC) and the Schlemm's canal as a less invasive filtration surgery.

In 1973, Mikhail Krasnov [1] reported successful, albeit temporary, IOP reduction by *puncturing ab interno* the TM with very short 693 nm laser pulses from a Q-switched pulsed ruby laser system. In the same year Hans Hager [2] published his trabeculo-puncture technique utilizing the Coherent model 800 continuous-wave (CW) 488+514 nm argon laser photocoagulator. Worthen and Wickham described their CW argon laser trabeculotomy in 1974 [3] and reported long-term benefits in a meaningful number of eyes 5 years later [4].

From the early experiences however, it became apparent that it was very difficult to drill holes in the TM with these types of lasers and almost impossible to keep them patent over a long term.

## Laser Trabeculoplasty with CW Lasers

In 1979 Wise and Witter described their "non-perforating" CW argon laser therapy for open-angle glaucoma (OAG) using a 50 μm spot laser beam to place 100 thermal burns

G. Dorin
Clinical Applications Development,
IRIDEX Corporation, 1212 Terra Bella Avenue,
Mountain View, CA 94043-1824, USA
e-mail: gdorin@iridex.com

evenly spaced over 360° pigmented TM [5]. This non-perforating technique was named argon laser trabeculoplasty (ALT) to reflect the authors' hypothesis that the IOP-lowering effect was attributable to mechanical forces, centripetal toward the visual axis, resulting from the reduction of trabecular ring's inner circumference due to thermal shrinkage of the sheets' collagen and to contraction of scar tissue at the burn sites, which pull open compressed subendothelial intertrabecular spaces and elevate collapsed TM sheets.

Gaasterland and Kupfer challenged this "mechanical" ALT's pressure-lowering hypothesis demonstrating that confluent CW argon laser burns in the TM of a rhesus monkey can elevate IOP and cause experimental glaucoma [6]. Other animal and human histologic studies did consistently show healing and scarring at the sites of CW laser thermal impacts, suggesting that perforating and non-perforating trabecular interventions with CW thermal lasers cannot create new permanent mechanical outflow pathways and that the reported long-term IOP-lowering benefits are most likely attributable to an enhanced outflow due to cellular and biochemical alterations resulting from the stress response to laser thermal injury. Ticho and Zauberman suggested a possible combination of mechanical and cellular mechanisms, observing that IOP was effectively lowered even when their attempt to create mechanical openings between the AC and the Schlemm's canal did not succeed or failed after a certain time of patency [7–9]. This seminal observation inspired the conceptual change that IOP can be also lowered without laser-created mechanical passages using low-intensity laser exposures capable of stimulating biological cellular transactional activities in TM endothelial cells.

Numerous studies and clinical trials [10–15] tested the effectiveness of CW laser trabeculoplasty in various phases of the glaucoma management using different treatment protocols, laser parameters, laser wavelengths, and technique modifications to optimize clinical outcomes and minimize TM tissue scarring and side effects. These studies provided the evidence that laser trabeculoplasty administered with a CW laser (488 and 514 nm argon, 532 nm frequency-doubled neodymium-doped yttrium aluminum garnet (Nd:YAG), 810 nm diode) is a proven and cost-effective glaucoma therapy. Nevertheless, over the years, ALT became gradually underused, most likely due to the (a) availability of new effective medications, (b) surgeon's concerns over ALT's fading effect at various times after treatment [16], and (c) limited retreatment possibility due to scarring in the TM. According to a retrospective Canadian study [17], the number of annually performed laser trabeculoplasty procedures bottomed in 2001, when the trend reversed with a steep increase in 2002 with the introduction of selective laser trabeculoplasty (SLT).

## Trabeculoplasty with "Pulsed" Lasers

The availability of new "pulsed" laser technologies and a better understanding of the cellular and molecular changes inducible with CW and pulsed laser exposures prompted the development of less destructive LT techniques with the goal of achieving an IOP-lowering effect at least non-inferior to that of ALT with CW lasers, but without scarring and fewer complications, thus, with the potential for retreatments PRN (pro re nata) as it may be required in the long-term management of glaucoma patients.

Selective laser trabeculoplasty (SLT), titanium-sapphire laser trabeculoplasty (TLT), and micropulse laser trabeculoplasty (MLT) are three LT techniques that utilize three different "pulsed" laser technologies, each one producing different tissue interactions and thermodynamic effects, but most likely eliciting similar beneficial biological responses and similar IOP-lowering effects with negligible damage, no coagulation, and no scarring.

## Selective Laser Trabeculoplasty (SLT)

SLT utilizes a 3 ns laser pulse ($3 \times 10^{-9}$ s) from a 532 nm frequency-doubled Q-switched Nd:YAG laser. Since the duration of the laser pulse is shorter than the thermal relaxation time in the absorbing melanocyte, heat cannot escape causing adiabatic heating with selective photothermolysis of the melanin-laden TM cells. In such adiabatic thermal conditions, there is no thermal damage to nonpigmented and surrounding cells and no coagulative effects at the TM beams, but there can be some pigmentary dispersion from the lysis of melanin-laden cells that may cause postoperative pressure spikes especially in darkly pigmented eyes.

## Titanium-Sapphire Laser Trabeculoplasty (TLT)

TLT is performed with a 790 nm titanium-sapphire (Ti-Al$_2$O$_3$) laser that emits 7 μs ($7 \times 10^{-6}$ s) laser pulses, focused on a 200-μm-diameter spot and with pulse energy titrated for a visible endpoint of a mini-bubble or a burst of pigment. The 790 nm infrared wavelength has a relatively long penetration in the TM and can affect deep structures in the juxtacanalicular region and the inner wall of the Schlemm's canal, which are the putative primary site of aqueous humor outflow's resistance.

## Micropulse Laser Trabeculoplasty (MLT)

MLT is performed with a 810 nm, or 577 nm, or 532 nm semiconductor laser operated in the MicroPulse mode, with a train of 100 (or 200 or 300) μs laser pulses, each one spaced by a relatively long thermal relaxation time resulting in 5 (10 or 15) % duty cycle (DC).

Figure 7.1 illustrates the tissue interactions differences with continuous-wave (CW) and MicroPulse laser emissions. In standard CW laser trabeculoplasty (i.e., ALT), the typical treatment endpoint is a readily visible blanching burn. An intraoperative visible burn requires a sudden high temperature rise (>30 °C above baseline temperature) which is lethal to the targeted tissue. Heat spreads by conduction toward adjacent cooler tissues, which are reached by the equilibrating and decaying thermal wave at a lower, but still lethal, temperature. More distant surrounding tissue, reached by the thermal wave at a lower sublethal temperature, remains viable and capable of thermal stress response that alters the gene expression profile with intracellular biological factors that are restorative and regenerative.

In MicroPulse laser trabeculoplasty (MLT), a visible burn endpoint is not desired and is carefully avoided using the micropulse emission mode with low duty cycles: the low temperature rise induced in the targeted tissue by each low-energy micropulse is sublethal and cannot produce a visible burn (subvisible-threshold treatment). Thus, the targeted tissues remain viable and capable of biological responses. Furthermore, in MLT, the low temperature gradient re-equilibrates to baseline temperature within a short distance, limiting and confining the therapeutic photothermal effect to the tissue directly targeted by the laser. For this reason, and conversely to conventional CW ALT that must be applied spacing the burns, MLT is normally performed with contiguous large spot applications over the TM, a novel laser treatment paradigm that is made possible by the absence of iatrogenic damage and scarring effects.

In an experimental study on human RPE cells in vitro, it has been demonstrated that micropulse laser exposures at subthreshold and sublethal doses that do not impair cells' viability can alter the gene expression profile in several pathways, with 25 % or more of the genes being affected (K.G. Csaky, 2011; personal communication, paper submitted for publication).

Table 7.1 summarizes the typical parameters used in various laser trabeculoplasty techniques performed with CW and pulsed lasers [18–24]. Unlike ALT with CW lasers, LT

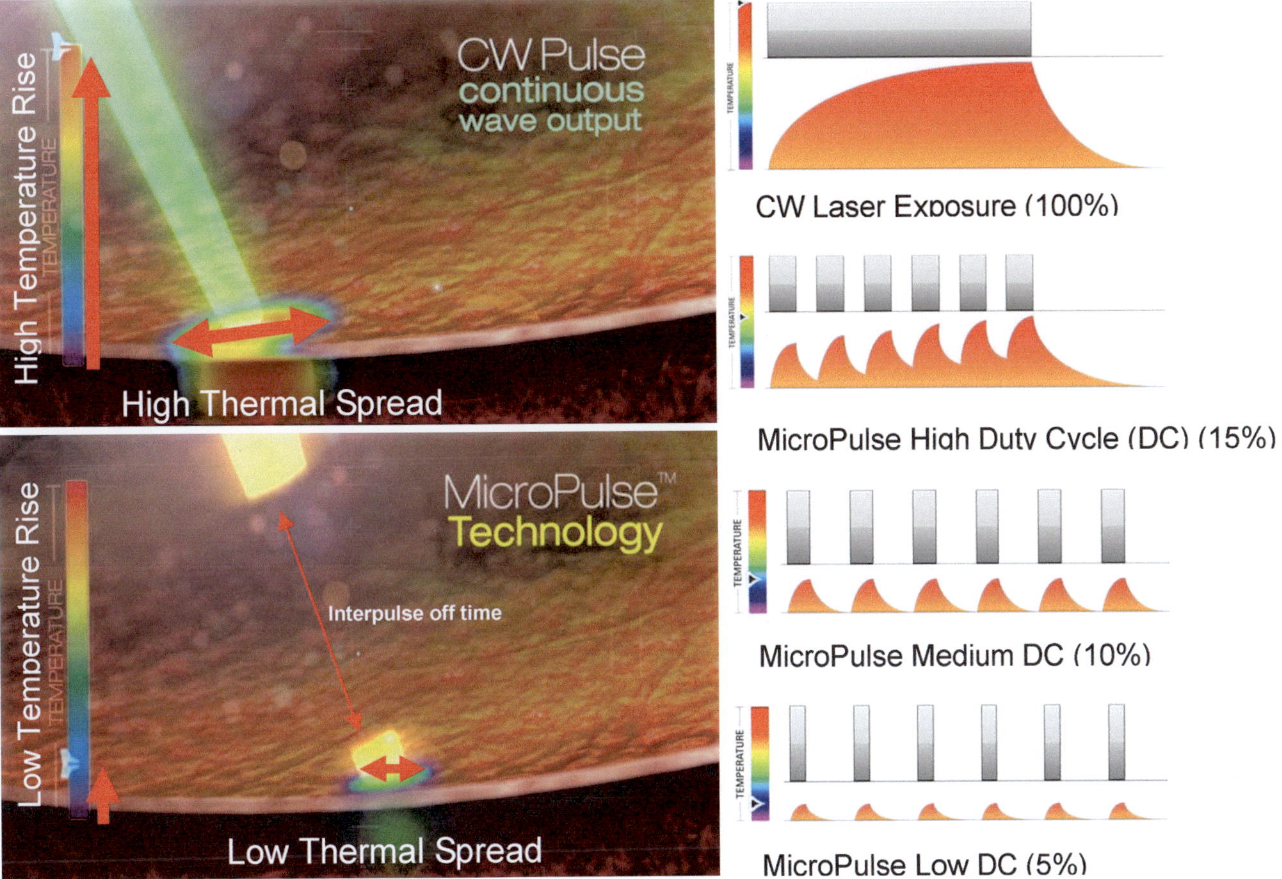


**Fig. 7.1** Tissue interactions with continuous-wave (*CW*) and MicroPulse laser emission

performed with pulsed lasers does not produce tissue coagulation and scarring and has the potential to be repeated PRN. Among the three LT techniques with pulsed lasers, MLT uses the lowest laser irradiance which effectively avoids bubble formation and inflammation and leaves the eye quiet with no need for post-op medications.

In all LT techniques, with CW or pulsed lasers, the beneficial IOP reduction is most likely due to at least one common mechanism of action: a cellular biological cascade activated by the stress response to different laser-induced thermodynamic stimuli, photothermal injury in ALT, selective photothermolysis in SLT, photoacoustic bubble formation in TLT, and sublethal photothermal protein denaturation in MLT.

## Contact Transscleral Cyclophotocoagulation (TSCPC) of the Ciliary Processes with CW Laser over the Pars Plicata

Cyclodestruction of the ciliary processes has long been practiced for the management of refractory glaucoma utilizing different destructive techniques such as diathermy, cryotherapy, xenon arc light, 1,064 nm Nd:YAG laser, and in our days, the 810 nm diode laser cyclophotocoagulation.

The goal of cyclophotocoagulation is to lower intraocular pressure (IOP) by reducing the amount of aqueous humor produced in the ciliary processes by secreting epithelial cells and ultra-filtrating fenestrated capillaries. In transscleral cyclophotocoagulation (TSCPC), the 810 nm diode laser CW energy is applied 1.2 mm posteriorly to the limbus and directed over the pars plicata to induce a lethal thermal rise in laser-absorbing pigmented epithelial cells of the ciliary processes. The heath originated within the targeted pigmented cells spreads coagulating adjacent cells and closing nearby capillaries, affecting the aqueous-producing ciliary processes without destroying the ciliary body itself.

Conventionally, TSCPC is performed with local anesthesia (2 % lignocaine given as peribulbar or retrobulbar injection) or general anesthesia. The G-Probe is held parallel to the visual axis with the shorter edge next to the anterior border of the limbus so that the laser beam is directed 1.2 mm posterior to the limbus over the pars plana and ciliary processes. Transillumination may be used to direct the laser in myopic and post-corneal transplant eyes, in which the ciliary processes may be found more posteriorly than expected. Usually, the treatment consists of 18–20 applications over 270°, sparing the 90° temporal quadrant, and using CW laser

**Table 7.1** Typical parameters used in various laser trabeculoplasty techniques performed with continuous-wave and with pulsed lasers

Continuous-wave and pulsed laser trabeculoplasty techniques
Treatment parameters within the range considered typical for average patients

| Characteristics and parameters | Units | CW laser trabeculoplasty | | Pulsed laser trabeculoplasty | | |
|---|---|---|---|---|---|---|
| | | ALT [18–20] | DLT [18–20] | SLT [19, 20] | MLT [21–23] | TLT [24] |
| Type of laser | –/– | Argon (or CW FD Nd:YAG) | Diode laser in CW mode | Q-switched FD Nd:YAG Laser | Diode laser in micropulse mode | Titanium-sapphire laser |
| Laser wavelength | nm | 488/514 (or 532) | 810 | 532 | 810 | 790 |
| Contact gonio lens (Laser magnification) | –/– | Goldmann 3-mirror lens (1.08×) | Ritch trabeculoplasty (0.71×) | Latina laser gonio lens (1.0×) | Latina laser gonio lens (1.0×) | Goldmann 3-mirror lens (1.08×) |
| (Spot diameter in air) Spot diameter at tissue | µm | (50) 54 | (75) 53 | (400) 400 | (300–200) 300–200 | (200) 216 |
| Laser power | W | 0.4–0.7 | 0.6–1.0 | $200–400 \times 10^3$ | 2 | $4.29–7.14 \times 10^3$ |
| Laser irradiance | W/cm$^2$ | $20–36 \times 10^3$ | $30–50 \times 10^3$ | $160–320 \times 10^6$ | $2.83–6.37 \times 10^3$ | $13.7–54.5 \times 10^6$ |
| Laser pulse length | s | 0.1 | 0.1–0.2 | $3 \times 10^{-9}$ | $300 \times 10^{-6}$ | $7 \times 10^{-6}$ |
| Exposure duration | s | 0.1 | 0.1–0.2 | $3 \times 10^{-9}$ | 0.2 | $7 \times 10^{-6}$ |
| Number of laser pulses | # | 1 | 1 | 1 | 100 | 1 |
| Duty factor | % | 100 | 100 | 100 | 15 0.3 ms ON + 1.7 ms OFF | 100 |
| Laser energy per pulse and per application site | J | $40–70 \times 10^{-3}$ | $60–200 \times 10^{-3}$ | $0.6–1.2 \times 10^{-3}$ | $0.6 \times 10^{-3}$/pulse $60 \times 10^{-3}$/ application | $30–50 \times 10^{-3}$ |
| Laser fluence per pulse | J/cm$^2$ | $2.0–3.6 \times 10^3$ | $3.0–10 \times 10^3$ | 0.5–1.0 | 0.85–1.91 | 81.9–136.5 |
| Number of applications and placement over the TM | # | 50 (or 100) spaced over 180° (or 360°) | 50 (100) spaced over 180° (360°) | 50 (or 100) confluent over 180° or 360° | 66–100 (132–200) confluent over 180° (360°) | 50 adjacent, but not overlapping spots over 180° |
| Treated fraction (%) of the TM circumference | –/– | 6.5–13 % | 6.5–13 % | 50 % (or 100 %) | 50 % or 100 % | 27 % |
| Total energy per eye | J | 2.0–7.0 | 3.0–20.0 | $30–120 \times 10^{-3}$ | 3.96–12.0 | 1.5–2.5 |
| Expected endpoint | –/– | Blanching (mild) to bubbles (intense) | Blanching to no visible reaction (in lightly pigmented TM) | No visible tissue reaction to small bubbles | No visible tissue reaction | Visible tissue reaction with mini-bubbles or burst of pigment |

emission of 1.25 W for 4.0 s (5.0 J) in highly pigmented eyes and 1.5 W for 3.5 s (5.25 J) in lightly pigmented Caucasian eyes. Postoperatively, the eye is patched for 1–6 h, and topical cycloplegic and steroids are applied four times a day and tapered as the inflammation subsides. Preoperative antiglaucoma medications are continued (except miotics) and tapered, depending on the intraocular pressure (IOP).

Successful IOP reduction and control is achieved when the production of aqueous humor is lowered to balance and not exceed the overall outflow capabilities of the eye.

TSCPC with the CW 810 nm laser delivered through the G-Probe is an effective IOP-lowering procedure, relatively noninvasive compared to filtration surgery and to drainage devices, with no risk of infection, and it is technically easy to learn and straightforward to perform. However, it is a destructive procedure, requires retrobulbar or peribulbar anesthesia, and can be associated with complications such as uveitis, phthisis bulbi, hypotony, transient hyphema and exudates in the anterior chamber, severe visual loss, and necrotizing scleritis. For these reasons, historically TSCPC has been utilized as a last-ditch effort in glaucomatous eyes that are refractory or nonresponsive to conventional pharmacological and surgical treatment options and with little remaining vision.

Advances in treatment modalities, such as the switch to slow coagulation techniques with lower CW power and longer exposure [25] and the use of the transillumination-guidance pioneered by Steven Vold for increased targeting precision, have allowed to improve the outcomes and significantly reduce tissue trauma, postoperative inflammatory response, complications, and amount of pain associated with the procedure.

Furthermore, the publication of long-term TSCPC results in eyes with ambulatory vision [26] and in eyes with good vision [27] showing outcomes similar to those of trabeculectomy and tube shunts [28] have encouraged many surgeons to consider TSCPC as a viable earlier treatment option for a wider patient population, including eyes with moderate to severe glaucoma.

More recently, MicroPulse laser emission has been used in place of conventional CW emission to perform lighter and nondestructive TSCPC treatments directed over the pars plana and further reduce tissue trauma, postoperative inflammation, complications, and pain [29, 30].

## Contact Transscleral MicroPulse Cyclophotostimulation (TSµpCPS) over the Pars Plana: A Nondestructive Cyclo-Treatment to Lower Intraocular Pressure

The observation that CW-TSCPC lowers IOP when the laser beam is directed 1.2 mm from the limbus over the pars plicata, as well as when it is applied at 3–4 mm posterior to the limbus over the pars plana, supports the assumption that there may exist aqueous-producing cells and capillaries further posterior to the ciliary processes than assumed. This assumption appears corroborated by the results of the endo-photocoagulation EPC-plus treatment protocol, which have shown that a further decrease of IOP can be obtained by extending the laser-blanching applications to areas posterior to the ciliary processes.

Furthermore, several clinicians have postulated the possibility that laser interactions with pars plana structures could also increase the uveoscleral outflow.

In an animal study in cynomolgus monkey eyes with tracer particles perfused in the anterior chamber, Liu and coworkers [31] demonstrated that contact TSCPC directed at the pars plana 3.0 mm posterior to the limbus decreased IOP and also resulted in tracer particles being present in the suprachoroidal space. Conversely, when contact TSCPC was directed at the pars plicata 1.0 mm posterior to the limbus, IOP decreased as well, but no tracer particles were found in the suprachoroidal space. The authors suggested that the IOP reduction after TSCPC at the pars plicata may be due to the reduction of aqueous secretion, whereas the IOP reduction after TSCPC at the pars plana may also enhance the uveoscleral outflow into the suprachoroidal space.

Tan et al. [29] reported that a TSCPC performed with an 810 nm diode laser in the MicroPulse emission mode over the pars plana resulted in clinically significant IOP reduction, comparable with conventional TSCPC with CW laser emission, but with markedly less postoperative pain and complications and with a prompter IOP reduction (as early as 1 day post treatment), which was attributed to the possibility of an enhanced uveoscleral outflow.

This possibility has prompted the hypothesis that IOP reduction after transscleral cyclo laser treatment can occur through different pathways with distinct or combined mechanisms:

- The treatment over the pars plicata would target the photocoagulation of epithelial cells with closure of surrounding capillaries and this ablation of the ciliary processes is thought to reduce the production of aqueous humor.
- The treatment over the pars plana would activate changes in extracellular matrix that would decrease the resistance in the uveoscleral outflow. In addition, the concomitant photothermal spread would promote two concomitant IOP-lowering mechanisms: the relaxation of the ciliary muscle, which would further increase the uveoscleral flow, and the coagulation of posteriorly located aqueous-secreting cells, which would reduce their aqueous humor production.

The possibility of differently addressing and titrating multiple IOP-lowering mechanisms represents an important option in the management of different types of glaucoma.

With conventional TSCPC, the IOP-lowering effect has been found to be directly related to the area of treated tissue, but so are the risk of complications and side effects. If TSCPC treatment could be titrated to be therapeutically effective with the minimum possible side effects and complications, greater effects could be achieved by treating more tissue and/or longer glaucoma management could be possible with more treatments as needed. MicroPulse dosing of laser emission has been shown capable of inducing therapeutic benefit without iatrogenic tissue damage in the treatment of retinovascular diseases as well as in IOP lowering with MicroPulse laser trabeculoplasty (MLT) and with micropulse TSCPC.

## Early Reports with MicroPulse Transscleral Pars Plana Cyclophotocoagulation (MP-TSppCPC)

At the National University Hospital in Singapore (Paul T.K. Chew and coworkers), MicroPulse diode laser contact transscleral photocoagulation over the pars plana was found to significantly reduce IOP in the majority of patients at 1 week postoperatively, with less but still significant effect at 12 weeks [32].

Likewise, in a prospective pilot study of 16 eyes of 16 patients, MP-TSppCPC was found to safely lower IOP, at least during the first 3 weeks after treatment. There was less pain during and after the procedure, minimal inflammation, but less degree of IOP lowering as compared to conventional TSCPC, and this may not necessarily be sustained [33].

**Table 7.2** Mean IOP reduction from MP-TSppCPC with the P2P probe

| Time point | Mean IOP (mmHg) | Mean IOP reduction (%) |
| --- | --- | --- |
| Pre-op baseline | 37.1±9.5 | 0.0 % |
| 1 day post-op | 28.7±10.8 | 24.0±17.1 |
| 1 week post-op | 25.6±9.7 | 30.9±18.7 |
| 1 month post-op | 22.2±7.0 | 38.2±19.6 |
| 3 months post-op | 22.9±8.9 | 35.4±24.2 |
| 6 months post-op | 23.7±9.7 | 37.6±19.4 |

The mean IOP reduction reported in a prospective study presented at the World Glaucoma Congress in July 2007 (Poster # P428), which included 23 eyes of 21 patients with uncontrolled glaucoma (age 62.9±20.3 years) that received MP-TSppCPC with the P2P probe, is summarized in Table 7.2.

Treatment success, defined as a 30 % or more reduction of IOP from baseline or a final IOP of less than 21 mmHg at the sixth month follow-up visit, was 38 % at 1 day, 57 % at 1 week, 76 % at 1 month, 80 % at 3 months, and 69 % at 6 months, as illustrated in Fig. 7.2.

None of the patients had hypotony or loss in their best corrected visual acuity.

One patient, who responded with good IOP reduction to MP-TSppCPC, required evisceration at 1 month after the treatment due to corneal perforation secondary to infected bullous keratopathy: remarkably, at the histopathological examination, no sign of laser-induced lesion or tissue alteration attributable to MP-TSppCPC could be found by the pathologist.

To validate this initial experience with MP-TSppCPC, a randomized comparison trial was conducted at the National University Hospital in Singapore by Paul T.K. Chew and coworkers aimed at comparing micropulse TSCPC versus continuous-wave TSCPC effects on patients with refractory, end-stage glaucoma [30]. Both transscleral treatments resulted effective in lowering IOP, but a safer and more sustained treatment effect was achieved with micropulse TSCPC.

In essence, the overall experience with micropulse TSCPC at the NUH in Singapore on patients with refractory glaucoma and poor vision can be summarized as follows:

(a) Remarkable acute IOP-lowering effect.

(b) Response with IOP reduction is very rapid: can be seen at day 1 compared to 1 week with the conventional G-Probe, probably due to less inflammation.

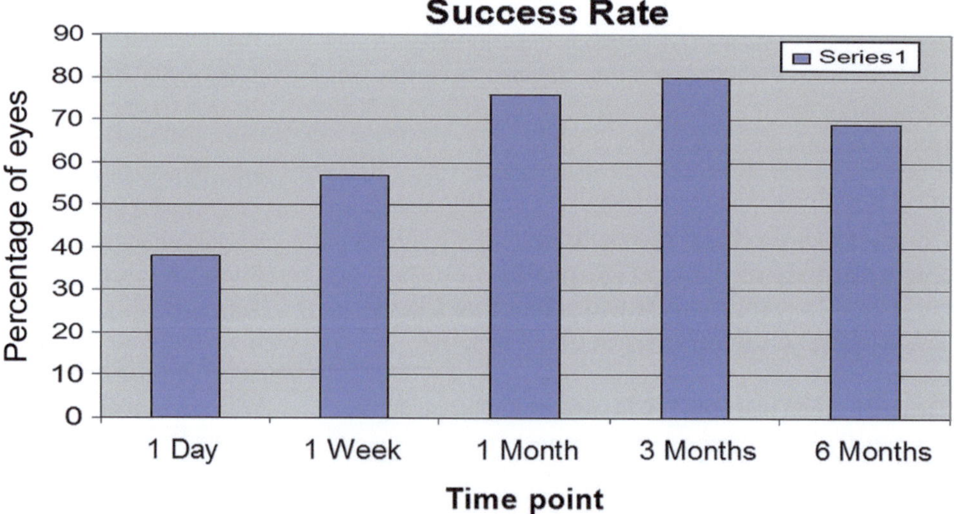


**Fig. 7.2** None of the patients had hypotony or loss in their best corrected visual acuity

(c) Less overall intraoperative pain. However, there is still some intraoperative pain and the use of peribulbar block is recommended.

(d) Much less chemosis (swelling of the conjunctiva).

(e) Less inflammation on day 1 post-op. Eyes are normally quiet.

(f) No postoperative pain/discomfort (much less pain at day 1 compared to conventional CW G-Probe).

(g) IOP reduction persists at the 18th month.

## Synoptic Summary

- Continuous-wave transscleral cyclophotocoagulation (CW-TSCPC) with the G-Probe is an effective therapy option to lower IOP, but it is a destructive procedure associated with side effects and complications.
- For this reason, CW-TSCPC with the G-Probe is normally used for cases resistant to conventional glaucoma management and it is not commonly considered at earlier stages of the disease.
- CW-TSCPC with the G-Probe is believed to lower the IOP by reducing the production of aqueous humor through the destruction of the ciliary body; however, many authors have suggested that it may also work by stimulating IOP-lowering mechanisms other than destruction of tissue.
- The relatively long laser exposure durations used with CW-TSCPC favor the spread of nonlethal decaying heat toward adjacent tissues, including the pars plana and suprachoroidal structures, and this may affect the uveoscleral outflow.
- Uveoscleral outflow is a significant drainage path in humans, and its contribution to overall drainage depends on patient age, health, and other conditions.

  The uveoscleral outflow is decreased by contraction (pilocarpine) and increased by relaxation (atropine) of the ciliary muscle. Thus, changing the tone of the ciliary muscle may redistribute aqueous humor between the conventional and uveoscleral outflow routes. Prostaglandins decrease the intraocular pressure by increasing the uveoscleral outflow. Two mechanisms seem to contribute to this effect: relaxation of the ciliary muscle and changes in extracellular matrix, causing decreased resistance in the uveoscleral outflow routes.
- A new contact probe, called the pars plana or P2-Probe, has been designed to radially deliver IR laser energy over the pars plana at 3–4 mm posterior to the limbus.
- The P2-Probe delivering nondestructive micropulse laser irradiation can photothermally affect the target tissue and lower IOP without tissue destruction. This is the goal of micropulse transscleral pars plana cyclophotocoagulation or MP-TSppCPC.

- MP-TSppCPC is not intended to and will not replace CW-TSCPC with the G-Probe for the destruction of ciliary body in the treatment of patients with refractory and neovascular glaucoma.
- MP-TSppCPC with the P2-Probe will most likely be used to lower IOP in patients in less advanced stages of glaucoma and with good vision by activating IOP-lowering mechanisms other than destruction of ciliary epithelium.
- MP-TSppCPC with the P2-Probe administered at *higher duty cycles* may also play a role as a gentler and effective cyclodestructive technique, with less damage and side effects.

## References


1. Krasnov MM. Laseropuncture of the anterior chamber angle in glaucoma. Am J Ophthalmol. 1973;75:674–8.
2. Hager H. Besondere mikrochirurgische Eingriffe. II. Erste Erfahrungen mit dem Argon-Laser-Gerat 800. Klin Monatsbl Augenheilkd. 1973;162:437–50.
3. Worthen DM, Wickam MG. Argon laser trabeculotomy. Trans Am Acad Ophthalmol Otolaryngol. 1974;78:OP371–5.
4. Wickam MG, Worthen DM. Argon laser trabeculotomy: long-term follow-up. Ophthalmology. 1979;86:495–503.
5. Wise JB, Witter SL. Argon laser therapy for open-angle glaucoma. A pilot study. Arch Ophthalmol. 1979;97:319–22.
6. Gaasterland D, Kupfer C. Experimental glaucoma in the rhesus monkey. Invest Ophthalmol. 1975;14:455.
7. Ticho U, Zauberman H. Argon laser application to angle structures in glaucoma. Arch Ophthalmol. 1976;94:61–4.
8. Ticho U, Cadet JC, Mahler J, et al. Argon laser trabeculotomies in primates: evaluation by histological and perfusion studies. Invest Ophthalmol. 1978;17:667–74.
9. Ticho U. Laser applications to the angle structures in animal and in the human glaucomatous eye. Adv Ophthalmol. 1977;34:201.
10. Glaucoma Laser Trial Research Group. The Glaucoma Laser Trial (GLT) and glaucoma laser trial follow-up study: 7. Results. Am J Ophthalmol. 1995;120:718–31.
11. Musch DC, et al., for the CIGTS Study Group. The collaborative initial glaucoma treatment study. Study design, methods, and baseline characteristics of enrolled patients. Ophthalmology. 1999;106:653–62.
12. Lichter PR, et al., for the CIGTS Study Group. Interim clinical outcomes in the collaborative initial glaucoma treatment study comparing initial treatment randomized to medications or surgery. Ophthalmology. 2001;108:1943–53.
13. Heijl A, et al., for the Early Manifest Glaucoma Trial Group. Reduction of intraocular pressure and glaucoma progression. Results from the Early Manifest Glaucoma Trial. Arch Ophthalmol. 2002;120:1268–79.
14. Leske MC, et al., for the Early Manifest Glaucoma Trial Group. Factors for glaucoma progression and effect of treatment. The Early Manifest Glaucoma Trial. Arch Ophthalmol. 2003;121:48–56.
15. Ederer F, Gaasterland DA, Dally LG, Kim J, VanVeldhuisen PC, Blackwell B, Prum B, Shafranov G, Allen RC, Beck A, AGIS Investigators. The Advanced Glaucoma Intervention Study 13. Comparison of treatment outcomes within race 10 years results. Ophthalmology. 2004;111(4):651–64.
16. Shigleton BJ, Richter CU, Dharma SK, et al. Long-term efficacy of argon laser trabeculoplasty. A 10-year follow-up study. Ophthalmology. 1993;100:1324–9.

17. Rachmiel R, Trope GE, Chipman ML, et al. Laser trabeculoplasty trends with the introduction of new medical treatments and selective laser trabeculoplasty. J Glaucoma. 2006;15(4):306–9.

18. American Academy of Ophthalmology. Committee on Ophthalmic Procedures Assessment. Laser trabeculoplasty for primary open-angle glaucoma. Ophthalmology. 1996;103(10):1706–12.

19. Park CH, Latina MA, Schuman JS. Developments in laser trabeculoplasty. Ophthalmic Surg Lasers. 2000;30(4):315–22.

20. Olivier MMG. Glaucoma laser treatment: where are we now? Tech Ophthalmol. 2004;2(3):118–23.

21. Fea AM, Bosone A, Rolle T, et al. Micropulse diode laser trabeculoplasty (MDLT): a phase II clinical study with 12 months follow-up. Clin Ophthalmol. 2008;2(2):247–52.

22. Ingvoldstad DD, Krishna R, Willoughby L. Micropulse diode laser trabeculoplasty versus argon laser trabeculoplasty in the treatment of open angle glaucoma. Invest Ophthal Vis Sci. 2005;46:ARVO E-Abstract 123.

23. Fea AM, Dorin G. Laser treatment of glaucoma: evolution of laser trabeculoplasty techniques. Tech Ophthalmol. 2008;6(2):45–52.

24. Goldenfeld M, Melamed S, Simon G, Ben Simon GJ. Titanium:sapphire laser trabeculoplasty versus argon laser trabeculoplasty in patients with open-angle glaucoma. Ophthalmic Surg Lasers Imaging. 2009;40:264–9.

25. Gaasterland DE. Diode laser cyclophotocoagulation. Technique and results. Glaucoma Today. 2009;7(2):35–8.

26. Wilensky JT, Krammer J. Long-term visual outcome with transscleral laser cyclotherapy in eyes with ambulatory vision. Ophthalmology. 2004;111:1389–92.

27. Ansari E, Gandhewar J. Long-term efficacy and visual acuity following transscleral diode laser photocoagulation in cases of refractory and non-refractory glaucoma. Eye. 2007;21(7):936–40.

28. Gedde SJ, Sciffman JC, Feuer WJ, et al. Three-year follow-up of the tube versus trabeculectomy study. Am J Ophthalmol. 2009;148(5):670–84.

29. Tan AM, Chockalingam M, Aquino MC, et al. Micropulse transscleral diode laser cyclophotocoagulation in the treatment of refractory glaucoma. Clin Experiment Ophthalmol. 2010;38:266–72.

30. Aquino MC, Tan AW, Xiang L, et al. Micropulse versus continuous wave transscleral diode cyclophotocoagulation in the treatment of refractory glaucoma: a randomized comparison trial. (submitted for publication).

31. Liu GJ, Mizukawa A, Okisada S. Mechanism of intraocular pressure decrease after contact transscleral continuous-wave Nd:YAG laser cyclophotocoagulation. Ophthalmic Res. 1994;26(2):65–79.

32. Ho CL, Wong EYM, Chew PTK. Effect of diode laser contact transscleral pars plana photocoagulation on intraocular pressure in glaucoma. Clin Exper Ophthalmol. 2002;30:343–7.

33. Ho CL. Micropulse diode transscleral cyclophotocoagulation. Asian J Ophthalmol. 2002; nos 3,4, 2001 Supplement.

# Excimer Laser Trabeculostomy (ELT): An Effective MIGS Procedure for Open-Angle Glaucoma

Michael S. Berlin, Marc Töteberg-Harms, Edward Kim, Iris Vuong, and Ulrich Giers

Elevated intraocular pressure (IOP) in most open-angle glaucoma is due to an obstruction of aqueous outflow thought to be localized predominantly at the juxtacanalicular trabecular meshwork (TM) and the inner wall of Schlemm's canal (SC). There have been multiple surgical attempts to directly treat this pathology by creating channels to connect the anterior chamber to SC. Various iterations have included mechanical drilling techniques, thermal laser and alternative thermal cautery techniques, and a variety of tube implants with the common goal of bypassing this increased outflow resistance. However, the majority of these techniques concurrently or subsequently create sufficient adjacent tissue disruption to eventuate in inflammatory healing responses adequate to overcome the benefits of the procedures, resulting in mid-term or long-term failures. To overcome these known causes of failure, technologies and techniques for the purpose of creating such channels were sought which did not cause scar tissue formation. The requirements include minimal tissue disruption during the process of creating the openings and channels which are of adequate size and number to enable outflow but not so large as to alter the aqueous composition.

The excimer laser trabeculostomy (ELT) concept utilizes a 308-nm xenon chloride excimer laser to provide a precise and essentially nonthermal approach to improve outflow in a manner which does not provoke a healing response. ELT is a procedure performed via a clear corneal incision, sparing conjunctiva, in which direct visualization of the target tissue via a goniolens or an endoscope provides immediate feedback to the surgeon. ELT, when compared to the more invasive glaucoma surgical procedures such as trabeculectomy, is almost as efficacious in both IOP-lowering and decreasing pressure-lowering medication use, while being far less traumatic. The sparing of conjunctiva is a major advantage of this technique, because success rates of a subsequent trabeculectomy, if ever necessary, would not be compromised. This microinvasive glaucoma surgery (MIGS) procedure, another option in the armamentarium for the glaucoma surgeon, has a high safety profile, rapid stabilization, and clinical verification of long-term efficacy with minimal impact on quality of life. It may also become a replacement option for topical glaucoma medicinal therapies eliminating their associated cost, compliance issues, and side effects from their long-term use.

M.S. Berlin, MD, MS (✉)
Glaucoma Institute of Beverly Hills, Jules Stein
Eye Institute, UCLA, 8733 Beverly Blvd.,
Suite 301, Los Angeles, CA 90048, USA
e-mail: berlin@ucla.edu

M. Töteberg-Harms, MD
Department of Ophthalmology, University Hospital Zurich,
Frauenklinikstrasse 24, Zurich 8091, Switzerland
e-mail: marctoeteberg@aol.com

E. Kim, BA • I. Vuong
Glaucoma Institute of Beverly Hills, 8733 Beverly Blvd.,
Suite 301, Los Angeles, CA 90048, USA
e-mail: ehkim36@gmail.com; irisvuong@gmail.com

U. Giers, MD
Augen-klinik OWL, Detmold, Elisabethstrasse 85,
32756 Detmold, Germany
e-mail: ugiers@doc4eye.de

## What Are MIGS Procedures and Where Do They Fit in Glaucoma Treatment Paradigms?

The invasive procedure and lifestyle altering sequelae of trabeculectomy limit the use of this procedure to later stage and recalcitrant glaucoma patients. Issues regarding medication costs, compliance, and toxicity of preservatives suggest medicinal therapeutic options also have limitations. Thus, there remains an unmet patient need for treatments that could effectively treat mild to moderate glaucoma. In recent years, several MIGS procedures have been developed to address these limitations of traditional treatment options. All have advantages and disadvantages, but no current technique fulfills all requirements which are (1) ab interno microincision, (2) minimal trauma, (3) efficacy, (4) high safety profile, and (5) rapid recovery [1].

J.R. Samples, I.I.K. Ahmed (eds.), *Surgical Innovations in Glaucoma*,
DOI 10.1007/978-1-4614-8348-9_8, © Springer Science+Business Media New York 2014

1. MIGS procedures use an ab interno micro-incisional approach through a clear corneal incision of less than 2 mm, which spares the conjunctiva and thus prevents significant external scarring, allowing future unaffected conjunctival surgery, if needed. This also allows for direct visualization of anatomic landmarks to optimize placement of a device, incision or excision within the angle and is easily combined with cataract surgery. Furthermore, a micro-incision facilitates the intra-operative maintenance of the anterior chamber, retention of normal ocular anatomy, minimizes changes in refractive outcome, and adds to procedural safety.

2. MIGS procedures are minimally traumatic to the target tissue, with negligible disruption of normal anatomy and physiology. Devices are biocompatible and ideally enhance physiologic outflow pathways.

3. MIGS procedures must be effective in both lowering IOP and reducing medication use.

4. MIGS procedures are characterized by an extremely high safety profile. Many MIGS procedures are less efficacious when compared to more invasive glaucoma surgeries such as trabeculectomy with antimetabolites or glaucoma drainage devices. However, this compromise in efficacy is balanced by their low-risk profile. MIGS procedures are associated with a decreased incidence of serious complications that are often associated with other glaucoma surgeries including hypotony, choroidal effusions, suprachoroidal hemorrhage, anterior chamber shallowing, corneal decompensation, cataract formation, diplopia, and bleb-related complications such as bleb dysesthesia and endophthalmitis.

5. MIGS procedures have a rapid recovery with minimal impact on the patient's quality of life.

In conclusion, MIGS procedures fit for mild do moderate glaucoma cases, in which an IOP in low to mid teens is sufficient. In addition, a reduction in IOP lowering medication is desired. The safety profile of the procedure as well as a rapid recovery is important.

## Previous Meshwork Surgeries and Their Disadvantages

Current MIGS procedures can successfully bypass the TM in order to create direct flow from the anterior chamber into SC unlike earlier attempts to address this anatomic pathology, which often failed. Procedures utilizing mechanical devices and lasers to perforate the TM have been shown to adequately bypass the outflow obstruction for the short term but have been unsuccessful in the long term due to the amount of adjacent tissue damage related to the nature of the technique or device. The adjacent tissue damage evokes a healing response which eventually closes the channels. As laser technology evolved, each new laser was applied for this purpose, but none enabled long-term patent openings. Krasnov et al. showed moderate success using a ruby laser (943 nm) to perform "trabeculopuncture" [2]. Other laser trabeculopuncture attempts including Hager's [3] use of an argon laser (488 + 514 nm) and Fankhauser's [4] use of a neodymium:yttrium-aluminum-garnet (Nd:YAG) laser (continuous wave 1,064 nm) have also been unsuccessful due to scarring. These and other laser trabeculopuncture attempts also limit prospective options for subsequent procedures [5, 6] should they become necessary as they induce destruction of local tissue and scar formation of adjacent tissue, often involving large regional areas. In addition, with large openings and markedly increased outflow, the compositional alterations of the aqueous would supplement the tissue destructive healing responses.

Following these initial attempts using lasers ab interno to perforate TM or to create full-thickness sclerostomies, Wise et al. determined that a continuous wave, essentially long pulsed argon laser (488 + 514 nm) could successfully modify the TM to increase outflow without perforation. Their argon laser trabeculoplasty (ALT) procedure effectively lowered IOP, but it functioned by creating thermal damage to the target tissue, causing coagulative necrosis of the TM [7]. In contrast to ALT, laser trabeculoplasty (LTP) is now more commonly performed with solid-state (532, frequency-doubled Nd:YAG) and diode (810 nm) lasers. Studies comparing efficacy of these thermal lasers demonstrate minimal differences in efficacy, longevity, or repeatability.

The efficacy of LTP in lowering IOP has been well documented in the literature [8–10]. However, long-term studies have shown that the IOP-lowering efficacy of LTP decreases over time, from 77 % success rate at 1 year, to 49 % at 5 years, and finally, to 32 % at 10 years [11]. Additionally, because of the significant TM scarring caused by ALT, repeat treatments are not recommended and have not proven successful clinically [12]. LTP causes thermal coagulative damage to the uveoscleral meshwork, disruption of the trabecular beams, and heat damage to the surrounding collagen fibers. This thermal damage is in part responsible for the inflammatory response, scarring of the TM tissue, peripheral anterior synechiae, and IOP spikes sometimes observed in eyes which have undergone LTP [13].

In contrast to the diffuse thermal effects of argon, solid-state, and diode laser with relatively long pulse durations in the range of 0.1 s, recent advances in LTP utilize lasers with shorter pulse durations of 3–10 ns. Selective laser trabeculoplasty (SLT), based on the principle of selective photothermolysis, relies on selective absorption of short laser pulses to generate and spatially confine heat to pigmented targets within TM cells [14, 15]. SLT uses a Q-switched, frequency-doubled 532-nm Nd:YAG laser. Q-switching of the laser allows for an extremely brief and thus high-powered light pulse to be delivered to the target tissues. The short duration of the pulse is critical in preventing collateral damage to the surrounding tissues [16]. The mechanisms of the pressure effects following ALT, LTP, and SLT which alter but do not perforate TM are yet undetermined.

Preserving the TM may become more important in the near future, as surgical techniques are developed to operate directly on SC or the juxtacanalicular TM. Thermal LTP would preclude the use of the newer MIGS procedures in these patients, as their TM and adjacent tissues, including SC would be likely to have been damaged. Once methods of pre-operative evaluations of the patency of the required outflow pathways are clinically useful, such patients can be better evaluated as candidates for MIGS procedures.

## The Concept of ELT

Ultraviolet excimer laser photoablation enables the precise removal of targeted tissue with meticulous local and adjacent temperature control to prevent thermal damage to surrounding tissues, exemplified by the use of 193-nm excimer lasers for corneal surface ablation, which facilitates successful refractive surgery. However, the 193-nm wavelength, although precise and non-tissue damaging, is not readily transmissible via fiber optics and can therefore not be used for intracameral procedures. In contrast, 308-nm excimer laser generated light is amenable to fiber-optic transmission and, after extensive preclinical experimentation, became the wavelength of choice for non-thermal, precisely targeted ab interno fistulizing procedures [17]. The applications of this non-thermal, ab interno, fiber-optic-delivered energy evolved, initially from full-thickness sclerostomy, creating a bleb via an ab interno approach, subsequently to trabeculostomy, once the parameters of the target tissue anatomy[1] [18, 19], localization of SC, and ablation rates for this wavelength in this tissue were determined and idealized to enable a successful procedure to bypass TM and juxtacanalicular TM obstructions allowing and improving physiological outflow directly into SC.

Initial in vitro experiments led to animal trials [20]. In a study of the effects of 308-nm excimer laser energy applied ab interno to the limbal sclera of rabbit eyes, long-term decreases in IOP were achievable. The use of this 308-nm wavelength, unlike that of earlier trials with thermal lasers, enables laser-tissue interactions with significant advantages. This excimer laser is less likely to evoke a cicatricle response in the TM or sclera than those seen in trials using visible or infrared lasers, which cause thermal tissue damage and subsequent healing responses. In addition, there is minimal exposure of adjacent tissue to radiation enabled by direct contact of the laser energy to the target tissue via the fiber-optic delivery system. With evidence that TM and scleral tissue could be successfully removed without adjacent tissue damage, without subsequent scar formation or channel closure, and with ablation accuracy which would enable precise targeting of TM, juxtacanalicular TM, and the inner wall of SC without perforating the outer wall of SC, these studies formed the basis for the development of the current ELT technology and techniques [21].

## ELT Technique

ELT, first used clinically in 1997 by Vogel and Lauritzen, treats the pathology responsible for most open-angle glaucoma by decreasing the outflow resistance at the juxtacanalicular TM and the inner wall of SC [22]. It is performed with a short-pulsed (80 ns) 308-nm xenon chloride (XeCl) excimer laser which delivers photoablative energy to precisely remove the tissue which obstructs aqueous outflow with minimal thermal damage to adjacent tissue [23]. ELT surgery is performed as an outpatient procedure, under topical, peribulbar, or retrobulbar local anesthesia. Following a paracentesis and stabilization of the anterior chamber with a viscoelastic agent, the surgeon introduces a fiber-optic probe, which is advanced across the anterior chamber to contact the TM (Fig. 8.1). Probe placement is controlled by direct observation using either a goniolens or an endoscope. Four to ten channels are created into SC (Fig. 8.2). The probe is then removed, the viscoelastic agent is replaced by balanced salt solution, and the patient is monitored postoperatively. Most commonly the probe insertion is superotemporal and the laser channels inferonasal. Variations include spacing the channels over both inferior quadrants, creating temporary hypotony following removal of the probe to enable enumeration of the number of patent channels into SC by observing an induced retrograde blood reflux followed by repressurization, among others. The blood reflux is a common but inconsequential occurrence (Fig. 8.3). To date no studies have shown benefit from treatment in more than one quadrant. As no single protocol has been established, each surgeon tends to create their own technique. In spite of these numerous variations, the outcomes are remarkably similar.

By means of the essentially non-thermal photoablation using the specified laser parameters, ELT evaporates human tissue, denaturing the organic structures without producing undesirable marginal necrosis [24]. ELT excises the TM, the juxtacanalicular TM, and the inner wall of SC without damaging the outer wall of SC or the collector channels [25]. No filtering fistula or bleb is created [21, 26, 27].

---

[1]Target tissue anatomic considerations to minimize healing responses must specifically address minimizing trauma to the outer wall of SC. The outer wall endothelium contains fibroblasts, whereas the inner wall endothelium does not. Thus, avoiding trauma to the outer wall and thereby not stimulating a fibroblast response is paramount to the successful maintenance of outflow. Another anatomic consideration is the space between the inner and outer walls of SC, which can be less than 20 μm. The accuracy of the tool used to enter the inner wall such that it does not disturb the outer wall must be of this same scale. The ablation precision of 308 nm on this tissue, unlike that of lasers and devices utilized in earlier attempts to fistulize SC, facilitates the non-thermal and accurate tissue removal which thereby enables the ELT procedure's efficacy.

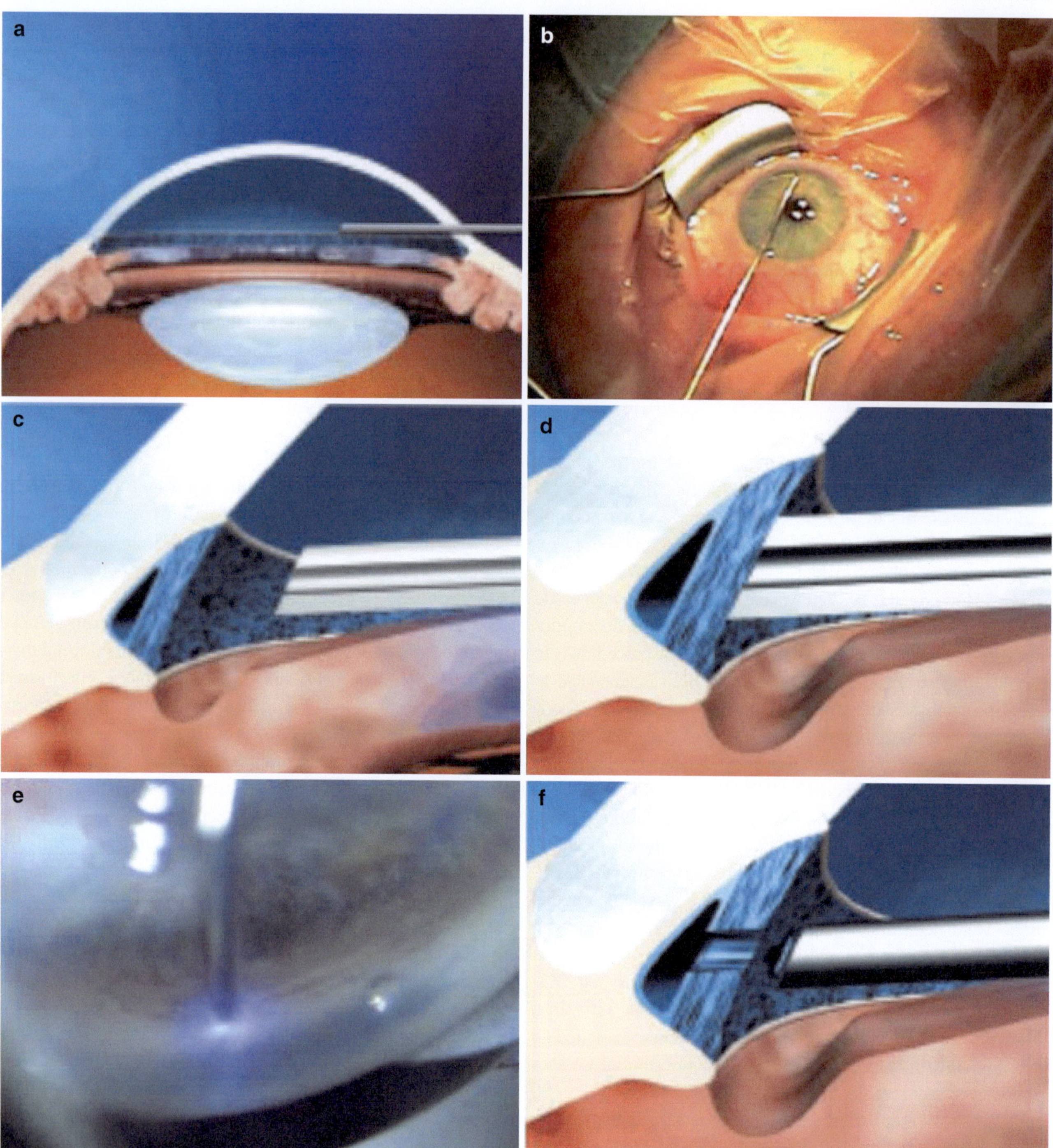

**Fig. 8.1** Drawings and photos of the excimer laser trabeculostomy procedure. The laser fiber is introduced into the anterior chamber through a clear cornea incision (**a**) and advanced across the anterior chamber (**b**) to the trabecular meshwork of the opposite quadrant (**c**). When the fiber tip is in contact with or slightly compresasing the trabecular meshwork laser pulses are initiated (**d**). Tissue fluorescence produced by each UV laser pulse can be visualized gonioscopicly (**e**). A series of laser channels of approx. 0.2mm diameter each enabels flow from the anterior chamber to Schlemm's canal (**f**). **a**, **c-d**, and **f**: Peschke GmbH, Waldshut-Tiengen, Germany; **b** and **e**: U. Giers

## Technical Aspects of Performing an ELT Procedure

The current ELT procedure is performed with an AIDA XeCl laser (TUI-Laser AG, Germering, Germany) in the following manner:

1. The laser is automated to internally calibrate and control the output fluence in accordance with the manufacturer's specifications. Unlike solid-state lasers, this XeCl gas laser requires a short "warm up" time during which the output energy is stabilized before use.

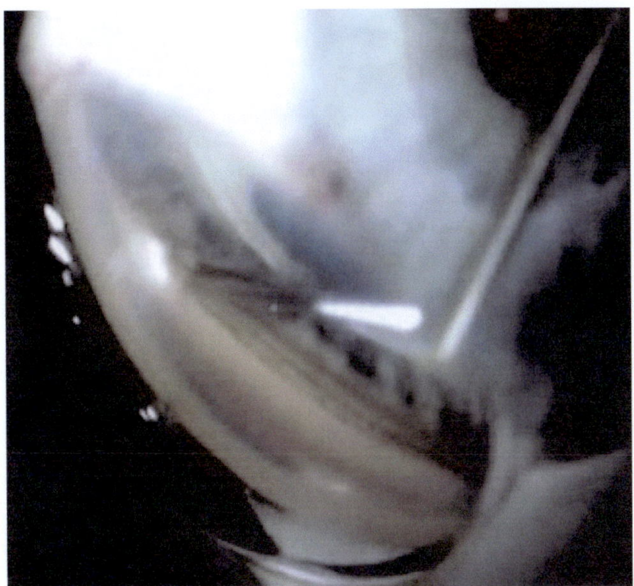

**Fig. 8.2** Gonioscope view/IOP high=SC not visible (U. Giers)

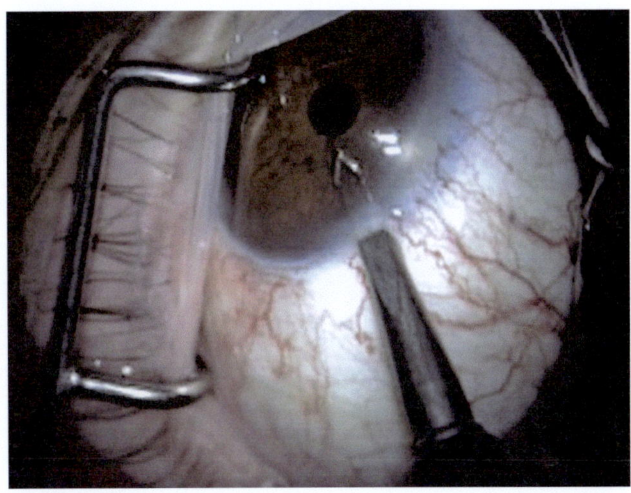

**Fig. 8.4** Paracentesis in the superotemporal perilimbal cornea (U. Giers)

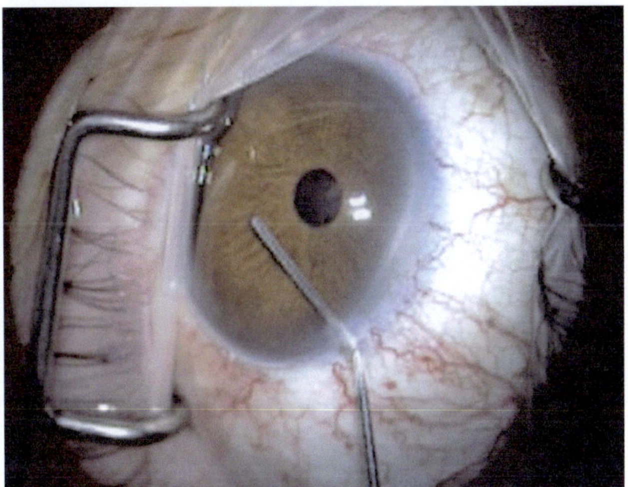

**Fig. 8.5** Viscoelastic agent is introduced (U. Giers)

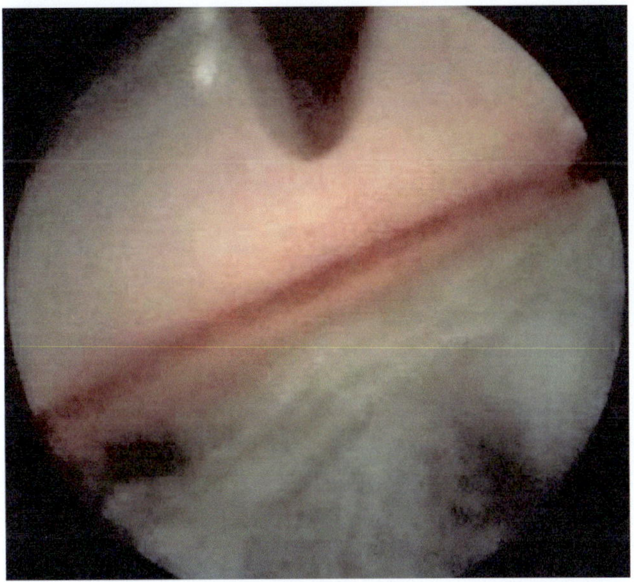

**Fig. 8.3** Endoscopic view/IOP low=SC visible, blood filled (U. Giers)

2. The sterile, non-reusable fiber-optic delivery system is coupled to the laser. The output beam is then adjusted at the fiber tip to ensure suprathreshold fluence for tissue ablation at the fiber tip. The console includes a power meter to enable this calibration which is performed prior to each procedure, similar to the tuning of a phaco handpiece before use.

3. Topical, peribulbar, or retrobulbar local anesthesia is administered. In ELT alone, topical pilocarpine 2 % is used preoperatively to constrict the pupil. In phakic patients this may also assist in protecting the lens. Alternatively, intracameral Miochol (acetylcholine 10 mg/ml) may be used.

4. A 1 mm paracentesis is created in the superotemporal perilimbal cornea 2 o'clock for left eyes and 10 o'clock for right eyes, or in combined cataract and ELT procedures, the previously created phaco-tunnel may be used in a similar fashion (Fig. 8.4).

5. A viscoelastic agent (Healon) fills the anterior chamber through the paracentesis. Depending on the surgeons' preference, the IOP may be unchanged or increased by this injection, enabling or precluding visualization of SC by blood reflux (Fig. 8.5).

6. The laser probe is inserted into the anterior chamber through the paracentesis (Fig. 8.6) and is advanced to the opposite chamber angle via gonioscopic (using the surgeon's preferred goniolens) or endoscopic visualization (Fig. 8.7). The ELT fiber may be attached coaxial with an endoscope, or a second paracentesis endoscopic view may be utilized.

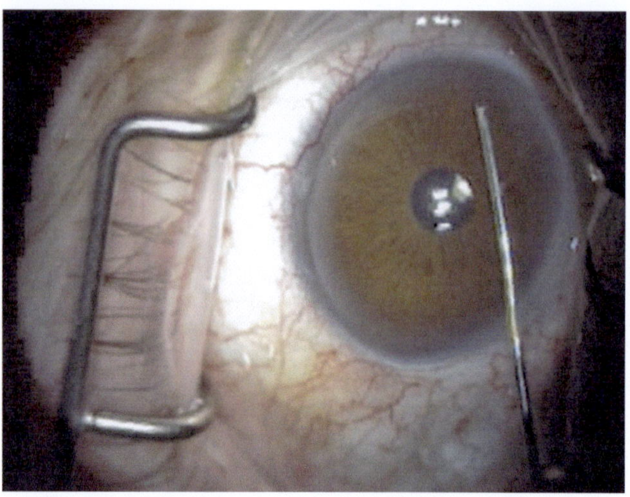

**Fig. 8.6** Laser probe is inserted through the paracentesis to cross the anterior chamber (U. Giers)

7. The fiber tip is centered on the pigmented TM and advanced to be in contact with the TM. SC is targeted whenever visible, or surgeons are advised to alternate placement of the fiber to anterior, mid, and posterior TM regions to assure some of the channels will, in fact, enter into SC. The number of pulses which controls the penetration depth is fixed, similar to the penetration depth control in LASIK. Perforation of the inner wall of SC into SC depends, therefore, on its distance from the fiber tip which can be variable depending on the angle of placement and the amount of pressure on the fiber. The calculation of this distance was determined in numerous preclinical experiments [28, 29]. Thus, the most common protocol consists of ten probe placement sites on TM, a percentage of which is likely to enter SC.

8. The laser is activated, delivering laser pulses at 20 Hz per treatment site. Each pulse converts the tissue at the fiber tip into gas. This gas may be seen exiting around the fiber tip during each ablation (Fig. 8.8).

9. As the channel is created, pulse by pulse, an opening is created from the anterior chamber into SC through photoablation of the TM, the juxtacanalicular TM and the inner wall of SC. As soon as the outflow obstruction at the fiber tip is removed as SC is entered, the pathway for the gas, previously retrograde around the fiber, becomes anterograde, entering SC. In theory, this product-of-ablation gas is then assumed to dilate SC, pushing the outer wall away and concurrently dilating the adjacent surrounding collector channels. This concept of the product-of-ablation gas dilation of SC and collector channels is termed "pneumatic canaloplasty." Once adequate imaging devices are developed to visualize this process in real time, this theory can be validated.

10. The probe tip is then repositioned such that additional channels are created.

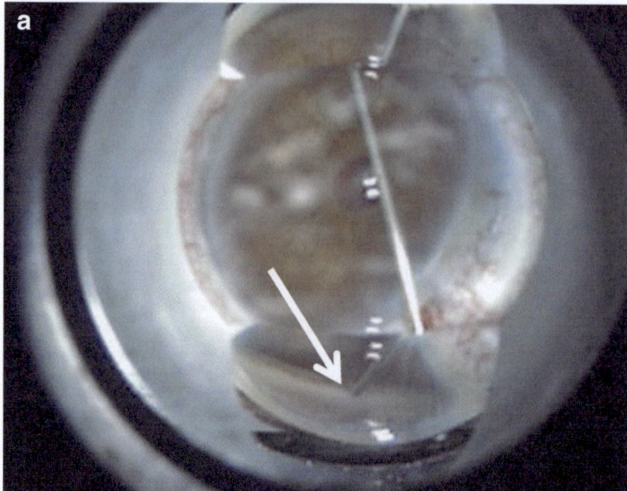

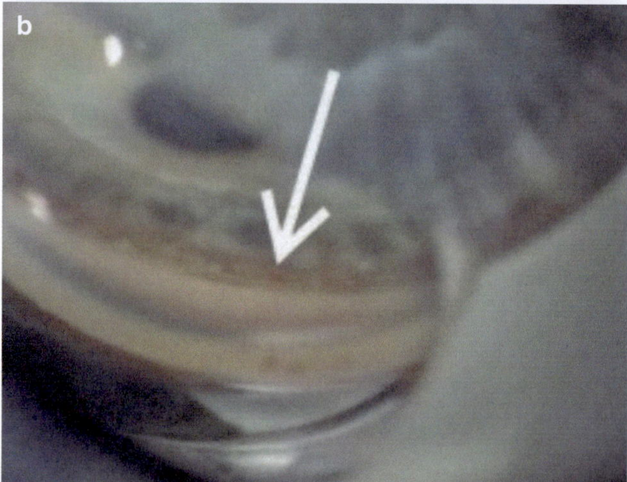

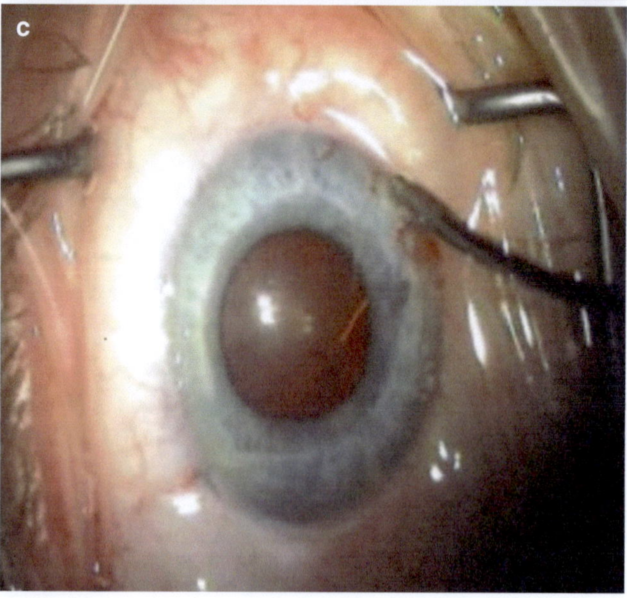

**Fig. 8.7** (**a**) Gonioscopic view of ELT probe in contact with TM (*white arrow*). (**b**) Blood in Schlemm's canal (*arrow*) verifies appropriate targeting and depth, gonioscopic view (**c**) Induced blood reflux verifies success and enables documentation of number of successful channels into Schlemm's canal (U. Giers)

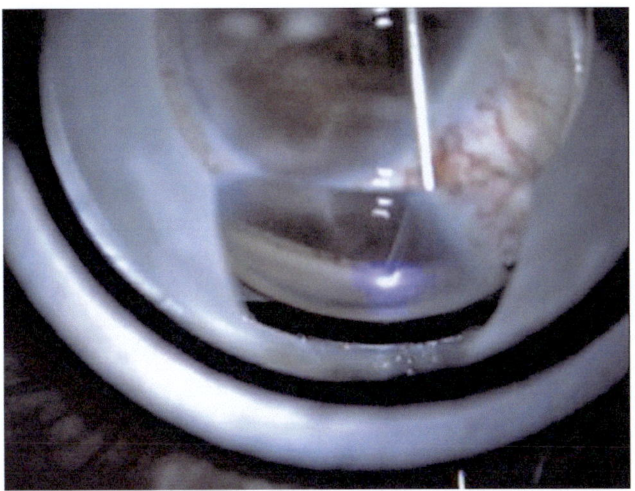

**Fig. 8.8**  In this series of chanels created tissue fluorescence is visible during a UV laser pulses creating the next channel. (U. Giers)

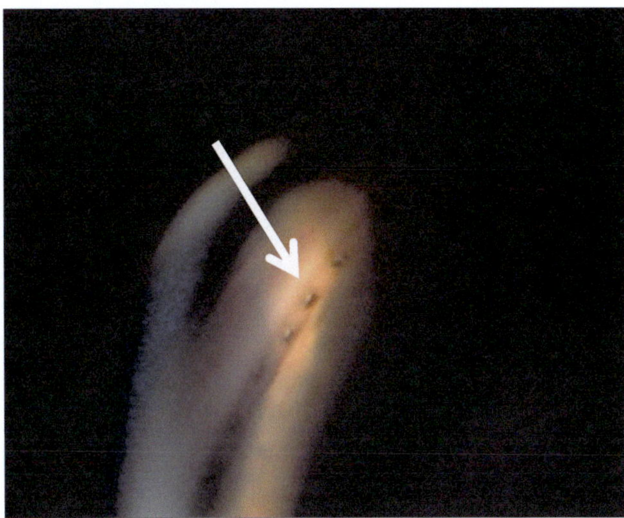

**Fig. 8.10**  Patent trabeculostomy channels into SC (*arrow*) documented 2.5 years after ELT (U. Giers)

4.  In the rare case of an anterior chamber inflammatory reaction, mydriatic eye drops may be added and the topical steroid can be intensified by surgeon's preference.

    Most surgeons discontinue all antiglaucoma medications after the procedure. However, preoperative antiglaucoma medication may be continued and later reduced dependent on the postoperative IOP. When medications are reduced, IOP should be monitored carefully on a regular basis.

## After ELT

Ideally, the patients are monitored postoperatively with gonioscopy in addition to IOP and the findings documented as to the number of sites noted patent. In the cases that have been followed in this manner, channels are documented to remain patent years after the ELT procedure, and in some of these patients, goniolens "pumping" can induce blood to appear at the channels, further confirming the patency of these channels into SC (Figs. 8.10 and 8.11).

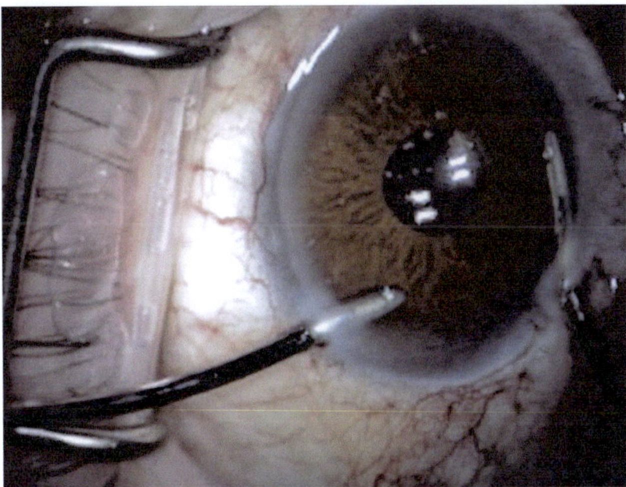

**Fig. 8.9**  Viscoelastic is exchanged for BSS (U. Giers)

11.  The probe is removed from the anterior chamber.
12.  The viscoelastic agent is exchanged for BSS with irrigation/aspiration, coaxial or bimanual (Fig. 8.9).
13.  The anterior chamber can be monitored for the number of and location of patent trabeculostomy sites by blood reflux from SC during a period of iatrogenic temporary hypotony during the viscoelastic agent/fluid exchange.

Postoperative topical ophthalmic medication regimens are individualized by surgeon, most include:

1.  A combination of steroid and antibiotic eye drops or ointment is administered immediately at the end of the procedure.
2.  The operated eye is shielded or patched, and the patient is released once stable, similar to after phacoemulsification.
3.  The operated eye is usually treated with a topical fixed combination of steroid (dexamethasone 0.1 %) and antibiotic eye drops qid for 1 week and then tapered over 3 weeks.

## ELT Enables Pneumatic Canaloplasty

Another potential benefit of ELT is that it enables pneumatic canaloplasty. Both endoscopic and gonioscopic views of ELT have revealed gas bubble formation in the tissue and in the anterior chamber as a result of photoablation of the TM tissue. When the ablation penetrates the outflow obstruction, gas is able to enter SC through the newly formed openings in the TM. The pressure of this gas has been proposed to localized dilate SC and collector channels to improve aqueous outflow, thereby lowering IOP. Observing gas bubbles exiting the adjacent openings confirms continuity of flow from SC.

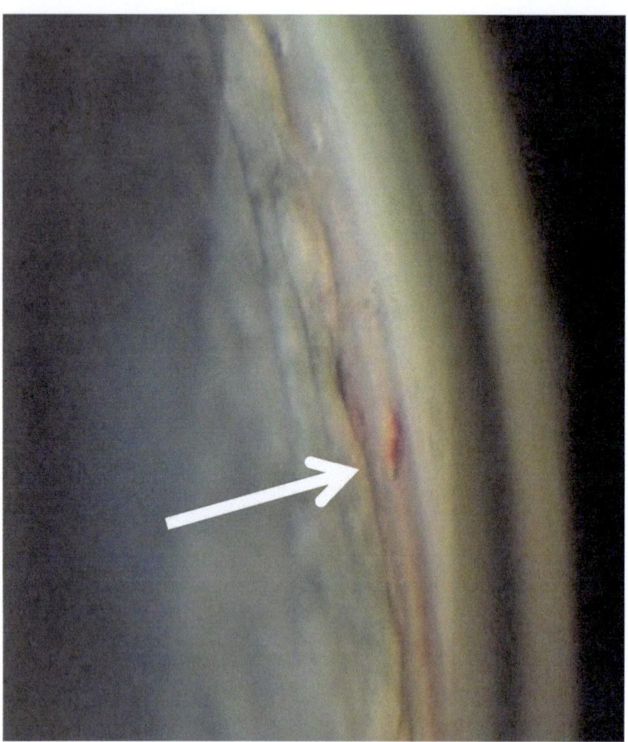

**Fig. 8.11** Blood Reflux at the patent opening of a laser channel (*white arrow*) from SC induced by "pumping" the goniolens 3 years after ELT (U. Giers)

This hypothesis has yet to be confirmed via real-time imaging or histologic studies. Real-time imaging and post-mortem histologic studies – in addition to histologic studies after ELT to evaluate the long-term changes which occur subsequent to this procedure – will enable better understanding of the effects and effectiveness of the current procedure and enable suggestions for modifications to potentially further improve the outcomes (Fig. 8.12).

## ELT as a MIGS Procedure

To date the study with the largest sample size was published in 2006 by Pache et al. [30]; included were 135 eyes with open-angle glaucoma or ocular hypertension after ELT alone or ELT combined with phacoemulsification. The follow-up was 1 year. Separately two subgroups (subgroup 1 with IOP >22 mmHg at baseline and subgroup 2 with IOP ≤21 mmHg at baseline) were analyzed. Success (IOP ≤21 mmHg, 20 % reduction from baseline, antiglaucoma medications (AGM) ≤ baseline, and no subsequent IOP-lowering surgery) was for ELT alone in SG1 57 % (baseline IOP: 27.9±3.9 mmHg; IOP at 1 year f/u: 19.3±5.5 mmHg) and in SG2 41 % (baseline IOP: 20.2±1.1 mmHg; IOP at 1 year f/u: 17.6±3.3 mmHg) and for ELT combined with phacoemulsification, in SG1 91 % (baseline IOP: 26.4±2.8 mmHg; IOP at 1 year f/u:

16.7±2.8 mmHg) and in SG2 52 % (baseline IOP: 19.6±1.1 mmHg; IOP at 1 year f/u: 16.3±2.2 mmHg). Hence, IOP reduction by ELT appears to be effective in both groups, but much more effective in eyes with higher baseline IOP. This finding has been confirmed by a later study [31].

Wilmsmeyer et al. investigated the outcome after ELT alone (70 eyes) versus ELT combined with phacoemulsification (60 eyes) after a follow-up of 2 years in patients with open-angle glaucoma or ocular hypertension [32]. They found a higher reduction of IOP after the combined procedure (IOP reduced from 24.1±0.7 mmHg to 16.8±1.0 mmHg at 2 years after ELT alone vs. reduced from 22.4±0.6 mmHg to 12.6±1.5 at 2 years after combined ELT. AGM use did not significantly change).

Babighian et al. found comparable results in an ELT study with 2 years follow-up of 21 eyes with open-angle glaucoma [33]. Success (IOP decrease 20%with no additional medication, or IOP-lowering surgery) rates were 54 % and IOP was reduced from 24.8±2.0 mmHg at baseline by 7.9±0.1 mmHg at 2 years.

Töteberg-Harms et al. were the first to show simultaneous IOP reduction and reduction of antiglaucoma medication after combined ELT (IOP changed from 25.33±2.85 at baseline to 16.54±4.95 at 1 year, while medications were reduced from 2.25±1.26 at baseline to 1.46±1.38 at 1 year) [34]. Complete success (IOP <21 mmHg, IOP reduction ≥20 %, without antiglaucoma medications, and no subsequent IOP-lowering surgery) in their study population was 21.4 % and qualified success (same as complete success but additional antiglaucoma medications were not excluded) 64.3 % at 1 year.

Berlin et al. investigated 46 eyes after combined ELT with a follow-up of 5 years [35]. They showed that IOP was lowered (from 25.5±6.3 at baseline to 15.9±3.0 at 5 years) and antiglaucoma medications were reduced (from 1.93±0.87 at baseline to 0.93±1.12 at 5 years) and that this effect remained stable over the entire follow-up of 5 years.

In conclusion, currently published data demonstrates that ELT can reduce IOP and lower antiglaucoma medication simultaneously for up to 5 years. The combined procedure, ELT plus phacoemulsification, appears to be more effective than ELT alone, and the amount of IOP lowering seems to be dependent on baseline IOP and is more effective in eyes with higher baseline IOP.

ELT has shown favorable outcomes in comparison to other outflow procedures (Fig. 8.13). Although ELT, as a laser treatment for glaucoma, is likely to be considered with other glaucoma laser treatments, it is not at all comparable in laser/tissue interaction effects. When compared to office laser treatments, patients undergoing SLT achieved up to a 27 % postoperative decrease in IOP but a negligible decrease in medications. Patients undergoing ALT had similar results, with a maximum of 23.5 % postoperative decrease in IOP and negligible decreases in medications.

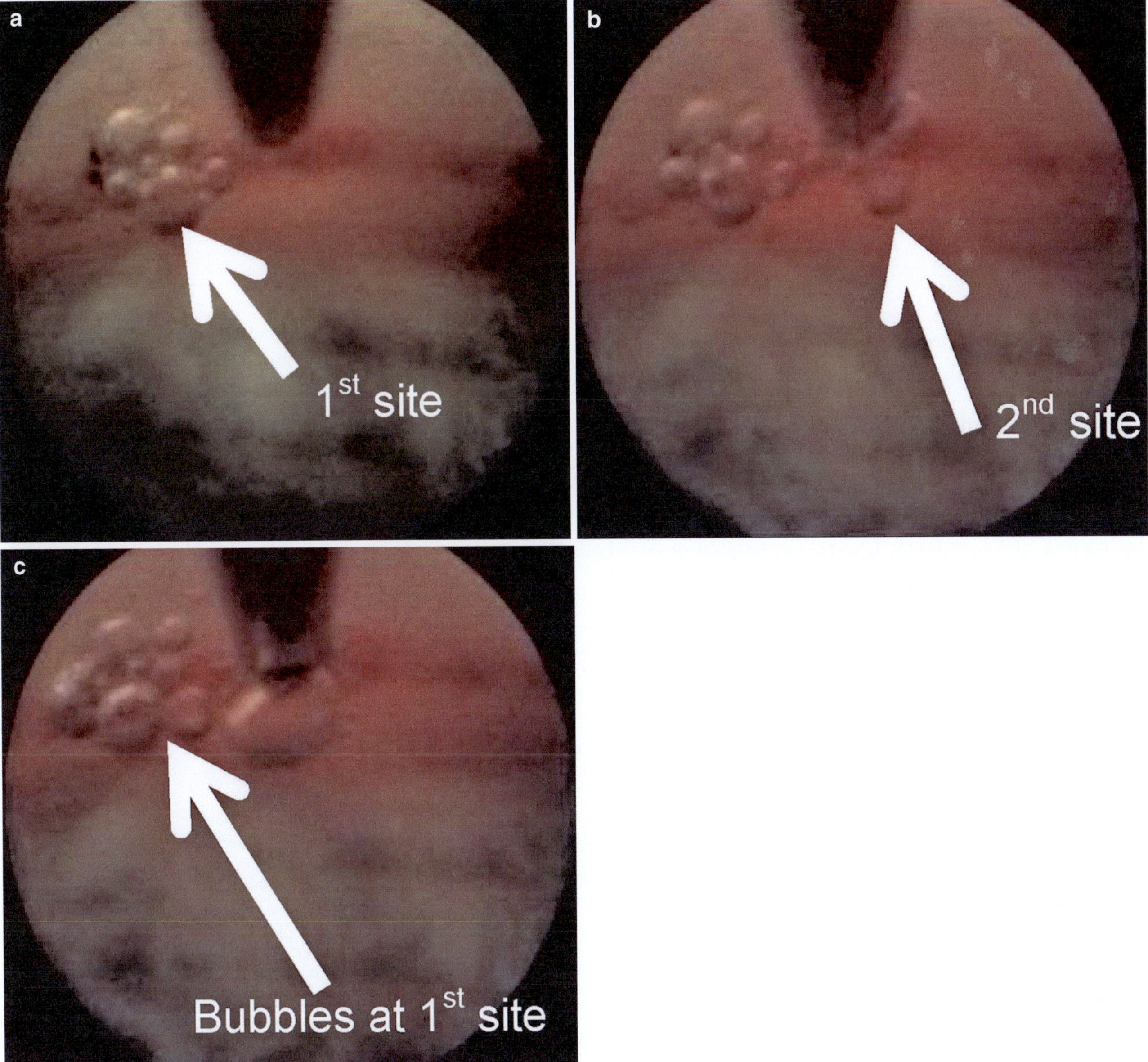



**Fig. 8.12** Photos of the ELT procedure demonstrating pneumatic canaloplasty: (**a**) Coaxial endoscopic view. (**b**) As the second channel is created into SC, (**c**) bubble expansion is observed at the first ELT site confirming channel patency into SC at both sites (J. Funk, Zurich, Switzerland)

ELT as an invasive surgical procedure has also shown favorable outcomes when compared to studies of other MIGS procedures. Patients undergoing clear cornea phacoemulsification followed by ab interno gonioscopically guided implantation of one iStent® achieved an IOP decrease of 21.4 % and a medication decrease of 75 % 1 year postoperative. Patients undergoing phacoemulsification cataract extraction combined with Trabectome achieved IOP decreases of up to 31.1 % and medication decreases of 41.7 %.

Of most relevance is the finding that ELT has shown comparable long-term IOP-lowering results (decrease of 38.6 % after 5 years) to significantly more invasive and risk inherent traditional OR surgeries, trabeculectomy and tube shunt procedures. Though trabeculectomy has demonstrated IOP decreases of 57.1 % and medication decreases of up to 90 %, when comparing the data obtained in the Collaborative Initial Glaucoma Treatment Study (CIGTS) on trabeculectomy patients, the 5-year postoperative ELT intraocular pressure measurements at all time points averaged 1 mm higher than those in the 300 patients who underwent trabeculectomy documented in CIGTS. In addition, the intraoperative complication rate of trabeculectomy was 12 %, and the 1 month postoperative complication rate was 50 % versus ELT intraoperative and postoperative complication rates of 0 % [36, 37].

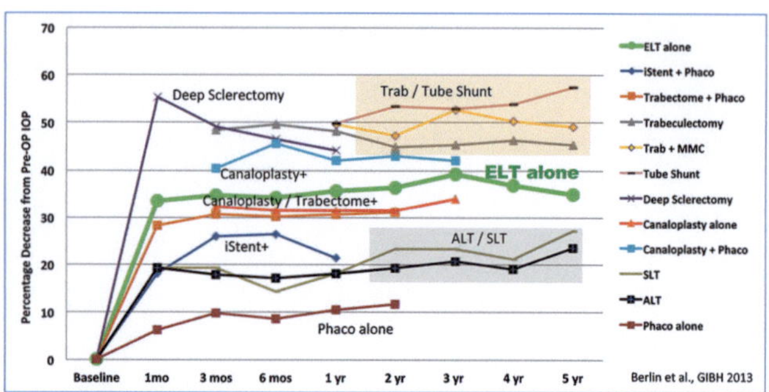


**Fig. 8.13** Comparison of various outflow procedures based on the results of exemplary studies.[35–44]

## Limitations and Next Generation

Feedback from leading surgeons who have performed over 2,000 ELT procedures have identified several limitations of the current ELT technique. The next generation of devices, called Guided ELT, is currently under development and is aimed to address the feedback from reporting surgeons. New sensors are being produced to better enable the surgeon to locate SC and TM and to automate the control of the laser, whereas currently tactile contact under observation provides surgeon feedback as to the amount of pressure applied to the meshwork. Furthermore, additional system controls assist in guiding the surgeon as to the depth of tissue removal and number of laser pulses required to penetrate the inner wall of SC with automated detectors and with imaging, especially real-time imaging. The progression of spectral-domain optical coherence tomography development in recent years shows promising abilities to meet these needs.

### Conclusion

ELT is a safe and effective method to reduce both IOP and medication use with minimal complications in most patients with open-angle glaucoma. It is less invasive relative to the methodologies currently being practiced and thus reduces many postoperative issues, including patient discomfort, number of postoperative visits required to assure adequacy and stability, and especially the long-term risks of filtering procedures. By essentially eliminating the damaging and healing response inducing thermal effects and tissue trauma seen with other laser and device procedures, ELT enables the lowering of IOP on a long-term basis. Furthermore, due to the minimal tissue trauma associated with UV tissue photoablation, only a few, small channels into SC have proven adequate to control the IOP. Unlike trabeculectomy, ELT preserves the integrity of the meshwork and SC, which restores the natural outflow without the creation of blebs or invasive foreign body implants. ELT is an important adjunct to cataract surgery, allowing physicians to address two pathologies in one surgical intervention without cutting the conjunctiva.

ELT has been approved for use in the European Union and Switzerland since 1998. Thousands of ELT procedures have been successful in lowering and maintaining lower IOP for years (Fig. 8.13). Currently, clinical studies are pending in both Canada and the United States. We look forward to a better future for our glaucoma patients and especially for their children.

## References

1. Saheb H, Ahmed II. Micro-invasive glaucoma surgery: current perspectives and future directions. Curr Opin Ophthalmol. 2012;23(2):96–104. doi:10.1097/ICU.0b013e32834ff1e7. Review. PubMed PMID: 22249233.
2. Krasnov MM. Laseropuncture of anterior chamber angle in glaucoma. Am J Ophthalmol. 1973;75:674.
3. Hager H. Besondere mikrochirurgische Eingriffe. 2. Teil. Erste Erfahrungen mit dem Argon-Laser-Geraet 800. Klin Monatsbl Augenheilkd. 1973;162:437–50.
4. Van der Zypen E, Fankhauser F, Bebie H, Marshall J. Changes in the ultrastructure of the iris after irradiation with intense light. A study of long-term effects after irradiation with argon ion. Nd:YAG and Q-switched ruby laser. Adv Ophthalmol. 1979;39:59–180.
5. Beckman H, Kinoshita A, Rota AN, et al. Transscleral ruby laser irradiation of the ciliary body in the treatment of intractable glaucoma. Trans Am Acad Ophthalmol Otolaryngol. 1973;46:423.
6. Beckman H, Sugar HS. Neodymium laser cyclocoagulation. Arch Ophthalmol. 1973;90:27.
7. Wise JB. Long-term control of adult open angle glaucoma by argon laser treatment. Ophthalmology. 1981;8:197.
8. Glaucoma Laser Trial Research Group. The Glaucoma Laser Trial (GLT) and glaucoma laser trials follow-up study. 7. Results. Am J Ophthalmol. 1995;120:718.
9. Odberg T, Sandvik L. The medium- and long-term efficacy of primary argon laser trabeculoplasty in avoiding topical medication in open-angle glaucoma. Acta Ophthalmol Scand. 1999;77:176–81.
10. Heijl A, et al. Reduction of IOP and glaucoma progression: results from the early manifest glaucoma trial. Arch Ophthalmol. 2002; 120:1268.
11. Shingleton BJ, et al. Long-term efficacy of argon laser trabeculoplasty: a 10-year follow-up study. Ophthalmology. 1998;100:1324.
12. Damji K, et al. Selective laser trabeculoplasty vs. argon laser trabeculoplasty: a prospective clinical trial. Br J Ophthalmol. 1995; 83:718.
13. Latina MA, Gulati V. Selective laser trabeculoplasty: stimulating the meshwork to mend its ways. Int Ophthalmol Clin. 2004;44:93.
14. Jacobi PC, Dietlein TS, Krieglstein GK. Prospective study of ab externo erbium:YAG laser sclerostomy in humans. Am J Ophthalmol. 1997;123:478.
15. Iwach AG, et al. Update on the subconjunctival THC:YAG (holmium) laser sclerostomy ab externo clinical trial: a 4-year report. Ophthalmic Surg Lasers. 1996;27:823.
16. Latina MA, Park C. Selective targeting of trabecular meshwork cells: in vitro studies of pulsed and CW interactions. Exp Eye Res. 1995;60:359.
17. Maguen E, Martinez M, Grundfest W, Papaioannou T, Berlin M. Excimer laser ablation of the human lens at 308 nm with a fiber delivery system. In: XXVI world congress of the International College of Surgeons, Milan, 3–9 July 1988.
18. Tripathy RC. Ultrastructure of Schlemm's canal in relation to aqueous outflow. Exp Eye Res. 1968;7:335–41.
19. Holmberg A. Schlemm's canal and the trabecular meshwork. An electron microscopic study of the normal structure in man and monkey (*Cercopithecus aethiops*). Doc Ophthalmol. 1965;19:339.

20. Berlin MS, Rajacich G, Duffy M. Excimer laser photoablation in glaucoma filtering surgery. Am J Ophthalmol. 1987;103: 713–714.3.

21. Huang S, Yu M, Feng G, Zhang P, Qiu C. Histopathological study of trabeculum after excimer laser trabeculectomy ab interno. Yan Ke Xue Bao. 2001;17(1):11–5.

22. Vogel M, Lauritzen K. Selective excimer laser ablation of the trabecular meshwork. Clinical results. Ophthalmologe. 1997;94(9): 665–7.

23. Jahn R, et al. Macroscopic and microscopic findings after excimer laser treatment of different tissue. J Clin Laser Med Surg. 1992; 10:413.

24. Neuhann T, Scharrer A, Haefliger E. Excimer laser trabecular ablation ab interno (ELT) in the treatment of chronic open-angle glaucoma, a pilot study. Ophthalmochirugie. 2001;13:3.

25. Laurtizen K, Vogel M. Trabecular meshwork ablation with excimer laser – a new concept of therapy for glaucoma patients. Invest Ophthalmol Vis Sci. 1997;38:826.

26. Walker R, Specht H. Theoretical and physical aspects of excimer laser trabeculotomy (ELT) ab interno with the AIDA laser operating at a wavelength of 308 nm. Biomed Tech (Berl). 2002; 47:106.

27. Kaufmann R, Hibst R. Pulsed Er:YAG and 308 nm UV excimer laser: an in vitro and in vivo study of skin-ablative effects. Laser Surg Med. 1989;9:132.

28. Berlin MS. Excimer laser applications in glaucoma surgery. Ophthalmol Clin North Am. 1988;1:255.

29. Berlin MS, et al. Excimer laser photoablation in glaucoma filtering surgery. Am J Ophthalmol. 1984;103:713.

30. Pache M, et al. Laser surgery for glaucoma: excimer-laser trabeculotomy. Klin Monbl Augenheilkd. 2006;223(4):303–7.

31. Töteberg-Harms M, Hanson JV, Funk J. Cataract surgery combined with excimer laser trabeculotomy to lower intraocular pressure: effectiveness dependent on preoperative IOP. BMC Ophthalmol. 2013 Jun 24;13:24. doi:10.1186/1471-2415-13-24. PubMed PMID: 23799932; PubMed Central PMCID: PMC3724507.

32. Wilmsmeyer S, et al. Excimer laser trabeculotomy: a new, minimally invasive procedure for patients with glaucoma. Graefes Arch Clin Exp Ophthalmol. 2006;244:670–6.

33. Babighian S, et al. Efficacy and safety of ab interno excimer laser trabeculotomy in primary open-angle glaucoma: two years of follow-up. Ophthalmologica. 2006;220:285–90.

34. Töteberg-Harms M, et al. One-year results after combined cataract surgery and excimer laser trabeculotomy for elevated intraocular pressure. Ophthalmologe. 2011;108(8):733–8.

35. Berlin MS, Kleinberg L, Stodtmeister R, Spitz J, Giers U. The IOP lowering efficacy of excimer-laser-trabeculostomy in open angle glaucoma patients remains consistent over 5 years. Poster session presented at: 23rd annual meeting of the American Glaucoma Society, San Francisco, 1–3 Mar 2013.

36. Stodtmeister R, Kleinberg L, Berlin M, Pillunat L, Giers U. Excimer laser trabeculostomy: 5-year follow-up. Abstract submitted for: the 111th congress of the German Association of Ophthalmologists, Berlin, 19–22 Sept 2013.

37. Jampel HD, Musch DC, Gillespie BW, et al., the CIGTS Study Group. Perioperative complications of trabeculectomy in the Collaborative Initial Glaucoma Treatment Study (CIGTS). Am J Ophthalmol. 2005;140:16–22.

# Laser Therapies: Cyclodestructive Procedures

Toshimitsu Kasuga, Guofu Huang, and Shan C. Lin

## Introduction

Cyclodestructive procedures are usually reserved for cases of glaucoma that are refractory to medical therapy and outflow surgeries and in eyes that have little or no visual potential. Cyclodestruction has been carried out by various methods including surgical excision [1], diathermy [2–4], ultrasound [5–7], cryotherapy [8–12], and laser [13–43]. Laser cyclophotocoagulation (CPC) has now become the principle method for surgically reducing aqueous inflow. The delivery of laser energy through the sclera may be performed by either the noncontact or contact method. In the noncontact approach, a slit lamp is employed to apply laser energy through the conjunctival/scleral surface. A contact lens is often applied to keep the eyelids open and blanch the conjunctiva. The focus of energy delivery is 1–1.5 mm behind the limbus and is offset from the aiming beam so that maximal therapeutic effect is at the level of the ciliary body. The potential benefits of the noncontact over the contact approach may include a more precise focus of laser energy on the ciliary body. More recently, contact CPC has gained favor as a preferred method for treating refractory cases of glaucoma.

A newer method to directly photocoagulate the ciliary body under endoscopic guidance—known as endoscopic CPC (ECP)—has become an increasingly important weapon in the glaucoma surgeon's armamentarium for the treatment of refractory glaucomas [44–53] and may have distinct advantages over the transscleral approach in eyes with visual potential. A classification of the modern techniques and lasers to achieve cyclodestruction is provided in Table 9.1 along with laser treatment parameters.

## Indications

### Transscleral Cyclophotocoagulation

TCP is an effective procedure for reducing intraocular pressure (IOP). It is usually performed after medications and filtration surgeries have been tried and have failed. TCP is a valuable option in eyes suffering from severe forms of glaucoma, such as neovascular or traumatic, typically with end-stage disease and significant loss of visual acuity. However, diode TCP has been successfully employed as a primary surgical procedure [54–57] and has been used in eyes with good visual acuity [40]. In fact, studies evaluating diode TCP as a primary surgery had good results both in open-angle and in angle-closure glaucomas, with few, if any, serious complications [55–57].

### Endoscopic Cyclophotocoagulation

As in TCP, ECP is indicated in glaucomas uncontrolled by medical treatment and/or filtering surgery [44–53]. It has been used in primary open-angle, pseudoexfoliation, neovascular, post-penetrating keratoplasty, pediatric, and angle-closure glaucomas [52]. ECP has been used as a primary glaucoma surgery in conjunction with cataract extraction [43–45] and also with tube shunt [58]. In fact, eyes with relatively intact central visual acuity may be appropriate candidates for ECP [43–45]·

T. Kasuga, MD
Department of Ophthalmology, University of California, 0730, 10 Koret Street, San Francisco, CA 94133-0730, USA

Department of Ophthalmology, Juntendo University School of Medicine, Tokyo, Japan

G. Huang, MD, PhD
Department of Ophthalmology, University of California, 0730, 10 Koret Street, San Francisco, CA 94133-0730, USA

State Key Laboratory of Ophthalmology, Zhongshan Ophthalmic Center, Sun Yat-sen University, Guangzhou, China

S.C. Lin, MD (✉)
Department of Ophthalmology, University of California, 0730, 10 Koret Street, San Francisco, CA 94133-0730, USA
e-mail: lins@vision.ucsf.edu

J.R. Samples, I.I.K. Ahmed (eds.), *Surgical Innovations in Glaucoma*, DOI 10.1007/978-1-4614-8348-9_9, © Springer Science+Business Media New York 2014

**Table 9.1** Laser treatment parameters for cyclophotocoagulation

| Type | Power/energy | No. of shots | Extent of area treated (degree) | Avoid 3 and 9 o'clock position |
|---|---|---|---|---|
| Noncontact TCP (Nd:YAG) | 7–8 W for 0.02 s | 24–32 (8 per quadrant) | 270–360 | Yes |
| Contact TCP (Nd:YAG) | 7–9 W for 0.7 s | 17–20 | 270 | Yes |
| Contact TCP (diode) | 1–2 W for 1.5–2.5 s | 17–20 | 270 | Yes |
| ECP (diode) | 0.3–0.9 W | Not applicable | 180–360 | No |

However, because the intraocular pressure (IOP) lowering with ECP seems modest, eyes with very elevated pressures may be considered more appropriate for TCP, particularly if potential visual function is limited. In the situation of excessively high IOP with intact vision, filtration surgeries are still the procedures of choice. These recommendations are based, in part, on the experience of the authors, since there are no studies that directly compare ECP to TCP or trabeculectomy in a randomized, controlled fashion. In, summary, the indications for ECP and TCP are evolving as both procedures are being performed in clinical scenarios that traditionally have been treated by filtrating procedures.

## Methods for TCP and ECP

Some of the techniques described below reflect the authors' personal preferences on the basis of their experience.

## Transscleral Cyclophotocoagulation (TCP)

Clinically, two types of laser are used for TCP: neodymium/yttrium-aluminum-garnet (Nd:YAG) and diode.

Preoperatively, a retrobulbar injection is provided because the application of laser energy can be painful, and there may be postoperative pain. The anesthetic agent(s) can be 2 % lidocaine only or a 1:1 mixture of 4 % lidocaine and 0.75 % bupivacaine. Topical proparacaine or tetracaine is also applied before laser treatment. A lid speculum is usually placed for optimal exposure, and the patient is in the supine or reclined position. Transscleral illumination may be used to identify ciliary body positioning with respect to the limbus.

### Nd:YAG TCP

The Nd:YAG laser (Surgical Laser Technologies Inc., Malvern, PA., USA) was one of the first used to do TCP. The probe is rounded and the energy delivery is through the center. Placement of the center of the probe is 1–2 mm posterior to the limbus, which can be measured by calipers but is often estimated visually. Energy levels are started at about 7 W and 0.7 s and are titrated to avoid an audible "pop" that indicates overtreatment and explosion of the ciliary body tissue. A total of 17–20 spots are usually applied to treat 270°

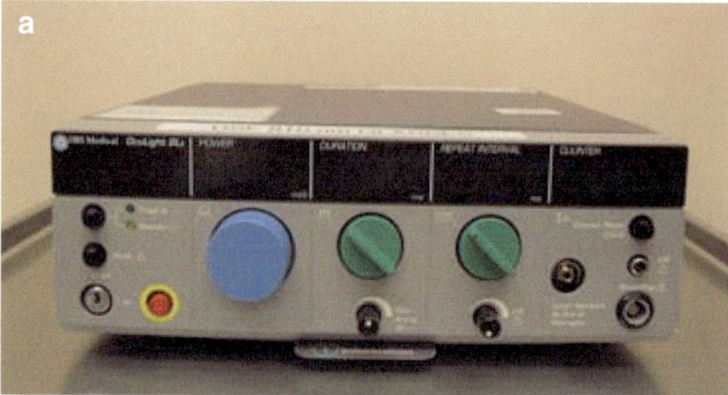

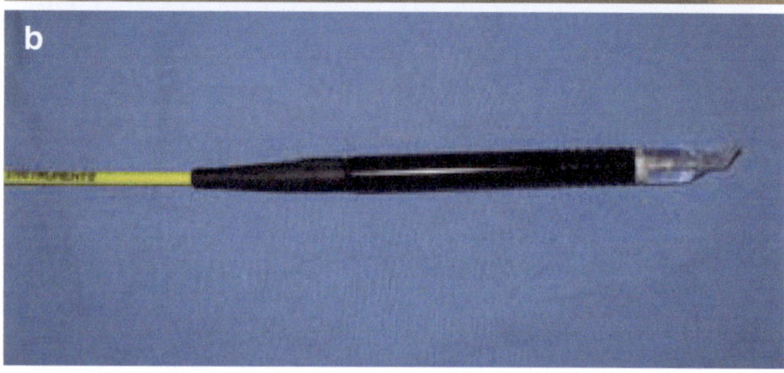

**Fig. 9.1** (**a**) Semiconductor diode laser (IRIS Oculight SLx, Iris Medical Inc., Mountain View, CA) for diode contact TCP. (**b**) "G-probe" handpiece for contact diode TCP

of ciliary processes, avoiding the 3 and 9 o'clock positions (Table 9.1).

After the procedure, atropine and dexamethasone ointments are applied and the eye is patched. The patch may be removed in the evening and glaucoma drops should be reinstituted. Prostaglandin analogs may be excluded in the short term if cystoid macular edema (CME) is a concern, and cholinergics should be temporarily discontinued to avoid increased inflammation. Postoperative prednisolone acetate 1 % is applied 4 times daily for 10–14 days and tapered according to inflammation.

### Diode TCP

The diode laser (IRIS Oculight SLx, Iris Medical Inc., Mountain View, CA, USA) (Fig. 9.1a) emits at 810 nm, and the probe has a tip shaped as a footplate (Fig. 9.1b). The heel of the footplate is placed adjacent to the limbus, and the laser tip is positioned 1.2 mm behind to be over the ciliary body. The laser tip, which protrudes 0.7 mm, should be applied firmly against the conjunctiva/sclera to help avoid conjunctival burn. The treatment principles are similar to the Nd:YAG laser. The initial energy settings are often about 1,000 mW with 2 s duration (Table 9.1). Lower energy levels can be used with longer durations. The 3 and 9 o'clock positions are avoided and a total of 17–20 shots are applied over approximately 270°. Energy is titrated to be just below that needed to achieve the "pop" sound. The number of treatment spots and avoidance of the 3 and 9 o'clock positions are similar to that for the Nd:YAG laser.

## Endoscopic Cyclophotocoagulation (ECP)

### Devices

The laser unit for ECP (Endo Optiks, Little Silver, NJ, USA) incorporates a diode laser that emits pulsed continuous-wave energy at 810 nm, a 175 W xenon light source, a helium-neon laser aiming beam, and video camera imaging, which can be recorded (Fig. 9.2a). All four elements are transmitted via fiber optics to an 18-gauge or 20-gauge probe (Fig. 9.2b), which is inserted intraocularly. The optimum focus for the laser is 0.75 mm from the probe tip, and the endoscope provides a 70° field of view. The main unit is compact and portable, with a maximum power output of 2.0 W. Controls for laser power and duration (up to 9.99 s) are adjustable on the console. The foot pedal controls laser firing with the actual duration of each treatment determined by how long the pedal is depressed.

### Techniques

The two main approaches to reach the ciliary processes are via a limbal or a pars plana entry. The limbal approach is preferred because anterior vitrectomy and associated risks for choroidal and retinal detachment are avoided. However, there are some cases that are more safely treated through the pars plana, for example, in aphakic eyes with posterior synechiae limiting access to the ciliary sulcus. In both situations, a retrobulbar block with lidocaine and bupivacaine is performed or general anesthesia can be considered in selective cases.

In the limbal approach, after dilation of the pupil with cyclopentolate 1 % and phenylephrine 2.5 %, a paracentesis is created and the anterior chamber is filled with viscoelastic agent, which is further used to expand the nasal posterior sulcus. This viscoelastic expansion of the posterior chamber allows for easier approach to the pars plicata with the ECP probe. A 2.2-mm or 2.5-mm keratome is then used to enter into the anterior chamber at the temporal limbus. After orientation of the probe image outside of the eye, the 18-gauge or 20-gauge probe is inserted through the incision and into the posterior sulcus. At this time, the ciliary processes are viewed on the monitor and treatment can begin. The laser is set at continuous wave and energy settings are 300–900 mW (Table 9.1). Approximately a 180° span of ciliary processes is photocoagulated (more area can be treated if a curved probe is used). Laser energy is applied to each process until shrinkage and whitening occur. Ciliary processes are

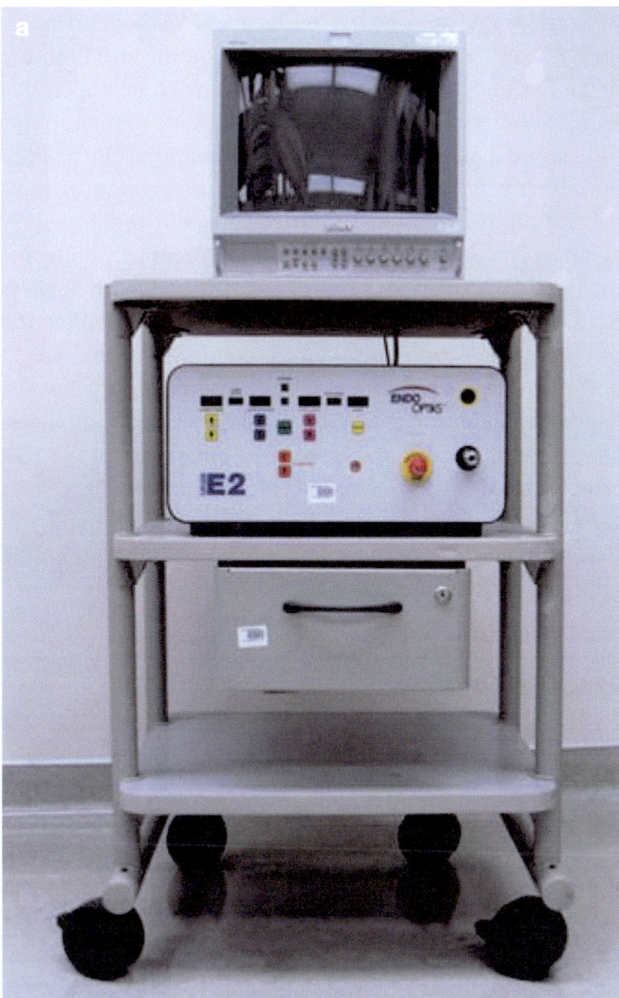

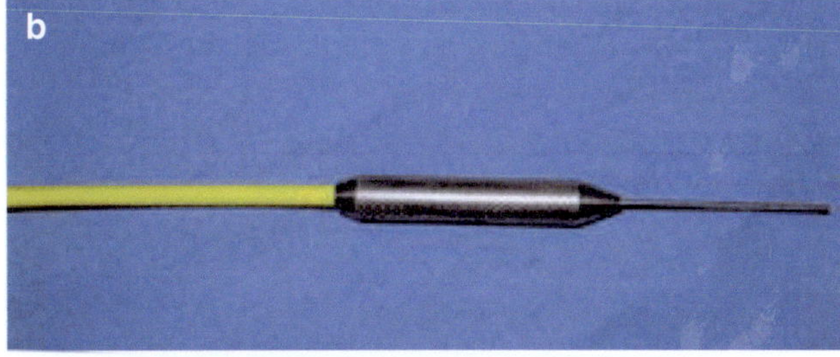

**Fig. 9.2** (**a**) ECP unit (Uram E2, Endo Optiks, Little Silver, NJ), including laser and monitor. (**b**) ECP probe (20 gauge)

treated individually or in a "painting" fashion across multiple processes. If excessive energy is used, the process explodes (or "pops") with bubble formation, leading to excessive inflammation and breakdown of the blood-aqueous barrier. After the nasal 180° of ciliary processes are treated, a separate incision is created at the nasal limbus in a similar fashion as above. The temporal processes are then photocoagulated for a total of up to 360°, if so desired. Typically, 180–360° are treated [46–48, 57]. The authors' preference is to treat 270–360° of processes. Before closure of the wounds, viscoelastic is removed from the anterior chamber with irrigation and aspiration.

In all patients, whether under local or general anesthesia, retrobulbar bupivacaine is administered before or at the end of the surgery to minimize postoperative pain. Sub-Tenon's injection of 1 mL of triamcinolone (40 mg/mL) is also given for inflammation. On postoperative day 1, patients are placed on a regimen of topical antibiotics, steroids, nonsteroidal anti-inflammatory agents, cycloplegics, and their preoperative glaucoma medications except for miotics and prostaglandin analogs because these may exacerbate intraocular inflammation or its sequelae. Antibiotics are discontinued after 1 week, and the steroids, nonsteroidal anti-inflammatory agents, and cycloplegics are tapered as inflammation subsides. Glaucoma medications are removed according to the IOP requirements. Administration of acetazolamide during the evening of surgery may be used to prevent a spike in IOP from underlying glaucoma, inflammation, or possible retained viscoelastic.

## Efficacy

### TCP

Both contact and noncontact TCP have been shown to be effective surgeries for treating refractory glaucoma in which medications and/or other surgeries have failed. Although definitions of success vary among reports, success rates for IOP control have been between 34 and 94 %, with mean follow-ups of up to 5.85 years [14–41].

The amount of energy used for diode TCP seems to correlate with treatment success without leading to a higher complication or vision loss rate [36–38]. In their meta-analysis of 47 eyes treated with diode TCP, Hauber and Scherer [37] found a direct, linear correlation between the success rate (IOP <22 mmHg) and total energy delivered. The risk of additional complications or vision loss was not increased. Murphy et al. [36] retrospectively examined the dose–response relation and found that there was a linear dose–response for the subset of neovascular glaucoma cases but not for the group as a whole. Although high pretreatment IOP and high mean energy per treatment episode seemed to be associated with hypotony, this was not statistically significant on multivariate analysis. Noureddin et al. [38] prospectively evaluated an aggressive protocol in 36 eyes. The relatively high treatment settings were kept constant (2,250 mW, 2,000 ms, and total of 28 shots), even if pops were achieved. The success rate (IOP <22 mmHg) was good (72 %), and there was relative preservation of vision without permanent complications. However, there are several studies which did not find a direct correlation between energy delivered and IOP outcome.

## ECP

One of the largest series on ECP was reported by our group at UCSF and included 68 eyes from 68 patients with refractory glaucoma of various diagnoses including primary open angle (16), congenital (12), chronic angle closure (11), aphakic/pseudophakic (10), uveitic (10), pseudoexfoliation/pigmentary (5), neovascular (2), and traumatic (2) [46]. With the exception of those undergoing combined cataract extraction and ECP, all of these patients had failed maximal medical therapy, and most had undergone one or more prior glaucoma surgeries. Eyes received between 180° and 360° of ciliary body treatment. The majority (56 eyes, 12 had concurrent cataract extraction) were treated through the limbal approach, whereas the others (12 eyes) were treated via pars plana incision. Seven percent had retreatment. The mean follow-up period was 12.9 months and the mean preoperative IOP was 27.7 mmHg. The mean IOP at last follow-up was 17.0 mmHg, yielding a mean reduction of 10.7 mmHg (34 % mean reduction). Glaucoma medication usage was reduced from an average of 3.0 preoperatively to 2.0 postoperatively. Success in controlling IOP <22 was 90 % at last follow-up.

Combined ECP with phacoemulsification cataract surgery has shown some promise in cases that are not refractory to maximal medical therapy [45–48]. Some studies on ECP have targeted childhood glaucomas [50–53]. As expected in pediatric cases, the success rate is not as high as in adult cases, and there is a greater risk for serious complications.

There are no studies directly comparing the results of ECP versus TCP. The lack of randomized trials may be related to the relatively different indications for each procedure.

## Complications

The complication rates after TCP varied significantly depending on the laser type, glaucoma diagnosis and severity, treatment protocol, and other factors [14–41]. Side effects include pain, vision loss, hyphema, anterior segment uveitis, cataract progression, hypotony, and phthisis. The outcome is typically less predictable than in other glaucoma surgeries, and there is often a substantial risk for significant vision loss [14–39]. In the more recent studies where TCP has been used as a primary surgery, the rates of serious complications seem to be none to few in number [40, 41, 54–57]. This may be related to the lower energy settings and the relatively higher proportion of primary open-angle glaucoma and less severe forms of glaucoma than in prior studies. In numerous studies, TCP has had significant rates of hypotony and/or phthisis, which may relate to its external approach. Greater energy is generally required to penetrate the sclera as compared with the endoscopic approach, which is a more selective ablation of the ciliary processes under direct visualization. Often there is overtreatment of the ciliary tissues and surrounding structures including the vasculature, the pars plana, and the iris root, all of which may potentially predispose to phthisis or hypotony. In addition, there have been several published reports of sympathetic ophthalmia (SO) after TCP [59–61]. Lam et al. [61] reported that the incidence of SO at their institution was 5.8 % (4 of 69) and 0.67 % (1 of 150) after noncontact and contact Nd:YAG CPC, respectively. Malignant glaucoma has also been reported after diode TCP [62, 63]. Recently, necrotizing scleritis has been reported after diode TCP [64, 65].

Complications associated with ECP included the following in the largest series [46] to date: fibrin exudate in 24 %, hyphema in 12 %, CME in 10 %, vision loss of 2 lines or greater in 6 %, and choroidal detachment in 4 %. Other reported serious complications include retinal detachment and hypotony, although most of these were in pediatric cases [50]. Although not reported in the literature, endophthalmitis and choroidal hemorrhage are potential severe complications, owing to the intraocular nature of the surgery.

## Summary

Both TCP and ECP are effective procedures for the treatment of glaucoma refractory to medical and/or prior surgical therapy. TCP is an extraocular procedure that has mainly been used as a "last resort" in eyes that had received prior filtration surgeries or that had very limited visual potential. However, more recently, there has been a trend toward using TCP as the primary surgery in eyes with relatively intact vision. ECP is an intraocular surgery that has also been used as a primary procedure—often combined with phacoemulsification cataract extraction—but should probably be considered almost exclusively in eyes that have good potential vision or that are the better-seeing eyes.

The major disadvantage of ECP is that it is an intraocular procedure with the attendant risks of penetrating surgeries. Endophthalmitis, choroidal hemorrhage, and retinal detachment are rare but remain potential complications. Therefore, although ECP may be a preferable surgery in cases of refractory glaucoma with relatively intact vision, it may not be recommended for eyes with very poor vision because it would unnecessarily expose them to such potential complications.

As TCP is increasingly employed as a primary surgical procedure for glaucoma, a prospective, randomized clinical trial comparing its safety and efficacy to ECP may be warranted.

## References


1. Bietti G. Surgical intervention on the ciliary body; new trends for the relief of glaucoma. JAMA. 1950;142:889–97.
2. Meyer SJ. Diathermy cauterization of ciliary body for glaucoma. Am J Ophthalmol. 1948;31:1540–6.
3. Weekers L, Weekers R. Nonperforating thermometric cyclodiathermy in treatment of hypertensive uveitis. Arch Ophthalmol. 1948;39:509–17.
4. Walton DS, Grant WM. Penetrating cyclodiathermy for filtration. Arch Ophthalmol. 1970;83:47–8.
5. Coleman DJ, Lizzi FL, Driller J, et al. Therapeutic ultrasound in the treatment of glaucoma. I. Experimental model. Ophthalmology. 1985;92:339–46.
6. Wilensky JT. Staphyloma formation as a complication of ultrasound treatment in glaucoma. Arch Ophthalmol. 1985;103:1113.
7. Coleman DJ, Lizzi FL, Driller J, et al. Therapeutic ultrasound in the treatment of glaucoma. II. Clinical applications. Ophthalmology. 1985;92:347–53.
8. De Roetth Jr A. Cryosurgery for the treatment of advanced chronic simple glaucoma. Am J Ophthalmol. 1968;66:1034–41.
9. De Roetth Jr A. Cryosurgery for the treatment of advanced chronic simple glaucoma. Trans Am Ophthalmol Soc. 1968;66:45–61.
10. Bellows AR, Grant WM. Cyclocryotherapy in advanced inadequately controlled glaucoma. Am J Ophthalmol. 1973;75:679–84.
11. Bellows AR, Grant WM. Cyclocryotherapy of chronic open-angle glaucoma in aphakic eyes. Am J Ophthalmol. 1978;85:615–21.
12. Caprioli J, Strang SL, Spaeth GL, Poryzees EH. Cyclocryotherapy in the treatment of advanced glaucoma. Ophthalmology. 1985;92: 947–54.
13. Beckman H, Kinoshita A, Rota AN, Sugar HS. Transscleral ruby laser irradiation of the ciliary body in the treatment of intractable glaucoma. Trans Am Acad Ophthalmol Otolaryngol. 1972;76: 423–36.
14. Beckman H, Sugar HS. Neodymium laser cyclocoagulation. Arch Ophthalmol. 1973;90:27–8.
15. Devenyi RG, Trope GE, Hunter WH, Badeeb O. YAG transscleral cyclocoagulation in human eyes. Ophthalmology. 1987;94: 1519–22.
16. Devenyi RG, Trope GE, Hunter WS. Neodymium-YAG transscleral cyclocoagulation in rabbit eyes. Br J Ophthalmol. 1987;71: 441–4.
17. McAllister J, O'Brien C. Neodymium: YAG transscleral cyclocoagulation: a clinical study. Eye (Lond). 1990;4(Pt 5):651–6.
18. Hampton C, Shields MB, Miller KN, Blasini M. Evaluation of a protocol for transscleral neodymium: YAG cyclophotocoagulation in one hundred patients. Ophthalmology. 1990;97:910–7.
19. Wright MM, Grajewski AL, Feuer WJ. Nd:YAG cyclophotocoagulation: outcome of treatment for uncontrolled glaucoma. Ophthalmic Surg. 1991;22:279–83.
20. Delgado MF, Dickens CJ, Iwach AG, et al. Long-term results of noncontact neodymium:yttrium-aluminum-garnet cyclophotocoagulation in neovascular glaucoma. Ophthalmology. 2003;110: 895–9.
21. Lin P, Wollstein G, Glavas IP, Schuman JS. Contact transscleral neodymium:yttrium-aluminum-garnet laser cyclophotocoagulation long-term outcome. Ophthalmology. 2004;111:2137–43.
22. Noureddin BN, Wilson-Holt N, Lavin M, et al. Advanced uncontrolled glaucoma. Nd:YAG cyclophotocoagulation or tube surgery. Ophthalmology. 1992;99:430–6; discussion 437.
23. Simmons RB, Shields MB, Blasini M, et al. Transscleral Nd:YAG laser cyclophotocoagulation with a contact lens. Am J Ophthalmol. 1991;15:671–7.
24. Echelman DA, Stern RA, Shields SR, et al. Variability of contact transscleral neodymium:YAG cyclophotocoagulation. Invest Ophthalmol Vis Sci. 1995;36:497–502.
25. Shields MB, Shields SE. Noncontact transscleral Nd:YAG cyclophotocoagulation: a long-term follow-up of 500 patients. Trans Am Ophthalmol Soc. 1994;92:271–83; discussion 283–7.
26. Brancato R, Giovanni L, Trabucchi G, Pietroni C. Contact transscleral cyclophotocoagulation with Nd:YAG laser in uncontrolled glaucoma. Ophthalmic Surg. 1989;20:547–51.

27. Schuman JS, Puliafito CA, Allingham RR, et al. Contact transscleral continuous wave neodymium:YAG laser cyclophotocoagulation. Ophthalmology. 1990;97:571–80.

28. Schuman JS, Jacobson JJ, Puliafito CA, et al. Experimental use of semiconductor diode laser in contact transscleral cyclophotocoagulation in rabbits. Arch Ophthalmol. 1990;108:1152–7.

29. Schuman JS, Bellows AR, Shingleton BJ, et al. Contact transscleral Nd:YAG laser cyclophotocoagulation. Midterm results. Ophthalmology. 1992;99:1089–94; discussion 1095.

30. Mankowska A, Zagorski Z, Kawa P, Mackiewicz J. Diode laser transscleral cyclo-photo-coagulation. Klin Oczna. 1999;101:103–4.

31. Rotchford AP, Jayasawal R, Madhusudhan S, et al. Transscleral diode laser cycloablation in patients with good vision. Br J Ophthalmol. 2010;94:1180–3.

32. Spencer AF, Vernon SA. "Cyclodiode": results of a standard protocol. Br J Ophthalmol. 1999;83:311–6.

33. Pucci V, Tappainer F, Borin S, Bellucci R. Long-term follow-up after transscleral diode laser photocoagulation in refractory glaucoma. Ophthalmologica. 2003;217:279–83.

34. Schlote T, Grub M, Kynigopoulos M. Long-term results after transscleral diode laser cyclophotocoagulation in refractory posttraumatic glaucoma and glaucoma in aphakia. Graefes Arch Clin Exp Ophthalmol. 2008;246:405–10.

35. Leszczynski R, Gierek-Lapinska A, Forminska-Kapuscik M. Transscleral cyclophotocoagulation in the treatment of secondary glaucoma. Med Sci Monit. 2004;10:CR542–8.

36. Murphy CC, Burnett CA, Spry PG, et al. A two centre study of the dose–response relation for transscleral diode laser cyclophotocoagulation in refractory glaucoma. Br J Ophthalmol. 2003;87:1252–7.

37. Hauber FA, Scherer WJ. Influence of total energy delivery on success rate after contact diode laser transscleral cyclophotocoagulation: a retrospective case review and meta-analysis. J Glaucoma. 2002;11:329–33.

38. Noureddin BN, Zein W, Haddad C, et al. Diode laser transcleral cyclophotocoagulation for refractory glaucoma: a 1 year follow-up of patients treated using an aggressive protocol. Eye (Lond). 2006; 20:329–35.

39. Kosoko O, Gaasterland DE, Pollack IP, Enger CL. Long-term outcome of initial ciliary ablation with contact diode laser transscleral cyclophotocoagulation for severe glaucoma. The Diode Laser Ciliary Ablation Study Group. Ophthalmology. 1996;103:1294–302.

40. Ansari E, Gandhewar J. Long-term efficacy and visual acuity following transscleral diode laser photocoagulation in cases of refractory and non-refractory glaucoma. Eye (Lond). 2007;21:936–40.

41. Youn J, Cox TA, Herndon LW, et al. A clinical comparison of transscleral cyclophotocoagulation with neodymium: YAG and semiconductor diode lasers. Am J Ophthalmol. 1998;126:640–7.

42. Lee PF. Argon laser photocoagulation of the ciliary processes in cases of aphakic glaucoma. Arch Ophthalmol. 1979;97:2135–8.

43. Lee PF, Shihab Z, Eberle M. Partial ciliary process laser photocoagulation in the management of glaucoma. Lasers Surg Med. 1980;1:85–92.

44. Uram M. Ophthalmic laser microendoscope ciliary process ablation in the management of neovascular glaucoma. Ophthalmology. 1992;99:1823–8.

45. Uram M. Combined phacoemulsification, endoscopic ciliary process photocoagulation, and intraocular lens implantation in glaucoma management. Ophthalmic Surg. 1995;26:346–52.

46. Chen J, Cohn RA, Lin SC, et al. Endoscopic photocoagulation of the ciliary body for treatment of refractory glaucomas. Am J Ophthalmol. 1997;124:787–96.

47. Gayton JL, Van Der Karr M, Sanders V. Combined cataract and glaucoma surgery: trabeculectomy versus endoscopic laser cycloablation. J Cataract Refract Surg. 1999;25:1214–9.

48. Lindfield D, Ritchie RW, Griffiths MF. "Phaco-ECP": combined endoscopic cyclophotocoagulation and cataract surgery to augment medical control of glaucoma. BMJ Open. 2012;2:pii: e000578.

49. Lima FE, Magacho L, Carvalho DM, et al. A prospective, comparative study between endoscopic cyclophotocoagulation and the Ahmed drainage implant in refractory glaucoma. J Glaucoma. 2004;13:233–7.

50. Neely DE, Plager DA. Endocyclophotocoagulation for management of difficult pediatric glaucomas. J AAPOS. 2001;5: 221–9.

51. Plager DA, Neely DE. Intermediate-term results of endoscopic diode laser cyclophotocoagulation for pediatric glaucoma. J AAPOS. 1999;3:131–7.

52. Al-Haddad CE, Freedman SF. Endoscopic laser cyclophotocoagulation in pediatric glaucoma with corneal opacities. J AAPOS. 2007;11:23–8.

53. Carter BC, Plager DA, Neely DE, et al. Endoscopic diode laser cyclophotocoagulation in the management of aphakic and pseudophakic glaucoma in children. J AAPOS. 2007;11:34–40.

54. Egbert PR, Fiadoyor S, Budenz DL, et al. Diode laser transscleral cyclophotocoagulation as a primary surgical treatment for primary open-angle glaucoma. Arch Ophthalmol. 2001;119:345–50.

55. Kramp K, Vick HP, Guthoff R. Transscleral diode laser contact cyclophotocoagulation in the treatment of different glaucomas, also as primary surgery. Graefes Arch Clin Exp Ophthalmol. 2002;240: 698–703.

56. Lai JS, Tham CC, Chan JC, Lam DS. Diode laser transscleral cyclophotocoagulation as primary surgical treatment for medically uncontrolled chronic angle closure glaucoma: long-term clinical outcomes. J Glaucoma. 2005;14:114–9.

57. Grueb M, Rohrbach JM, Bartz-Schmidt KU, Schlote T. Transscleral diode laser cyclophotocoagulation as primary and secondary surgical treatment in primary open-angle and pseudoexfoliative glaucoma. Long-term clinical outcomes. Graefes Arch Clin Exp Ophthalmol. 2006;244:1293–9.

58. Francis BA, Kawji AS, Vo NT, et al. Endoscopic cyclophotocoagulation (ECP) in the management of uncontrolled glaucoma with prior aqueous tube shunt. J Glaucoma. 2011;20:523–7.

59. Bechrakis NE, Muller-Stolzenburg NW, Helbig H, Foerster MH. Sympathetic ophthalmia following laser cyclocoagulation. Arch Ophthalmol. 1994;112:80–4.

60. Edward DP, Brown SV, Higginbotham E, et al. Sympathetic ophthalmia following neodymium:YAG cyclotherapy. Ophthalmic Surg. 1989;20:544–6.

61. Lam S, Tessler HH, Lam BL, Wilensky JT. High incidence of sympathetic ophthalmia after contact and noncontact neodymium:YAG cyclotherapy. Ophthalmology. 1992;99:1818–22.

62. Muqit MM, Menage MJ. Malignant glaucoma after phacoemulsification: treatment with diode laser cyclophotocoagulation. J Cataract Refract Surg. 2007;33:130–2.

63. Azuara-Blanco A, Dua HS. Malignant glaucoma after diode laser cyclophotocoagulation. Am J Ophthalmol. 1999;127:467–9.

64. Shen SY, Lai JS, Lam DS. Necrotizing scleritis following diode laser transscleral cyclophotocoagulation. Ophthalmic Surg Lasers Imaging. 2004;35:251–3.

65. Ganesh SK, Rishi K. Necrotizing scleritis following diode laser trans-scleral cyclophotocoagulation. Indian J Ophthalmol. 2006;54: 199–200.

# CO$_2$ Laser-Assisted Deep Sclerectomy

**10**

Alon Skaat and Shlomo Melamed

Lowering the intraocular pressure (IOP) is one of the main treatment goals in the management of glaucoma patients, aiming to arrest the characteristic progressive optic neuropathy and prevent the expected irreversible visual field loss [1, 2]. This goal may be achieved by either medical, laser, or surgical modalities.

Surgical treatment is usually indicated when glaucomatous optic neuropathy worsens or visual field damage progresses despite laser trabeculoplasty or maximally tolerated medical therapy.

Trabeculectomy is the most common surgical approach to reduce IOP in glaucoma patients. Trabeculectomy is considered effective in many cases but is associated with a variety of complications, such as shallow anterior chamber [3] due to overfiltration, hypotony maculopathy, choroidal detachment or hemorrhage, hyphema, aqueous misdirection, cataract, or endophthalmitis [4–6]. Most of these complications are due to the fact that the surgery is invasive and involves penetration of the AC. Other procedures such as glaucoma drainage devices (GDD) which shunt aqueous from the AC to the posterior sub-conjunctival space may be also associated with similar complications like hypotony, diplopia, tube extrusion, and infection [7, 8].

The non-penetrating deep sclerectomy (NPDS) procedure, ab externo filtration procedure, first described by Krasnov [9] and Walker [10] at 1964, was aimed to prevent

these complications. The procedure includes unroofing of Schlemm's canal and exposure of the juxtacanalicular trabeculum in order to allow effective fluid percolation [11], while the AC is not penetrated. This procedure was suggested to have a higher safety profile as compared to trabeculectomy [12, 13] with almost similar success in controlling IOP compared to trabeculectomy [3, 14–16].

One of the main drawbacks of the procedure is its technical difficulty. In the manual NPDS procedure, a deep scleral flap is first dissected and then a second scleral layer is cut out, leaving an exposed thin layer of trabecular meshwork and Descemet's membrane. Fluid percolation through the remaining tissue is the desired outcome of the procedure. However, since the scleral tissue needs to be dissected manually to more than 95 % of its depth (leaving a residual intact layer of only several tens of microns), inadvertent perforation is a frequent complication. These perforations in manual NPDS occur in about 30–50 % of the cases in the early stages of the learning curve of the procedure [17]. In the case of perforation, the procedure may be converted to a conventional trabeculectomy; however, the high rates of perforation limit the use of the manual deep sclerectomy as a treatment procedure. On other hand, while the risk of perforation is relatively high, if the tissue is not cut deep enough, the filtration may not be effective, and the intraocular pressure will not be reduced to the desired level. Therefore, in order to achieve good clinical results, this procedure requires high surgical skills and experience with a long learning curve. For that reason, the manual NPDS was adopted only by a minority of surgeons and did not gain a wide popularity in spite of its advantages [18] which include less frequent flattening of the anterior chamber, less choroidal detachments, and reduced inflammation due to the avoidance of penetrating the anterior chamber.

Many modifications, such as yttrium aluminum garnet (YAG) laser goniopuncture, placing spacer under the flap, and antimetabolite applications, improved the efficacy of the procedure, however not yet to the level of a wide acceptance [18].

In order to improve the clinical outcomes, attempts to use laser technology in the NPDS have been studied. The purpose


A. Skaat, MD (✉)
New York Eye & Ear Infirmary,
321 East 13 St. (Apt 10A), New York, NY 10003, USA

The Sam Rothberg Glaucoma Center, Goldschleger
Eye Institute, Sheba Medical Center, Tel Aviv
University, Tel Hashomer, Ramat Gan 52621, Israel
e-mail: skaatalon@gmail.com

S. Melamed, MD
The Sam Rothberg Glaucoma Center, Goldschleger
Eye Institute, Sheba Medical Center, Tel Aviv
University, Tel Hashomer, Ramat Gan 52621, Israel
e-mail: melamed.shlomo@gmail.com



J.R. Samples, I.I.K. Ahmed (eds.), *Surgical Innovations in Glaucoma*,
DOI 10.1007/978-1-4614-8348-9_10, © Springer Science+Business Media New York 2014

was based on the laser's properties that include reduced collateral tissue damage and ability to achieve isolated subsurface surgical effect in the sclera [19].

Attempts to use femtosecond laser [20], argon fluoride excimer laser [21], and erbium/YAG laser [22, 23] were reported in the literature although none of these attempts have been demonstrated in continuing clinical trials.

As opposed to the lasts, the $CO_2$ laser seemed to have several advantages.

The unique characteristic of the $CO_2$ laser is its effectiveness in ablating only dry tissues (therefore its common use in general and plastic surgeries). This inherent characteristic is due to the fact that the far-infrared radiation of this laser (wavelength of 10,600) is absorbed in water and thus is ineffective when applied over wet tissues. Applying $CO_2$ laser energy on the dried scleral tissue over the trabecular meshwork then results in a localized ablation of the sclera up until the point at which fluid begins to percolate through the thinned wall of the anterior chamber. Once percolation begins, further laser application is ineffective, and thus, further tissue ablation does not occur. In this fashion, tissue ablation is "automatically" halted when the desired endpoint of the procedure is achieved [24].

The use of these unique characteristics in NPDS was first described by Assia et al. [24, 25]. The OT-135 system ("IOPtiMate"; IOPtima Ltd., Ramat Gan, Israel), which was developed for this purpose, includes a Beam Manipulator System conjugated with an "off-the-shelf" $CO_2$ laser (Fig. 10.1). This system enables deep tissue ablation with minimal risk of perforation. As such, it offers an alternative to the manual NPDS, making the procedure simpler and less surgeon dependent [26]. The new technique was called CLASS – $CO_2$ laser-assisted deep sclerectomy.

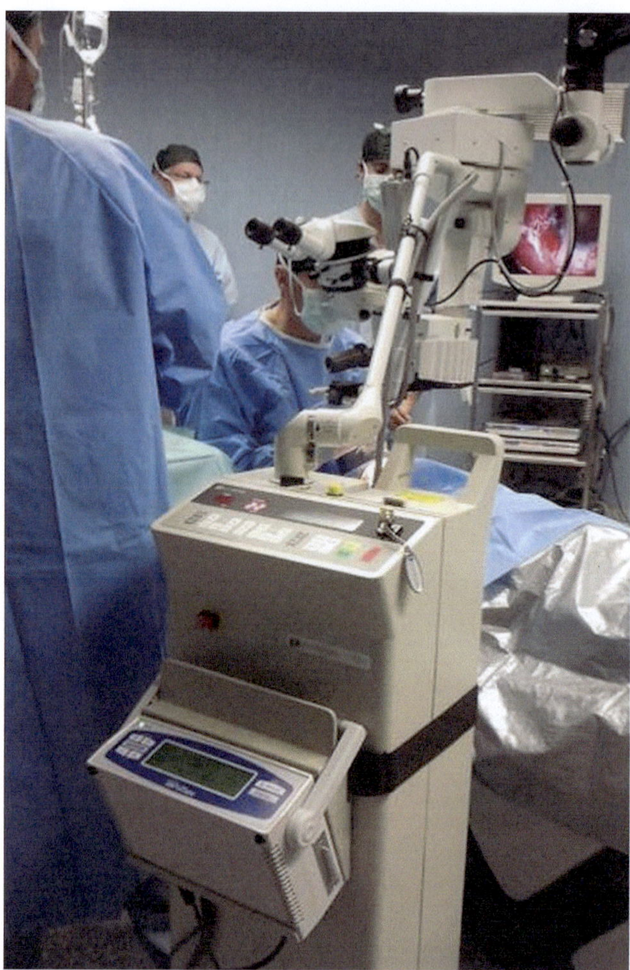

**Fig. 10.1** CLASS OT-135 system ("IOPtiMate"; IOPtima Ltd., Ramat Gan, Israel) consists of a Beam Manipulator System conjugated with a $CO_2$ laser

## CLASS: Surgical Procedure

The procedure is performed under sub-conjunctival anesthesia with 2 % lidocaine without epinephrine. The perilimbal conjunctiva and Tenon's capsule are dissected. A half-thickness $5 \times 4$ mm superior scleral flap is fashioned with a crescent knife. A red laser (HeNe) aiming beam is used to mark the scanning area boundaries, with four clear red dots at the corners. Scan dimensions (width and length) can be changed within the range of 1–4 mm. Initially a wide scan area is used to repeatedly remove layers of sclera until a percolation zone can be readily identified. The $CO_2$ laser is repeatedly applied with time intervals of 2–3 s between applications to allow percolation to take place and be detected until sufficient percolation zone of at least 3 mm in region length is clearly evident. The scleral flap is then repositioned and sutured with 10-0 nylon sutures. Figure 10.2 demonstrates the CLASS steps.

## Preclinical and Clinical Studies

The preclinical studies (which took place at Goldschleger Eye Research Institute, Sheba Medical Center, Israel; at the Laboratory for Intraocular Microsurgery and Implants, Meir Medical Center, Kfar Saba, Israel; and at the Center for Research on Ocular Therapeutics and Biodevices, Storm Eye Institute, Medical University of South Carolina, USA) were performed on varied experimental models [25]: enucleated pig eyes, live rabbit eyes, and human cadaver eyes. Scleral ablation and aqueous percolation were repeatedly achieved in all models. Histology in each case demonstrated deep scleral craters with thin intact sclera-corneal tissue layer at the ablation area (Fig. 10.3), while the neighboring structures (including sclera, cornea, iris base, and ciliary body) remained undamaged. The results of these experiments indicated that CLASS is a safe and effective procedure for achieving effective fluid percolation.

**Fig. 10.2** CLASS – surgical procedure steps

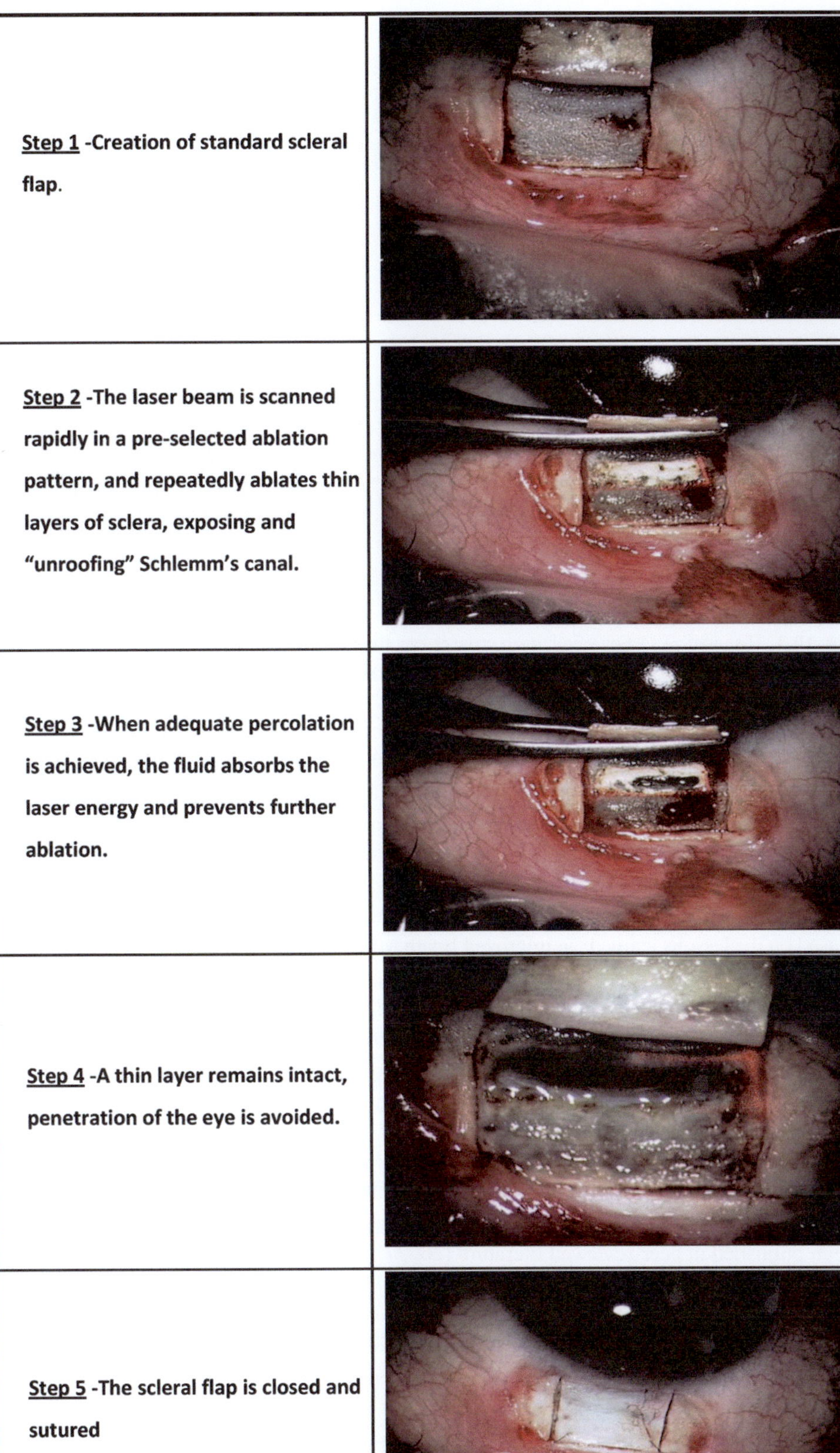

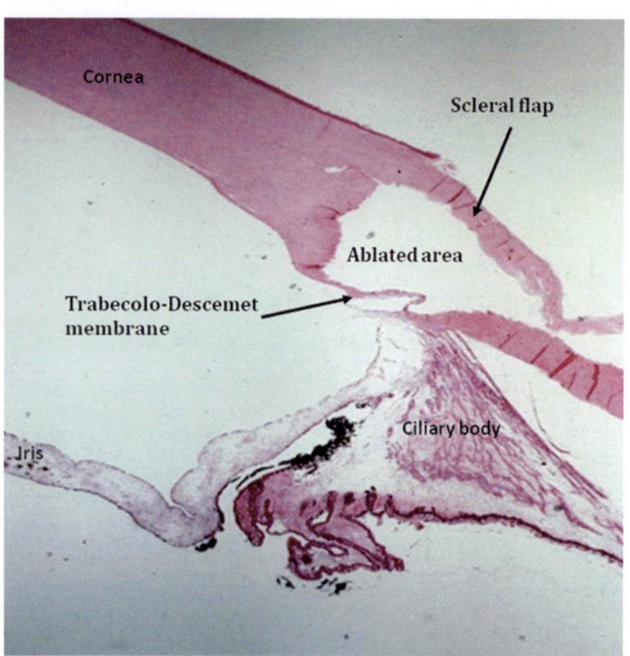



**Fig. 10.3** Histological section of a human cadaver eye after CLASS. A half depth scleral flap covers a residual thin intact layer overlying the trabecular meshwork and peripheral Descemet's membrane

Most of the experiments used prior models of the system (OT-133 and OT-134 "IOPtiMate"; IOPtima Ltd., Ramat Gan, Israel) which were involved with several drawbacks, such as an excessive charring and a tissue coagulation around the treated area, which cause early fibrosis, adhesions, and surgery failure, as reported previously in sporadic cases [24, 25]. Based on the lessons learned, an improved Beam Manipulator System version (OT-135) (Fig. 10.1) was developed using a higher power laser with the ability to diminish localized heating and tissue photocoagulation, increase the control on the ablation process, and minimize the adverse effects to neighbor tissues.

The preclinical experiments have led the way to multicenter clinical trials to come.

Up to now, the technology was clinically tested in several multicenter and multinational studies. Some have already been published in peer-reviewed literature [26, 27].

Studies were done in nine sites: Israel, Tel Hashomer (Prof. Melamed and Dr. Skaat); Israel, Kfar Saba (Prof. Assia and Dr. Geffen); Mexico, Mexico City (Dr. Gil); India, Madanapalle (Dr. Naveen); Russia, Moscow (Dr. Anisimova); Italy, Ancona (Dr. Mariotti); Spain, Valencia (Dr. Muñoz); Swiss, Genève (Dr. Shaarawy); and Swiss, Lausanne (Dr. Mermoud).

A total number of 111 patients with either primary open-angle glaucoma (POAG) or exfoliative glaucoma (PEXG) who were candidates for primary glaucoma filtration surgery were included in the studies. Inclusion and exclusion criteria are shown in Table 10.1. Demographic data is shown in

Table 10.2. Comprehensive ophthalmologic examination was performed before and at intervals of 1 day, 1 week, and 1, 3, 6, 12, and 24 months after the surgical procedure. The examination included assessment of best-corrected visual acuity, IOP measurement using Goldmann applanation tonometry (average of three repeated measurements taken at the same time of the day ±1 h), slit-lamp examination, optic disc evaluation, and posterior pole examination. Patients also underwent gonioscopy and assessment of central corneal thickness (average of three repeated measurements). Intraoperative and postoperative complications were documented. The incidence of intraoperative macro-perforations, defined as perforations accompanied by iris prolapse or anterior chamber swallowing or both, was also recorded.

"Complete success" was defined as IOP values measure at the 12-month endpoint, ranging between 5 and 21 mmHg, and IOP reduction equal to or more than 20 % as compared to baseline IOP without additional hypotensive medications or repeat filtration surgery. The same outcome, but including also subjects who required hypotensive medications postoperatively, was defined as "qualified success." Failure was defined as an IOP value lower than 5 and higher than 21 mmHg, IOP reduction of less than 20 % as compared to baseline IOP, severe loss of vision, or the need to undergo additional glaucoma surgery.

The preoperative IOP of 25.7±5.25 mmHg (mean±SD) dropped to 13.5±3.7 mmHg at 6 months, to 13.6±4.04 mmHg at 12 months, and to 13.5±3.05 mmHg at 24 months postoperatively, yielding average IOP reductions at 6, 12, and 24 months of 12.4±6.52 mmHg (47 %), 12.2±7.03 mmHg (54 %), and 14.8±8.12 mmHg (52 %), respectively ($P<0.001$).

The IOP measurements from the preoperative stage up to 24 months postoperatively are shown in Fig. 10.4.

Complete success was achieved by 64 and 52 % of the patients at 12 and 24 months, respectively, whereas qualified success was achieved by 86 and 80 % of the patients at 12 and 24 months, respectively.

Preoperative use of hypertensive medications per patient dropped from an average of 2.3 ± 1.2 to 0.5 ± 0.84 at 12-month visit ($P<0.001$) and to 0.4±0.75 at 24-month visit.

Shallow diffuse blebs were observed in all cases. No needling procedures, YAG laser goniopuncture, suture lysis, or 5FU injections were needed.

No device malfunctions were reported.

Choroidal detachment was reported in four cases (from which two cases were needed surgical interventions). No other major complications (such as hypotony maculopathy, aqueous misdirection, or endophthalmitis) were reported. There were minor postoperative complications, which were all transient within few weeks, and are shown in Table 10.3.

The use of mitomycin-C (MMC) a well-known drug used during the initial stages of glaucoma surgery to prevent the scarring and fibrosis of the filtering bleb, was left to the

**Table 10.1** CLASS studies inclusion and exclusion criteria

**Inclusion criteria**

1. Patient age 18 years or older
2. Patient must have primary open-angle glaucoma or pseudoexfoliative glaucoma in the study eye; diagnosis is based on glaucomatous optic neuropathy, Shaffer angle of +2, and visual field defect attributed to glaucoma (at least two consecutive abnormal visual field test results, defined as a pattern SD (PSD) outside the 95 % normal confidence limits and/or glaucoma Hemifield Test (Carl Zeiss Meditec, Inc.))
3. Treated eye must be phakic or pseudophakic eye with no ocular disorder or ocular diseases but cataract and no prior surgical intervention in study eye but cataract surgery with clear corneal incision and trabeculoplasty performed >3 months ago
4. Patient is indicated for filtration surgery
5. Presence of ocular hypertension, defined as an intraocular corrected pressure (IOP) $\geq$21 mmHg in the study eye while on maximal tolerated medications.[a] This IOP level of above or equal 21 mmHg must be verified and recorded in the most recent two consecutive measurements (but not taken on the same day) prior to operation
6. Best-corrected visual acuity (BCVA) better than 20/200 in the fellow eye
7. Optic neuropathy is attributed exclusively to glaucoma

[a]Patients on maximal tolerated medications refer to those patients who cannot or will not use medications due to cost issues, memory problems, difficulty of instillation, or inability to tolerate medications

**Exclusion criteria**

1. Diagnosis of glaucoma other than primary open-angle glaucoma or pseudoexfoliative glaucoma
2. History of previous intraocular surgery in the study eye, referring to but not limited to glaucoma filtering surgery (penetrating and non-penetrating), laser gonioplasty, corneal transplant, and history of any other laser ocular procedures except for laser trabeculoplasty surgery
3. Laser trabeculoplasty surgery within the last 3 months in the study eye
4. Study eye is aphakic
5. Patients with previous cataract extraction with scleral tunnel and or conjunctival incision in the study eye
6. Proliferative or severe nonproliferative retinopathy in either eye
7. Eyes with (dilated) pupil diameter of less than 2 mm in the study eye
8. Discernable congenital anomaly of the anterior chamber angle in the study eye
9. Patients with neuropathy other than glaucoma in the study eye
10. Patient with RVO (retinal vein occlusion) or RAO (retinal artery occlusion) in the study eye
11. History of prior vitrectomy or vitreous hemorrhage (VH) in the study eye
12. Patient with media opacification which may interfere with optic nerve evaluation in the study eye
13. Patient with ocular malformations such as microphthalmia in the study eye
14. Patient with concurrent inflammatory/infective eye disorder (e.g., episcleritis, scleritis) in the study eye
15. Patient with any sign of past or present uveitis (anterior/posterior)
16. Patient with known allergy to the study medications
17. Patient with severe systemic disease or disabling conditions such as chronic renal failure requiring dialysis, severe and disenabling neurological disease, and post organ transplants
18. Patient participating in another clinical trial or participation in another clinical trial is <3 months
19. Patient is pregnant or breastfeeding

**Table 10.2** Demographic data of CLASS group

|  |  | $n$ | % |
|---|---|---|---|
| Total number of patients |  | 111 |  |
| Mean age $\pm$ SD |  | 69.3 $\pm$ 1.2 |  |
| Mean age at diagnosis $\pm$ SD |  | 64.2 $\pm$ 1.3 |  |
| *Gender* | Male | 62 | 55.9 |
|  | Female | 49 | 44.1 |
| *Race* | African | 2 | 1.8 |
|  | Caucasian | 82 | 73.9 |
|  | Hispanic | 14 | 12.6 |
|  | Indian | 13 | 11.7 |
| *Glaucoma type* | Primary open angle | 85 | 76.6 |
|  | Pseudoexfoliative | 26 | 23.4 |

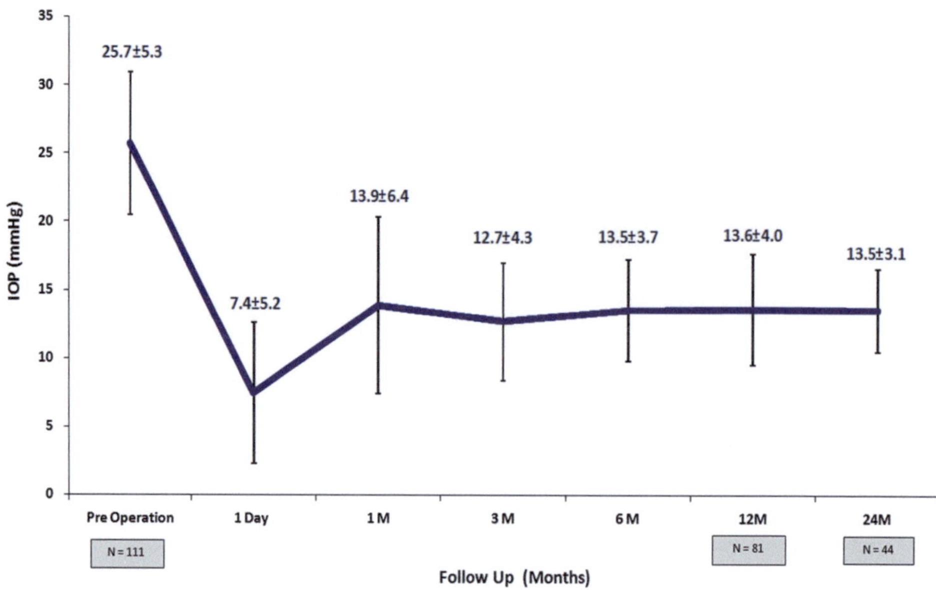

**Fig. 10.4** Cumulative IOP±SD measurements from the preoperative stage up to 24 months postoperatively



**Table 10.3** Summary of minor complications

| Complications | N (%) |
|---|---|
| Hypotony | 2.7 |
| Wound leak | 4.5 |
| Chorodial effusion/detachment | 3.6 |
| Hyphema | 3.6 |
| Iris prolapse/incarceration | 6.3 |
| Dry eye/keratitis | 0.9 |

surgeon's discretion and was applied eventually in 93 % of the cases at a concentration of 0.04 % for 60 s. This use is based on a recent publications and meta-analysis [28] which demonstrated that intraoperative use of MMC in non-penetrating glaucoma surgeries is associated with greater IOP-lowering efficacy, with statistically significant differences in IOP reduction after 1 year postoperatively.

## Summary

CLASS procedure utilizes the unique physical properties of the $CO_2$ laser and its ability to ablate dry tissue with almost complete absorption of the energy by percolating aqueous humor. By this, it protects deeper tissues like trabecular meshwork from the laser energy and enables an accurate dissection of the scleral wall and unroofing of the Schlemm's canal without penetrating the anterior chamber (making this procedure practically an extraocular procedure). It has an excellent safety and efficacy profile and enables the surgeon and patient to enjoy the advantages of NPDS without its major complications and with a very short learning curve only.

## References


1. The Advanced Glaucoma Intervention Study (AGIS): 7. The relationship between control of intraocular pressure and visual field deterioration. The AGIS Investigators. Am J Ophthalmol. 2000;130(4):429–40.
2. Musch DC, Gillespie BW, Lichter PR, et al. Visual field progression in the collaborative initial glaucoma treatment study the impact of treatment and other baseline factors. Ophthalmology. 2009; 116(2):200–7.
3. Cillino S, Di Pace F, Casuccio A, et al. Deep sclerectomy versus punch trabeculectomy with or without phacoemulsification: a randomized clinical trial. J Glaucoma. 2004;13(6):500–6.
4. Edmunds B, Thompson JR, Salmon JF, Wormald RP. The national survey of trabeculectomy. III. Early and late complications. Eye (Lond). 2002;16(3):297–303.
5. Stalmans I, Gillis A, Lafaut AS, Zeyen T. Safe trabeculectomy technique: long term outcome. Br J Ophthalmol. 2006;90(1):44–7.
6. Ang GS, Varga Z, Shaarawy T. Postoperative infection in penetrating versus non-penetrating glaucoma surgery. Br J Ophthalmol. 2010;94(12):1571–6.
7. Patel S, Pasquale LR. Glaucoma drainage devices: a review of the past, present, and future. Semin Ophthalmol. 2010;25(5–6): 265–70.
8. Melamed S, Ben Simon GJ, Goldenfeld M, Simon G. Efficacy and safety of gold micro shunt implantation to the supraciliary space in patients with glaucoma: a pilot study. Arch Ophthalmol. 2009;127(3): 264–9.
9. Krasnov MM. Sinusotomy in glaucoma. Vestn Oftalmol. 1964;77: 37–41.
10. Walker WM, Kanagasundaram CR. Surgery of the canal of Schlemm. Trans Ophthalmol Soc U K. 1964;84:427–42.
11. Sourdille P, Santiago PY, Villain F, et al. Reticulated hyaluronic acid implant in nonperforating trabecular surgery. J Cataract Refract Surg. 1999;25(3):332–9.
12. Sarodia U, Shaarawy T, Barton K. Nonpenetrating glaucoma surgery: a critical evaluation. Curr Opin Ophthalmol. 2007;18(2): 152–8.
13. Chiselita D. Non-penetrating deep sclerectomy versus trabeculectomy in primary open-angle glaucoma surgery. Eye (Lond). 2001;15(Pt 2):197–201.

14. Zimmerman TJ, Kooner KS, Ford VJ, et al. Trabeculectomy vs. nonpenetrating trabeculectomy: a retrospective study of two procedures in phakic patients with glaucoma. Ophthalmic Surg. 1984;15(9):734–40.

15. Hondur A, Onol M, Hasanreisoglu B. Nonpenetrating glaucoma surgery: meta-analysis of recent results. J Glaucoma. 2008;17(2):139–46.

16. Mendrinos E, Mermoud A, Shaarawy T. Nonpenetrating glaucoma surgery. Surv Ophthalmol. 2008;53(6):592–630.

17. Khaw PT, Siriwardena D. "New" surgical treatments for glaucoma. Br J Ophthalmol. 1999;83(1):1–2.

18. Assia EI. Non penetrating filtration surgery with CO2 laser. In: Garg A, Rosen E, editors. Instant clinical diagnosis in ophthalmology – glaucoma. St. Louis: Jaypee Brothers Medical Publisher LTD; 2009. p. 292–7.

19. Chai D, Chaudhary G, Mikula E, et al. In vivo femtosecond laser subsurface scleral treatment in rabbit eyes. Lasers Surg Med. 2010;42(7):647–51.

20. Bahar I, Kaiserman I, Trope GE, Rootman D. Non-penetrating deep sclerectomy for glaucoma surgery using the femtosecond laser: a laboratory model. Br J Ophthalmol. 2007;91(12):1713–4.

21. Argento C, Sanseau AC, Badoza D, Casiraghi J. Deep sclerectomy with a collagen implant using the excimer laser. J Cataract Refract Surg. 2001;27(4):504–6.

22. Klink T, Schlunck G, Lieb WE, et al. Long-term results of Erbium YAG-laser-assisted deep sclerectomy. Eye (Lond). 2008;22(3):370–4.

23. Pallikaris IG, Kozobolis VP, Christodoulakis EV. Erbium: YAG laser deep sclerectomy: an alternative approach to glaucoma surgery. Ophthalmic Surg Lasers Imaging. 2003;34(5):375–80.

24. Assia EI, Rotenstreich Y, Barequet IS, et al. Experimental studies on nonpenetrating filtration surgery using the CO2 laser. Graefes Arch Clin Exp Ophthalmol. 2007;245(6):847–54.

25. Ton Y, Geffen N, Kidron D, et al. CO2 laser-assisted sclerectomy surgery part I: concept and experimental models. J Glaucoma. 2012;21(2):135–40.

26. Geffen N, Ton Y, Degani J, Assia EI. CO2 laser-assisted sclerectomy surgery, part II: multicenter clinical preliminary study. J Glaucoma. 2012;21(3):193–8.

27. Geffen N, Assia EI, Melamed S. Laser-assisted techniques for penetrating and nonpenetrating glaucoma surgery. Dev Ophthalmol. 2012;50:96–108.

28. Cheng JW, Cai JP, Li Y, Wei RL. Intraoperative mitomycin C for nonpenetrating glaucoma surgery: a systematic review and meta-analysis. J Glaucoma. 2011;20(5):322–6.

# Part III

# Ultrasound Technologies

Florent Aptel and Philippe Denis

## Introduction

To-date, elevated intraocular pressure (IOP) is the only proven treatable risk factor of glaucoma [1–3]. IOP is the result of a balance between the production of the aqueous humor by the ciliary epithelium and its elimination by the trabecular and uveoscleral pathways. All treatments for glaucoma can therefore have two mechanisms of action: reducing aqueous humor production via the partial destruction or medical inhibition of the ciliary body and facilitating the evacuation of aqueous humor out of the eye medically or by filtering surgery. The recommended steps for lowering the IOP are usually topical medications first, followed by incisional surgery, and then cyclodestructive procedures [4]. Medical treatment failure is common, often due to lack of compliance of the patients in using the prescribed therapy. For this reason, surgical procedures are frequently performed. Filtering surgeries often fail due to the healing processes at the incision site. Over the long term, almost one-third to one-half of glaucoma surgeries fail because of this healing process [5]. In case of glaucoma that is refractory to conventional filtering surgery, partial physical destruction of the ciliary body may be considered (cyclodestructive procedures). Although diode laser transscleral cyclophotocoagulation is currently the clinical standard, many other methods and energy sources for destroying the ciliary processes have been investigated, resulting in coagulation necrosis of the ciliary body following heating (laser, microwave) or freezing (cryotherapy) [6–13]. All these methods have two major drawbacks which limit their use. Firstly, they are nonselective of the organ to be treated, often resulting in damage to the adjacent structures and ocular inflammation. Laser energy is mainly absorbed by the pigmented tissues and therefore can also damage the iris and the choroid. Cryotherapy and cyclodiathermy also result in a large area of treatment having unpredictable dimensions. Secondly, these methods have an unpredictable dose-effect relationship, which prevents accurate prediction of the treatment effect. Undertreatment leads to insufficient IOP reduction, and repeat treatment may be required. Overtreatment may lead to a major drop in intraocular pressure and ocular atrophy (ocular phthisis, definitive loss of visual acuity, and ocular pain). Published studies report a 6–64.3 % risk of visual acuity decrease, 0.5–37.5 % risk of ocular phthisis, 12.4–27 % risk of chronic inflammation, 2–6 % risk of corneal dystrophy, 10–35 % risk of cataract formation, and 12.9–80 % risk of failure 1 year after the procedure [6–13]. As a result, these cyclodestructive methods are currently reserved for treatment of refractory glaucoma. They do not represent an alternative that can be proposed as second-line treatment if medical treatment fails.

Therapeutic ultrasound, although less well known than ultrasound for diagnostic imaging, has become a topic of growing interest in ophthalmology. High-intensity focused ultrasound (HIFU) for the treatment of glaucoma is one of the main areas of research and potential clinical applications. The specific advantage of HIFU, particularly when compared to laser, is that the energy can be focused through optically opaque media, especially through the sclera which is a strongly light-scattering medium, and that energy deposition and tissue heating at the focus site do not depend on tissue pigmentation, which may vary greatly, particularly in the ciliary body. HIFU is therefore a possible method for partial coagulation of the ciliary body and, hence, reducing IOP.

To overcome the drawbacks of the current and past methods of cyclodestruction and taking advantage of recent breakthroughs in the field of high-intensity focused ultrasound

F. Aptel, MD, PhD (✉)
Department of Ophthalmology, University Hospital
of Grenoble, Boulevard de la Chantourne, CHU Grenoble,
Grenoble F-38043, France
e-mail: faptel@chu-grenoble.fr

P. Denis, MD, PhD
Department of Ophthalmology, University Hospital of Lyon,
Hôpital de la Croix-Rousse, 103, grande rue de
la Croix-Rousse, Lyon 69004, France
e-mail: philippe.denis@chu-lyon.fr

J.R. Samples, I.I.K. Ahmed (eds.), *Surgical Innovations in Glaucoma*,
DOI 10.1007/978-1-4614-8348-9_11, © Springer Science+Business Media New York 2014

(HIFU) technology, a new HIFU device was recently developed by physicians, scientists, and a start-up company, the aim being to achieve a selective and precise destruction of the ciliary body, sparing the adjacent ocular structures [14–17]. The aim of this chapter is to present an overview of the interest of HIFU for cyclocoagulation and to detail the mechanisms of action, technical procedure, and clinical results of the recently developed device.

## Historical Perspectives: Ultrasonic Cyclocoagulation

Ultrasonic coagulation of the ciliary body using HIFU has been studied since the late 1980s [18–28], and a commercially available device (Sonocare Therapeutic Ultrasound System Model, Sonocare Inc., Ridgewood, NJ) was marketed [18–28].

### The Sonocare: Experimental Studies

The first HIFU device for the treatment of glaucoma was developed in the 1980s by Lizzi et al. (Riverside Research Institute, NY) and Coleman et al. (Cornell University Medical College, NY), and a commercially available system was marketed by a spin-off company (The Sonocare CST-100 Therapeutic Ultrasound System, Sonocare Inc, Ridgewood, NJ) and was one of the first HIFU devices approved by the Food and Drug Administration. The Sonocare was composed of an electronic control unit and a transducer assembly supported by an articulated arm. The transducer assembly was composed of a focused ultrasound transducer for the therapy, a central A-mode diagnostic transducer to determine the distance to the target organ ($z$), and a fiber-optic module to determine the position on the surface of the sclera ($x$, $y$). The therapy transducer was a 1.46-mm-thick PZT-4 spherical shell, with a fundamental frequency of 1.5 MHz, operating at its third harmonic, i.e., about 4.5 MHz. For animal studies, the transducer diameter was 42 mm, with a focus of 90 mm and a focal zone having a 14.9-mm axial length and 0.6-mm transverse focal width at its third harmonic [18]. Exposure durations varied from 1 to 5 s and intensity levels from 100 to 2,000 W/cm$^2$ at the focal point. A fluid coupling bath of saline heated at 37 °C was made by sticking a plastic sheet to the skin. The distance and the placement of the transducer from the eye were determined with the diagnostic transducer and the optic fiber. Once the correct distance was determined and the focal zone of the transducer was positioned, a single application of energy was performed. The transducer was then moved for each of the approximately six applications.

In the first published animal study, Coleman et al. treated, using the parameters mentioned above, 14 rabbit eyes in which ocular hypertension was induced by an injection of alpha-chymotrypsin and then compared over 3 months the treated eyes to ten controls and seven receiving a mock treatment [18]. Ten of the fourteen treated eyes demonstrated an initial IOP reduction. In six of these ten eyes, IOP further increased and remained near the level of the controls, whereas in the remaining four, IOP was sustained below the intraocular pressure of the controls. Histological examinations – light and transmission electron microscopy – performed at varying times showed localized thinning of the sclera with intact conjunctiva and focal disruption of the ciliary epithelium. The scleral lesions were very highly localized with immediate disruption of the collagen fibers of the sclera gradually replaced by fibrils, which were smaller in diameter and which were produced by activated fibroblasts. According to the authors, this study demonstrated two mechanisms of action: reduced aqueous production because of ciliary epithelium destruction and enhanced outflow through the thinned sclera.

In a further study performed in rabbit and pig eyes and also in human eyes enucleated after treatment (nonfunctional and painful eyes), histological examinations also showed a cleavage between the sclera and the ciliary body, suggesting a third mechanism of action, which is an enhanced outflow via the uveoscleral pathway (outflow of aqueous between the sclera and the choroids until transscleral venous system) [22].

### The Sonocare: Human Studies

Several clinical studies have been conducted with Sonocare, and these have suggested that ultrasound cyclodestruction was an effective method, with favorable results in terms of IOP reduction [19–21, 23–27]. The transducer used in humans was also a 1.46-mm-thick PZT-4 spherical shell operating at its third frequency (4.5 MHz) but with a diameter of 80 mm, a focus of 90 mm, and a focal zone having a 3.0-mm axial length and 0.4-mm transverse focal width at its third harmonic. Exposure duration varied from 1 to 5 s and intensity levels from 800 to 4,800 W/cm$^2$. In the first published clinical study, Coleman et al. treated 42 eyes (7 congenital glaucomas, 13 primary open-angle glaucomas, and 22 secondary glaucomas) with the abovementioned parameters and obtained an IOP of 25 mmHg or less in 83 % of patients with a minimum 3-month follow-up period [19]. Maskin et al. achieved a 38.4 % reduction in intraocular pressure 8 months after the cyclodestructive procedure in 158 eyes with refractory glaucoma [26]. Sterk et al. achieved a 42.2 % reduction in IOP 3–4 months after the procedure in 44 eyes with refractory glaucoma [27]. Denis and Valtot obtained satisfactory IOP control in 75.2 % of cases 3 months after treatment of 62 eyes with failed trabeculectomy. The success rate was higher in phakic eyes compared to pseudophakic or aphakic eyes (82 % versus 68 %) [24].

## Limitations

The Sonocare was not fully convenient to use and handle. The transducer was bulky, heavy, and attached to an articulated arm which had to be positioned manually using a light source and A-scan imaging probe. It had a fluid coupling bath of heated saline that had to be set up by sticking a plastic sheet to the patient's skin. Because the correct distance and position have to be checked before each burst, the procedure was rather lengthy. To address this, a second model without articulated arm was proposed, allowing a freehand insonification. Later, a balloon touch transducer technique that eliminated the saline water bath was also developed [28].

Treatable complications such as IOP spikes following the procedure were frequently reported. Severe complications such as scleral thinning or perforation have been rarely described, especially encountered in congenital and pediatric glaucoma [18, 19, 25]. Other complications such as inflammation, chronic uveitis, cataract formation, and decrease of visual acuity were also sometimes reported. A review of the published studies shows complication rates of 9.5–43 % (decrease of visual acuity), 9.5–22 % (chronic uveitis), 5–13 % (corneoscleral burns), and 1.4–4 % (ocular phthisis) [19–21, 23–27]. Because of these complications and the development of diode laser transscleral photocoagulation, the use of HIFU for cyclodestruction was gradually abandoned in the mid-1990s.

## High-Intensity Focused Ultrasound

### Definition and Characteristics

Sound is made up of cyclic pressure waves produced by the mechanical vibration of a support material and propagated through the elasticity of the medium. Ultrasound is a cyclic sound pressure wave with a frequency greater than 20 kHz. The pressure variations, that is to say the periodic alternation of overpressure and depression, are displaced in the propagation medium. By contrast, the molecules or atoms of the medium do not move but oscillate only a few nanometers around their initial position. Longitudinal or transverse waves correspond to molecules or atoms moving in the same direction or perpendicular to the wave, respectively. In biological tissue, the ultrasonic waves are essentially of longitudinal type.

The propagation velocity of ultrasound in a medium is independent of frequency and depends on the mechanical properties of the medium, in particular its density and

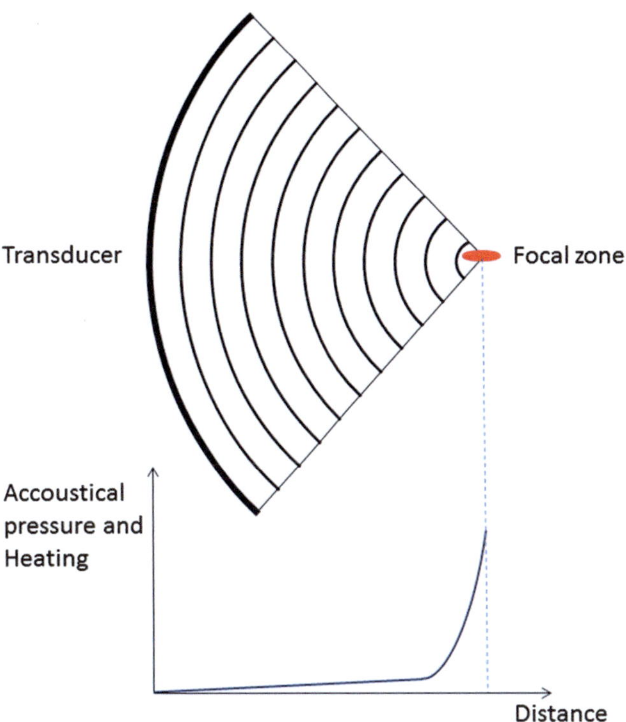



**Fig. 11.1** High-intensity ultrasound beam focusing with induced increased acoustical pressure, energy absorption, and tissue heating

compressibility. In soft tissue, the ultrasound propagation velocity is about 1,550 m/s. During the propagation of a wave in a homogeneous soft tissue, the intensity of the wave decreases gradually. Several phenomena may contribute to the gradual attenuation of the ultrasonic wave: the divergence of the beam, resulting in a decrease in energy per unit area; the scattering of the beam, resulting in a "scattering" multidirectional ultrasonic waves; the beam propagation as waves not longitudinal; and the absorption of the beam, resulting in a conversion of the ultrasonic energy into heat. In nonhomogeneous tissue, ultrasonic waves can further be more or less partially reflected by the interfaces formed by the differences in acoustic properties of the media.

When the intensity and focusing of the ultrasonic beam are adequate to obtain sufficient beam absorption, thereby heating to coagulate biological tissue, we talk of high-intensity focused ultrasound (HIFU). Focus can concentrate the energy of the ultrasonic beam in a small volume of space called the focal spot. Focusing can be obtained from a curved piezoelectric transducer or by using multiple transducers oriented so as to cross the ultrasonic beams (mechanical focusing). All points of the curved transducer or transducers are adequately oriented and excited simultaneously. The propagation of ultrasonic waves leads to a maximum sound intensity at the focal volume, located at the geometric center of the arc formed by the transducer (Fig. 11.1). The shape of the focal volume depends on the radius of curvature of the transducers.

Focusing can also be obtained by time-shifted activation of transducers located in the same plane, by delaying the activation of the piezoelectric elements central with respect to those located on the periphery (electronic focusing).

## Biological Effects of High-Intensity Focused Ultrasound

In biological tissue, the periodic changes in pressure may result in biochemical, cellular, or tissue effects through three main mechanisms: the thermal effect related to the absorption of the ultrasonic energy, the mechanical effect related to periodic movements, and a cavitation effect due to the formation of gas microbubbles in the tissues.

The main effect involved with high-intensity focused ultrasound is the thermal effect due to energy absorption. The absorbed energy causes a rise of temperature. Induced heating depends on many factors and can range from a rise of a few degrees to a significant rise causing coagulation necrosis almost instantaneously. The absorption is defined as the phenomenon of conversion of the ultrasonic energy (mechanical energy) to heat (thermal energy) which is transferred to the medium which it crosses through. Two main mechanisms contribute to the absorption of ultrasonic waves, the phenomena of friction and relaxation. The passage of an ultrasonic wave in a medium induces movements of particles and therefore frictional forces opposed to these movements. The acoustic wave loses energy due to the friction, and energy is transferred to the tissues in the form of heat. The relaxation phenomena are related to the transfer of energy to the tissues occurring during a finite time. The ultrasonic wave transmits mechanical energy to tissues as it passes through. If the duration of return to equilibrium is different from the transit time of the ultrasonic wave in this element, the energy compensation is out of phase with respect to the ultrasonic wave which is then reduced. There is then a peak of the absorption coefficient corresponding to a frequency called relaxation.

## Comparison to Laser

Compared with the laser, a specific advantage of ultrasound is that the energy can be focused through nonoptically transparent media with controlled energy absorption which reduces the effect on the adjacent tissues. Therefore, energy absorption and tissue heating in front and behind the focal zone are very limited to negligible. A very small focal point can be achieved deep in tissue. Similarly, energy deposition and tissue heating at the focal site do not depend on tissue pigmentation, which may vary greatly, particularly in the eye (ciliary body, iris, choroid). Finally, when compared to a non-focused laser, such as the diode laser that is used for cyclophotocoagulation, focused ultrasound can be used to heat and treat a well-defined and adjustable tissue volume at any depth or location.

## Mechanisms of Action

A circular device including multiple transducers was proposed to achieve a rapid, selective, and one-step coagulation of the ciliary body, without displacement of the device during the procedure [14–17]. The device placed on the eye is composed of two parts. A coupling cone made of polymer is placed in direct contact with the eye, allowing good placement of the transducers in terms of centering and distance (Fig. 11.2). A ring containing six active piezoelectric transducers is then inserted in the top of the coupling cone. The ring is about 30 mm in diameter and 15 mm high. Each of the six transducers is a segment of a 10.2-mm radius cylinder with a 4.5-mm width and a 7-mm length (active surface area of approximately 35 mm$^2$). The focal volume of each transducer has approximately an elliptic cylinder shape, with an axial length of about 1 mm (major section of the ellipse), a transverse focal width of about 0.1 mm (minor section of the ellipse), and a lateral focal width of about 3.5 mm (height of the elliptic cylinder). During the exposure time of insonification, the heat generated in the area of the focal volume propagates in all directions around, leading to a heated volume which is proportional to the time of exposure. The heated volume is bigger than the focal volume and can be accurately set to a target volume according to the exposure time (Fig. 11.3). The six transducers are placed at regular intervals on the circumference of the ring and oriented to create a focal zone consisting of six elliptical cylinder-shaped spots. A high operating frequency of 21 MHz is used. A control module allows to select some parameters of the treatment (e.g., number of sectors to be activated, duration of exposure) and automatically sets other parameters for each piezoelectric crystal to obtain a homogeneous focal volume (power and frequency) and then sequentially activates each sector.

## Animal Experiments

In the published pilot animal study designed to evaluate the feasibility and safety of the method, 18 healthy adult New Zealand white rabbits were treated with the abovementioned device [14]. The coupling cone was placed directly in contact with the surface of the eye and used to obtain good and reproducible placement of the transducers in terms of alignment with the optical axis and distance from the sclera. The ring-shaped device was then inserted into the coupling cone, and the cavity was filled with 5 mL of saline solution. Six eyes of six rabbits were treated with the six transducers activated, six

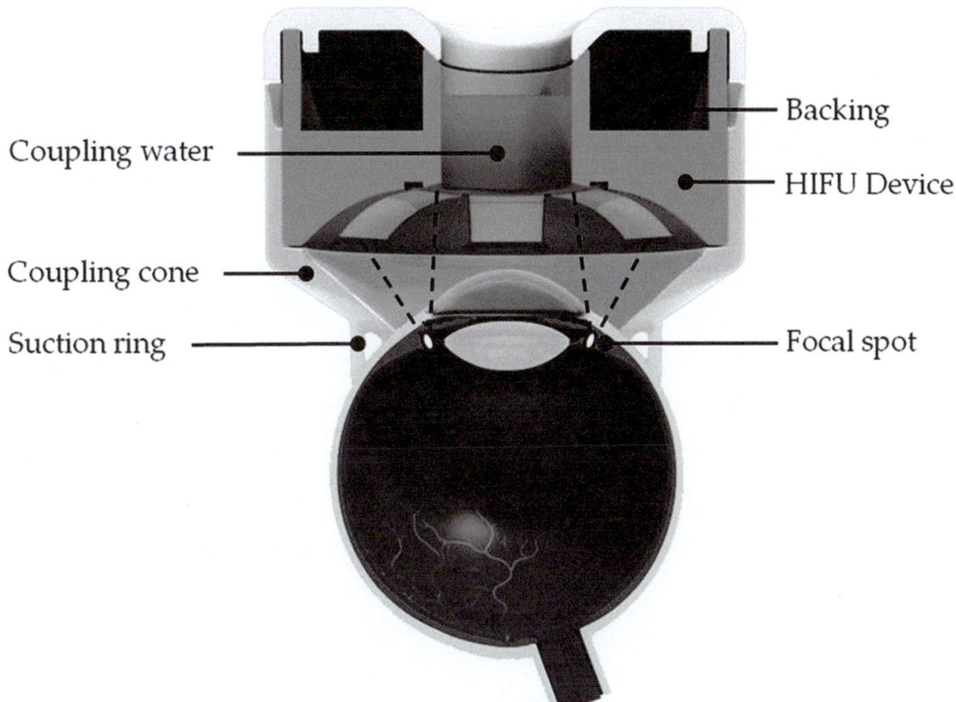



**Fig. 11.2** Cross section of the device. The cavity is filled with saline serum to allow ultrasound propagation. The ultrasound beam focusing into the ciliary body is represented by *dotted lines* (Charrel et al. [15])

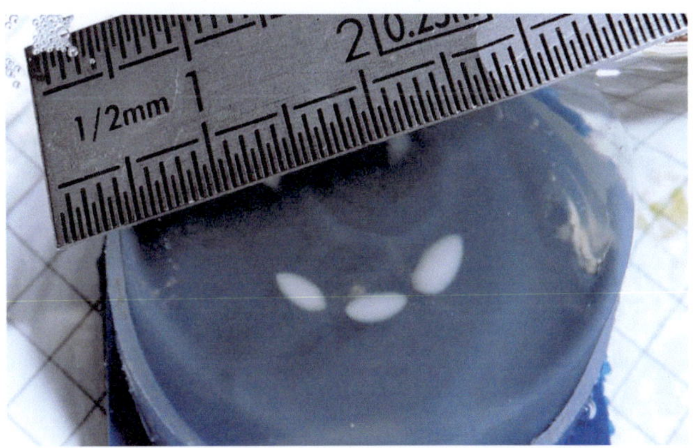



**Fig. 11.3** Heated zones produced after insonification in thermosensitive gel around the focal zones after several seconds of exposure

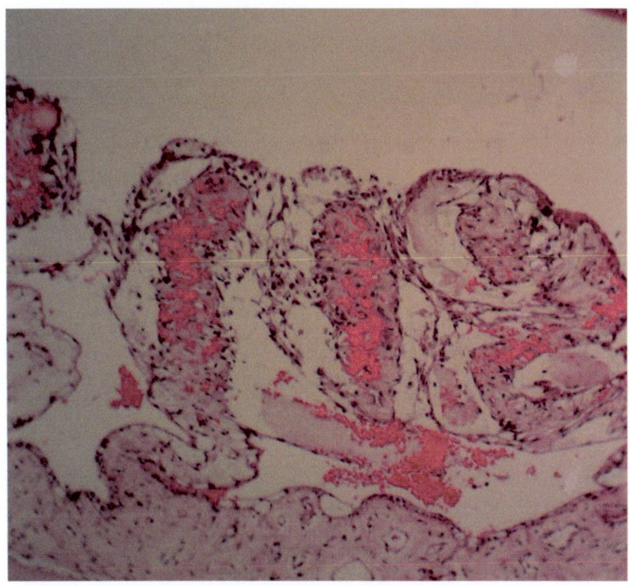

**Fig. 11.4** Photomicrographs showing ciliary processes with coagulation necrosis, loss of the bilayered epithelium, distension of the stromal collagen fibers, and hemorrhage (magnification ×40)

eyes of six rabbits with five of the six transducers activated, and six eyes of six rabbits with four of the six transducers activated. The rabbits were followed for 28 days with regular IOP measurement and ophthalmic examinations (day 0 before treatment, days 1, 7, 15, 21, and 28) and then sacrificed to perform histological examinations of the treated eyes. In the treated eyes, intraocular pressure changes ranged from −16.6 mmHg (−55.3 %) at day 28 to −8.9 mmHg (−29.7 %) at day 7 in eyes with six transducers activated, from −4.7 mmHg (−25.5 %) at day 28 to −1.4 mmHg (−7.6 %) at day 21 in eyes with five transducers activated, and from −7.9 mmHg (−28.1 %) at day 28 to +2.0 mmHg (+7.1 %) at day 7 in eyes with four transducers activated.

## Aqueous Production Reduction

Histological examinations performed in the treated rabbits found a selective and circumferentially distributed coagulation necrosis of the ciliary processes and ciliary body [14] (Figs. 11.4 and 11.5). Maximum intensity was consistently observed in the deepest regions of the ciliary processes,

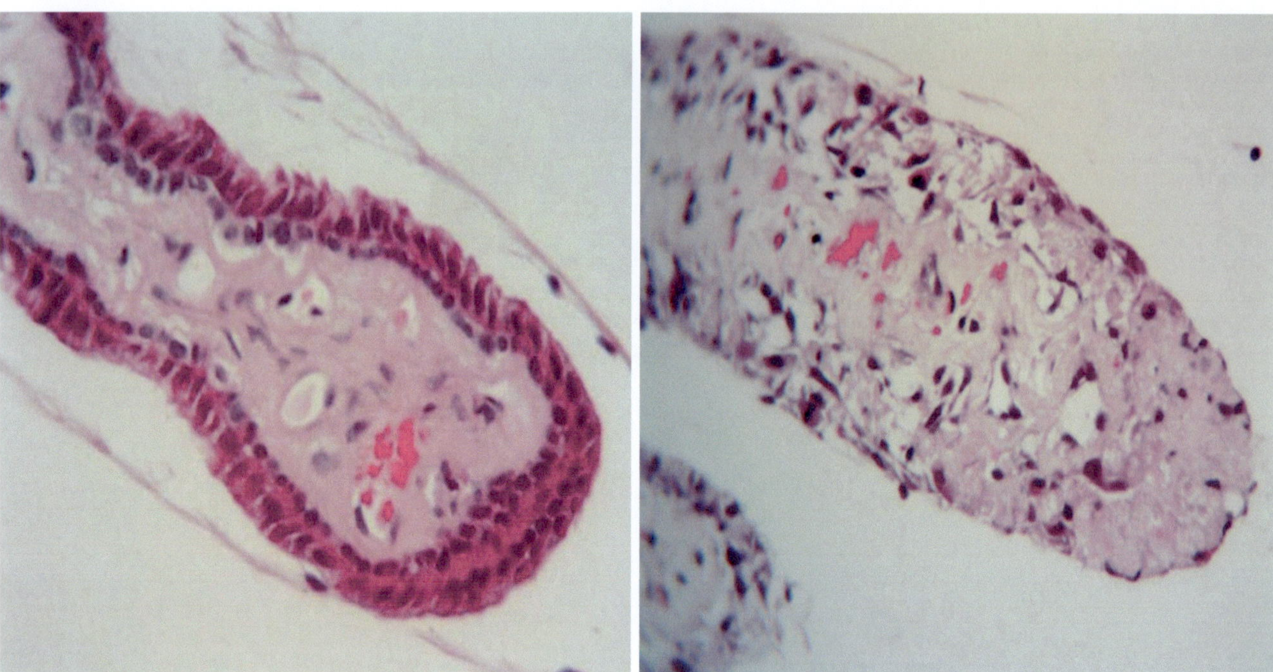

**Fig. 11.5** High-magnification photomicrograph showing details of necrotic ciliary processes with loss of ciliary epithelium, vascular congestion, and distension of the stromal collagen fibers (*right*) and intact ciliary processes (*left*) (magnification ×120)

whereas the rostral and caudal regions were less affected. In the affected regions, the distal and intermediate parts of the ciliary processes showed acute inflammatory and necrotic changes ranging from stromal edema (marked distension of collagen fibers) and vascular congestion (distension of vascular lumens by erythrocytes) to coagulation necrosis with loss of surface epithelium and hemorrhage. The bilayered epithelium was degenerated or necrotic and sloughed off in the distal parts of the most affected areas. The inflammatory cellular reaction was very limited, with a very small number of macrophages, lymphocytes, plasma cells, polymorphonuclear cells, and giant cells. The sclera across from all treated areas appeared normal with no signs of thinning or necrosis.

Histological examinations performed months after the treatment showed involution of the ciliary processes, with short or absent ciliary processes covered by a non-bilayered epithelium and composed of dysmorphic and probably nonfunctional cells (Fig. 11.6).

Scanning electron microscopy performed in treated animals shows lesions spatially limited to five to eight adjacent ciliary processes (Fig. 11.7) for each area of single ultrasound exposure. In the days following the insonification, the volume of the ciliary processes is increased. A few weeks after, scanning electron microscopy shows involution and atrophy of the treated ciliary processes. In the first days following the insonification, higher-magnification images show a smooth membrane likely corresponding to the basal membrane without

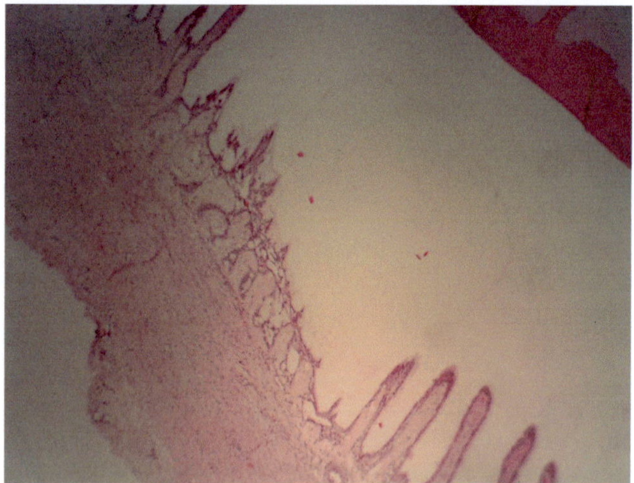

**Fig. 11.6** Photomicrographs showing the evolution of treated ciliary processes and ciliary body 3 weeks after sectorial insonification (magnification ×10)

any residual epithelial cells. By contrast, images of the adjacent untreated areas show a normal ciliary epithelium, with ciliary processes covered by numerous epithelial cells (Fig. 11.8). Fibrin deposits are usually very limited or absent.

Vascular corrosion casting: light microscopy and scanning electron microscopy of vascular corrosion cast performed after intravascular injection of methacrylate resin show focal

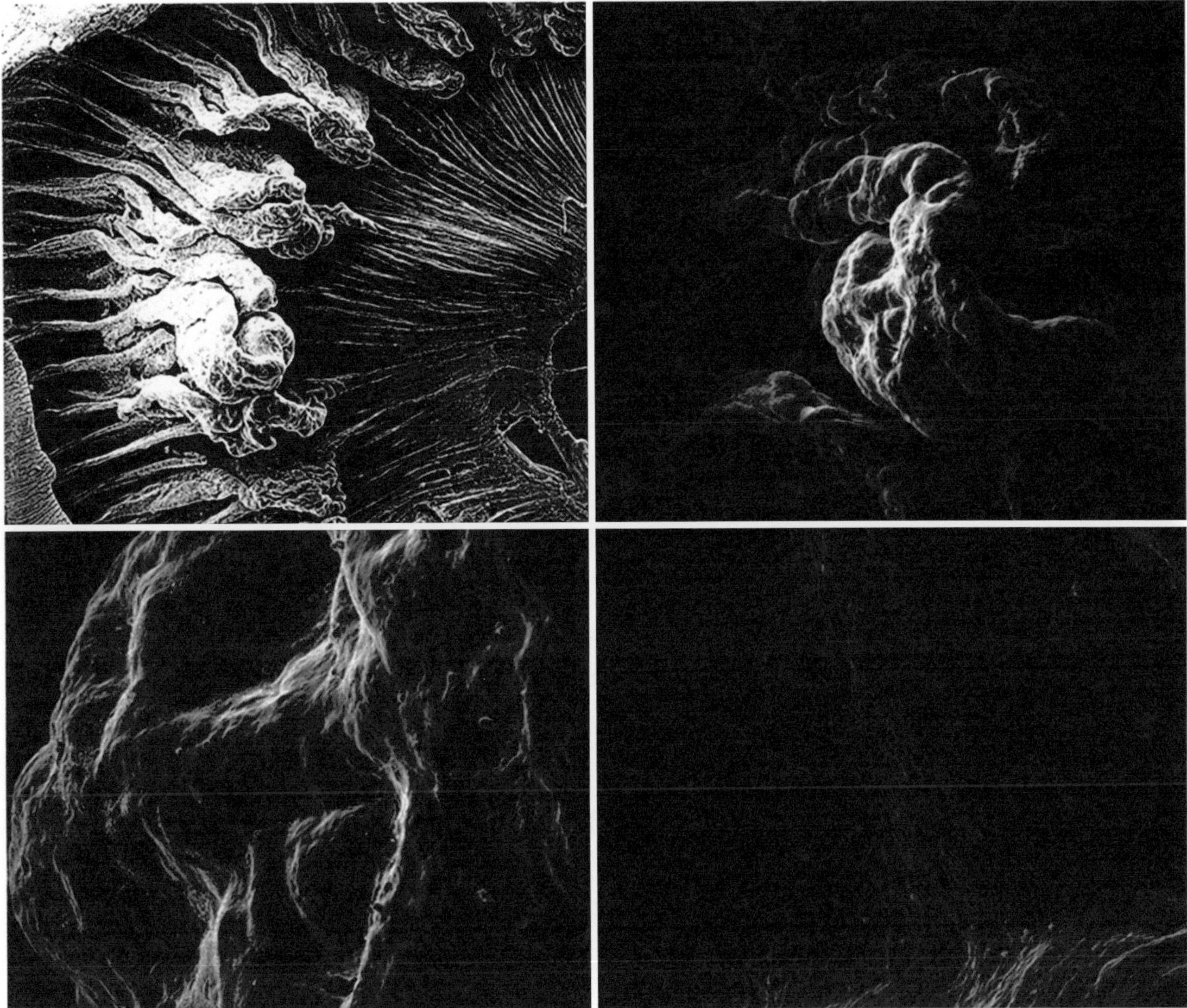

**Fig. 11.7** Scanning electron microscopy showing details of treated ciliary processes: same location at ×40 (*top left*), ×104 (*top right*), ×500 (*bottom left*), and ×4,000 (*bottom right*) magnification

interruption of the ciliary body microvasculature (Fig. 11.9). Vascular defect was limited to the treatments areas with dimensions comparable to those of lesions observed with light or scanning electron microscopy. The major and minor arterial iris circles appeared undamaged. The three-dimensional architecture of the microvasculature of the untreated areas of ciliary body and ciliary processes also appeared intact.

## Aqueous Outflow Increase

In most animals treated, a fluid space could be seen between the sclera and the ciliary body and between the sclera and the choroid adjacent to treated areas but not adjacent to untreated areas

(Fig. 11.10). This aspect therefore likely corresponds to an area where the opening of the space should lead to an increase of the aqueous outflow via the uveoscleral pathway. This characteristic seems to be maintained over time in animals, likely indicating that it is due to tissue retraction or tissue microarchitecture changes rather than intraocular inflammation. Moreover, similar aspects were found in humans after treatment using ultrasound biomicroscopy (Fig. 11.11). In the pilot human study, cystic involution of the ciliary body was found in 9 of the 12 eyes, with multiple hypoechoic ovoid cystic cavities ranging from 0.05 to 0.15 mm in diameter and hyporeflective suprachoroidal fluid space in 8 of the 12 eyes [16]. Patients with hyporeflective suprachoroidal space had significantly lower IOP than those without visible suprachoroidal space.

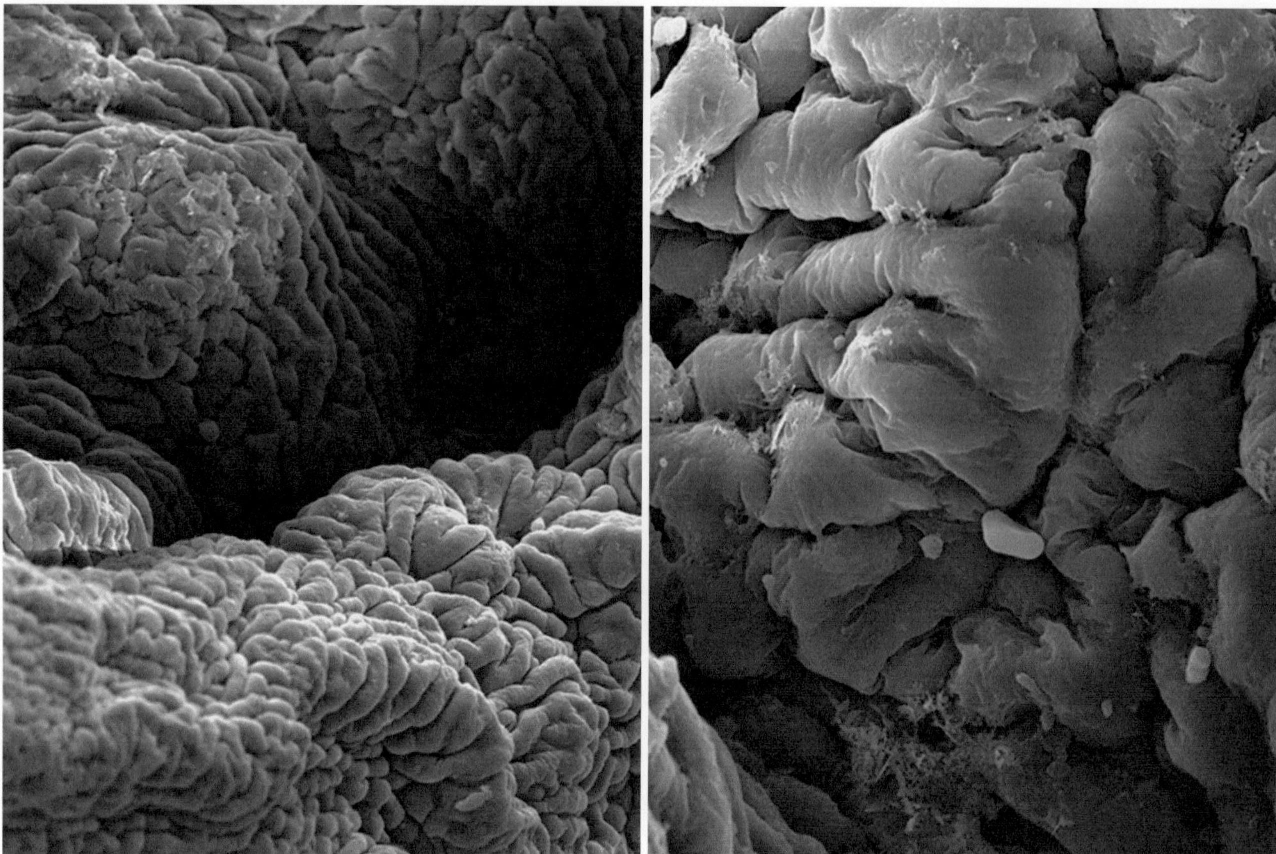

**Fig. 11.8** Scanning electron microscopy showing details of untreated adjacent ciliary processes: same location at ×400 (*left*) and ×2,000 (*right*) magnification

## Procedure

### Indications

The initial pilot study conducted with the device for ultrasound circular cyclocoagulation was performed in patients with refractory primary or secondary glaucoma (at least one previous incisional glaucoma surgery) and a limited residual visual acuity and visual field [16]. Patients included had primary open-angle glaucoma, neovascular glaucoma, congenital glaucoma, primary angle-closure glaucoma, and iridocorneal endothelial glaucoma. The second larger clinical trial conducted with the device was performed in patients with refractory primary open-angle glaucoma (at least one previous incisional glaucoma surgery) but possibly having a slightly altered visual field [29]. As detailed below, results between these two studies in terms of efficacy (mean IOP reduction and rate of responders) and safety were very similar. At the time of writing this chapter, a third clinical trial was about to commence in patients with uncontrolled primary open-angle glaucoma with medical treatment and naïve of any glaucoma surgeries.

There are few theoretical contraindications to the procedure, including previous retinal detachment with scleral buckling, major scleral thinning, major buphthalmos or nanophthalmic eyes, and dislocated or sub-dislocated lens.

### Device

A coupling cone made of polymer is placed in direct contact with the eye allowing easy and accurate positioning of the transducers in terms of centering and distance. At the base of the coupling cone and externally, two suction holes allow the application of mild vacuum (150 mmHg) to the conjunctiva only without the risk of increasing IOP significantly during the procedure and enable the cone to maintain contact and position with the eye throughout the procedure. A 30-mm-diameter, 15-mm-high ring containing six active piezoelectric elements is inserted in the upper part of the coupling cone. The cavity created between the eye, the cone, and the probe (4 mL) is filled through the central aperture of the device with room-temperature saline solution (Fig. 11.12).

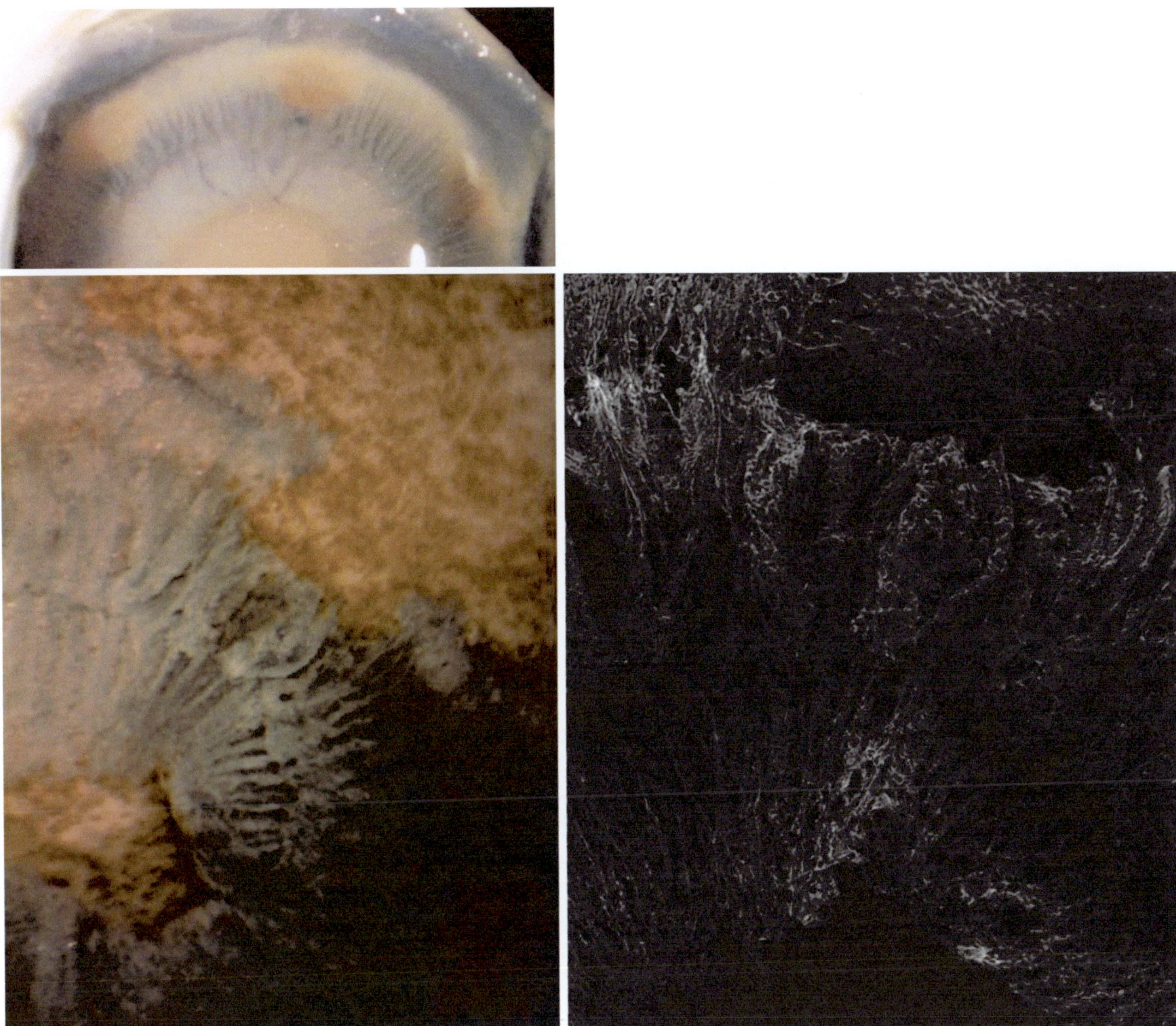

**Fig. 11.9** Light (*left*) and scanning electron microscopy (*right*) of vascular corrosion cast performed after intravascular injection of methacrylate resin, before tissue dissolution (*above*) and after tissue dissolution (below *left* and *right*) showing focal defect of the ciliary body microvasculature

Each of the six transducers is a segment of a 10.2-mm radius cylinder with a 4.5-mm width and a 7-mm length (active surface area, approximately 35 mm²). The six transducers are located at regular intervals on the upper and lower circumference of the ring, avoiding the nasal and temporal meridians, and are oriented to create a focal zone consisting of six regularly distributed elliptical cylinder-shaped volumes. Four different ring diameters are available. Depending on the diameter, the six elliptical cylinder-shaped volumes are centered on a 10.0-, 11.0-, 12.0-, or 13.0-mm-diameter circle (Fig. 11.13). In each patient, the ring model whose focal zones actually matched the ciliary body is determined by high-resolution imaging of the anterior segment using preferably ultrasound biomicroscopy (UBM). The location of the focal zones is simulated from the UBM images, allowing to choose the model that best targets the ciliary body (Fig. 11.14). Anterior segment optical coherence tomography images can also be used to estimate the diameter although the ciliary body is not usually visible. White-to-white diameter and axial length anatomical parameters can also be used to estimate the required diameter, thereby avoiding dependence on preoperative imaging. These two parameters are significantly and strongly correlated to the UBM measurements done to estimate the diameter to be used.

The ring is connected to a control module, which allows each sector to be sequentially activated according to a program defined by the operator.

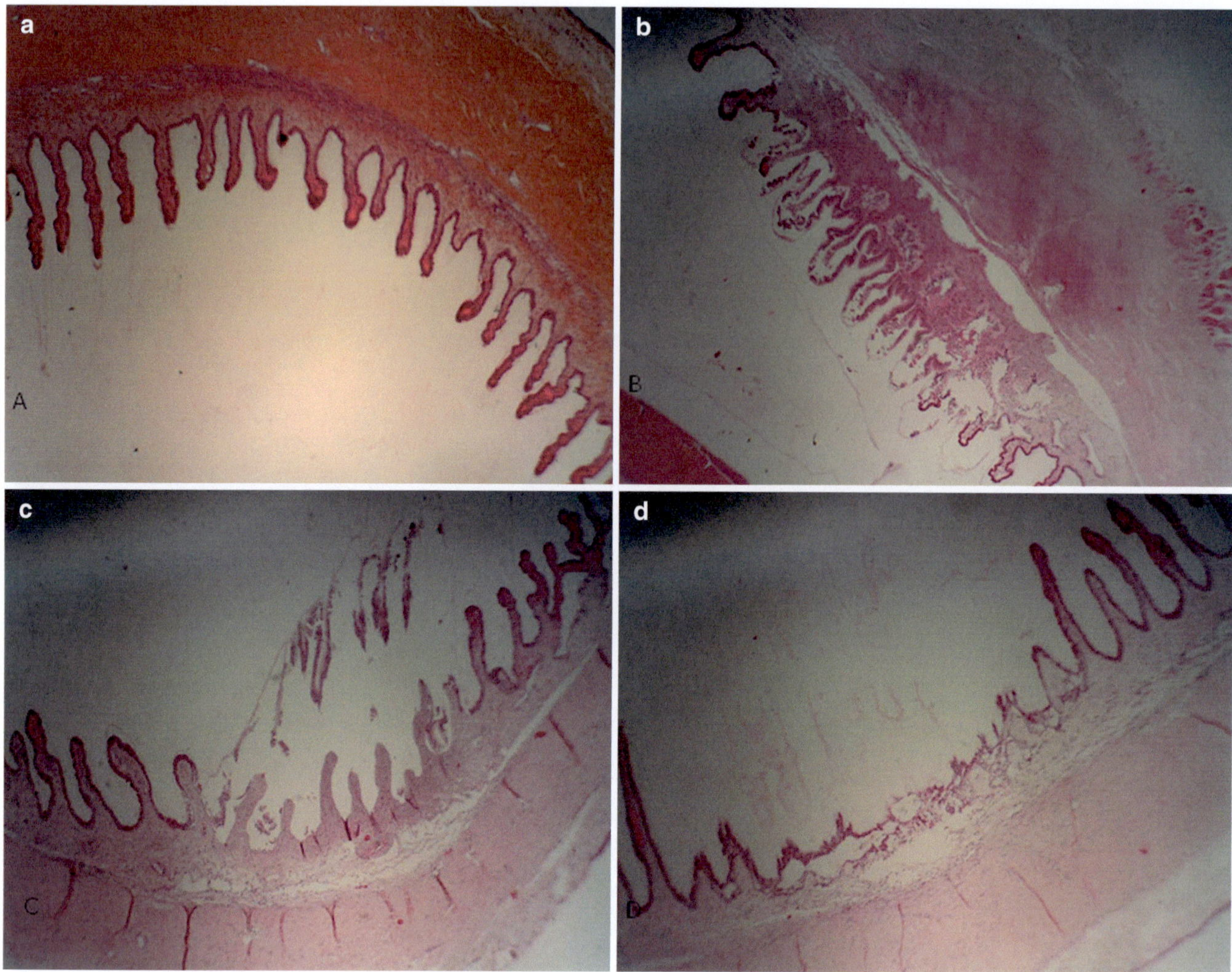

**Fig. 11.10** Photomicrographs showing a fluid space between the sclera and the ciliary body adjacent to a treated sector demonstrating ciliary process coagulation necrosis and loss of ciliary epithelium, 2 h (**b**), 5 days (**c**), and 3 weeks (**d**) after insonification (**a**, control) (magnification ×20)

## Anesthesia

Most of the procedures conducted to-date were performed under general or regional (peribulbar or retrobulbar) anesthesia. Regional anesthesia seems to be a particularly adapted choice of anesthesia to perform ultrasonic circular cyclocoagulation. It should be mentioned that in this case the injection should be performed with caution so as to avoid the occurrence of chemosis. A large chemosis may prevent proper positioning of the device and lead to a defocus of the focal zone and an ineffective or irregular targeting of the ciliary body as the simulations performed using UBM images to choose the probe diameter assume the conjunctiva is of average thickness.

Topical anesthesia has also been used in some patients. In this case, most of the patients felt pain, but only during activation of the transducers, not between each shot or after the procedure. A good way to perform ultrasonic circular cyclocoagulation under topical anesthesia avoiding pain was successfully experimented by injecting intravenously and concomitantly to the procedure a small amount of short-acting opioid receptor agonists such as remifentanil, making the procedure painless without deep sedation or delayed drug action.

## Technique

Depending on the operator choice, the activation time varied from 4 to 6 s for each transducer, with a rest time of 20 s between each sector shot. The procedure is therefore about 2 min long.

By virtue of the coupling cone designed to position and center the device and of the vacuum system which allows to maintain the device well centered and in contact with the eye, the procedure is rather easy to perform with a very short learning curve.

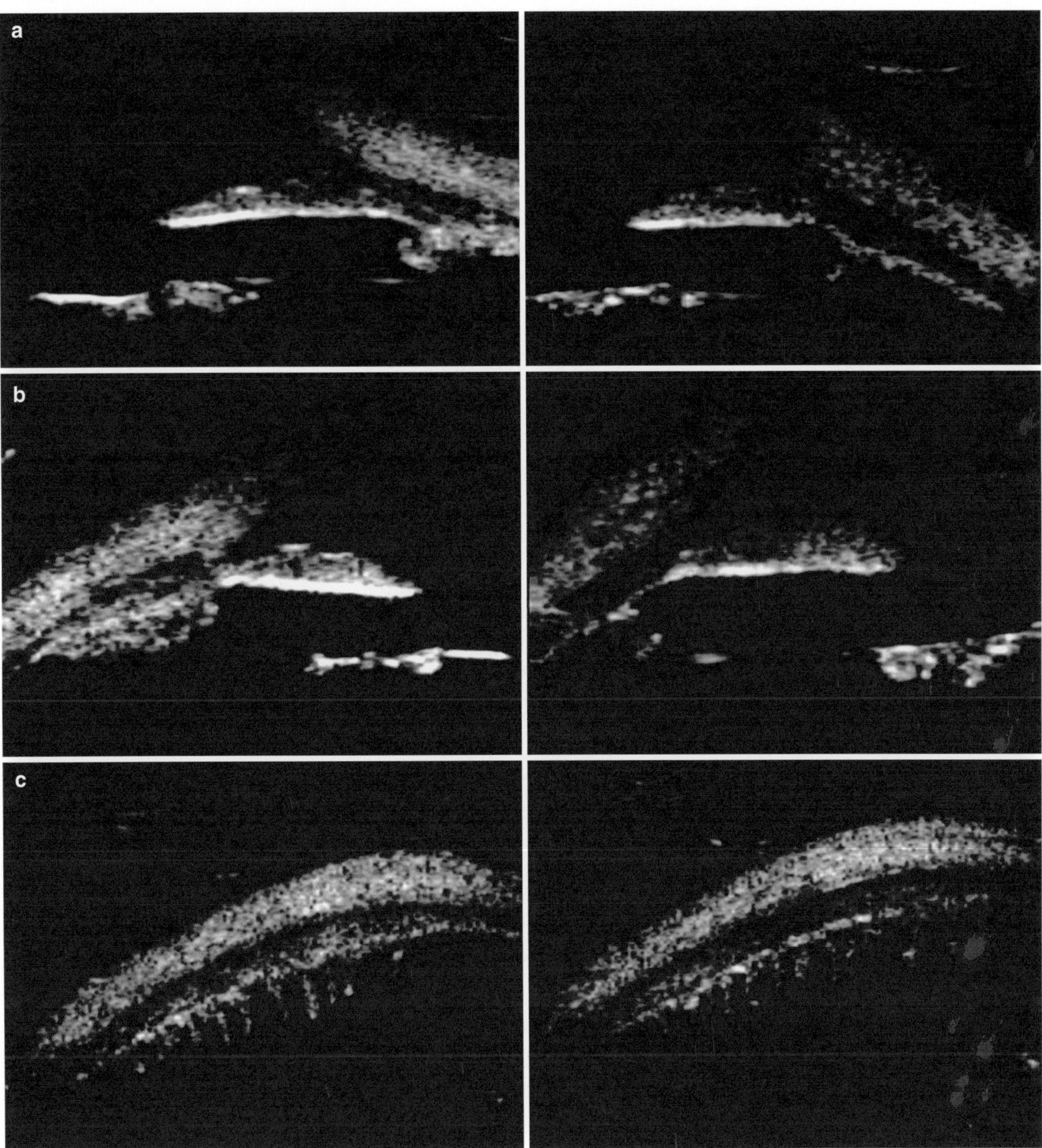

**Fig. 11.11** 50-MHz UBM before (*left*) and 1 month after (*right*) ultrasonic circular cyclocoagulation in a pseudophakic patient with refractory primary open-angle glaucoma. (**a**) Radial 90° meridian section. (**b**) Radial 145° meridian section. (**c**) Transverse section centered on the 90° meridian. Note the cystic involution of the treated ciliary body and the hyporeflective suprachoroidal fluid space (Aptel et al. [16])

## Postoperative Care

Medical treatment: As the post-procedure inflammation is limited, patients can be treated postoperatively with a rather low dose of topical steroidal or nonsteroidal anti-inflammatory drugs, for example, dexamethasone three or four times a day for 4 weeks. Preoperative hypotensive medication is usually maintained unchanged during the first 1 or 2 months and then decreased depending on the IOP reduction.

Follow-up: Because of the lack of major ocular inflammation and IOP spikes (see Outcomes section, below),

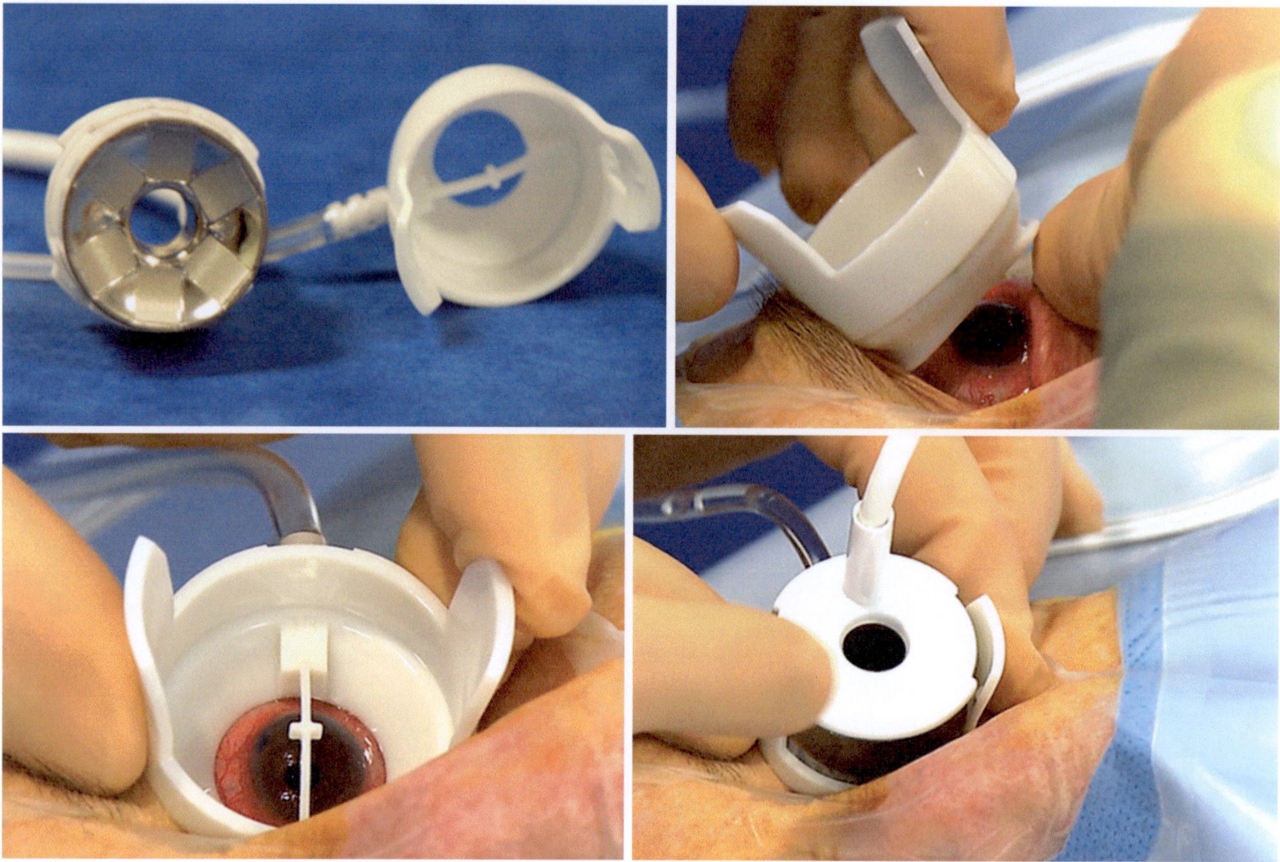

**Fig. 11.12** Coupling cone and therapeutic probe with the six piezoceramic transducers (*top left*). Positioning of the coupling cone under the lids (*top right*). Centering of the coupling cone relative to the pupil and the limbal-scleral ring (*bottom left*). Insertion of the probe in the coupling cone (*bottom right*)

a standard follow-up protocol is adequate (1 day, 1 week, 1 month, and then biannual monitoring).

## Outcomes

Efficacy: In the pilot study conducted in patients with refractory and very advanced glaucoma, twelve patients were enrolled and followed during at least 1 year [16]. No complications occurred during the treatment. IOP was significantly reduced ($p<0.01$) from a mean preoperative value of $37.9 \pm 10.7$ mmHg to a mean postoperative value of $27.3 \pm 12.4$, $25.2 \pm 11.3$, $25.2 \pm 7.7$, $24.8 \pm 9.8$, and $26.3 \pm 5.1$ mmHg at 1 day, 1 week, and 1, 3, and 6 months, respectively, and to a mean value of $24.7 \pm 8.5$ at the last follow-up visit. An IOP reduction of 33.9 % was obtained at the last follow-up visit. Surgical success (defined by an IOP reduction greater than or equal to 20 % and an IOP more than 5 mmHg) was obtained in 10 of 12 patients (83.3 %) at the last visit.

In the first multicenter study conducted in about 60 patients with primary open-angle glaucoma, a first group of patients were treated with a 4-s exposure time for each shot and a second group of patients with a 6-s exposure time [29].

IOP was significantly reduced in both groups ($p<0.05$), from a mean preoperative value of $28.6 \pm 4.7$ mmHg in group 1 and $28.1 \pm 8.6$ mmHg in group 2 to a mean value of $16.1 \pm 2.8$ mmHg in group 1 and $16.7 \pm 4.4$ mmHg in group 2 at the last follow-up. Success (IOP reduction >20 % and IOP >5 mmHg) was achieved in 67 % eyes of the group 1 with an average IOP decrease of 44 % and in 71 % eyes of the group 2 with an average IOP decrease of 40 %.

Tolerability and safety: In the pilot study, no major intra- or postoperative complications occurred. Superficial punctate keratitis occurred in three patients and central superficial corneal ulceration in one patient. All patients presented prior corneal conditions: corneal ulceration occurred in a patient with congenital glaucoma and moderate corneal edema, and superficial punctate keratitis occurred in patients with congenital glaucoma, iridocorneal endothelial syndrome, and neovascular glaucoma, all having mild to moderate corneal edema before the treatment.

None of the patients encountered IOP spikes or major IOP increases in the early follow-up (IOP>baseline IOP+10 mmHg in the first 7 days). Clinical examinations showed little or no signs of intraocular inflammation. Visual acuity remained statistically unchanged.

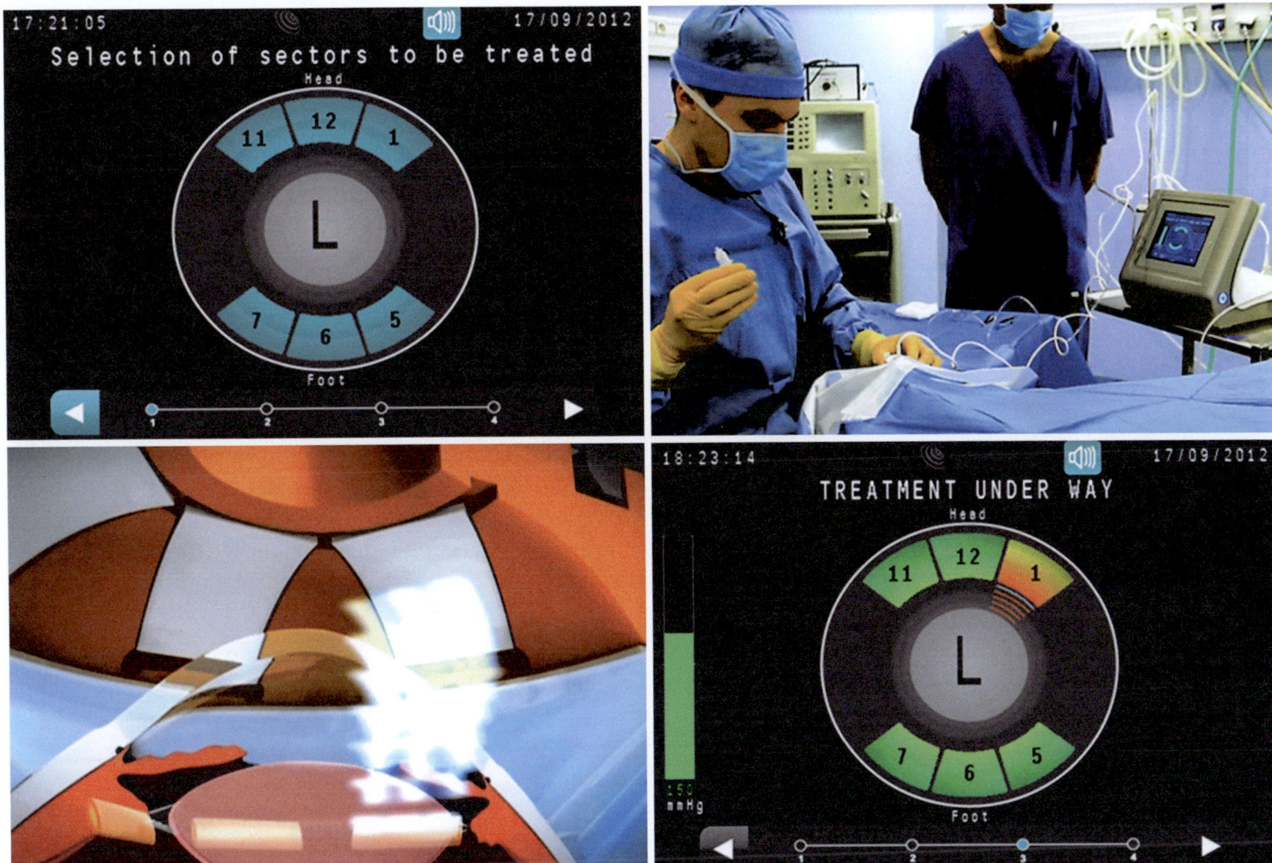


**Fig. 11.13** Choice of the number and position of the sectors to be activated (*top left*). Filling the device with saline solution and commencing the procedure (*top right*). Figured ultrasound beam during a sector shot (*bottom left*). Screen of the control module allowing the surgeon to check the progress of the procedure (sector one is being activated) (*bottom right*)

In the first multicenter study, no IOP spikes occurred just after the procedure or during the follow-up. Four patients were retreated with HIFU ($n=3$) or diode laser ($n=1$) due to lack of efficacy. Superficial punctuate keratitis occurred in eight patients. Transient macular edema occurred in one patient at 1 month with complete and spontaneous recovery at 2 months. Visual acuity remained statistically unchanged.

Retreatment: Some patients having an IOP response insufficient to reach the target IOP were retreated in the multicenter study. The six transducers were activated, and the orientation of the device was unchanged (no rotation); however, the diameter of the probe used for the second treatment was different from that used for the first treatment allowing to treat a more anteriorly or posteriorly located part of the ciliary body. IOP decrease was significant after the retreatment. However, it should be mentioned that only four patients were retreated with a limited duration of follow-up at the time of writing this chapter.

## Conclusions

IOP reduction by partial coagulation of the ciliary body using high-intensity focused ultrasound was first proposed in the late 1980s and resulted in the development and marketing of the Sonocare device. Several clinical studies were performed in patients with refractory glaucoma. Overall, the method seemed to be effective, providing a significant reduction in IOP. Despite these inherent advantages, the Sonocare was gradually abandoned in the mid-1990s, probably due, in part, to the complexity of using the system and also to the improvement of diode laser cyclophotocoagulation. Taking advantage of recent advances in the field of HIFU, a miniaturized device allowing selective, reproducible, and minimally invasive ciliary body coagulation was recently developed [14–17].

In animals, histological examination showed segmental coagulation necrosis of the ciliary body and ciliary processes with the loss of the bi-stratified epithelium and edema and vascular congestion of the ciliary stroma. These findings are consistent with those of previous studies in which transscleral or endoscopic diode or Nd:YAG laser cyclophotocoagulation was performed. By contrast, regeneration of the treated ciliary processes was not observed after HIFU treatment. Previous studies have shown that the ciliary epithelium may regenerate after laser cyclophotocoagulation resulting in restoration of aqueous humor secretion. The regeneration process is probably related to the recolonization of an intact

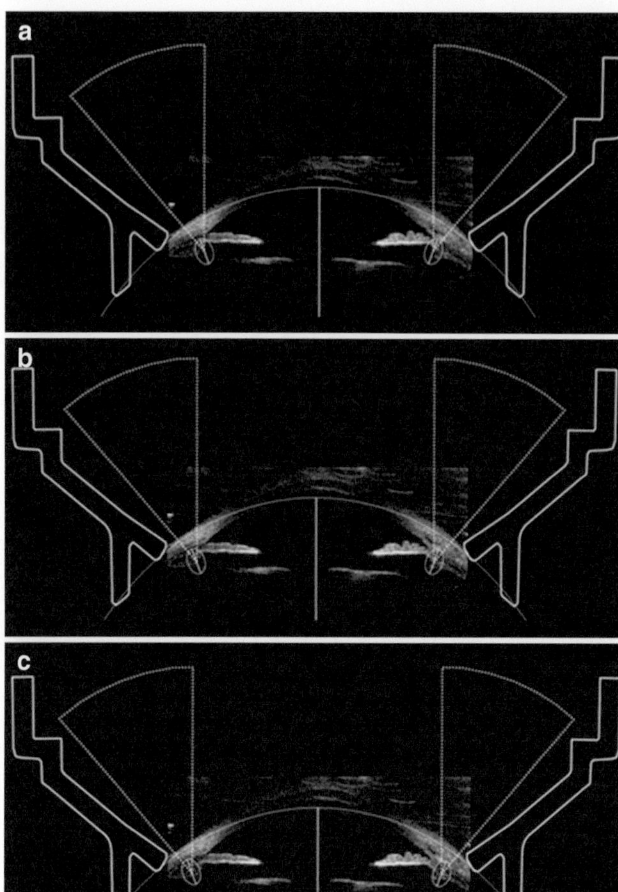

**Fig. 11.14** Location of the focal zones of the small- (**a**), middle- (**b**), and large (**c**)-diameter ring simulated on the UBM images. In this example, the larger-diameter model that better targets the ciliary body was chosen (Aptel et al. [16])

basement membrane by epithelial cells from basal and undestroyed areas of the ciliary processes. With HIFU cyclocoagulation, heating is probably greater – up to 80 °C – and is sufficient to completely destroy the basement membrane.

In about two-thirds of the animals treated, a fluid space could also be visualized between the sclera and the ciliary body and between the sclera and the choroid, likely corresponding to an increase of the aqueous outflow by the uveoscleral pathway. This aspect seems to be maintained over time in animals, likely indicating that it is due to tissue retraction or tissue microarchitecture change rather than intraocular inflammation. Moreover, similar aspects were found in humans after treatment using ultrasound biomicroscopy.

A first clinical pilot study, for which the main objectives were to assess the feasibility and safety of this new method of treatment, was conducted from March 2010. The destruction of the ciliary body using HIFU delivered by miniaturized transducers appears to be an effective and well-tolerated method of reducing intraocular pressure in patients with refractory glaucoma. An average IOP reduction of about 40 % was achieved at the last follow-up visit. A second multicenter study evaluating the long-term efficacy and safety of this procedure on a larger number of patients having less advanced primary open-angle glaucoma has produced very similar results. Similar studies are currently conducted in three European countries.

As the tolerability and safety profile of this new method of cyclocoagulation is very good, it seems logical to compare this new method to filtering surgery as a second-line treatment, after medical treatment. At the time of writing this chapter, a third clinical trial is about to commence in patients with primary open-angle glaucoma uncontrolled with medical treatment and naïve of any glaucoma surgery. Similarly, a randomized prospective clinical trial should be conducted to directly compare the efficacy of HIFU cyclocoagulation with that of trabeculectomy in the forthcoming months. These studies should help to define the indications and place of this new method of treatment.

## References


1. Weinreb RN, Khaw PT. Primary open-angle glaucoma. Lancet. 2004;363:1711–70.
2. Kass MA, Heuer DK, Higginbotham EJ, Johnson CA, Keltner JL, Miller JP, et al. The ocular hypertension treatment study: a randomized trial determines that topical ocular hypotensive medication delays or prevents the onset of primary open-angle glaucoma. Arch Ophthalmol. 2002;120:701–13.
3. Leske MC, Heijl A, Hussein M, Bengtsson B, Hyman L, Komaroff E. Early manifest glaucoma trial group. Factors for glaucoma progression and the effect of treatment: the early manifest glaucoma trial. Arch Ophthalmol. 2003;121:48–56.
4. American Academy of Ophthalmology preferred practice patterns. Primary open-angle glaucoma. San Francisco: American Academy of Ophthalmology; 2010. Available at: http://one.aao.org/CE/PracticeGuidelines/PPP.aspx?sid=ca9ec1b5-2567-4e85-96f6-b6540e5ac5a1.
5. Nouri-Mahdavi K, Brigatti L, Weitzman M, Caprioli J. Outcomes of trabeculectomy for primary open-angle glaucoma. Ophthalmology. 1995;102:1760–9.
6. Hamard P, Gayraud JM, Kopel J, Valtot F, Quesnot S, Hamard H. Treatment of refractory glaucomas by transscleral cyclophotocoagulation using semiconductor diode laser. Analysis of 50 patients followed up over 19 months. J Fr Ophtalmol. 1997;20:125–33.
7. Al-Ghamdi S, al-Obeidan S, Tomey KF, al-Jadaan I. Transscleral neodymium:YAG laser cyclophotocoagulation for end-stage glaucoma, refractory glaucoma, and painful blind eyes. Ophthalmic Surg. 1993;24:526–9.
8. De Roetth Jr A. Cryosurgery for the treatment of glaucoma. Trans Am Ophthalmol Soc. 1965;63:189–204.
9. Maus M, Katz LJ. Choroidal detachment, flat anterior chamber, and hypotony as complications of neodymium: YAG laser cyclophotocoagulation. Ophthalmology. 1990;97:69–72.
10. Uram M. Ophthalmic laser microendoscope ciliary process ablation in the management of neovascular glaucoma. Ophthalmology. 1992;99:1823–8.

11. Kosoko O, Gaasterland DE, Pollack IP, Enger CL. Long-term outcome of initial ciliary ablation with contact diode laser transscleral cyclophotocoagulation for severe glaucoma: the Diode Laser Ciliary Ablation Study Group. Ophthalmology. 1996;103:1294–302.

12. Sabri K, Vernon SA. Scleral perforation following trans-scleral cyclodiode. Br J Ophthalmol. 1999;83:502–3.

13. Vernon SA, Koppens JM, Menon GJ, Negi AK. Diode laser cycloablation in adult glaucoma: long-term results of a standard protocol and review of current literature. Clin Experiment Ophthalmol. 2006;34:411–20.

14. Aptel F, Charrel T, Palazzi X, Chapelon JY, Denis P, Lafon C. Histologic effects of a new device for high-intensity focused ultrasound cyclocoagulation. Invest Ophthalmol Vis Sci. 2010;51(10):5092–8. Epub 2010 May 19.

15. Charrel T, Aptel F, Birer A, Chavrier F, Romano F, Chapelon JY, Denis P, Lafon C. Development of a miniaturized HIFU device for glaucoma treatment with conformal coagulation of the ciliary bodies. Ultrasound Med Biol. 2011;37(5):742–54.

16. Aptel F, Charrel T, Lafon C, Romano F, Chapelon JY, Blumen-Ohana E, Nordmann JP, Denis P. Miniaturized high-intensity focused ultrasound device in patients with glaucoma: a clinical pilot study. Invest Ophthalmol Vis Sci. 2011;52(12):8747–53.

17. Aptel F, Lafon C. Therapeutic applications of ultrasound in ophthalmology. Int J Hyperthermia. 2012;28(4):405–18. doi:10.3109/02656736.2012.665566. Review.

18. Coleman DJ, Lizzi FL, Driller J, Rosado AL, Chang S, Iwamoto T, et al. Therapeutic ultrasound in the treatment of glaucoma. I. Experimental model. Ophthalmology. 1985;92:339–46.

19. Coleman DJ, Lizzi FL, Driller J, Rosado AL, Burgess SE, Torpey JH, et al. Therapeutic ultrasound in the treatment of glaucoma. II. Clinical applications. Ophthalmology. 1985;92:347–53.

20. Burgess SE, Silverman RH, Coleman DJ, Yablonski ME, Lizzi FL, Driller J, et al. Treatment of glaucoma with high-intensity focused ultrasound. Ophthalmology. 1986;93:831–8.

21. Valtot F, Kopel J, Haut J. Treatment of glaucoma with high intensity focused ultrasound. Int Ophthalmol. 1989;13:167–70.

22. Valtot F, Kopel J, Le Mer Y. Principles and histologic effects of the treatment of hypertension with focused high-intensity ultrasound. Ophtalmologie. 1990;4:135–7.

23. Haut J, Colliac JP, Falque L, Renard Y. Indications and results of Sonocare (ultrasound) in the treatment of ocular hypertension. A preliminary study of 395 cases. Ophtalmologie. 1990;4:138–41.

24. Valtot F, Denis P. The treatment of failed trabecular surgery in glaucoma with ultrasound (Sonocare). Ophtalmologie. 1990;4:142–4.

25. Silverman RH, Vogelsang B, Rondeau MJ, Coleman DJ. Therapeutic ultrasound for the treatment of glaucoma. Am J Ophthalmol. 1991;111:327–37.

26. Maskin SL, Mandell AI, Smith JA, Wood RC, Terry SA. Therapeutic ultrasound for refractory glaucoma: a three center study. Ophthalmic Surg. 1989;20:186–92.

27. Sterk CC, vd Valk PH, van Hees CL, van Delft JL, van Best JA, Oosterhuis JA. The effect of therapeutic ultrasound on the average of multiple intraocular pressures throughout the day in therapy-resistant glaucoma. Graefes Arch Clin Exp Ophthalmol. 1989;227:36–8.

28. Polack PJ, Iwamoto T, Silverman RH, Driller J, Lizzi FL, Coleman DJ. Histologic effects of contact ultrasound for the treatment of glaucoma. Invest Ophthalmol Vis Sci. 1991;32:2136–42.

29. Aptel F, Denis P, Rouland JF, Nordmann JP, Lachkar Y, Renard JP, Sellem E, Baudouin C, Bron A. Ultrasonic circular cyclo coagulation in patients with primary open-angle glaucoma: preliminary results of a multicenter clinical trial. Presented at ARVO 2012, Nice, France.

# Therapeutic Ultrasound for Glaucoma (TUG)

Donald Schwartz

## Advantages of Ultrasound in the Treatment of Glaucoma

The use of ultrasound to treat glaucoma has a number of specific advantages over current treatment modalities that have become more apparent over time.

Pharmaceutical agents have a multitude of side effects: hyperemia, allergy, potential for respiratory or cardiac events, fat atrophy, etc. There is the additional problem with costs and also with decreased cost of generics with quality control issues. The issue of *compliance* with pharmaceutical agents is problematic. It is plagued with issues of forgetfulness, inability to squeeze the bottle, poor drop placement, etc.

The laser offers an attractive alternative to the use of pharmaceuticals. But the laser requires a slit-lamp bio-microscope to be able to see the meshwork as treatment is given. In addition the positioning of some patients is difficult due to neck problems or stature or other considerations. The opening of the angle, iris synechiae, and the size of the palpebral aperture all can figure into whether the procedure may be easily administered. Repeatability is limited with the laser and the cost of the laser must also be considered. If not the laser, are there other means of "tickling" the trabecular meshwork with any other entity that could trigger beneficial biochemical changes?

The use of therapeutic ultrasound for glaucoma (TUG) has the potential for offering a repeatable, comfortable method for intraocular pressure control. It was perceived that such a gentle treatment might last for 6 months, but it has been found that it usually lasts longer. A slit lamp is not needed, and visualization of the anterior chamber is not required. The depth of the chamber is not a hindrance to treatment. As a direct result of the ability to perform the procedure without the need for a slit lamp, the device has the potential for miniaturization and portability. This portability has very significant implications for use in third world countries where pharmaceuticals are not a viable option, and the number of ophthalmologists to treat glaucoma surgically is insufficient.

Ultrasound had been used in the recent past to treat glaucoma as a means of cyclodestruction [8, 9, 20–24, 43]. The TUG model of glaucoma treatment is an outflow treatment. Ultrasound has three specific properties that offer some means of enhancing outflow: sonomechanical, local hyperthermia, and integrin triggering. The TUG device was designed to utilize the localized hyperthermia effect of focused ultrasound. But if heat is the only criterion for the treatment, why not just apply a heating element to the eye?

The application of a warm or hot probe to the outside of the eye will, by necessity, require a tip hotter than that of the ultrasound. In order to reach the 42.5 or 43.0 °C within the eye, it must be hotter than that on the surface. A temperature above 45° would lead to pain and necrosis. The energy of the ultrasound may be focused to a position apart from the tip and beyond where the application of the tip might lead to cell destruction.

As noted above, ultrasound offers additional advantages for the potential for sonomechanical effect and a direct effect on triggering integrins that may allow an additional effect of enhancing the cytokine cascade.

## Cataract Surgery and the Decrease in Intraocular Pressure

Those of us old enough to remember intracapsular cataract surgery may recall that when we approach that surgery, we did not have the same confidence that it would lead to a decrease in intraocular pressure (IOP) as we do today.

D. Schwartz, MD, OD, MPA, MOpt
Department of Ophthalmology,
Long Beach EyeCare Associates,
2650 Elm Ave 108, Long Beach, CA, USA
e-mail: dschwartz@eyesonix.com

**Electronic supplementary material** Supplementary material is available in the online version of this chapter at http://dx.doi.org/10.1007/978-1-4614-8348-9_12. Videos can also be accessed at http://www.springerimages.com/videos/978-1-4614-8347-2

J.R. Samples, I.I.K. Ahmed (eds.), *Surgical Innovations in Glaucoma*,
DOI 10.1007/978-1-4614-8348-9_12, © Springer Science+Business Media New York 2014

In fact a study by Radius in 1984 [7] revealed that a slight increase in IOP was found after intracapsular cataract surgery.

More recently the expectation that routine cataract surgery might actually benefit our patients with glaucoma and indeed might even be proposed as a method of decreasing the IOP was certainly in contrast to the experience with intracaps. There is no question that such is the case with narrow-angle glaucoma, but now some are advocating for cataract surgery with only minimal cataract as a surgery with benefits for open-angle glaucoma [1–5, 57]. What has changed during this time? The change in cataract surgery to phacoemulsification using ultrasound appears to be coexistent with the finding of a decrease in the IOP following cataract surgery [1–6].

Underlying much of the recent literature supporting the finding of decreasing IOP after cataract surgery [66] is an assumption that this decrease is a result of an increase in the opening of the anterior chamber angle [18, 58, 65]. This assumption, although convenient, was in conflict with the findings of a slight increase in IOP after cataract surgery when an intracapsular cataract surgery was performed. Wasn't the angle opened up as much with an intracapsular cataract surgery as with phaco? When studies have been performed to verify if there were correlation between the increase in the angle architecture and the decrease in pressure, this was not found [18, 58, 65, 66]. The correlation between the decrease in preoperative intraocular pressure and postoperative pressure was found with the severity of the preoperative pressure, but not with a change in the angle or depth of the chamber [6, 18].

The point of most resistance to the outflow of aqueous humor is considered to be in the juxtacanalicular portion of the trabecular meshwork [32–34, 36–42].

The juxtacanalicular portion of the trabecular meshwork is the most distal portion of the meshwork. Would an increase in the angle therefore lead to an increase in aqueous exit through the juxtacanalicular portion of the trabecular meshwork?

If the increase in the angle is not the reason for the decrease in pressure, and there is acceptance that cataract surgery is able to somehow lead to a decrease in pressure, what has changed since intracapsular surgery? The most important starting point to consider is the advent of the use of ultrasound in removing the nucleus of the lens. Could the various effect of ultrasound within the confines of the anterior segment of the eye lead to an unanticipated but beneficial side effect of lowered intraocular pressure? [14, 15].

In 2006 I began to consider that there was an unanticipated beneficial effect of ultrasound in leading to a decrease in IOP. If the specific nature of this effect could be determined and refined, could this lead to the development of a new technique to treat glaucoma?

Throughout the latter months of 2006, I began to familiarize myself with the effects of ultrasound with potential for leading to a decrease in pressure. I also had to delve into the biochemistry of glaucoma and how ultrasound might have an effect on the various pathways that were becoming known.

Although photographs of the histology of the trabecular meshwork after ALT and SLT laser treatment are markedly different [59], it was interesting to consider that the laser effect in both was from triggered biochemical cascades rather than a change in the microarchitecture of the meshwork.

Ultrasound for the treatment of glaucoma was not a completely new concept. In the 1980s Jackson Coleman and group developed an ultrasound instrument to treat refractory glaucoma [9, 20–24] (Sonocare system CST 100). Their instrument was designed to use HIFU (high-intensity focused ultrasound) 20 kW/cm$^2$ to ablate the ciliary body [20]. This instrument has fallen into disfavor due to significant side effects.

There are three potential mechanisms of ultrasound that had some possible means of leading to a decrease in pressure. These mechanisms were not mutually exclusive: (1) sonomechanical or vibratory effect of ultrasound [10, 25, 26, 28–30, 32], (2) thermal effect [19], and (3) mechanism of triggering a cellular integrin response [11, 12].

In Sweden Bjorn Svedbergh worked on a device using non-focused ultrasound to treat glaucoma. His work centered on the sonomechanical effect of ultrasound and its use was aimed at a vibratory cleansing of the trabecular meshwork. Private communications reveal that this led to a significant decrease in IOP (20 %) in 26 % of those treated lasting for 1 year.

To study the sonomechanical effect, I evaluated the additional effect of ultrasound that might be present beyond the flushing effect of irrigation and aspiration during cataract surgery. The anterior chambers of five different pig eyes were filled with 2 μm size fluorescein-labeled microspheres. Irrigation and aspiration of the anterior chamber was then performed. The position of the movement of the microspheres through the outflow path of the porcine eyes in those with ultrasound turned on in the anterior chamber was compared with microphotographs to those that only had irrigation and aspiration. The movement of the microspheres through the outflow was further in the eyes with ultrasound (Fig. 12.1).

The movement of the microspheres was gratifying with ultrasound, but it also became apparent that in order for the sonomechanical effect to be substantial, there had to be a simultaneous irrigation of fluid. In addition such a device had a substantial potential for cataract formation in the phakic eye. Furthermore, I was concerned about the sonomechanical mechanism of ultrasound which had the capacity to increase from "aqueous streaming" to significant "cavitation" effect and additional tissue destruction.

# Sonomechanical ultrasound effect

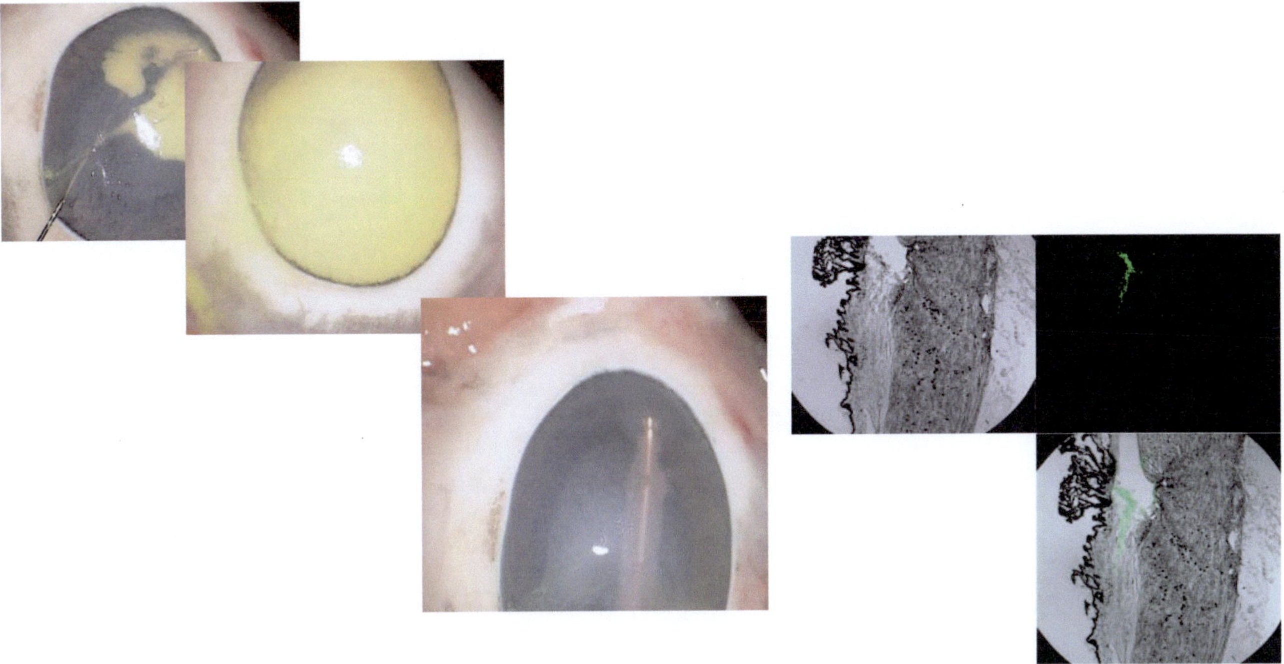

**Fig. 12.1** Fluorescein-dyed microspheres appearance in outflow after intraocular ultrasound in pig eye

Attention was then directed to the thermal effect of ultrasound. The literature reporting on the thermal effects of ultrasound was primarily focused on orthopedic or oncologic processes and treatments [44–56, 61–64]. These areas of interest and work seemed to offer substantial possibilities, for very often the processes involved a triggering of cytokine activity by the thermal effects of ultrasound in the orthopedic literature. In the oncology literature there was a great deal of interest in the use of either local or whole-body hyperthermia to trigger beneficial inflammatory responses [60–62].

A further literature search revealed a paper by Schuman et al. [13]. that reported the finding of specific inflammatory cytokines in eyes after cataract surgery. This paper proposed that the decrease in IOP after cataract surgery might be due to these cytokine findings.

This paper along with the proposed mechanism of action of SLT [27, 35, 36] and the potential for localized hyperthermia by ultrasound might offer another means of triggering a beneficial cytokine cascade quite analogous to the laser but with a different energy source.

Further review of the literature was done. This time the specific purpose was to find the maximum temperature that could be attained without leading to cell death or pain. Various sources reported that cell death and/or pain began at 45 °C [63, 64]. I also reviewed the literature to find the temperature pattern where inflammatory cytokines were triggered. This temperature was approximately 42.5 °C. This

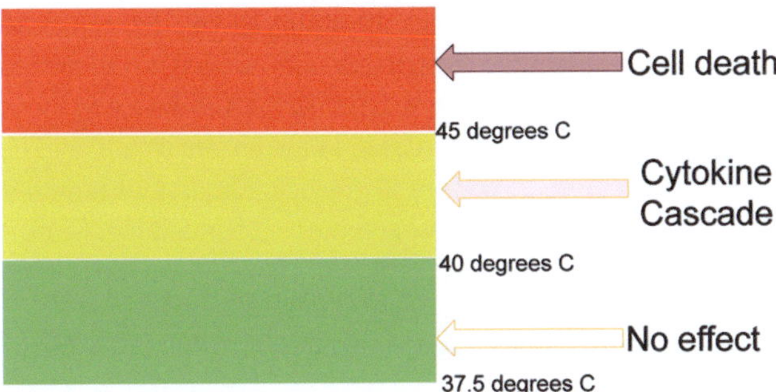


**Fig. 12.2** Hyperthermia and cell cytokine cascade

seemed to indicate that there was a "sweet spot" of a range of a few degrees where the elevated temperature could trigger cytokines but not lead to cell death or pain (Fig. 12.2).

If an ultrasound could be produced that could be used to create a localized, controlled limited hyperthermia, I needed to determine such a power and frequency. Because of the potential for damage in such a small temperature range and the close proximity of vulnerable tissue, I chose to work with a focused ultrasound. I was unsure of the power, but I knew that whatever the power was, it had to be able to produce a sustained temperature of 43 or so degrees centigrade.

**Fig. 12.3** Evolution of handpiece for ultrasound treatment

## Evolution of the prototype Hand piece

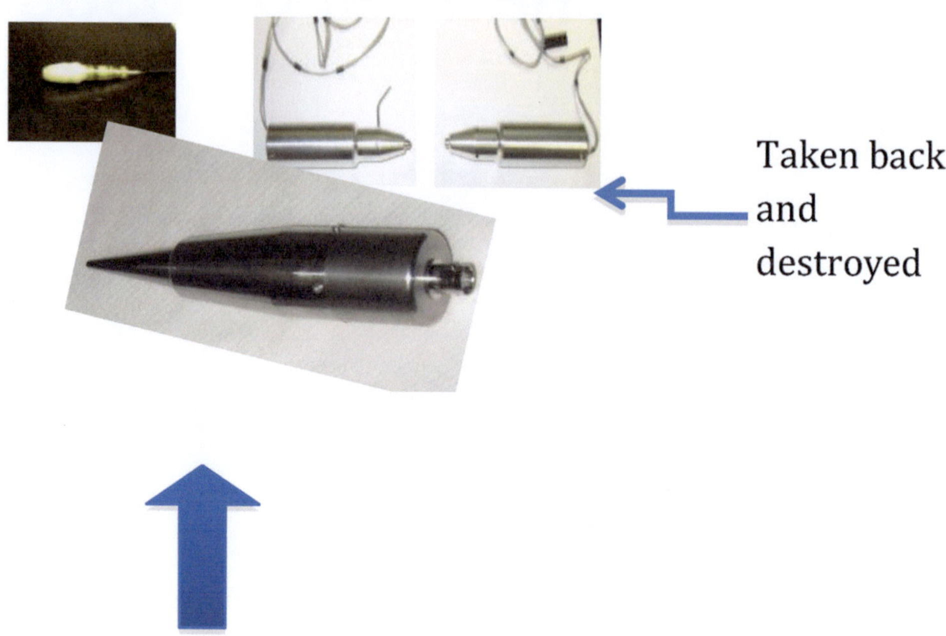


Clinical work began with this one

## AAO Las Vegas 2006

I met with an ultrasound designer/builder on the exhibit floor of the Academy meeting. I had no idea of the proper frequency (ultrasound starts at 20 KHz and extends into the millions). He suggested one million as the proper frequency for my needs. I had him build the device with the ability to vary the power so that I could determine how much was needed to attain the proper temperature. I told him that I needed the device to focus the power at a point 1 mm in front of the tip. He agreed and he started the project. I received the device. Excitedly I turned it on….I heard nothing…..I saw nothing ….I felt nothing. I called him; I was disappointed and told him. He told me to hook it up to my oscilloscope. I didn't have a G.D… oscilloscope!!

I decided to return to what was obvious. If phacoemulsification had the capacity to produce the effect then that was the frequency that I could use. I went looking for a company that could produce an ultrasound with enough power, to be focused and be in the range of 50 KHz. I found such a company about 25 miles from my office. The engineer/owner was about 75 years old and was quite interested in my device. He told me he could build my device without charge, but he wanted first refusal to produce it. I agreed. He built two versions of slightly different frequencies.

I set up a laboratory through my hospital. I plugged in the device. I obtained pig eyes, made a small incision at the limbus, and inserted a micro-thermometer wire into the trabecular meshwork. I placed the tip of the handpiece against the limbus and aimed the tip at the position of the temperature wire. I was

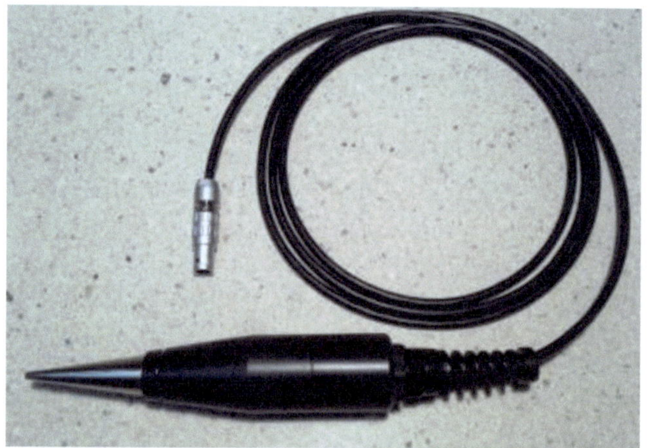

## Most recent hand piece

**Fig. 12.4** Latest "TUG" handpiece

looking for a temperature rise of approximately 6 °C. I worked with these two devices, but I found that there was some variability in effect depending on the angle of application and the amount of pressure applied during the treatment. The owner of the ultrasound company came to the lab to offer assistance. He offered to take the handpieces back and rework them to improve the design. It was over a month of calls when he finally answered and returned my calls. He told me he was too old to see much value in pursuing what would probably be many years before a product would be marketed. He didn't want to be part of such a long-time venture (Figs. 12.3 and 12.4).

**Fig. 12.5** Temperature increase with various power setting for early in vitro studies

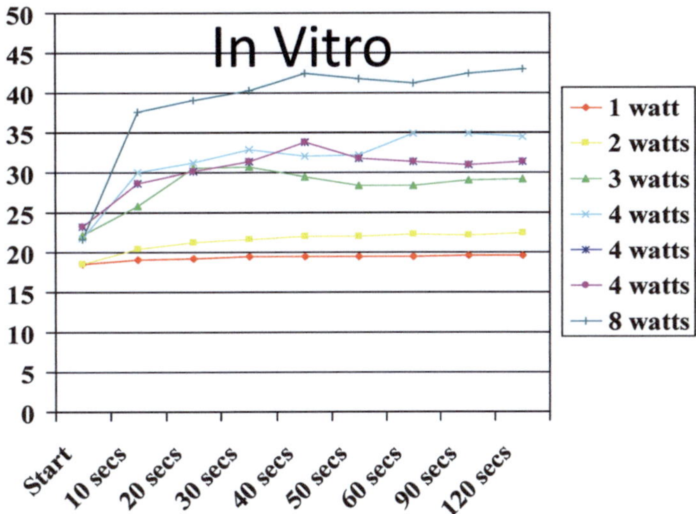


He destroyed the handpieces and used the parts in other devices he had sold. I tried to pay him to build more prototypes, but he never returned my calls or letters.

I went back to the search for another company to build the prototypes. I found one that could and would build them. I bought two, one of 40 KHz and one of 60 KHz. These prototypes had a function generator where I could vary the frequency to tune the handpiece, a power amplifier to get me to enough energy to deliver, and the handpieces that produced focused ultrasound into the meshwork. I set out to find the proper amount of power to raise the temperature by 6° (Fig. 12.5).

The earliest in vitro testing was to determine the increase in temperature from the ambient room temperature. Once I found the right combination, I purchased a used water bath on eBay to warm up some pig eyes to basal temperature of 37.5 °C. I repeated the studies until I could find the correct power and frequency and application pressure to raise the temperature to 43° and maintain the temperature for 25 s. It typically took 20 s of application of the ultrasound to reach the temperature. On one of the testing days, I accidentally placed the power setting at about five times maximum and blew out the core of the 60 K handpiece. I continued all of my subsequent work with the 40 KHz handpiece (there was no difference in the findings of the two handpieces up until it blew out).

Once I determined the settings that worked in the in vitro model, I arranged for in vivo work on the porcine eye.

## Porcine Study

Treatments were performed in eyes with matching controls at various powers around the power settings that worked on the in vitro work. Trained veterinary ophthalmologists performed a careful analysis of the eyes, which were sent on to the university for analysis. Unfortunately, there was no final report filed by the researcher, but in a meeting with the pathologist, it was reported that there was only minimal inflammation except in the case of the application of a power that was twice the expected treatment power. It was also shown that when the application of the tip of the device was directly on the cornea with that higher power setting, there was evidence of a corneal burn. From that point forward the application of the tip has been always with a clear space between the cornea and the tip.

## Results

...Gross ocular observations are presented in Table 12.2. On Day 1, animals in Group A and B displayed no signs of ocular irritation or discomfort in either eye. The animal in Group C (No.66 exhibited mild conjunctival redness in both eyes on Day 2. The animal in Group d (No67) exhibited moderate conjunctival redness and discharge and mild chemosis in both eyes on Day 2....

## Rabbit Study

The study was then performed on the rabbit model with concentration on the power setting much more closely in line with that expected to be used for treatment. I was anxious to refine the treatment parameters, and I felt that using the rabbit (reputed to be much more sensitive to inflammatory stimuli), the findings would be more valuable. These studies revealed a mild inflammatory response in the external examination. The globes were then fixed and transported to an independent laboratory that sectioned and analyzed the tissue.

## Results

….All right eye sections had a lesion diagnosed as chronicactive inflammation, limbus (graded minimal to mild). The lesion was characterized by an infiltrate of mononuclear cells and polymorphonuclear cells near the limbus. The infiltrate was usually just under the conjunctiva (subconjunctival connective tissue) and extended towards or into the canal of Schlemm." "…….There were no changes observed in the cornea, sclera or ciliary body…..

## TUG.1

The next step was human clinical work. For such work I needed an oversight of an appropriate institutional review board; I began with the two institutions where I am affiliated, University of Southern California and University of California at Irvine. Because I am on the voluntary faculty, I could not be in charge of such research at either place. In addition I had some concerns that the intellectual property rights that I had paid so dearly for might be in some way transferred to the institutions. I decided to go with an independent, nonaffiliated board. This was actually an excellent decision, for the board meets very frequently, has many such projects, and can make decisions on almost a daily basis rather than waiting for a month between such committees in a university setting.

After reviewing my application to treat human eyes and the work that was done, the institutional review board (IRB) agreed that my device was an nonsignificant risk device. This finding meant that I did not have to have the full IDE review by the FDA for the study intended. The first treatments were performed on patients with blind eyes to simply determine the tolerability of the treatment. These treatments would be done with appropriate and necessary informed consent and with no expectation of any help with vision. I scoured my patient population in my practice and found very few who would meet the qualifications. I approached the local Braille Institute to find any potential subjects. I offered to pay money and transportation for the treatments. I found a total of 13 subjects who wished to be part of such a study.

The procedure up until it was first used had a cumbersome description and no name. I knew that in referring to the procedure that such procedures typically had a three-letter acronym to make it easier to recall. I played with the three words that were important, therapeutic, ultrasound, and glaucoma in various permutations, and felt that the procedure would best be called "TUG" for therapeutic ultrasound for glaucoma. It offered an easily remembered name, it had the three important words included and additionally it gave an impression of being a gentle method of treatment.

This study, TUG.1, was purely a tolerability study to determine if such a treatment and protocol was comfortable. The evaluations were performed pretreatment and posttreatment with symptoms of discomfort or pain reported to my clinical coordinator. In addition a slit-lamp examination was performed with evaluation of conjunctival hyperemia and anterior segment flare and cells.

On March 9, 2009, I treated the first patient with the device. He had been in Nicaragua and in 1986 had a bomb blow up in his face leaving him with no usable vision in his eye (Fig. 12.6).

He was excited about what I was doing, knew that there was no expectation of vision for the eye to be treated, and took it as a special badge of honor to be the very first person in the world to have ever been treated with the device. Coincidentally that date in 2009 was World Glaucoma Day.

A number of subjects were transported from the Braille Institute, and those of my own practice constituted the subjects for this first study. The procedure was tolerated easily with only mild irritation reported by the subject for the first day. These subjects were seen 2–3 h after treatment to check for any pressure spike, 1 day, 1 week, and monthly for 6 months. If there were more than mild irritation and more than mild conjunctival injection noted at slit lamp at the first day, the subject was given a topical nonsteroidal to use for a couple of days.

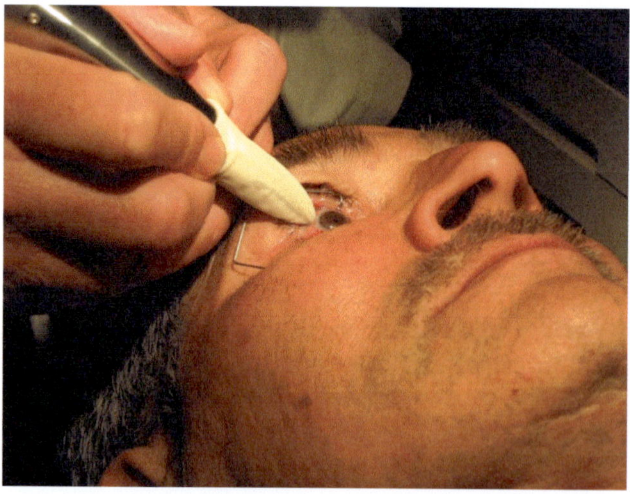

**Fig. 12.6** First human treatment with TUG device

The TUG.1 study revealed an easily tolerated procedure with very little subjective discomfort and only mild inflammatory reaction noted at slit lamp the first day. Although the IOP was not part of this initial study protocol, it was followed and did reveal a gratifying decrease.

Some of the nuances of the actual treatment protocol had to be addressed. How many treatment spots, how many seconds at each spot, how much pressure to exert against the eye, exactly how far from the limbus, how to tell how much pressure was being exerted, and what angle should the device be held against the eye? What if there was a scar that prevented treatment in a specific location? In addition there was the continuing difficulty of tuning the whole treatment apparatus.

Each time the device was used it had to be tuned. The tuning process involved setting the frequency to match the handpiece frequency that worked the best. Although the piezoelectric crystals were set for 40 KHz, it seemed to work best at 40.33 KHz once it was warmed up (Fig. 12.7).

Therefore, the function generator was set in the general range of 40 K and then dialed around the 40.33 K much like tuning a radio to be the best reception. And like a radio, there was frequently a slight drift that occurred. Constant monitoring of the frequency was required. The function generator therefore created a source for the power amplifier. This proper frequency with a small voltage was then fed into the power amplifier. This voltage output of the function generator needed to be tuned to the proper mVolt usually in the range of 100–115 mV. The amplifier allowed the power to be stepped up to a point where the handpiece was functional. On the power amplifier was a window that allowed monitoring of the power sent to the handpiece. This window showed two numbers: the first number was the power sent to the handpiece and the second was the "reflectance" back to the power amplifier. If they were equal, such as "3" and "3," that meant that there was no real power being used, and it was all reflected back to the amplifier. The best situation was that of the first number being

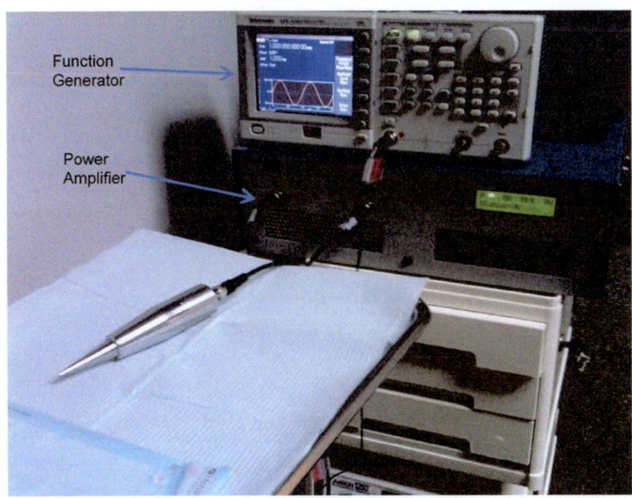


**Fig. 12.7** TUG apparatus used for early clinical studies

"3" or more and the second "0," ensuring that all of the power was being used by the handpiece and none reflected back. My assistant monitored these numbers as the treatments were performed. One difficulty with this "reflectance" window was that it was a digital readout and simply jumped from "3" to "4"; there was no "3.2" or "3.9." It was only whole integers in the readout, so I had to extrapolate. As I increased the function generator power knob, I could see the power window number jump to the next integer. I was able to determine the range within the "3" before it jumped to "4" and thereby found the function generator setting that would create approximately 3.5–3.75 W. Again my assistant would keep track of any variation caused by drift as the treatment was progressing. The tuning could take up to 45 min before the device was functional. The power amplifier had a moderately loud fan and loud humming sound, and it would gradually heat up the room, many times to an uncomfortable level.

## Method of Treatment

### Video (Video 12.1)

The subject was examined at slit lamp immediately before the treatment. A drop of tetracaine was placed in the eye to be treated. Then the subject was tilted back in the examination chair. A lid speculum was placed in the eye and the conjunctiva was marked with a marking pen. (The marking originally was to demarcate the 12 equally spaced treatment locations with 12 marks. In reality this simply became confusing. The eye is now marked with 4 lines demarcating 4 quadrants, and 3 treatments are performed within each treatment quadrant). An additional 4 % xylocaine gel was then used to over the limbal area and the cornea. This gel provides three functions. It adds additional anesthesia, it provides the contact gel for the ultrasound transmission, and it keeps the cornea moist throughout the procedure. The subject would be able to move his/her eye to expose the treatment location. I would be seated at the 12:00 position and begin treatment at the 1:00 position. The frequency, mV readings, and power amplifier readings were noted and followed by my assistant at each application of the handpiece to the eye. The "angle of attack" of the handpiece was 45° to the globe with the tip aimed deep to the center of the crystalline lens. This angle was chosen to place the focal point of the ultrasound within the trabecular meshwork. The tip is placed on the globe at the limbus with a small clear space from the cornea on the scleral side allowing approximately 0.5 mm from the cornea. The handpiece is then held firmly against the globe for the full 45 s. A timer with a countdown is used for this with the assistant counting off 10 s intervals. The amount of pressure against the globe is such that it is just enough to distort the corneal arc to become flat at the location of the application of the tip. This amount of pressure does not cause pain, and it is also enough to allow the globe to become mildly fixed to the tip as the seconds count off so that there is constant treatment. Occasionally the subject will report some discomfort. Moving the tip slightly toward one side or another from the location easily stops this. Less than 1 mm will move the tip away from any point of pain (positioning of the tip directly over the nerves is felt to be the cause of this discomfort). The subject will typically feel some warmth and a mild tingling during the course of the treatment.

## TUG.2

Once the TUG.1 series was followed over the 6 months without significant side effects and seen to be well tolerated, the IRB was approached again. This time a protocol was designed to evaluate the treatment on sighted eyes with glaucoma. These subjects were typically on medical treatment. Only one of the subjects' eyes was treated. The eye to be treated was randomized by coin flip. The non-treated eye continued on medication, whereas the treated eye had a washout by protocol before treatment (where the patient had an eye with previous pressures above 40 mmHg there was no washout). This series was of ten subjects. It was designed to verify the best treatment parameters and techniques to lead to a decrease in IOP. Those parameters were listed above in the Method of Treatment, but were refined within the TUG.2 group. This study was aimed at small changes in the number of seconds of application, the amount of pressure exerted against the globe, and trying to determine within the "integer" window of the power amplifier how to extrapolate to the very best power in W/cm$^2$.

The treatment was done as per the method above with some specific variables to be analyzed as to affect. The subjects were seen 2 h after the treatment for a pressure check to determine any spike. Then they were seen at 1 day, 1 week, 1 month, and then monthly for 6 months.

Subjective findings of discomfort and pain were noted by assistants on a scale of 1–4 with 4 being the worst. Objective findings of conjunctival injection, anterior chamber flare, and anterior chamber cell were noted by the physician (DS).

The measurement of the intraocular pressure was paramount during these early studies and always followed the same method. Before the physician came into the room, a tonopen was used to make five separate measurements of each eye. Then the Goldmann applanation tonometer (calibrated each week) was then used by the assistant. At this time the physician examined the patient and did his own Goldmann pressures. The tonopen measurements were then averaged and then this was averaged with the average of the two Goldmann measurements. It was felt in this manner that bias in measurements was mitigated as much as possible, with the single measurement by the investigator counting only one third against the two thirds of the digital tonopen and the assistant.

### TUG.2 Example (Fig. 12.8)

Subject #231 has been followed far beyond the original TUG.2 study.

He had undiagnosed glaucoma when first presented to the office in 2008. He was controlled on two medications since

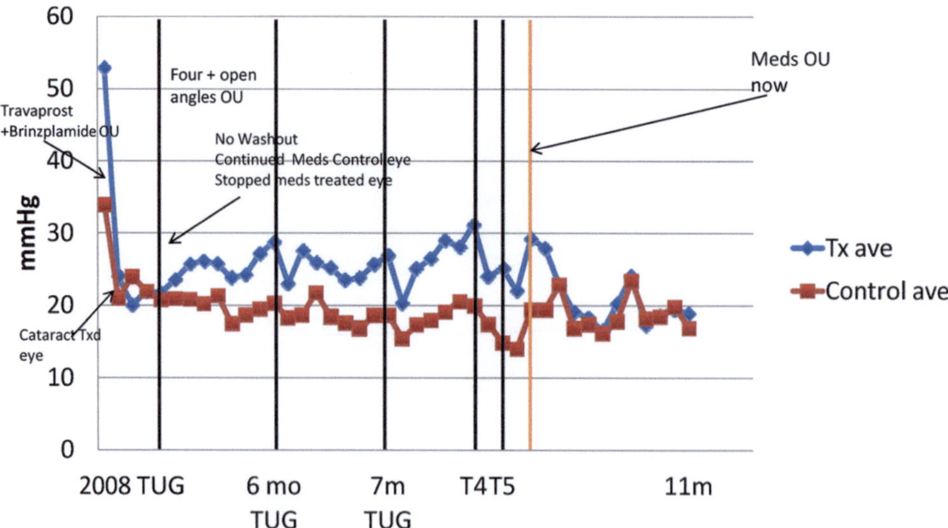



**Fig. 12.8** TUG.2 study with repeated treatments

2008 and then had cataract surgery in the eye that would later become the TUG treated eye. His anterior chamber angle was noted, even before cataract surgery as being 4+ deep. Because of the previous high pressure, I elected not to wash out the treatment eye to avoid a significant pressure spike. He was treated, but after 6 months the IOP was seen to be climbing toward 30 mmHg. He was treated again, and this lasted for an additional 7 months. After an additional 6 months, another treatment was given. At this point there was a question raised by the subject as to a potential benefit by two treatments close together to act as an additional effect rather than waiting for any pressure rise. A fifth treatment (T5) was then given only 1 month after the fourth treatment to see if such a quick succession of treatments might be even more beneficial. That strategy seemed to offer an additional effect, but then he wished to be off of the study follow-up schedule (he was seen 32 times between the first TUG treatment and the re-initiation of pharmaceutical treatment over an 18-month period). He is now 11 months after the reintroduction of medical treatment with both eyes with an IOP of 18 mmHg.

This particular subject reveals that multiple treatments are possible without deleterious effects on the resumption of medication. It also indicates that even with the potential for a very high IOP, the pressure could be controlled with repeated TUG treatments.

## TUG.3

The TUG.3 clinical study was designed with two branches. It is a prospective, randomized, and "controlled" study. The branches are (1) those who were either naïve to pharmaceutical treatment or who had not been on such treatment for at least 6 months prior to the TUG treatment and (2) subjects who were using pharmaceutical agents. Those who were on pharmaceutical agents had a washout of 1 month for the prostaglandin medications and one week for other medications prior to treatment.

A total of 26 patients were followed for the full year of the study (with many now followed over 3 years since the study was begun). There were 17 subjects who were on medication when brought into the study. There were 9 who were in the "naïve" group.

The baseline for the "naïve" group was an average of IOP of the two visits before the TUG treatment. For the pharmaceutical treatment group, the baseline was an average of the two previous visits while on medication prior to washout. This baseline comparison to medical control was chosen as the move to "comparative effectiveness" was being considered.

Besides the evaluation of the change in intraocular pressure, the study followed the subjective and objective effects of the treatment. The same symptoms and signs as followed in the TUG.2 study were followed in the TUG.3 study.

In comparing TUG.3 to TUG.2, there were differences in the washout and use of medication. As opposed to TUG.2, in TUG.3 the washout was in both eyes, but the treatment was only in one randomly chosen eye. If there were a significant difference in IOP, the higher pressure of the two was treated with the non-treated eye serving as what was considered the "control."

The toleration of the procedure was evaluated on a scale of 1–4 for both subjective symptoms and objective signs. An average of all 26 subjects was taken for these markers and is seen in graphs that follow (Figs. 12.9 and 12.10).

The effect on intraocular pressure is exemplified by the following subject #237 (Fig. 12.11).

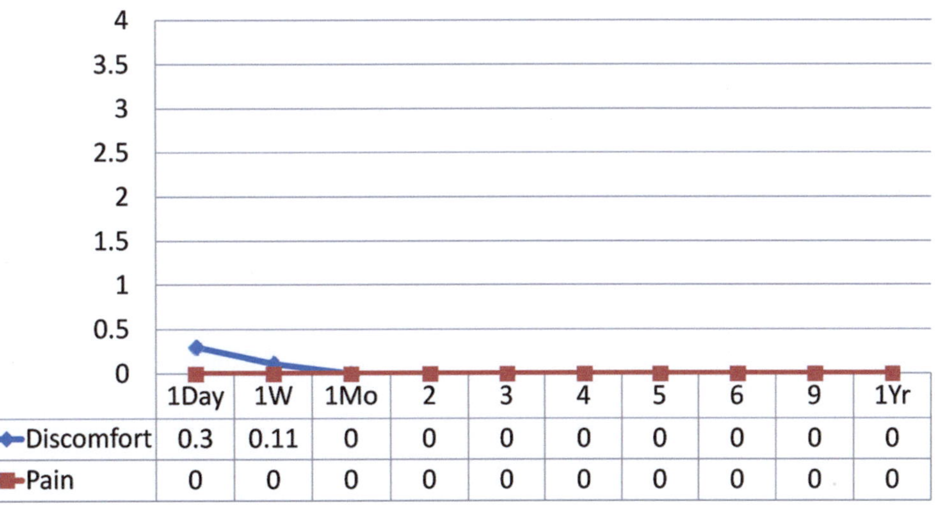



|  | 1Day | 1W | 1Mo | 2 | 3 | 4 | 5 | 6 | 9 | 1Yr |
|---|---|---|---|---|---|---|---|---|---|---|
| Discomfort | 0.3 | 0.11 | 0 | 0 | 0 | 0 | 0 | 0 | 0 | 0 |
| Pain | 0 | 0 | 0 | 0 | 0 | 0 | 0 | 0 | 0 | 0 |

**Fig. 12.9** Symptoms posttreatment

**Fig. 12.10** Signs posttreatment

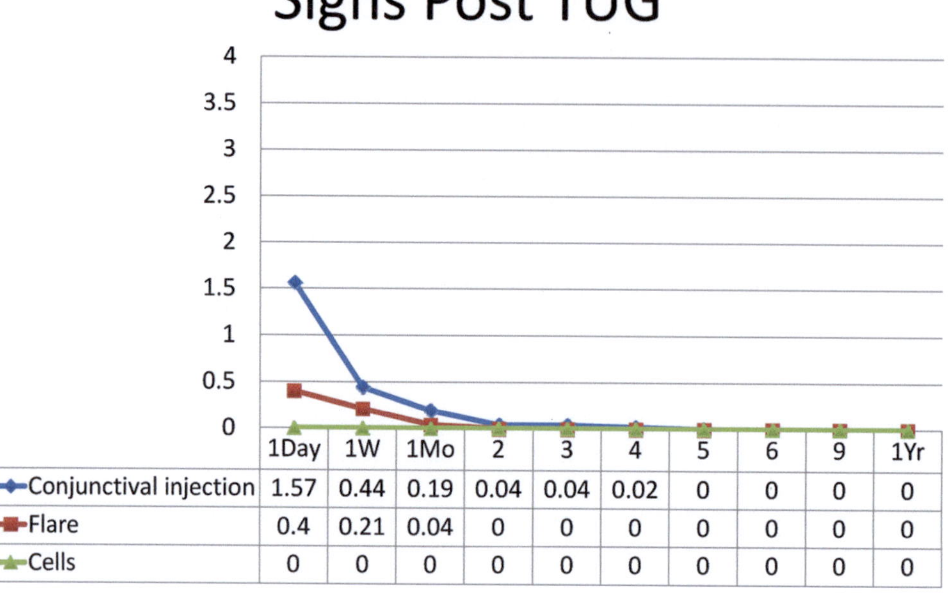



| | 1Day | 1W | 1Mo | 2 | 3 | 4 | 5 | 6 | 9 | 1Yr |
|---|---|---|---|---|---|---|---|---|---|---|
| Conjunctival injection | 1.57 | 0.44 | 0.19 | 0.04 | 0.04 | 0.02 | 0 | 0 | 0 | 0 |
| Flare | 0.4 | 0.21 | 0.04 | 0 | 0 | 0 | 0 | 0 | 0 | 0 |
| Cells | 0 | 0 | 0 | 0 | 0 | 0 | 0 | 0 | 0 | 0 |

**Fig. 12.11** TUG.3 Washout subject

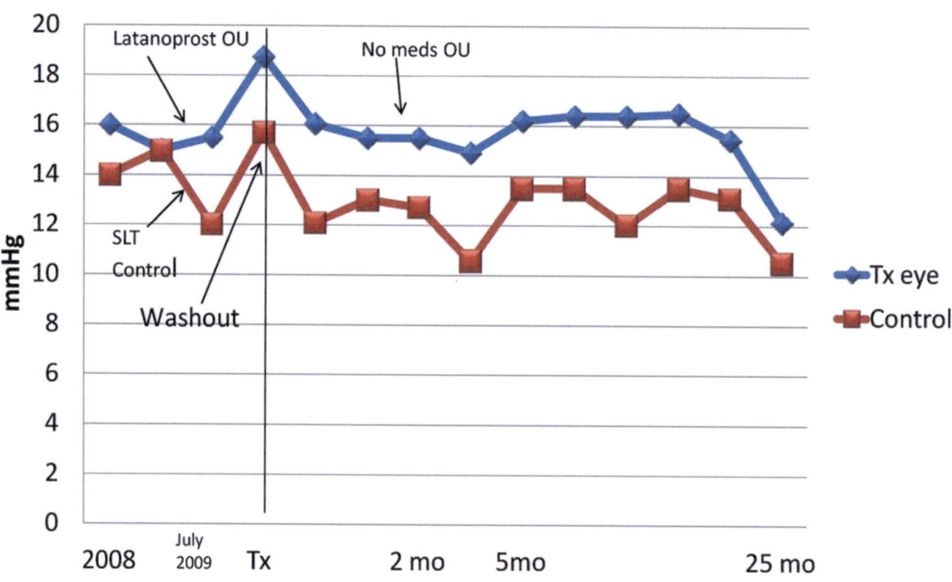



This subject with normotensive glaucoma had been on treatment with latanoprost since 2008. Because of worsening optic nerve cupping, he had an SLT in one (the non-TUG treated eye). At the initiation of the TUG treatment, he had a washout of the latanoprost for 1 month with an elevation in IOP. The washout was in both and shows an expected mild increase in IOP. Only one eye (treatment eye) was treated and then both eyes have been followed. Although the TUG.3 study only lasted for 1 year, he has been followed for over 2 years post-TUG treatment with the IOP at least comparable to that when he was on latanoprost. He has had only one TUG treatment, in one eye, which has lasted over 25 months with a pressure in each eye at least comparable to that when he was on bilateral latanoprost.

## A Bilateral Effect?

Additionally, as can be seen, there appear to be intraocular pressure changes in the non-treated eye. The IOP readings reflect a similar decrease in IOP in the non-treated (control) eye that shadows the effect in the treated eye. If the effect of the treatment were purely mechanical (such as a vibration that allowed clearance of debris from the meshwork) the effect would be expected to be present in only one eye. If the effect were an ablative technique that led to a decrease in IOP due to ciliary body injury, the effect would be expected to be seen in only the eye treated.

With the advent of SLT laser the consideration of the possible mechanism for bilateral IOP lowering seen with monocular treatment have been proposed. These potential mechanisms are based upon a triggering of cytokines, which then systemically effect the IOP, in turn by production of a matrix metalloproteinase enzyme and the induction of macrophages, which help to clear the path for aqueous exit from the eye. Because of this bilateral effect seen repeatedly in the TUG series of subjects, I feel that a similar, if not the same, mechanism of action is being triggered by the TUG and SLT.

## IOP Changes After TUG in Naïve Branch

In the group where there was no pharmaceutical control of pressure, a comparison was made to the IOP found on initial examination or, if two visits had occurred, to the average of these two pressures (Figs. 12.12 and 12.13).

It is well known that the IOP control is more difficult when treating normotensive glaucoma patients. With this in

**Fig. 12.12** Intraocular pressure effect on entire "naïve" group

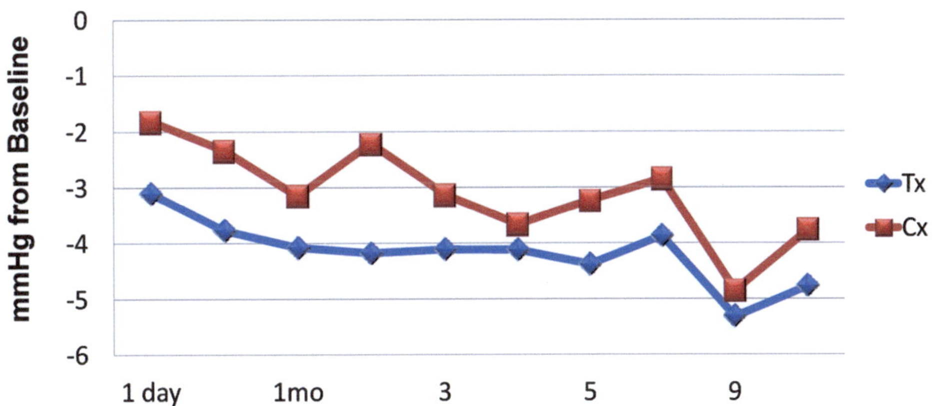


**Fig. 12.13** Intraocular pressure effect on naïve group without normotensive glaucoma subjects

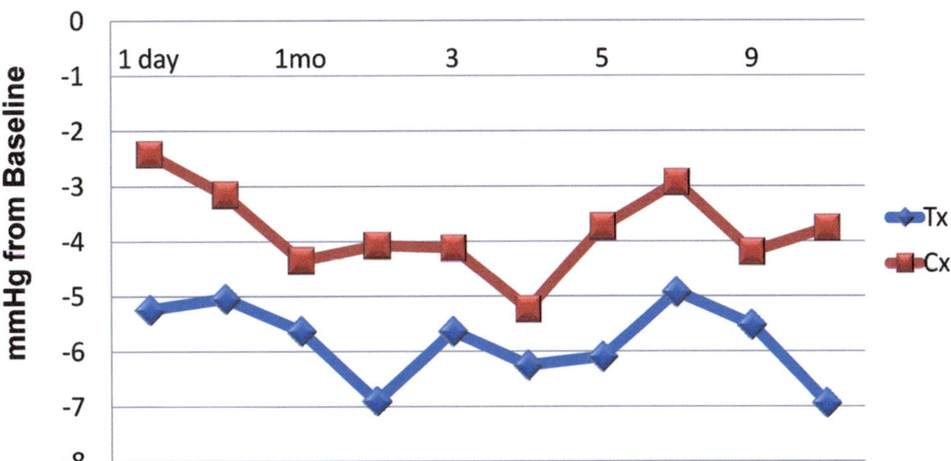

**Fig. 12.14** Comparison of intraocular pressure while on medication prior to washout to post-TUG treatment

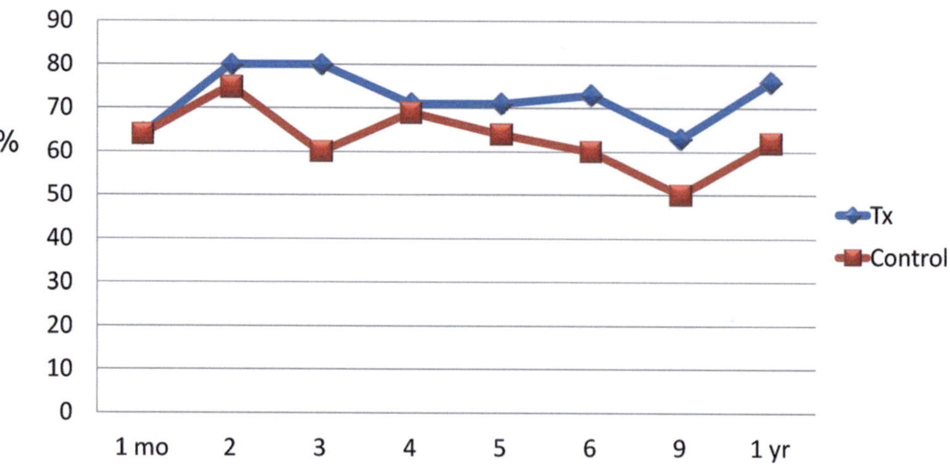



**Fig. 12.15** Unilateral glaucoma patient with return to medication and multiple treatments

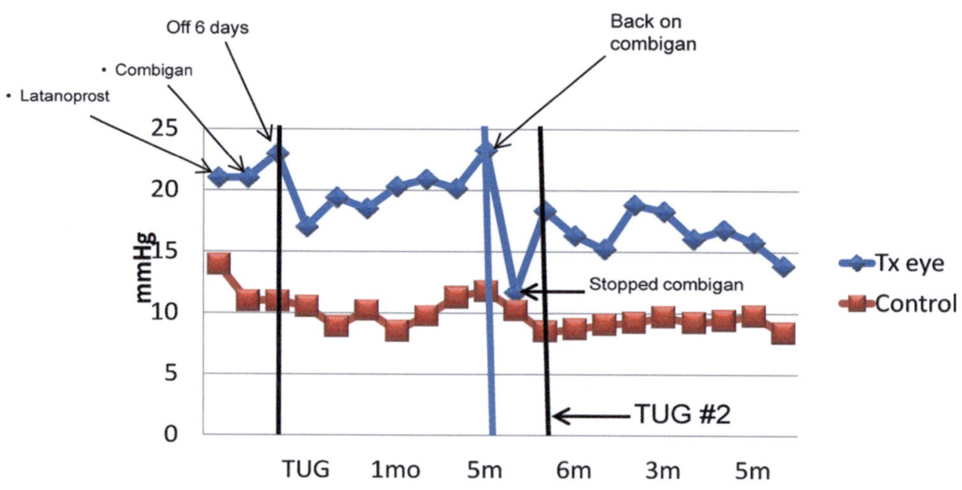



mind a second chart was designed to show the IOP change in those naïve patients whose pretreatment IOP was greater than 19.5 mmHg (non-normotensives).

IOP increased and they needed medication, but those exhibited typically more than a 25 % additional effect with the resumption of medication.

## Comparison of TUG to Previous Pharmaceutical Treatment

Over the 1-year time frame, a comparison was made of the IOP found after the TUG treatment to the average pressure on medication. An average of the comparison at each visit was then made to see what percentage was equal to (within 10 %) or better than the pharmaceutical control (Fig. 12.14).

Within this group of 17, there were 13 who only required one treatment to last the year. Two were dropped when their

## Specific Subjects (Fig. 12.15)

Subject #264 presented a number of unusual and instructive findings from the TUG studies. She has unilateral glaucoma and is very sensitive to some medications and allergic to others. She had been on latanoprost and then Combigan with IOP 21.5 with each one. A washout was performed, the IOP rose slightly, and TUG was performed. By 5 months the IOP was approaching the washout pressure. She was placed back on Combigan. The IOP

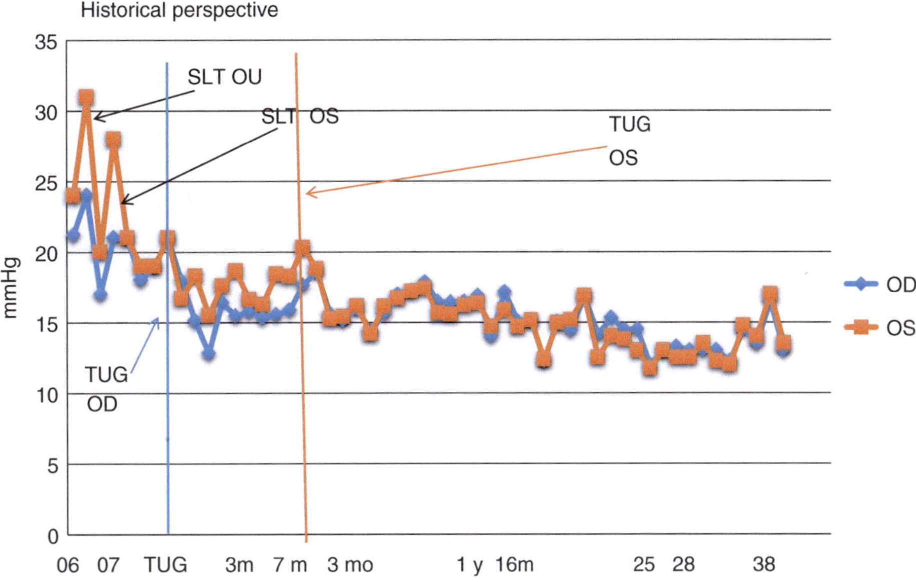


**Fig. 12.16** Naïve to medical treatment subject with sequential bilateral treatment

dropped to 11.5 when now on medication after the TUG. She was again bothered by injection from the medication. The Combigan was stopped and a second TUG was performed with an effect now off of medication lasting an additional 7 months. Whereas when originally seen on medication, the IOP was above 20, the IOP off medication after the second TUG was significantly better (Fig. 12.16).

Subject #259 was the first subject where a treatment was performed in each eye. He had previous SLT laser in 2006 in each eye and then a repeat in the left eye in 2007. His IOP was 19 in each eye but gradually rose to 21 in 2010 when TUG was considered. Both eyes were 21, and a coin flip determined the right eye was the first eye treated. There was good effect in the treated eye with a moderate decrease noted in the non-treated eye. At 7 months after the treatment, the non-treated eye intraocular pressure increased to 21. Treatment to the left eye was performed. As the graph reveals 25 months after the treatment of the second eye, both eyes had a pressure of 11.75. He has never been on any pharmaceutical agent for glaucoma. A previous SLT treatment has not been found to decrease the potential effect of the TUG treatment.

## Updated System

The 45 lb of equipment consisting of the function generator, the power amplifier, and handpiece has been reduced in size to 3″ by 5″ by 11″ and weight to 5 lb (not including the foot pedal). The unit is self tuning and quiet with internal checks for safety (Fig. 12.17).

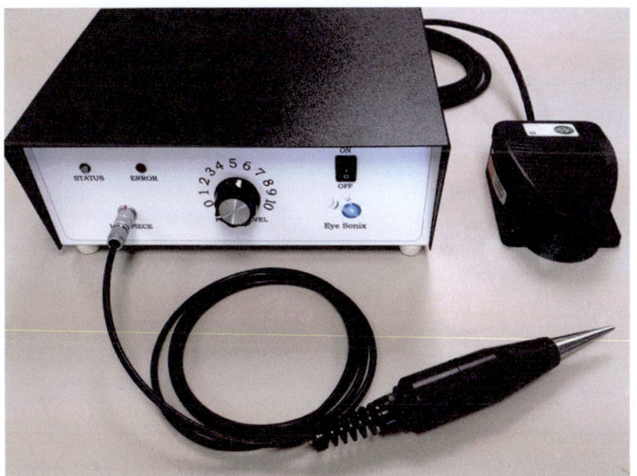

**Fig. 12.17** TUG treatment device, June 2013

### Conclusion

The use of ultrasound to treat glaucoma (TUG) has the potential for offering a novel way of treating IOP as an adjunct to medication or as initial therapy. It appears to be well tolerated and repeatable with a significant effect on IOP. Further studies with a multicenter clinical protocol are planned for validation of this method of glaucoma treatment.

## References

1. Poley BJ, Lindstrom RL, Samuelson TW. Long-term effects of phacoemulsification with intraocular lens implantation in normotensive and ocular hypertensive eyes. J Cataract Refract Surg. 2008;34(5):735–42.

2. Bowling B, Calladine D. Routine reduction of glaucoma medication following phacoemulsification. J Cataract Refract Surg. 2009;35(3):406–7.

3. Shingleton BJ, Laul A, Nagao K, Wolff B, O'Donoghue M, Eagan E, Flattem N, Desai-Bartoli S. Effect of phacoemulsification on intraocular pressure in eyes with pseudoexfoliation: single-surgeon series. J Cataract Refract Surg. 2008;34(11):1834–41.

4. Pohjalainen T, Vesti E, Uusitalo RJ, Laatikainen L. Phacoemulsification and intraocular lens implantation in eyes with open-angle glaucoma. Acta Ophthalmol Scand. 2001;79(3):313–6.

5. Mierzejewski A, Eliks I, Kałuzny B, Zygulska M, Harasimowicz B, Kałuzny JJ. Cataract phacoemulsification and intraocular pressure in glaucoma patients. Klin Oczna. 2008;110(1–3):11–7.

6. Issa SA, Pacheco J, Mahmood U, Nolan J, Beatty S. A novel index for predicting intraocular pressure reduction following cataract surgery. Br J Ophthalmol. 2005;89:543–6. doi:10.1136/bjo.2004.047662.

7. Radius RL, Schultz K, Sobocinski K, Schultz RO, Easom H. Pseudophakia and intraocular pressure. Am J Ophthalmol. 1984;97(6):738–42.

8. Silverman RH, Vogelsang B, Rondeau MJ, Coleman DJ. Therapeutic ultrasound for the treatment of glaucoma. Am J Ophthalmol. 1991;111(3):327–37. Erratum in: Am J Ophthalmol 1991;112(1):105.

9. Valtot F, Kopel J, Haut J. Treatment of glaucoma with high intensity focused ultrasound. Int Ophthalmol. 1989;13(1–2):167–70.

10. Feril LB Jr., Kondo T, Tachibana K, Ogawa R, Ogawa K. Biological effects of ultrasound: sonomechanical mechanism, and its implications on therapy and biosafety. Therapeutic ultrasound: 5th international symposium on therapeutic ultrasound; 2006;829. New York. Available from: http://proceedings.aip.org/proceedings

11. Zhou L, Maruyama I, Li Y, Cheng EL, Yue BY. Integrin transduction expression of integrin receptors in the human trabecular meshwork. Curr Eye Res. 1999;19(5):395–402.

12. Choi BH, Choi MH, Kwak MG, Min BH, Woo ZH, Park SR. Integrin transduction initiated by mechanical receptors of stretch activated channels mechanotransduction pathways of low-intensity ultrasound in C-28/I2 human chondrocyte cell line. Proc Inst Mech Eng H. 2007;221(5):527–35.

13. Wang N, Chintala SK, Fini ME, Schuman JS. Ultrasound activates the TM ELAM-1/IL-1/NF-kappaB response: a potential mechanism for intraocular pressure reduction after phacoemulsification. Invest Ophthalmol Vis Sci. 2003;44(5):1977–81.

14. Bradley JM, Kelley MJ, Rose A, Acott TS. Signaling pathways used in trabecular matrix metalloproteinase response to mechanical stretch. Invest Ophthalmol Vis Sci. 2003;44(12):5174–81.

15. Bradley JM, Kelley MJ, Zhu X, Anderssohn AM, Alexander JP, Acott TS. Effects of mechanical stretching on trabecular matrix metalloproteinases. Invest Ophthalmol Vis Sci. 2001;42(7):1505–13.

16. Prevent Blindness America. Available from: http://www.prevent-blindness.org.

17. Glaucoma Research Foundation. Available from: http://www.glaucoma.org.

18. Pradhan S, Wilkes M, Leffler CT, Pratt DC, Mahmood MA. Correlation of change in IOP with anterior chamber depth and angle after cataract surgery measured by anterior segment OCT. Poster presented at the American Society of Cataract and Refractive Surgery (ASCRS) meeting, San Francisco; 6 April 2009.

19. Floyd MS, Valentine JR, Olson RJ. Fluidics and heat generation of Alcon Infiniti and Legacy, Bausch & Lomb Millennium, and advanced medical optics sovereign phacoemulsification systems. Am J Ophthalmol. 2006;142(3):387–92.

20. Polack PJ, Iwamoto T, Silverman RH, Driller J, Lizzi FL, Coleman DJ. Histologic effects of contact ultrasound for the treatment of glaucoma. Invest Ophthalmol Vis Sci. 1991;32(7):2136–42.

21. Valtot F, Kopel J, Le Mer Y. [Principles and histologic effects of the treatment of hypertension with focused high-intensity ultrasound]. Ophtalmologie. 1990;4(2):135–7.

22. Coleman DJ, Lizzi FL, Driller J, Rosado AL, Chang S, Iwamoto T, Rosenthal D. Therapeutic ultrasound in the treatment of glaucoma. I. Experimental model. Ophthalmology. 1985;92(3):339–46.

23. Silverman RH, Vogelsang B, Rondeau MJ, Coleman DJ. Therapeutic ultrasound for the treatment of glaucoma. Am J Ophthalmol. 1991;111(3):327–37.

24. Coleman DJ, Lizzi FL, Silverman RH, Dennis Jr PH, Driller J, Rosado A, Iwamoto T. Therapeutic ultrasound. Ultrasound Med Biol. 1986;12(8):633–8.

25. Liton PB, Liu X, Challa P, Epstein DL, Gonzalez P. Induction of TGF-beta1 in the trabecular meshwork under cyclic mechanical stress. J Cell Physiol. 2005;205(3):364–71.

26. Liton PB, Luna C, Bodman M, Hong A, Epstein DL, Gonzalez P. Induction of IL-6 expression by mechanical stress in the trabecular meshwork. Biochem Biophys Res Commun. 2005;337(4):1229–36. Epub 2005 Oct 7.

27. Liton PB, Li G, Luna C, Gonzalez P, Epstein DL. Cross-talk between TGF-beta1 and IL-6 in human trabecular meshwork cells. Mol Vis. 2009;15:326–34. Epub 2009 Feb 11.

28. Kalapesi FB, Tan JC, Coroneo MT. Stretch-activated channels: a mini-review. Are stretch-activated channels an ocular barometer. Clin Experiment Ophthalmol. 2005;33(2):210–7.

29. Sato Y, Matsuo T, Ohtsuki H. A novel gene (oculomedin) induced by mechanical stretching in human trabecular cells of the eye. Biochem Biophys Res Commun. 1999;259(2):349–51.

30. Luna C, Li G, Liton PB, Epstein DL, Gonzalez P. Alterations in gene expression induced by cyclic mechanical stress in trabecular meshwork cells. Mol Vis. 2009;15:534–44. Epub 2009 Mar 11.

31. Mozaffarieh M, Flammer J. A novel perspective on natural therapeutic approaches in glaucoma therapy. Expert Opin Emerg Drugs. 2007;12(2):195–8.

32. WuDunn D. Mechanobiology of trabecular meshwork cells. Exp Eye Res. 2009;88(4):718–23. Epub 2008 Nov 24.

33. Acott TS, Kelley MJ. Extracellular matrix in the trabecular meshwork. Exp Eye Res. 2008;86(4):543–61. Epub 2008 Jan 25.

34. Tamm ER, Fuchshofer R. What increases outflow resistance in primary open-angle glaucoma? Surv Ophthalmol. 2007;52 Suppl 2:S101–4.

35. Kelley MJ, Rose A, Song K, Lystrup B, Samples JW, Acott TS. p38 MAP kinase pathway and stromelysin regulation in trabecular meshwork cells. Invest Ophthalmol Vis Sci. 2007;48(7):3126–37.

36. Bradley JM, Anderssohn AM, Colvis CM, Parshley DE, Zhu XH, Ruddat MS, Samples JR, Acott TS. Mediation of laser trabeculoplasty-induced matrix metalloproteinase expression by IL-1_ and TNF_. Invest Ophthalmol Vis Sci. 2000;41:422–30.

37. Kelley MJ, Rose AY, Song K, Chen Y, Bradley JM, Rookhuizen D, Acott TS. Synergism of TNF and IL-1 in the induction of matrix metalloproteinase-3 in trabecular meshwork. Invest Ophthalmol Vis Sci. 2007;48(6):2634–43.

38. Hosseini M, Rose AY, Song K, Bohan C, Alexander JP, Kelley MJ, Acott TS. IL-1 and TNF induction of matrix metalloproteinase-3 by c-Jun N-terminal kinase in trabecular meshwork. Invest Ophthalmol Vis Sci. 2006;47(4):1469–76.

39. Pang IH, Hellberg PE, Fleenor DL, Jacobson N, Clark AF. Expression of matrix metalloproteinases and their inhibitors in human trabecular meshwork cells. Invest Ophthalmol Vis Sci. 2003;44(8):3485–93.

40. Alexander JP, Acott TS. Involvement of the Erk-MAP kinase pathway in TNF alpha regulation of trabecular matrix metalloproteinases and TIMPs. Invest Ophthalmol Vis Sci. 2003;44(1):164–9.

41. Shearer T, Crosson CE. Activation of extracellular signal-regulated kinase in trabecular meshwork cells. Exp Eye Res. 2001;73(1): 25–35.

42. Samples JR, Alexander JP, Acott TS. Regulation of the levels of human trabecular matrix metalloproteinases and inhibitor by interleukin-1 and Dexamethasone. Invest Ophthalmol Vis Sci. 1993;34(12):3386–95.

43. Drews UW. Ultrasound treatment of glaucoma. Fortschr Ophthalmol. 1989;86(5):489–93.

44. Tarner IH, Müller-Ladner U, Uhlemann C, Lange U. The effect of mild whole-body hyperthermia on systemic levels of TNF-alpha, IL-1beta, and IL-6 in patients with ankylosing spondylitis. Clin Rheumatol. 2009;28(4):397–402.

45. Xie X, Shao X, Gao F, Jin H, Zhou J, Du L, Zhang Y, Ouyang W, Wang X, Zhao L, Zhang X, Tang J. Effect of hyperthermia on invasion ability and TGF-$\beta$1 expression of breast carcinoma MCF-7 cells. Oncol Rep. 2011;25(6):1573–9. doi:10.3892/or.2011.1240. Epub 2011 Mar 29.

46. Kramer G, Steiner GE, et al. Response to sublethal heat treatment of prostatic tumor cells and of prostatic tumor infiltrating T-cells. Prostate. 2004;58(2):109–20.

47. Lee CT, Zhong L, Mace TA, Repasky EA. Elevation in body temperature to fever range enhances and prolongs subsequent responsiveness of macrophages to endotoxin challenge. PlosOne. 2012;7(1):e30077. Epub 2012 Jan 10.

48. Morita Y, Oda S, Sadahiro T, Nakamura M, Oshima T, Otani S, Hirasawa H. The effects of body temperature control on cytokine production in a rat model of ventilator-induced lung injury. Cytokine. 2009;47(1):48–55. Epub 2009 May 8.

49. Baronzio G, Gramaglia A, Fiorentini G. Hyperthermia and immunity. A brief overview. In Vivo. 2006;20(6A):689–95. Radiotherapy Hyperthermia Department, Policlinico di Monza, Via Amati, 111, 20052, Italy. barongf@intercom.it.

50. Atanackovic D, Pollok K, Faltz C, Boeters I, Jung R, Nierhaus A, Braumann KM, Hossfeld DK, Hegewisch-Becker S. Patients with solid tumors treated with high-temperature whole body hyperthermia show a redistribution of naive/memory T-cell subtypes. Am J Physiol Regul Integr Comp Physiol. 2006;290(3):R585–94. Epub 2005 Oct 27. Department of Oncology/Hematology, University Medical Center Hamburg-Eppendorf, Martinistr. 52, 20246 Hamburg, Germany. D. Atanackovic@uke.uni-hamburg.de.

51. Yamashita N, Hoshida S, Otsu K, Taniguchi N, Kuzuya T, Hori M. Involvement of cytokines in the mechanism of whole-body hyperthermia-induced cardioprotection. Circulation. 2000;102(4): 452–7. First Department of Medicine, Osaka University Medical School and the Cardiovascular Division, Osaka, Japan.

52. Robins HI, Grosen E, Katschinski DM, Longo W, Tiggelaar CL, Kutz M, Winawer J, Graziano F. Whole body hyperthermia induction of soluble tumor necrosis factor receptors: implications for rheumatoid diseases. J Rheumatol. 1999;26(12):2513–6.

53. Haveman J, Geerdink AG, Rodermond HM. Cytokine production after whole body and localized hyperthermia. Int J Hyperthermia. 1996;12(6):791–800.

54. Katschinski DM, Wiedemann GJ, Longo W, d'Oleire FR, Spriggs D, Robins HI. Whole body hyperthermia cytokine induction: a review, and unifying hypothesis for myeloprotection in the setting of cytotoxic therapy. Cytokine Growth Factor Rev. 1999;10(2):93–7. University of Wisconsin, School of Medicine, Madison 53792, USA.

55. Robins HI, Kutz M, Wiedemann GJ, Katschinski DM, Paul D, Grosen E, Tiggelaar CL, Spriggs D, Gillis W, d'Oleire F. Cytokine induction by 41.8 degrees C whole body hyperthermia. Cancer Lett. 1995;97(2):195–201. University of Wisconsin Clinical Science Center, Madison, USA.

56. Shen RN, Hornback NB, Shidnia H, Wu B, Lu L, Broxmeyer HE. Whole body hyperthermia: a potent radioprotector in vivo. Int J Radiat Oncol Biol Phys. 1991;20(3):525–30. Dept. of Medicine (Hematology/Oncology), Indiana University School of Medicine, Indianapolis 46202.

57. Issa SA, Pacheco J, Mahmood U, Nolan J, Beatty S. A novel index for predicting intraocular pressure reduction following cataract surgery. Br J Ophthalmol. 2005;89:543–6.

58. Altan C, Bayraktar S, Altan T, Eren H, Yilmaz OF. Anterior chamber depth, iridocorneal angle width, and intraocular pressure changes after uneventful phacoemulsification in eyes without glaucoma and with open iridocorneal angles. J Cataract Refract Surg. 2004;30(4):832–8.

59. Noecker RJ, Kramer TR. Comparison of the acute morphologic changes after selective laser trabeculoplasty and argon laser trabeculoplasty in human eye. Invest Ophthalmol Vis Sci. 1998;39: S472.

60. Chang IA, Nguyen UD. Thermal modeling of lesion growth with radiofrequency ablation devices. BioMed Eng OnLine. 2004;3: 1–19.

61. Takahashi S, Tanaka R, Watanabe M, Takahashi H, Kakinuma K, Suda T, Yamada M, Takahashi H. Effects of whole-body hyperthermia on the canine central nervous system. Int J Hyperthermia. 1999;15(3):203–16.

62. Zhou Y-F. High intensity focused ultrasound in clinical tumor ablation. World J Clin Oncol. 2011;2(1):8–27.

63. van der Zee J. Heating the patient: a promising approach? Ann Oncol. 2002;13(8):1173–84.

64. Falk MH, Issels RD. Hyperthermia in oncology. Int J Hyperthermia. 2001;17(1):1–18.

65. Zhou AW, Giroux J, Mao AJ, Hutnik CM. Can preoperative anterior chamber angle width predict magnitude of intraocular pressure change after cataract surgery? Can J Ophthalmol. 2010;45(2): 149–53.

66. Shrivastava A, Singh K. The effect of cataract extraction on intraocular pressure. Curr Opin Ophthalmol. 2010;21(2):118–22.

# Part IV

# Internal Outflow Enhancement

# The iStent® MIGS Family: iStent®, iStent Inject®, and iStent Supra®



Richard A. Hill, David Haffner, and Lilit Voskanyan

## Introduction

Microinvasive glaucoma surgeries (MIGS) represent a fundamental shift in glaucoma surgical philosophy. MIGS are surgeries that exploit existing physiologic outflow pathways and create minimal morbidity postoperatively in patients. The surgeon is required to interact correctly with small anatomic functional structures in a minimally destructive manner. The pre-MIGS carry with them tremendous perioperative and postoperative morbidities. These morbidities vary from the severe, such as bleb-related endophthalmitis massive suprachoroidal hemorrhage, and difficult to treat strabismus to the less severe but debilitating, such as acceleration of cataract formation, filtering bleb dysesthesia, delayed return of visual function, or worsening of visual acuity. The beginning of the MIGS era looks promising in terms of control of intraocular pressure (IOP) with rapid visual rehabilitation and minimal perioperative and postoperative liabilities for our patients. All of these devices will evolve over time but it is of greatest importance that there is a shifting in philosophy (Fig. 13.1).

The restoration of function with minimal undesired effects is the goal of most surgeries. The first two Glaukos devices target trabecular outflow (iStent and iStent inject (Fig. 13.2), Glaukos Corporation, Laguna Hills, CA) [1–9]. The third in the series targets uveoscleral outflow (iStent Supra, Fig. 13.3). Over 4000 iStents have been placed in over 30 studies in the past 10 years [10–25].


R.A. Hill, MD (✉)
Orange County Glaucoma Inc., 1200 N. Tustin Ave, S. 240, Santa Anna, CA 92705, USA
e-mail: ocg@mac.com

D. Haffner
Vice President, Product Development, Glaukos Corp., 26051 Merit Circle, Suite 103, Laguna Hills, CA 92653, USA
e-mail: dhaffner@glauicos.com

L. Voskanyan, MD, PhD
Glaucoma, S.V. Malayan Eye Center, Fuchik's Street, 30, Orbbii Street; 4; app. 55, Yerevan, Arabkir 375028, Armenia
e-mail: lilitvosk@mail.rm


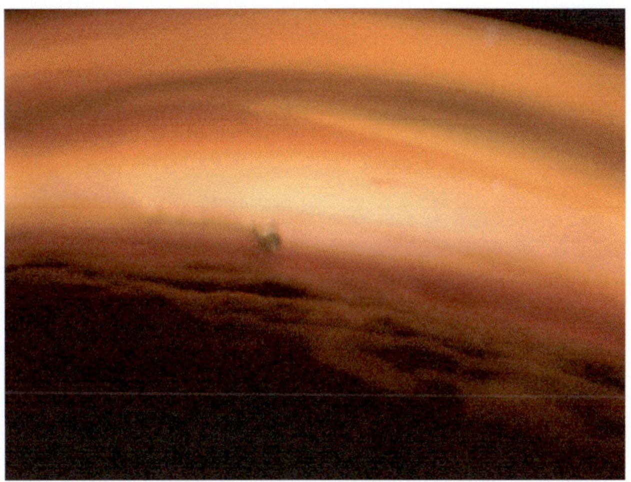

**Fig. 13.1** First human trabecular stent implant

## Glaukos iStent (Generation 1 (G1))

The Glaukos iStent device (Fig. 13.3) received FDA approval in June 2012. It is one of the smallest medical implants with a 1 mm body with an angular pointed tip and retention ridges that are arch-shaped and continue on to a tubular inlet device known affectionately as the "snorkel." The inner and outer diameters of the snorkel are 120 and 180 μm and the device is coated with Duraflo heparin to allow for self-priming of the device. The heparin is not intended for any pharmacologic purpose beyond priming. The body of the iStent is arch-shaped so that the slit-like canal of Schlemm can be stented open and the posterior wall containing the collector channels, tented maximally open. The device is made of medical grade titanium (6AL4V) and micro-machined to tolerances of less than 5 μm. The device comes in left and right eye


**Electronic supplementary material** Supplementary material is available in the online version of this chapter at http://dx.doi.org/10.1007/978-1-4614-8348-9_13. Videos can also be accessed at http://www.springerimages.com/videos/978-1-4614-8347-2



J.R. Samples, I.I.K. Ahmed (eds.), *Surgical Innovations in Glaucoma*, DOI 10.1007/978-1-4614-8348-9_13, © Springer Science+Business Media New York 2014

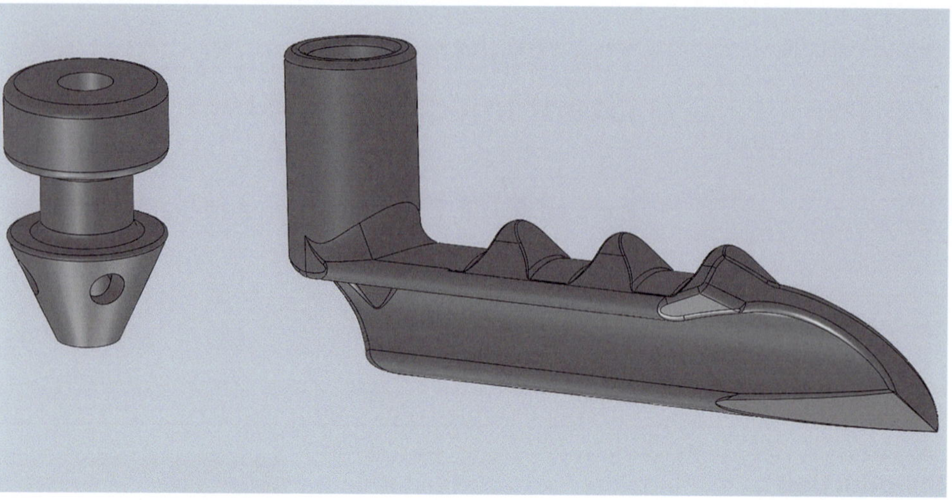

**Fig. 13.2** Glaukos iStent (Generation 1) and iStent inject (Generation 2) implants

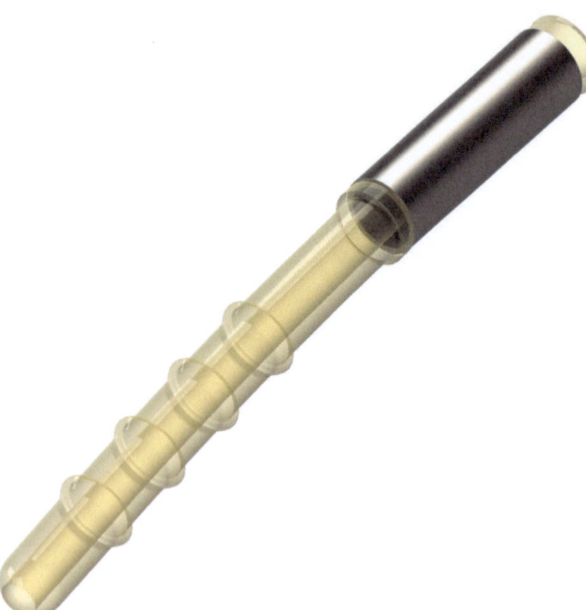

**Fig. 13.3** Glaukos iStent Supra implant (Generation 3)

There are many functions of the trabecular meshwork and Schlemm's canal that are not completely understood; however, one theory advanced by Murray Johnstone is that a pumping effect exists secondary to motion of the trabeculum induced by pressure changes from the cardiac cycle [26]. It is believed that preservation of the structural integrity of the meshwork and its dynamic abilities are important physiologies to be respected by surgical implants. Therefore, the Glaukos iStent was designed to be only 1 mm long and not to obviate any pumping mechanism that would occur with pressure shifts during the cardiac cycle. There has been discussion regarding circumferential flow of aqueous in Schlemm's canal. It has been demonstrated that the cannulation of the canal with tubing connected to a hypodermic syringe and with the application of tremendous pressure can force fluid circumferentially for large number of degrees. However, with physiologic pressures and the distribution of aqueous collector channels concentrated about the horizontal meridian, circumferential flow is most likely limited to a few clock hours, especially in the quadrants about the 3 and 9 o'clock position in eyes. A fortunate occurrence of nature is that the largest number of aqueous veins is inferior and nasal [26], corresponding to the locations in which the iStent is most easily placed. In terms of fine-tuning the placement further, the work of Doug Johnson, and that of Hann and Fautsch [4] has shown us that pigmentation occurs in the trabecular meshwork in areas that are overlying aqueous collector

versions (Fig. 13.4). The angled tip of the device allows for easy penetration through the trabecular meshwork and there is a small relief bevel to take the tip off contact with the inner layer of the Schlemm's canal.

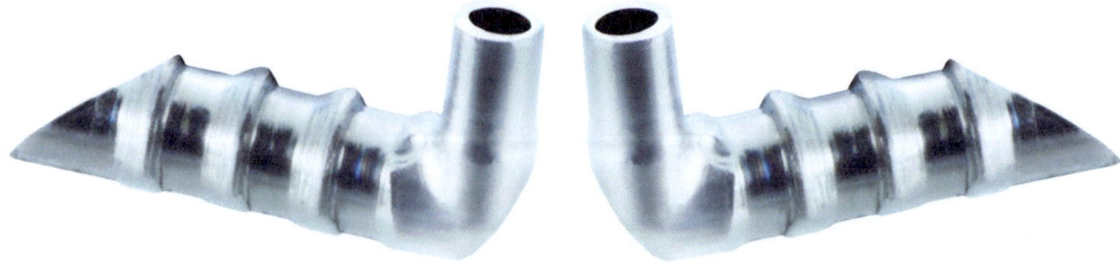

**Fig. 13.4** Glaukos iStent in left and right eye versions

channels. It is believed that this is an important marker for placement of the iStent and iStent inject devices.

Studies using a human anterior segment perfusion model have shown that the largest increase in outflow facility is with the placement of the first device. A smaller yet significant effect occurs with the placement of a second device. The placement of a third device offers only a small increase in outflow facility [1, 2]. When two stent implants are desired, the devices can be placed nasally and infranasally preferentially through pigmented areas of the trabecular meshwork. The device is placed with an applicator (Fig. 13.5) which uses sliding 26 gauge stainless steel tubing over a smaller diameter laser slotted tube which holds the device via the snorkel (Fig. 13.6). It was the intent that this applicator be able to reacquire any devices should the need occur. Devices are released after implantation by depressing a button on the top of the ergonomically designed applicator device.

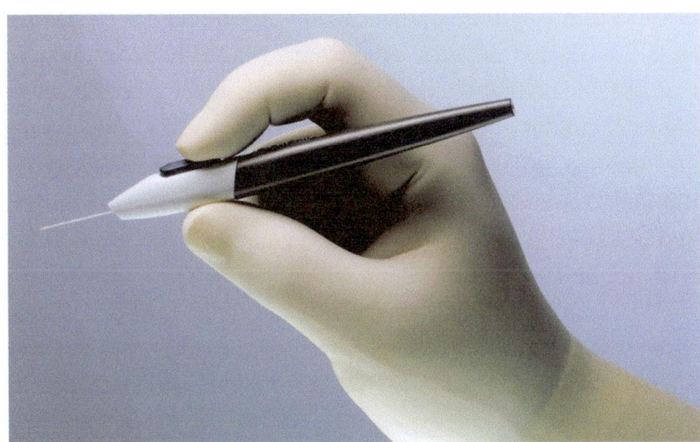

**Fig. 13.5**  Glaukos iStent applicator

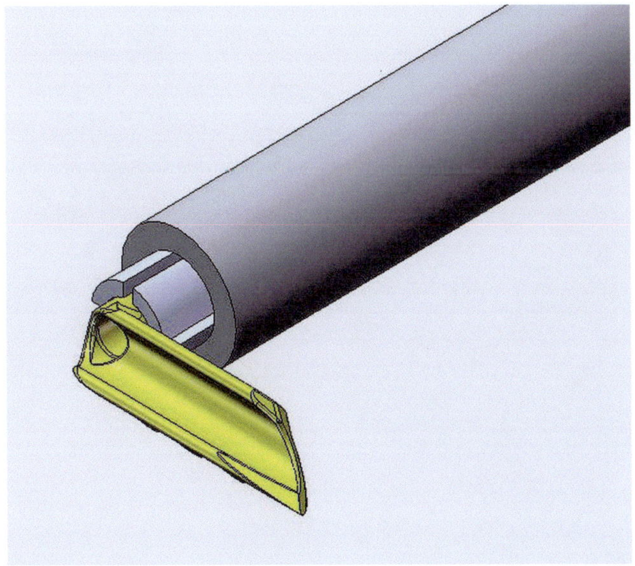

**Fig. 13.6**  Glaukos iStent applicator shown holding the iStent by the snorkel

## Implantation of the iStent

The implantation of the Glaukos iStent begins with gonioscopy in the clinic. The patient should be examined preoperatively for the practicality of the proposed surgery. If good anatomic landmarks do not exist or if there are other problems such as peripheral anterior synechiae (PAS), then this device will be of somewhat lessened value and its implantation difficult or impractical. Numerous authors have described various landmarks for accuracy in gonioscopy. In clinical practice, one can look for the parallelepiped of light obtained with a narrow high-intensity slit beam on gonioscopy. The terminus of this is always Schwalbe's line. Schwalbe's line is the landmark most likely visible even in cases of angle closure or narrow angles. Below the terminus of the parallelepiped of light is the trabecular meshwork. This may or may not contain pigmentation and may or may not have hyperpigmented zones. A more favorable situation would be the easy demarcation of the trabecular meshwork and the existence of hyperpigmented implantation sites. Scleral spur is often thought as the most reliable landmark but may not be visible in closed angles. The combination of Schwalbe's line and scleral spur can easily be identified. Even in cases of angle closure in which the trabecular meshwork can be demonstrated with Forbes compression gonioscopy, the iStent may be of use. In this situation, the angle would be opened and the iStent would be implanted after cataract surgery. The FDA approval and package labeling is for the iStent to be inserted after cataract removal and lens implantation. The implantation of this device theoretically could occur before cataract surgery. One first reason to implant before cataract surgery is that there may be a transient decrease in transparency of the tissue overlying the cataract wound. This is the tissue that the surgeon must view the filtering angle through to implant the device, and if this suffers in optical quality, then the implantation will be more difficult. This would be more likely to occur with very dense nuclei and extended phaco times. It is very important to obtain the proper visualization to implant this device. If one thinks about the location of the trabecular meshwork relative to other structures, it is clear that the filtering angle must be viewed parallel to the iris plane and not parallel to the peripheral corneal plane. Viewing across the corneal plane will not allow for visualization of the angle structures and most likely will not allow for the proper approach to the trabecular meshwork that would allow implantation of the G1 or G2 type devices. An important part of the visual access and visualization of the filtering angle is the surgical gonioscope that was developed with Ocular Instruments, Inc. (Bellevue, WA; Fig. 13.7). The gonioscope is available with multiple iterations of left handed (left hand held for right hand implantation), right handed (right hand held for left hand implantation), or universal model. The differences in models are the angle

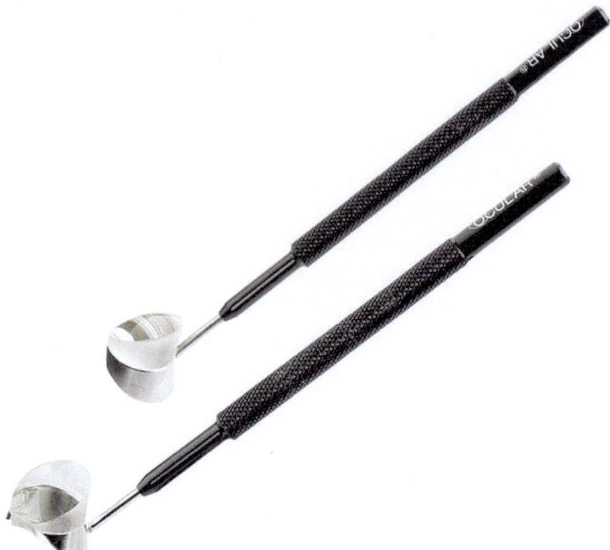

**Fig. 13.7** Hill Gonioprism by Ocular Instruments in left hand and right hand versions. There is a large cut out for surgical access and a large viewing area with ridges on the bottom of the stainless steel ring for holding eyes stable

that the handle comes off relative to the viewing surface. The gonioscope is held in the nondominant hand with the operator's hand resting alternately on either the patient's cheek or forehead for stability. In addition to visualization, the gonioscope also holds the eye in position and allows some back resistance to eye tissue being pushed away from the operator

during implantation and stabilization and/or further rotation of the eye. There are ridges on the metal surface holding the optics that also provide stabilization of the eye during implantation of these devices.

The gonioscope is autoclavable and meets all modern ambulatory care center (ACC) standards. After the patient's head is tilted away, the iStent is very carefully removed from the box sterile tray and visualized under the operating microscope. The patient's head is rotated away 30°–40° and the microscope tilted toward the surgeon (Fig. 13.8). In practice, any combination of tilting either the patient's head or microscope can be used to achieve the correct viewing plane based on compromises between surgeon and patient flexibility. The gonioscope is placed on the eye to assess the level of visualization achieved. If the surgeon is viewing slightly above the iris plane, all the angle structures will be visible. Once the correct viewing plane is achieved, the anterior chamber is filled with viscoelastic (Fig. 13.9). The device then is advanced through the corneal wound to the pupillary margin (Fig. 13.10) and then the gonioscope placed back on the eye (Fig. 13.11) so that the device can be advanced into the filtering angle under gonioscopic control (Fig. 13.12). This avoids any damage to iris or corneal endothelium. The device is implanted with the tip pointed inferiorly and comes in a left and right eye version. To improve ergonomics, some surgeons will implant a second iStent labeled from the opposite eye with the tip pointing superiorly. The angle of attack to the meshwork is important. This is not a flat type attack, but it is a low angle of attack (10°–15°, Fig. 13.13). This is sufficient

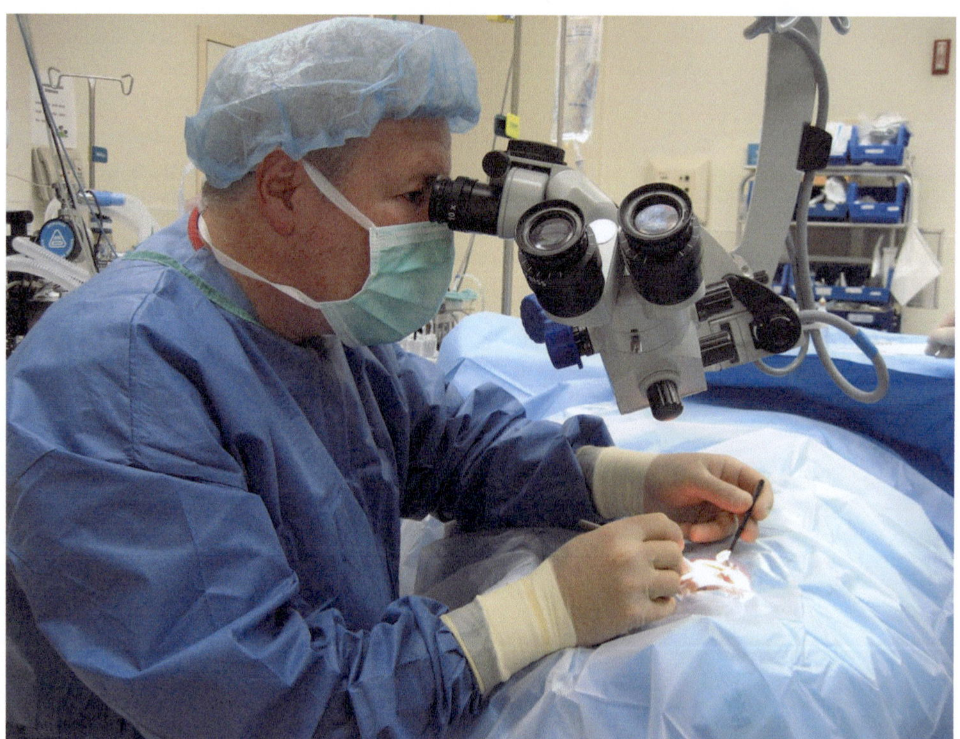

**Fig. 13.8** Surgical set up showing correct orientation of microscope and patient for viewing along the iris plane

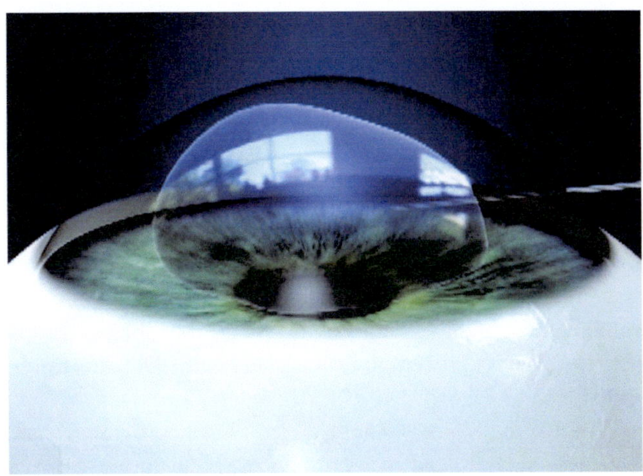

**Fig. 13.9** Filling the anterior chamber with viscoelastic

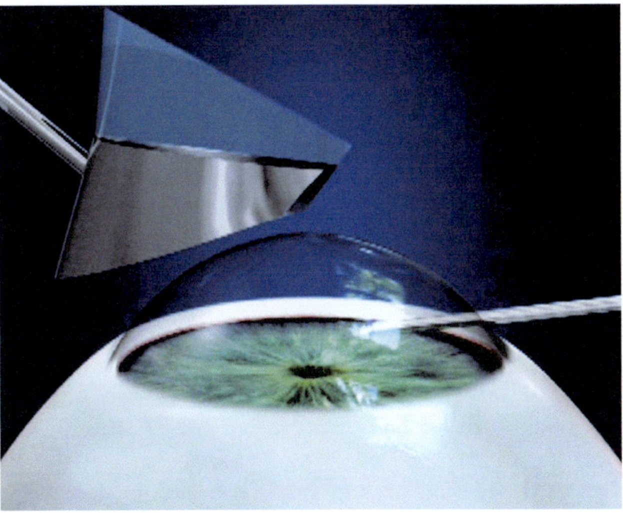

**Fig. 13.11** Placing the gonioscope on the cornea and advancing the implant to the trabecular meshwork

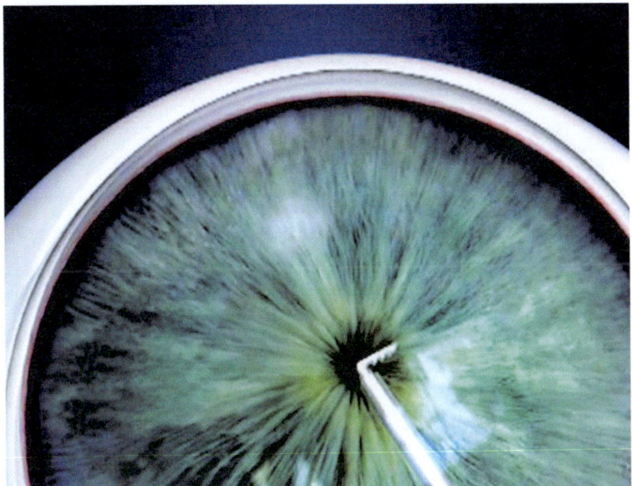

**Fig. 13.10** Advancing the implant through the corneal wound to the pupillary space

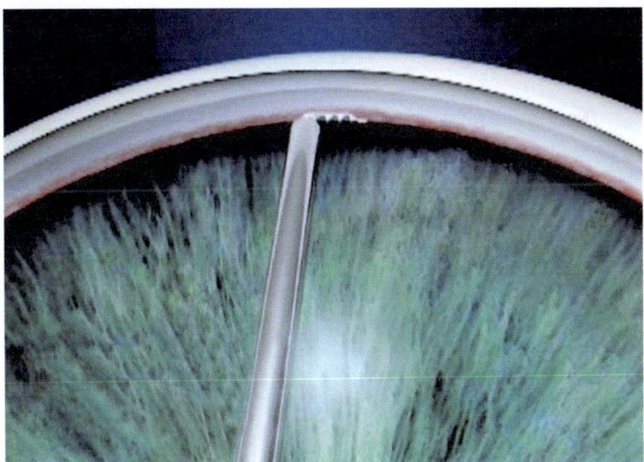

**Fig. 13.12** Setting up the correct angle of attack (10°–15°)

to engage the trabecular meshwork and pass the point of the device through the meshwork where it will most likely embed slightly in the posterior wall of Schlemm's canal. When this occurs, a solid resistance is felt. At this point in time, the device absolutely should not be advanced because this could damage the posterior wall of Schlemm's canal. Additionally, attempting advancement of the device after encountering resistance could cause the tip to abruptly release from the scleral wall and possibly damage the trabecular meshwork. After the initial penetration, the surgeon is advised to stop and lift slightly prior to further advancement of the device. This will align the body of the device with the lumen of Schlemm's canal. This movement is very similar to placement of an intravenous catheter. After the tip penetration, lift, and slide movements, the trabecular meshwork will be seen to cover the body of the device. When the snorkel meets the meshwork, the release button is pressed (Fig. 13.14). It is very important

not to have the device under tension and to have a smooth release. After release, the heel of the device is still slightly above the trabecular meshwork and the entire body of the device should be tapped gently or pushed over to seat the heel of the device (Fig. 13.15). There will often be seen a reflux of blood at this point in time or with removal of viscoelastic. This is expected as the Schlemm's canal is essentially venous sinus and the presence of this blood demonstrates to the operator successful implantation into the correct space. It also should be noted that the hypotony transiently introduced with the main incision and placement of viscoelastic will allow for blood to reflux into Schlemm's canal, and in cases where pigmentation of the meshwork is minimal, this may give a secondary (and only) clue to the operator regarding the location of the trabecular meshwork. This is shown in Video 13.1, courtesy of R. Hill, MD. The implantation of the iStent with

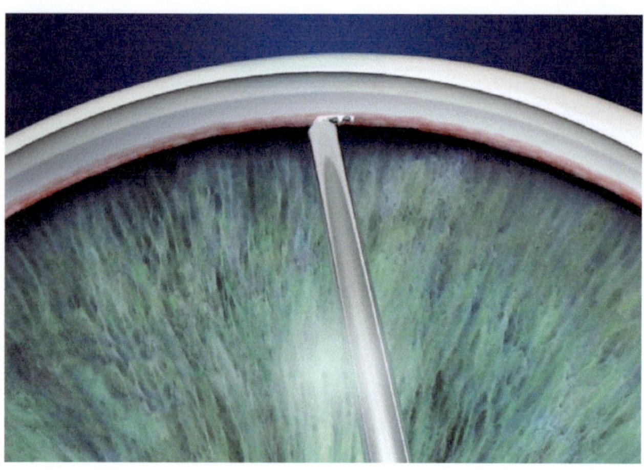

**Fig. 13.13** Penetrate, lift very slightly, and slide the implant into Schlemm's canal

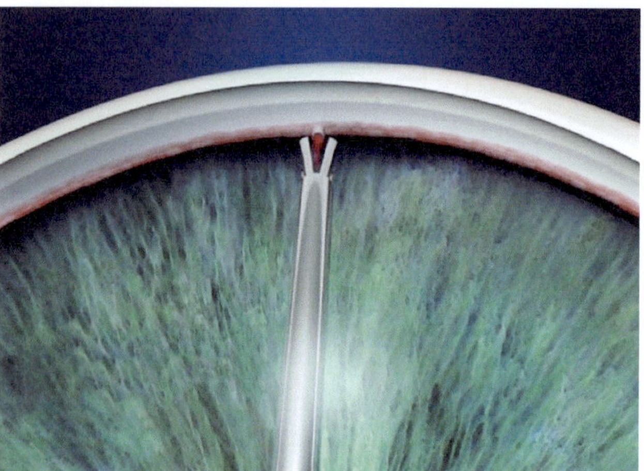

**Fig. 13.14** Under minimal tension, release the implant

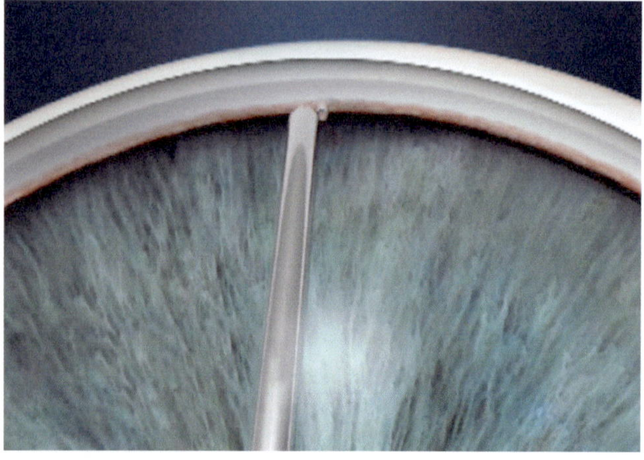

**Fig. 13.15** Gently tap or push over the implant so the heel of the device drops into the canal

heavily pigmented meshwork is shown nicely in Video 13.2, courtesy of I. Ahmed, MD. If the anterior chamber is over-inflated with viscoelastic, blood may be expressed out of Schlemm's canal and the canal flattened, making it more difficult to identify landmarks and insert the device into a collapsed canal. After the device is successfully implanted, the cataract surgery can occur after rotation of the patient's head and operating microscope. Videos 13.1 and 13.2 nicely illustrate the sequence of penetrate, lift, and slide core motions for implantation of the iStent device. The entire incorporation into the cataract procedure is illustrated in the Glaukos teaching video (13.3), courtesy of I. Ahmed, MD.

The United States pivotal trial for FDA approval involved 240 eyes randomized to receive one iStent during cataract surgery or cataract surgery alone. The primary efficacy measure was unmedicated IOP ≤21 mmHg at 1 year. The study showed that 72 % of the treatment group versus 50 % of the control group ($p < 0.001$) achieved this goal [19]. The results of other multiyear trials have also been published as abstracts by Tobias Neuhann (ESCRS Annual Meeting, Free Paper, 9/12/12), Jose Martinez-de-la-Casa (ESCRS Annual Meeting, Free Paper, 9/10/12), and Antonio M. Fea (ARVO Annual Meeting, Program 3731/Poster A197, May 8, 2012). In general, one iStent is appropriate for early to moderate glaucoma, as IOP is generally lowered to the 16–18 mmHg range with decreased medication burden. In addition to these single iStent studies, the effects of one, two, and three stents implanted as the sole procedure and administered one postoperative prostaglandin (G. Auffarth, Annual Meeting ESCRS, free paper, September 9, 2012) have also been studied in eyes not well controlled on two medications preoperatively. Eyes with multiple iStents achieved lower IOP compared to one iStent. A study of two iStents implanted as the sole procedure is also available. In 28 patients with 12-month follow-up (David Chang, ESCRS Annual Meeting, September 10, 2012), IOP dropped from a mean preoperative level of $20.7 \pm 2.1$ mmHg on one medication to $13.6 \pm 2.0$ mmHg at 12 months with 25 out of 28 patients on no medication. Similar findings were published by Belovay et al [11]. in a study of 47 patients undergoing cataract surgery with the implantation of 2 or 3 iStents. At one year follow-up, the mean overall IOP was 14.3 with a 74 % decrease in medications [11]. Risks and adverse events encountered in study groups were comparable to cataract surgery alone.

## iStent Inject (Generation 2 (G2))

The first-generation iStent device is a very useful device but does require a high level of surgical expertise in its implantation. The iStent inject device is currently investigational in

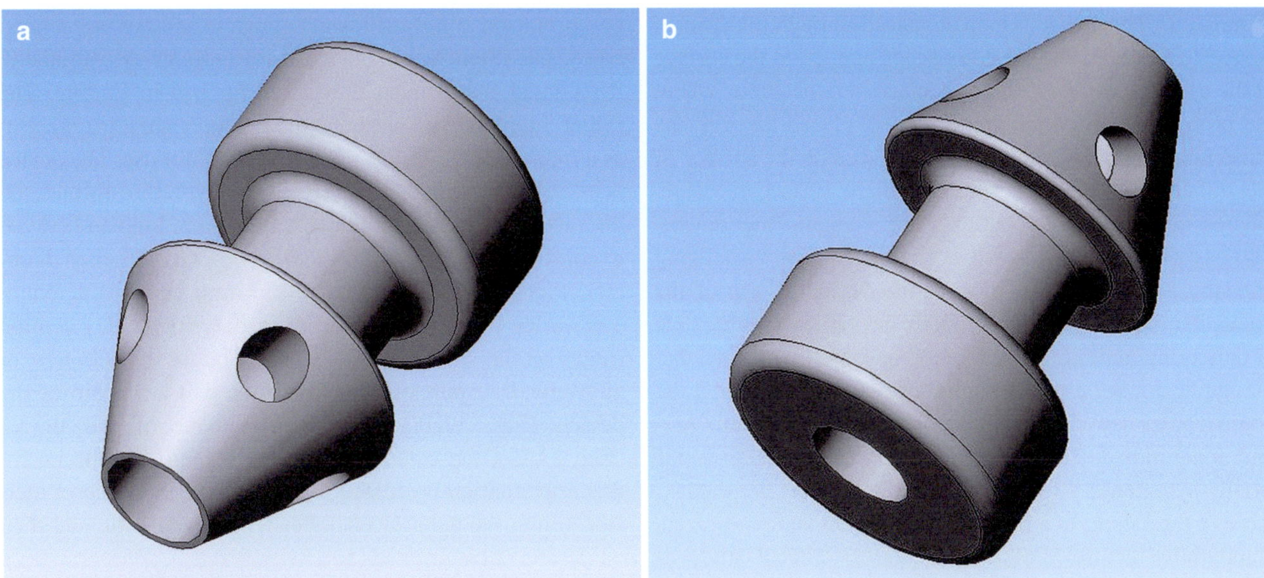

**Fig. 13.16** (**a**, **b**) Two view of the Glauckos iStent Inject (G2)

the United States but CE Marked for use in Europe. The G2 applicator/injector facilitates device placement in terms of numbers of degrees of freedom that need to be controlled for successful implantation. The iStent inject device is an axial symmetric device also constructed of medical grade titanium (6AL4V). It is 0.4 mm high with an outside diameter that varies between 0.2 and 0.3 mm. The main inlet diameter is 0.08 mm with 0.05 mm side flow lumens (Fig. 13.16a, b). It is somewhat conical in its wound entry side and is designed to utilize a high speed over the trocar-type implantation. This eliminates the steps of lifting, sliding, and tapping necessary for a successful implantation of the original iStent. During implantation, the cone-shaped end is driven into and through the trabecular meshwork. The meshwork will be stretched up over this cone and the device will be retained at the midportion via a recessed area. A small disc-like surface with a central canal will be seen postimplantation (Fig. 13.17). The aqueous inlet is along the central axis of this device and there are four exit points posteriorly located at an angle of 90° to the main channel. These are additional exits from the central channel lumen which would most likely be occluded by the posterior wall of Schlemm's canal. The device is inserted via applicator and driven at high speed. It is felt that a transient cavitation space is created, which allows for implantation of the head of the device and stretching of the trabecular meshwork over this head and the retention of the device through meshwork, which now grips the device around its waist. This device also preserves any pumping function of the meshwork. The implantation requires similar maneuvers initially to the G1 device in that the patient's head is tilted away from

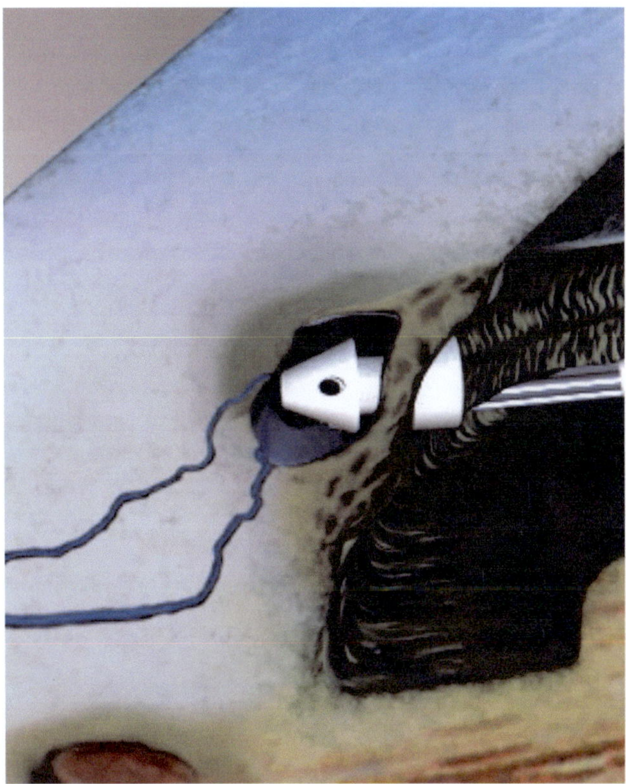

**Fig. 13.17** Glaukos iStent inject with anterior chamber side facing

the operator and the microscope is tilted toward the operator. After creation of the cataract wound, the gonioscope is placed on the eye to reconfirm successful optical viewing acquisition. The device is then advanced through the corneal wound to the pupil and the gonioscope applied to the surface of the eye. The device is then advanced into the angle, where the protruding tip of the guide wire is placed through the trabecular meshwork and the device placed on the surface of the trabecular meshwork with only light surface pressure. Depressing the release button then implants the device. Successful implantation will be confirmed by visualizing only the terminal disc portion of the device on top of the trabecular meshwork (Video 13.4). The applicator is capable of delivering multiple devices in a sequential manner, so that the applicator need not be withdrawn from the eye and the gonioscopic view disrupted. The corneal entry of this second-generation device is easier as the profile is smaller and is axially symmetric. Results with the iStent inject are comparable to the iStent. In a multicenter prospective randomized, comparative control (3:1; active/control) clinical study of 121 mild to moderate glaucoma patients taking 1–3 medications and having IOP ≤ 24 mmHg, patients underwent either two iStent inject implantations with cataract surgery or cataract surgery alone. Forty-two patients have reached two years follow-up. Efficacy endpoints were unmedicated IOP ≤ 18 mmHg (trial 1) or unmedicated IOP ≤ 21 mmHg with ≥ 20% decrease in IOP. At one year 72 % (18/25) had IOP ≤ 18 mmHg and IOP reduction ≥ 20% versus 24 % (4/17) of controls. At two years 68 % of the treatment group and 24 % of the control group achieved these outcomes. The reported safety profile was similar to cataract surgery alone (Carlos Buznego, ASCRS Annual Meeting, 2012, abstract 1238534).

## iStent Supra (Generation 3 (G3))

The third-generation Glaukos device is the iStent Supra®. This implant is designed to increase suprachoroidal outflow to lower IOP in cases where trabecular outflow is felt to be compromised or not sufficient enough to achieve target pressures. The iStent Supra device is currently investigational in the United States but CE Marked for use in Europe. The iStent Supra may be placed at the time of cataract surgery or as a freestanding surgery where approved for use. The device is made of Polyethersulfone (PES) for favorable bio-material interaction and minimal fibrosis. It is 4 mm long and curved to conform to the suprachoroidal space. It has a lumen diameter, which varies from 0.16 to 0.17 mm. The outside diameter varies from 0.3 to 0.4 mm in diameter with retention ridges on the surface of the device. The lumen is hollow to allow for transport of aqueous to the exit at the tip of the device (Fig. 13.18). In the placement of the device (Fig. 13.19), the cataract wound or wound appropriate for this implantation is created by first making a side port incision filling the anterior chamber with viscoelastic and then

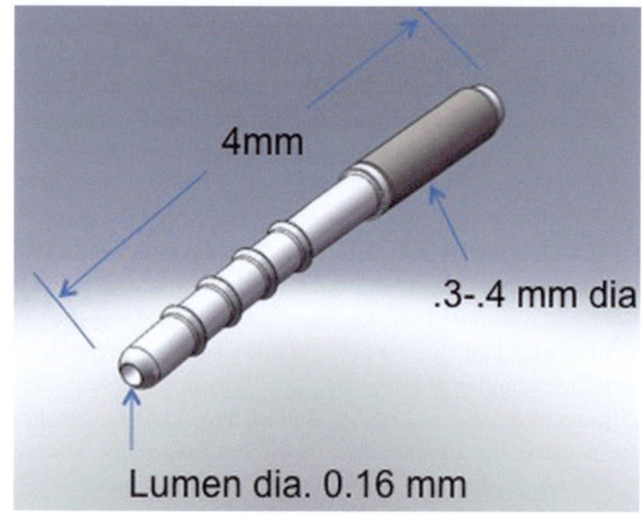


**Fig. 13.18** Glaukos iStent Supra® with dimensions

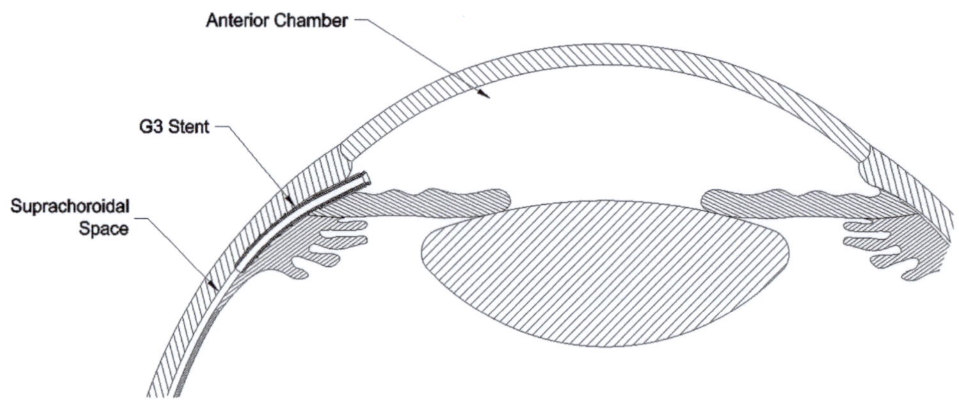


**Fig. 13.19** Drawing of Glaukos iStent Supra® after release from the trocar in site

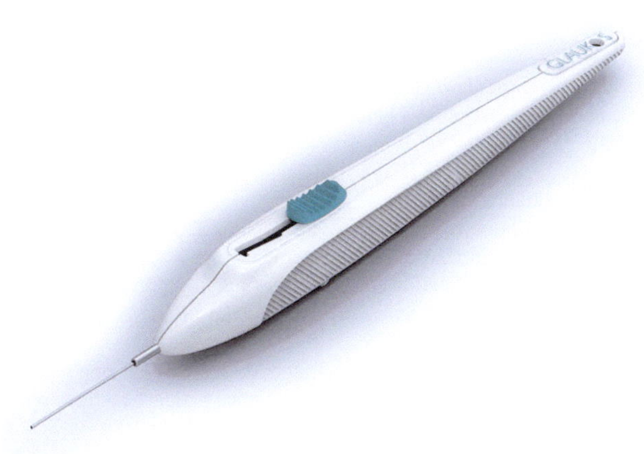

**Fig. 13.20** Glaukos iStent Supra® applicator

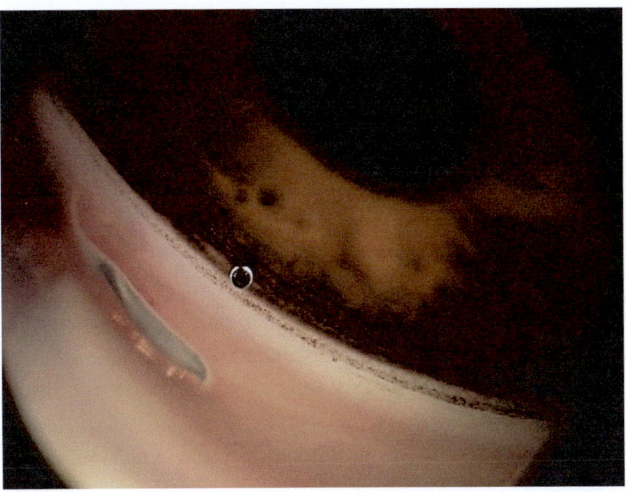

**Fig. 13.21**  Glaukos iStent Supra correctly placed

making the main entry wound. The patient's head is then tilted away slightly and the gonioscope applied to the eye to test the image acquisition. The visualization criteria for implantation of this device are not as critical as they are for the trabecular iStent devices. The entry site for implantation is not the trabecular meshwork, but is the uveal insertion site on the scleral spur. There are some advocates of suprachoroidal implants that advise that a gonioscope is optional during the implantation of this device. However, the surgical entry site should be visualized to prevent iris or corneal endothelial damage. After the creation of the wound and installation of viscoelastic and optical acquisition, the device inserter (Fig. 13.20) is advanced through the corneal wound. The device should be implanted to its appropriate depth and then released by sliding the button on the inserter button backward (Fig. 13.21; Video 13.5). This device is essentially the creation of a controlled cyclodialysis cleft with a stent. The iStent Supra or G3 is CE marked in Europe and undergoing an investigational device exemption (IDE) clinical registration trial in the United States. It can be implanted in phakic or pseudophakic eyes as a freestanding procedure (Video 13.6) or combined with cataract surgery and is usually reserved for more advanced OAG or to enhance IOP control in combination with trabecular stents. In terms of published results, one study of iStent Supra implantation as the sole procedure in 40 patients with OAG not well controlled on two medications (Eric Donnenfeld, ESCRS Annual Meeting, September 10, 2012) found that IOP dropped from a mean preoperative level of $20.8 \pm 2.2$ mmHg to $13.8 \pm 3.62$ mmHg at 12 months, and medications decreased from two to one. This compares favorably with trabeculectomy and aqueous drainage implants.

## Combination Therapy: iStent G1 or G2 + iStent Supra G3

The philosophy of the Glaukos MIGS type devices are that these devices can be titratable to patients' clinical situations and synergistic in effect by enhancing both uveoscleral outflow and trabecular outflow. There are analogous examples of synergism in medical therapy of this approach with the application of topical pharmaceuticals that increase outflow, either trabecular or uveoscleral, combined with drugs that decrease aqueous production. It was believed that this idea could be extended into a surgical application as well. This probably is best illustrated by one study in which 50 patients who had failed prior trabeculectomy on maximal medication therapy (refractory glaucoma) underwent implantation of two trabecular iStents, a single suprachoroidal iStent, and topical travoprost. At the time of this report, 6-month follow-up data was available for 30 patients. Preoperatively, mean medicated IOP was 22.9 mmHg (SD 3.4; range 18–36). Postoperatively, patients with 6-month follow-up data had a mean medicated IOP of 12.4 (SD 1.5) without reports of adverse events (Ike Ahmed and the MIGS Study Group, AGS Annual Meeting, 2013). The surgical results of the trabecular and suprachoroidal stents used in combination are remarkable and do compare well with trabeculectomy and aqueous drainage shunts in eyes that have failed trabeculectomy (refractory cases). The advantage of placing two MIGS devices of different functionalities is also very attractive based on the synergism utilized between trabecular outflow and uveoscleral outflow, as well as the rapid visual rehabilitation of the patients.

## Conclusions

The MIGS approach allows for tailoring of therapy during cataract surgery for a patient's clinical stage of disease.

In high-risk ocular hypertensive and early to moderate glaucoma patients, trabecular outflow (iStent Gen 1 and iStent inject, Gen 2) can be targeted with one or more iStents. In general, the implantation of one stent lowers IOP to the 16–18 mmHg range with decreased medication burden. The use of multistenting can drop IOP below 15 mmHg with decreased medical burden.

In moderate to more advanced disease, multiple trabecular iStents can be used, and suprachoroidal outflow may be enhanced by the primary or follow-up implantation of the iStent Supra, Gen 3. A single Gen 3 implant is capable of producing IOP below 15 mmHg and decreasing medical burden.

In advanced or refractory cases, the possibility of synergism utilizing trabecular stents in combination with suprachoroidal outflow devices has been studied and shown to be effective, producing IOP results well below 15 mmHg.

At the time of this writing, December 2013, only the iStent Gen 1 is FDA approved for use in patients undergoing cataract surgery in the United States. The iStent inject Gen 2 and iStent Supra, Gen 3 are currently in FDA NDA trials in the United States. The iStent Gen 1, iStent inject Gen 2, iStent Supra, Gen 3, are all CE marked for use in Europe. It is our hope that visual loss from bleb-related endophthalmitis will become of historical interest only and that MIGS continue to evolve and control glaucoma with a minimal creation of morbidity for our patients.

# References


1. Bahler C, Smedley G, Zhou J, Johnson D. Trabecular bypass stents decrease intraocular pressure in cultured human anterior segments. Am J Ophthalmol. 2004;138:988–94.
2. Bahler C, Hann C, Fjield T, et al. Second-generation trabecular meshwork bypass stent (iStent inject) increases outflow facility in cultured human anterior segments. Am J Ophthalmol. 2012;153:1206–13.
3. Fernández-Barrientos Y, Garcia-Feijoó J, Martinez de la Casa JM, et al. Fluorophotometric study of the effect of the Glaukos trabecular micro-bypass stent on aqueous humor dynamics. Invest Ophthalmol Vis Sci. 2010;51:3327–32.
4. Hann CR, Fautsch MP. Preferential fluid flow in the human trabecular meshwork near collector channels. Invest Ophthalmol Vis Sci. 2009;50(4):1692–7.
5. Ichhpujani P, Katz LJ, Gille R, Affel E. Imaging modalities for localization of an iStent®. Ophthalmic Surg Lasers Imaging. 2010;41:660–3.
6. Phares DJ, Smedley GT, Zhou J. Laminar flow resistance in short micro tubes. Int J Heat Fluid Flow. 2005;26:506–12.
7. Phares DJ, Smedley GT. A study of laminar flow of polar liquids through circular micro tubes. Am Inst Phys. 2004;16:1267–72.
8. Zhou J, Smedley GT. Trabecular bypass: effect of Schlemm canal and collector channel dilation. J Glaucoma. 2006;15:446–55.
9. Zhou J, Smedley GT. A trabecular bypass flow hypothesis. J Glaucoma. 2005;14:74–83.
10. Arriola-Villalobos P, Martinez-de-la-Casa J, Fernandez-Perez J, et al. Combined iStent trabecular micro-bypass stent implantation and phacoemulsification for coexistent open-angle glaucoma and cataract: a long-term study. Br J Ophthalmol. 2012. doi:10.1136/bjophthalmol-2011-300218.
11. Belovay GW, Naqi A, Chan BJ, Rateb M, Ahmed II. Using multiple trabecular micro-bypass stents in cataract patients to treat open-angle glaucoma. J Cataract Refract Surg. 2012;38:1911–7.
12. Buchacra O, Duch S, Milla E, Stirbu O. One-year analysis of the iStent trabecular microbypass in secondary glaucoma. Clin Ophthalmol. 2011;5:321–6.
13. Buznego C. Trabecular micro-bypass stent for glaucoma. Tech Ophthalmol. 2008;6:114–8.
14. Craven ER, Katz LJ, Wells JM, Giamporcaro JE. Cataract surgery with trabecular micro-bypass stent implantation in patients with mild-to-moderate open-angle glaucoma and cataract: Two-year follow-up. J Cataract Refract Surg. 2012;38:1339–45.
15. Fea AM. Phacoemulsification versus phacoemulsification with micro-bypass stent implantation in primary open-angle glaucoma. J Cataract Refract Surg. 2010;36:407–12.
16. Fea A, Dogliani M, Macetta F, et al. The trabecular bypass stent in a pseudophakic glaucoma patient: a 1-year follow-up. Clin Ophthalmol. 2008;2:931–4.
17. Morales-Fernandez L, Martinez-De-La-Casa J, Diaz Valle D, et al. Glaukos® trabecular stent used to treat steroid-induced glaucoma. Eur J Ophthalmol. 2011. doi:10.5301/ejo.5000073.
18. Nichamin LD. Glaukos iStent® trabecular micro-bypass. Middle East Afr J Ophthalmol. 2009;16:138–40.
19. Samuelson TW, Katz LJ, Wells JM, et al. Randomized evaluation of the trabecular micro-bypass stent with phacoemulsification in patients with glaucoma and cataract. Ophthalmology. 2011;118:459–67.
20. Spiegel D, Wetzel W, Neuhann T, Sturmer J, Hoh H, Garcia-Feijoo J, Martinez de la casa JM, Garcia-Sanchez J. Coexistent primary open-angle glaucoma and cataract: interim analysis of a trabecular micro-bypass stent and concurrent cataract surgery. Eur J Ophthalmol. 2009;19:393–9.
21. Spiegel D, Garcia-Feijoo J, Garcia-Sanchez J, Lamielle H. Coexistent primary open-angle glaucoma and cataract: preliminary analysis of treatment by cataract surgery and the iStent trabecular micro-bypass stent. Adv Ther. 2008;25:453–64.
22. Spiegel D, Wetzel W, Haffner DS, Hill RA. Initial clinical experience with the trabecular micro-bypass stent in patients with glaucoma. Adv Ther. 2007;24:161–70.
23. Spiegel D, Kobuch K. Trabecular meshwork bypass tube shunt: initial case series. Br J Ophthalmol. 2002;86:1228–31.
24. Traverso CE, Papadia M, Scotto R, Bagnis A. iStent® trabecular micro-bypass stent for open angle glaucoma. Expert Rev Ophthalmol. 2010;5:443–50.
25. Vandewalle E, Zeyen T, Stalmans I. The iStent® trabecular micro-bypass stent: a case series. Bull Soc Belge Ophtalmol. 2009;311:23–9.
26. Johnstone M, Annisa J, Martin E. Chapter 7: Aqueous veins and open angle glaucoma. In: Schacknow PN, Samples JR, editors. The Glaucomas. New York: Springer; 2010.

# Canaloplasty

**14**

Toby Yiu Bong Chan and Iqbal Ike K. Ahmed

Trabeculectomy, as initially described by Cairns in 1968, is still considered by many ocular surgeons as the gold standard of glaucoma surgery [1]. At around the same time, Molteno introduced the first tube shunt [2], which was subsequently followed by other glaucoma drainage devices including the Krupin and Ahmed valves and the Baerveldt drainage device [3–5]. These penetrating procedures achieve generous lowering of intraocular pressure (IOP) by way of nonphysiological passage from the anterior chamber (AC) to the subconjunctival space. However, their well-established efficacy come at the cost of significant risk of complications, including hypotony, bleb encapsulation and dysesthesia, overhanging or leaking bleb, blebitis, bleb fibrosis and failure, cataract formation or progression, and tube exposure or migration, as well as corneal decompensation [6, 7].

In light of this, there was desire for surgical alternatives that would allow enhancement of physiologic aqueous outflow while maintaining higher safety profiles. Ab externo approaches to "externalize" Schlemm's canal (SC) without full-thickness entry into the AC were initially described by Epstein and Krasnov in the 1960s [8, 9], but they only came into popularity in the 1990s in the form of non-penetrating procedures such as deep sclerectomy and viscocanalostomy [10–12].

More recently, a variation of these techniques, known as canaloplasty, was developed [13]. In the setting of glaucoma, SC may collapse as a result of reduced flow, due to increased resistance in its inner wall and trabecular meshwork (TM) [14]. Subsequent elevation in IOP may further compress SC, resulting in a vicious cycle. The main goal of canaloplsty (CP) is to re-expand SC and restore its patency. It involves placement of a nonabsorbable suture through the entire circumference of SC using a microcatheter, and the suture is tied down to generate a centripetal force. Tension from the suture may generate a pilocarpine-like effect by putting the TM on stretch, thereby enhancing outflow into SC and the collector channels [15]. As part of the procedure, viscodilation of SC (which has been postulated to create microperforations in the TM) and creation of a scleral lake may also contribute to further lowering of IOP [16, 17]. This chapter aims to review the technique and efficacy of CP.

## Instrumentation and Technique

CP utilizes a microcatheter that is 45 mm long, with a rounded 250-μm diameter tip and 200-μm diameter shaft (iScience International Inc.). It is made of a flexible polymer for atraumatic passage through SC and has a central wire that provides support and prevents kinking. On the proximal end of the microcatheter, one arm connects to a non-sterile laser-based light source which emits a red blinking light. This light is transmitted by optical fibers to the tip of the microcatheter, allowing visualization during passage in SC (Fig. 14.1). Another arm connects to a sterile screw-mechanism syringe, which allows controlled delivery of viscoelastic through a central lumen in the microcatheter to expand SC during passage.

In most cases, CP can be performed safely under topical anesthesia, although peribulbar or retrobulbar anesthesia may also be used. A superior approach is ideal to allow for coverage of a bleb by the upper lid in case one is formed, and also for less discomfort postoperatively. If a traction suture is used to improve exposure, it should be placed a few clock hours away from the surgical site to avoid obstruction of view into the AC and/or distortion of perilimbal anatomy.


T.Y.B. Chan, MD, FRCSC (✉)
Division of Ophthalmology, Department of Surgery,
McMaster University, Waterloo Regional Campus,
Suite 411, 564 Belmont Ave West,
Kitchener, ON, N2M 5N6 Canada
e-mail: toby.yb.chan@gmail.com

I.I.K. Ahmed, MD, FRCSC
Department of Ophthalmology and Vision Sciences,
University of Toronto, Toronto, ON, Canada
e-mail: ike.ahmed@utoronto.ca



J.R. Samples, I.I.K. Ahmed (eds.), *Surgical Innovations in Glaucoma*,
DOI 10.1007/978-1-4614-8348-9_14, © Springer Science+Business Media New York 2014

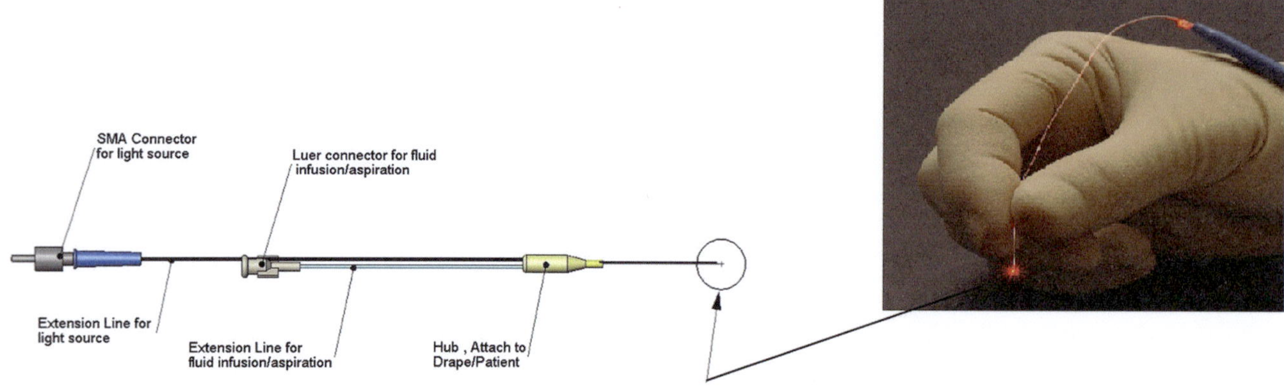


**Fig. 14.1** iScience canaloplasty microcatheter with laser-based fiber-optic light. Image courtesy of iScience Interventional Inc.

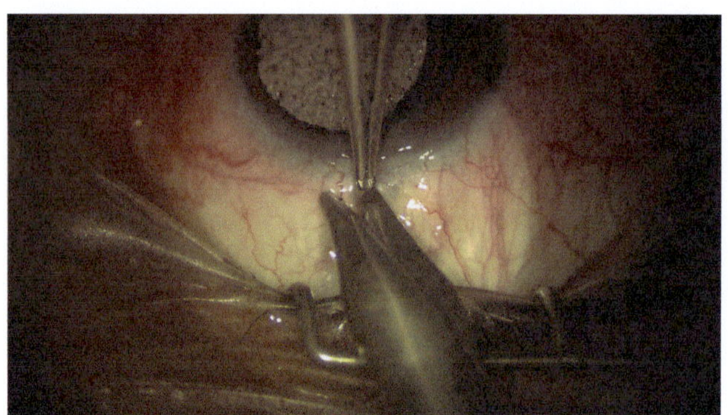

**Fig. 14.2** Localized peritomy leaving a small anterior skirt of conjunctiva at the limbus

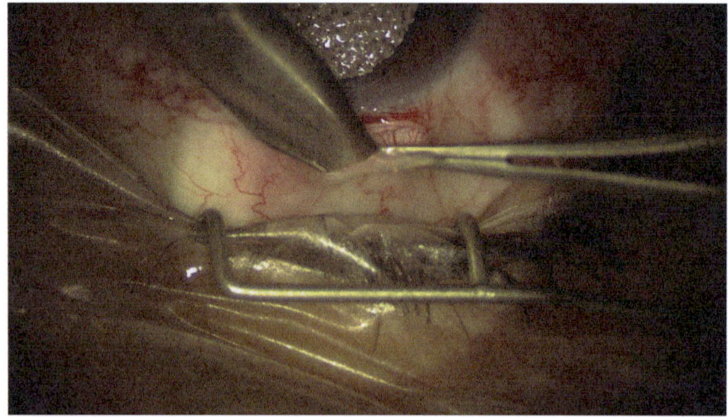

**Fig. 14.3** Blunt dissection posteriorly with Westcott scissors beneath Tenon's capsule

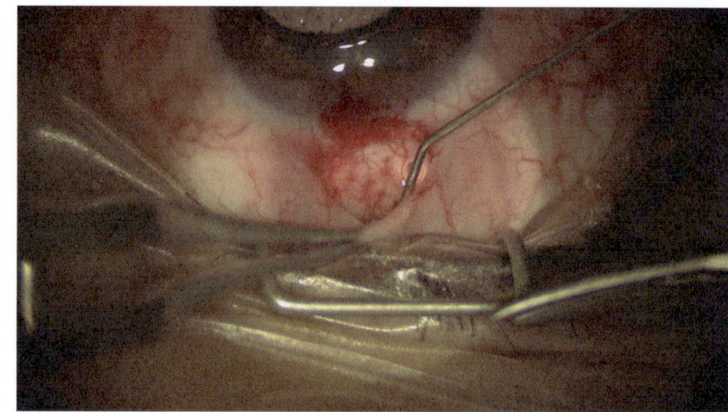

**Fig. 14.4** One percent plain Xylocaine is applied for further local anesthesia

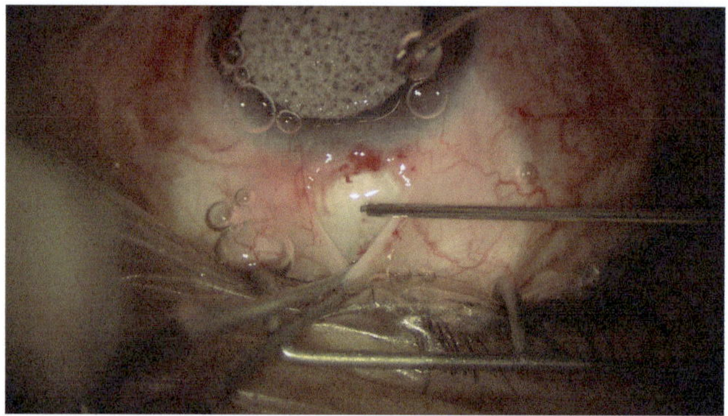

**Fig. 14.5** Light cautery is applied only as needed

A fornix-based peritomy is created using sharp-tipped Westcott scissors while leaving a small anterior skirt of conjunctiva at the limbus (Fig. 14.2). Blunt dissection is directed posteriorly to allow the posterior edge of the peritomy to be sufficiently relaxed for creation of scleral flap (Fig. 14.3). Location of ciliary veins should be considered when deciding where to perform the dissection. One percent plain Xylocaine is injected under Tenon's capsule to apply further

local anesthesia (Fig. 14.4). Cautery should be performed lightly only as needed, and avoiding these veins and collector channels (Fig. 14.5).

Given the high accuracy required to create the scleral flaps, diamond blades can be helpful in making incisions and dissections. A 5 mm×5 mm superficial scleral flap of parabolic shape (which in our experience provides good watertight closure) is outlined using a diamond trifacet

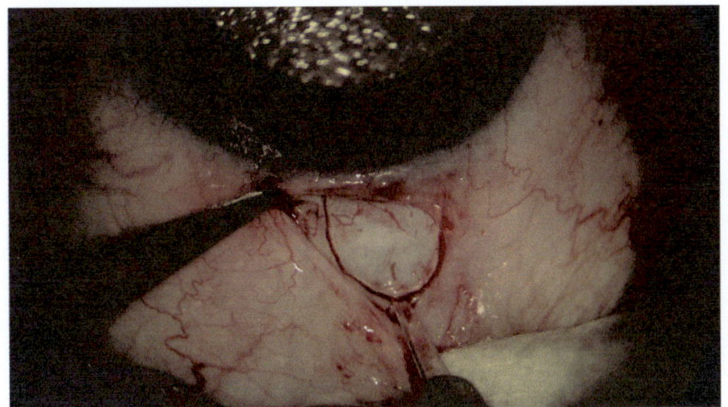

**Fig. 14.6** A diamond trifacet blade is used to outline a 5 mm×5 mm parabolic scleral flap

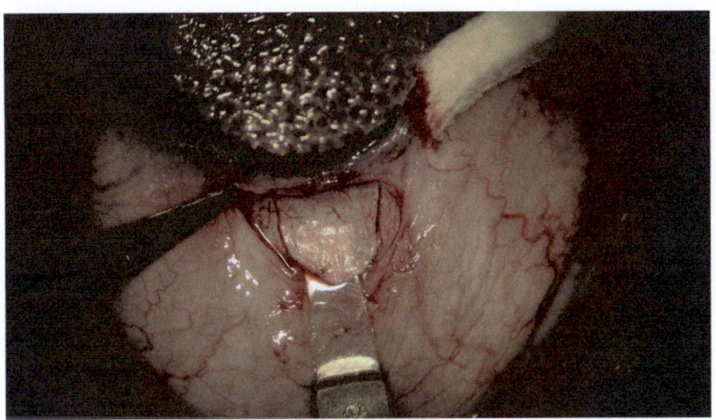

**Fig. 14.7** A diamond crescent blade is used to dissect at a depth of approximately one-third of the full scleral thickness to create the superficial scleral flap

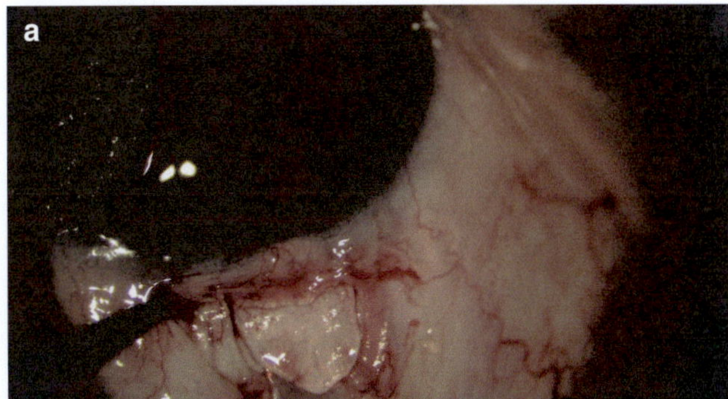

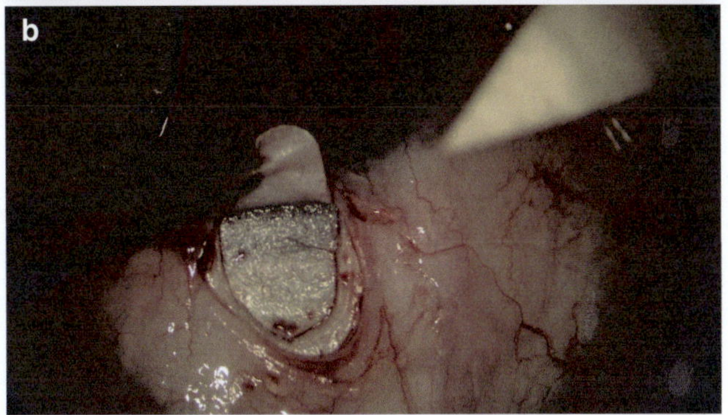

**Fig. 14.8** Dissection is carried forward (**a**) until it reaches the clear cornea (**b**)

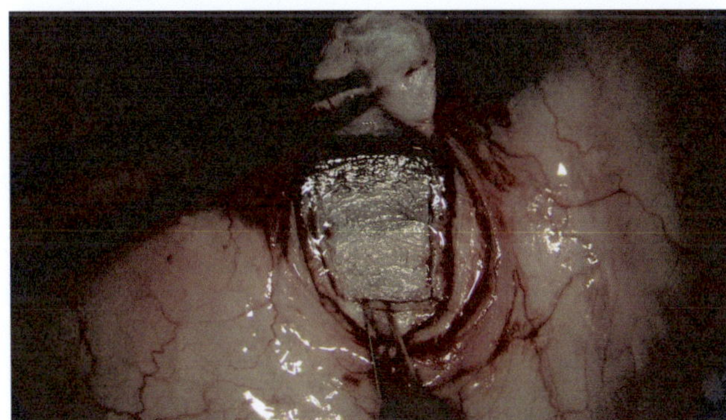

**Fig. 14.9** A deep scleral flap is outlined using the diamond trifacet blade

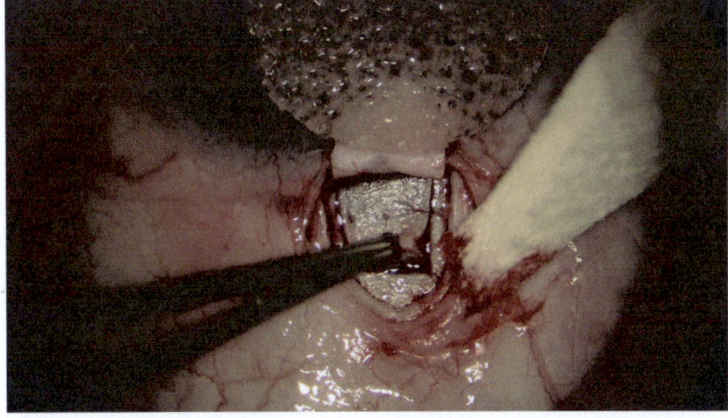

**Fig. 14.10** Suprachoroidal space is reached at the posterior edge of the deep scleral flap. This will facilitate identification of the depth required for creation of the deep flap

blade (Fig. 14.6). The flap is then fashioned with a diamond crescent knife at about one-third scleral thickness (200–300 μm) (Fig. 14.7), dissecting 1–2 mm into clear cornea (Fig. 14.8).

Then under high magnification, again using the diamond trifacet blade, a deep flap is outlined from 1 mm inside the posterior edge of the superficial flap (Fig. 14.9). This deep flap is also fashioned using the diamond crescent blade, but now at 90 % scleral thickness, leaving only about 100 μm of sclera covering the choroid (one may cut down into suprachoroidal space just at the back end of the flap to allow better determination of the required depth) (Fig. 14.10). At the desired depth, you should see irregular scleral fibers with an underlying purple hue coming from the choroid (Fig. 14.11). Sometimes a full-thickness dissection may inadvertently occur, in which case care must be taken to restart a new tissue plane leaving behind a thin layer of scleral bed. If dissection is too deep, then one risks penetration into the choroid or even the vitreous; yet if it is too superficial (more often the case), when dissection reaches the limbus, one may pass right over SC into clear cornea without exposing the canal (where it becomes even more difficult to reestablish a new plane or flap). Creation of a good deep scleral flap exposing

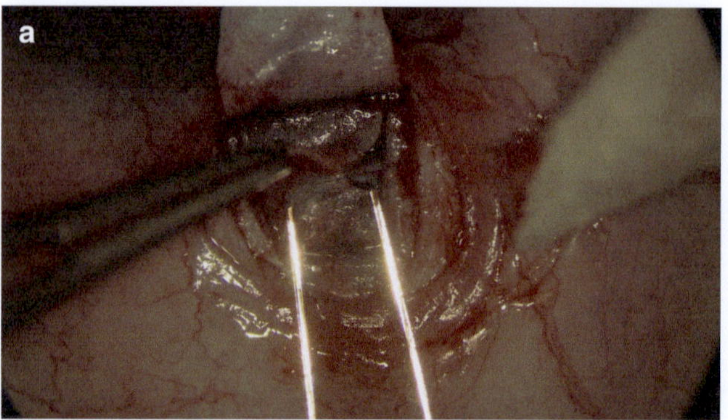

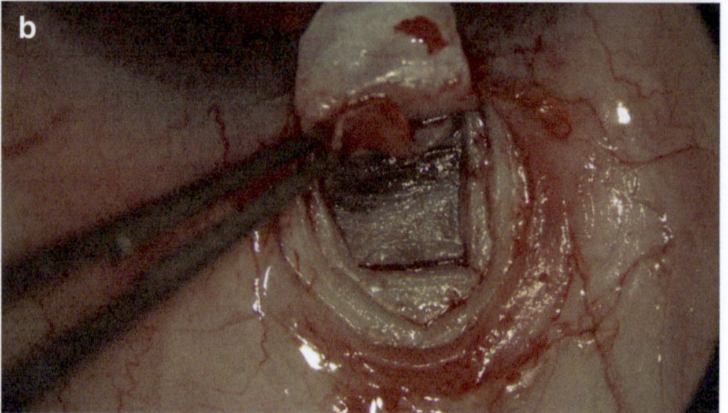

**Fig. 14.11** The diamond crescent blade is used to fashion the deep scleral flap (**a**). At the desired depth, the thin remaining scleral bed has a light purple hue coming from the underlying choroid (**b**)

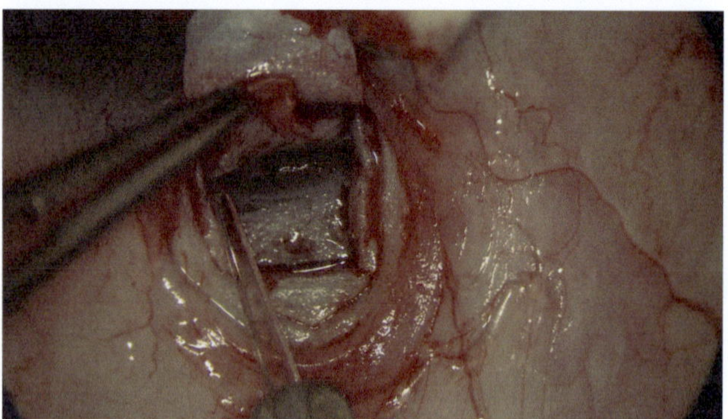

**Fig. 14.12** Careful dissection is performed to unroof Schlemm's canal at the base of the scleral flap

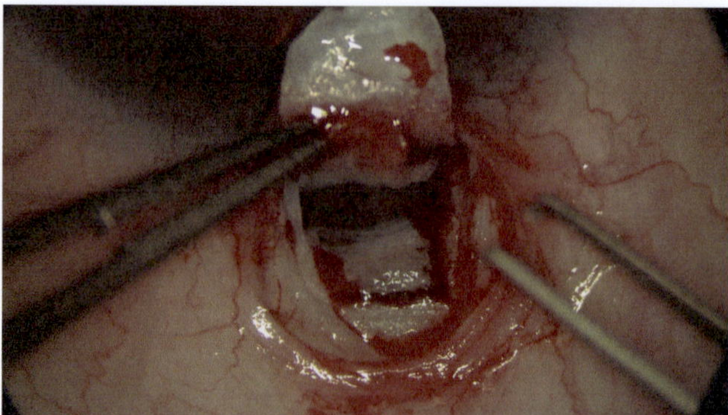

**Fig. 14.13** Once Schlemm's canal is reached, slow percolation of aqueous and reflux hemorrhage from the canal can be visualized

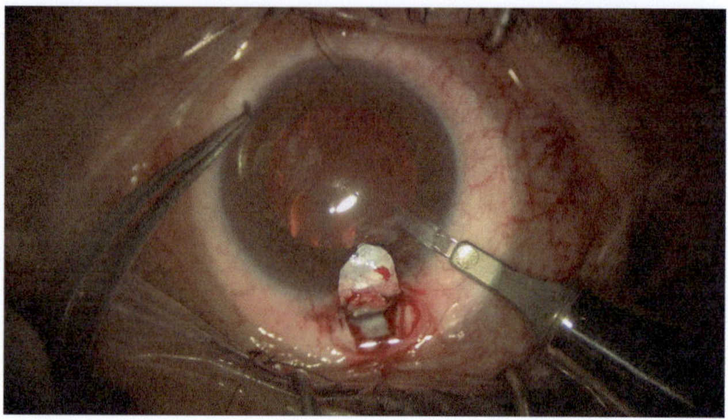

**Fig. 14.14** A paracentesis is made with the diamond trifacet blade at least a couple of clock hours away from the surgical site. This will decompress the anterior chamber and prevent bulging of Descemet's membrane at the base of the scleral flap

SC is thus likely the most technically challenging step of CP. Identification of proper anatomical landmarks is crucial, and this step must be performed under high magnification. This is particularly true when dissection reaches the base of the flap at the limbus, where unintentional penetration into the AC can occur. If that is the case, which would be evident with a gush of aqueous coming from the AC, one can convert to a penetrating procedure (trabeculectomy).

The deep flap is carried anterior enough when one sees scleral fibers changing from random to organized circumferential arrangement parallel to the limbus. At this point the scleral spur is reached. One may then either slowly and carefully dissecting forward to unroof SC (Fig. 14.12) or simply use a pair of toothed forceps to lift the deep flap up to expose fibers of the outer wall of SC at the base of the flap. Good exposure is confirmed when one sees aqueous percolating through SC, or blood reflux from cut ends of SC (Fig. 14.13).

A paracentesis is then made through the clear cornea away from the surgical site (Fig. 14.14). This would allow IOP to drop gradually to almost single digits, and thus preventing bulging of Descemet's membrane and the inner wall of SC. One should ensure gradual entry and retraction of the blade while making the paracentesis, so as to avoid sudden decompression of the eye which would risk sudden shallowing of the AC and/or intraoperative hemorrhage. This is particularly true if the reason of choosing CP (a non-penetrating procedure) instead of a penetrating procedure was because the eye is prone to such issues.

The deep flap is advanced forward for another 1 mm into the clear cornea, where further advancement only requires little force as it gets into the plane between Descemet's membrane and the corneal stroma. The trabeculo-Descemet's window (TDW) is thereby fashioned. To allow better advancement and exposure of TDW, one may use the diamond trifacet blade to gently create vertical relaxing incisions into the clear cornea at the lateral edges of the flap (with the cutting edge of the blade facing you, thus reducing the chance of penetration into the AC) (Fig. 14.15).

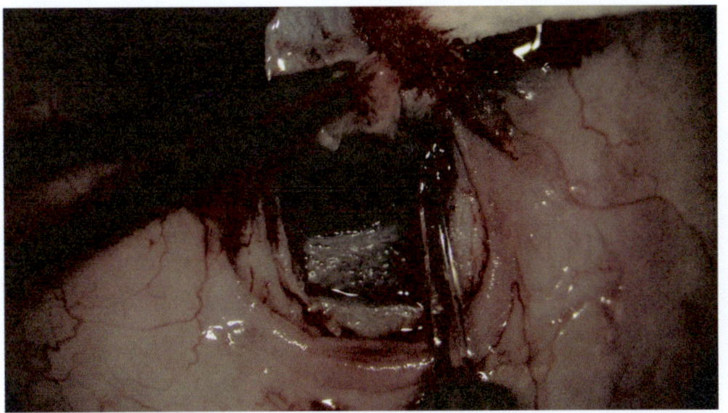

**Fig. 14.15** Relaxing incisions are made with the diamond trifacet blade at the lateral edges of the base of the deep scleral flap. One has to be careful to avoid inadvertent penetration through Descemet's membrane and enter the anterior chamber

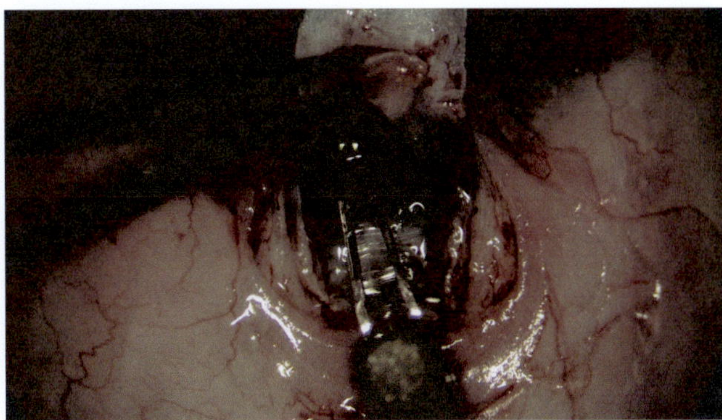

**Fig. 14.17** The diamond trifacet blade is used to mark and score the base of the deep scleral flap (but not the superficial flap)

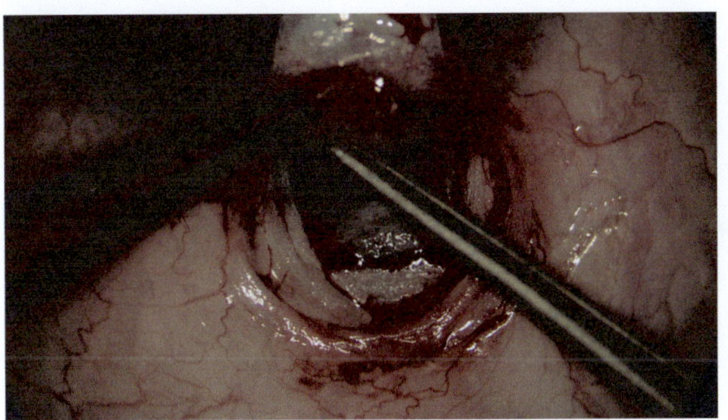

**Fig. 14.16** Forceps may be used to gently strip away any overlying scleral fibers and/or the walls of Schlemm's canal

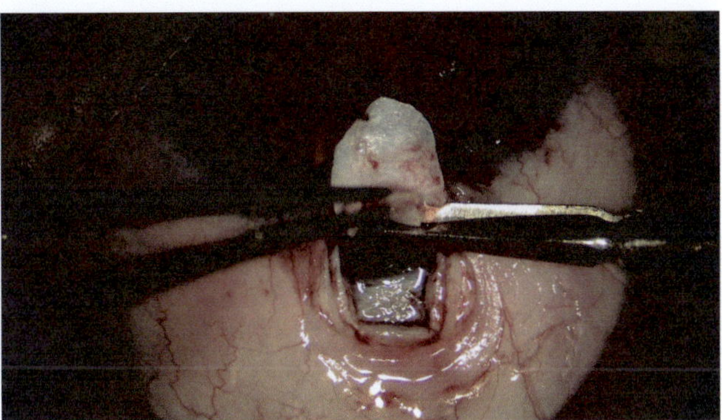

**Fig. 14.18** Vannas scissors are used to excise the deep scleral flap. This will facilitate a space beneath the superficial flap after closure, acting as the intrascleral lake

One may use a pair of Mermoud forceps to delicately strip the inner wall of SC away to further increase aqueous percolation (Fig. 14.16). Surgical sponges such as Weck-cel (Medtronic, Minneapolis, Minnesota) can be used to carefully push down on Schwalbe's line and Descemet's membrane to separate corneal stroma from TDW. However, any excessive downward pressure or sudden movement may easily perforate TDW and cause inadvertent penetration into the AC. Thus, we recommend moistening the tip of the Weck-cel prior to use, as it will reduce the rigidity of the tip when it is placed on the TDW, allowing a "soft touch." Once a satisfactory TDW is created, the trifacet diamond blade can be used to score the underside of the base of the deep scleral flap (Fig. 14.17). A pair of Vannas scissors is then used to excise the deep flap (Fig. 14.18), allowing formation of scleral lake in its place later on.

The two cut ends of SC can now be intubated with a special 150-μm diameter viscocanalostomy cannula (Grieshaber, Switzerland) (Fig. 14.19), through which a cohesive high viscosity viscoelastic such as Healon GV (Advanced Medical Optics Inc., Santa Ana, California) is injected to widen the ends of SC for easier entry of the microcatheter. The iScience microcatheter can be secured to the drape with Steri-strips (3M, St. Paul, Minnesota). Using two non-toothed forceps, the catheter is passed into one of the cut ends of SC and is advanced for

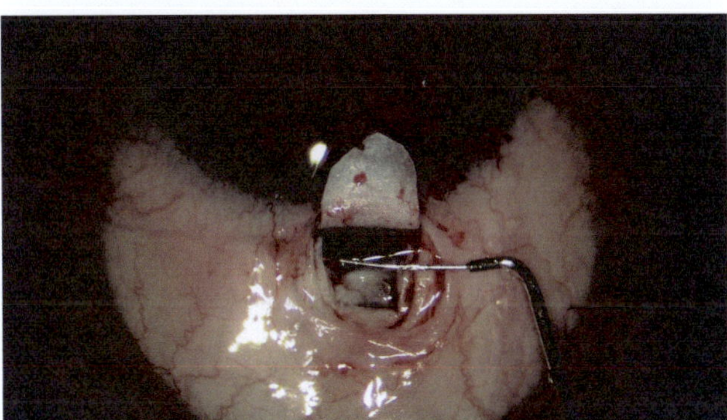

**Fig. 14.19** The viscocanalostomy cannula is used to inject cohesive viscoelastic into the cut ends of Schlemm's canal, thus dilating the entry site for the microcatheter

360° until the tip emerges from the other cut end of the canal (Fig. 14.20). During passage, one must pay attention to any resistance or false passage into the suprachoroidal space by observing the blinking red light at the leading tip of the microcatheter. If strong resistance or false passage is encountered, one should stop pushing further, retract, and reattempt with scleral depression at the site of resistance, or simply pull out and try passage in the opposite direction through the other cut end of SC.

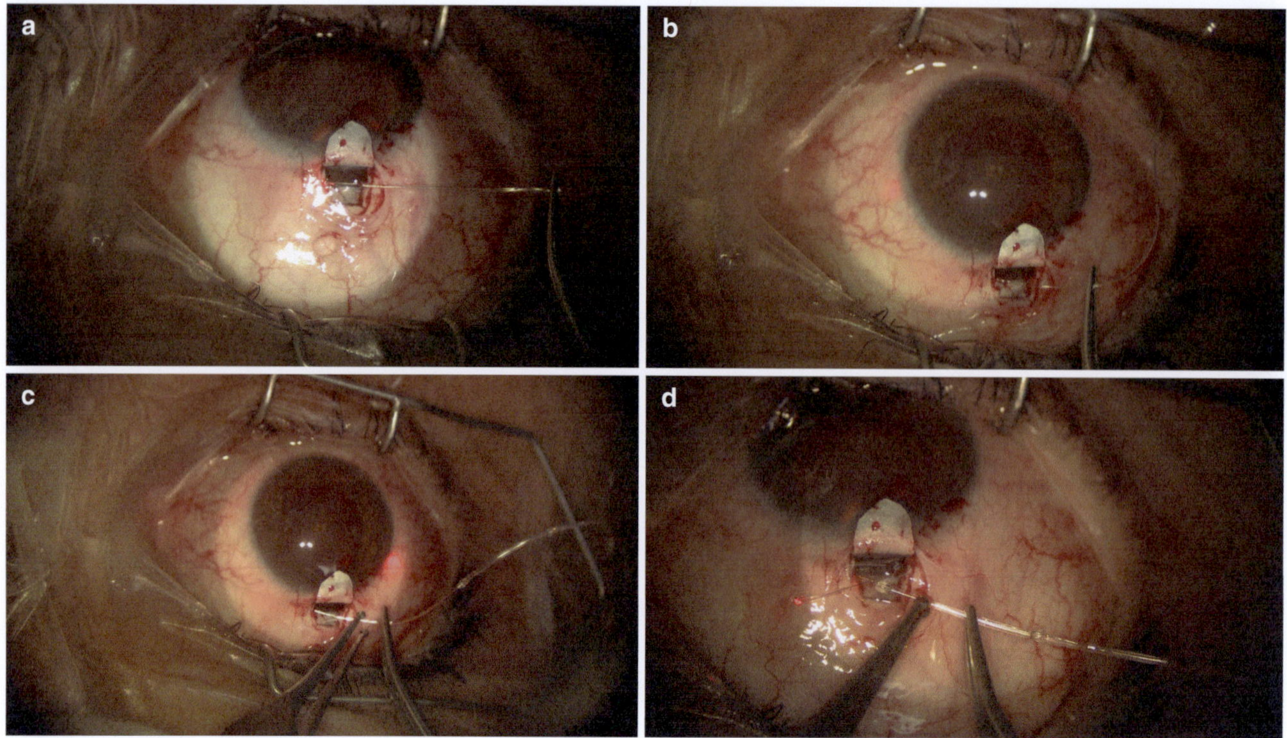

**Fig. 14.20** The microcatheter is inserted into Schlemm's canal using non-toothed forceps (**a**). A blinking red light can be visualized behind the sclera, indicating the leading tip of the catheter during passage (**b, c**). The catheter is passed though Schlemm's canal for its entire circumference, until the tip emerges from the other end of the canal (**d**)

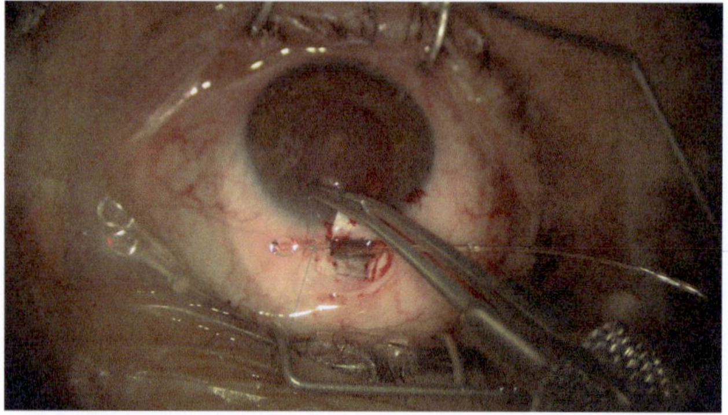

**Fig. 14.21** A 10-0 Prolene suture is tied on itself to the tip of the microcatheter

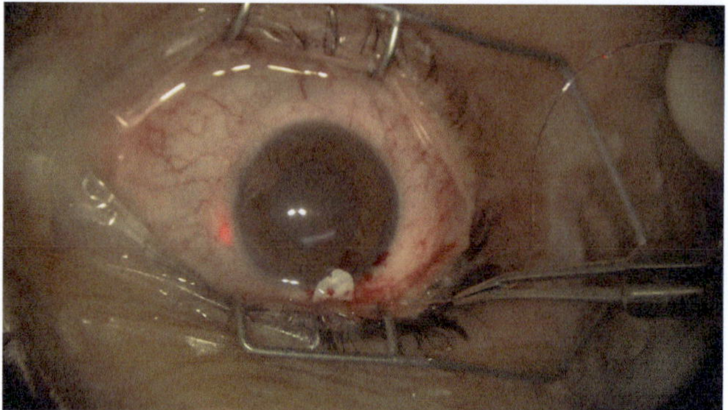

**Fig. 14.22** The microcatheter, now with the Prolene suture tied to its tip, is retracted through the entire circumference of Schlemm's canal. Again the blinking red light indicates the location of the catheter's tip

Once the catheter has passed 360° and the tip emerges, a 10-0 Prolene suture (polypropylene) with needles cut off is tied around the shaft of the device near its tip (by tying the two loose ends to the loop) (Fig. 14.21). The microcatheter is then withdrawn slowly in the reverse direction to which it was passed (Fig. 14.22); meanwhile viscoelastic is injected into SC using the screw mechanism by a surgical assistant. One must avoid injecting excessive viscoelastic which can cause Descemet's detachment (approximately 1/8th turn of the screw for every 2 clock hours of passage is recommended). Reflux of blood into the AC can be expected during passage or withdrawal of catheter. Once the entire catheter is removed (Fig. 14.23), the 10-0 Prolene suture is released from the catheter tip using Westcott scissors. By now there

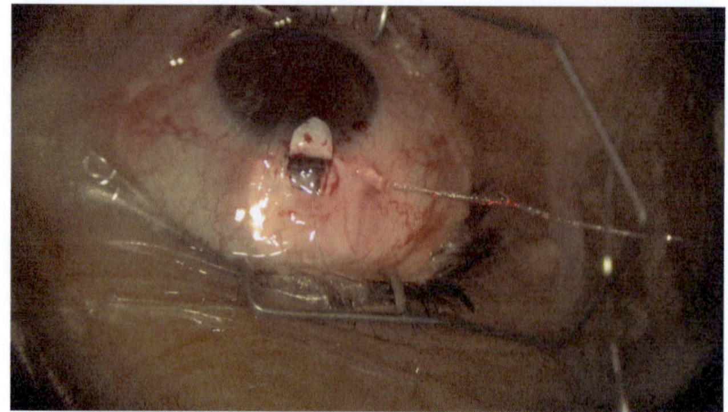

**Fig. 14.23** The entire microcatheter is externalized, with the 10-0 Prolene suture now remaining within the canal

should be 2 single 10-0 Prolene sutures in SC with 4 loose ends exposed. After confirming the corresponding ends, each suture is tied to itself with a slip knot (Fig. 14.24) with a back-and-forth movement in SC known as "flossing." Suture tension is adjusted such that one sees a small indentation of TDW by the suture, which should sit anteriorly in SC – this is confirmed by pulling the knot posteriorly until it is barely able to reach the scleral spur (Fig. 14.25). More tension of

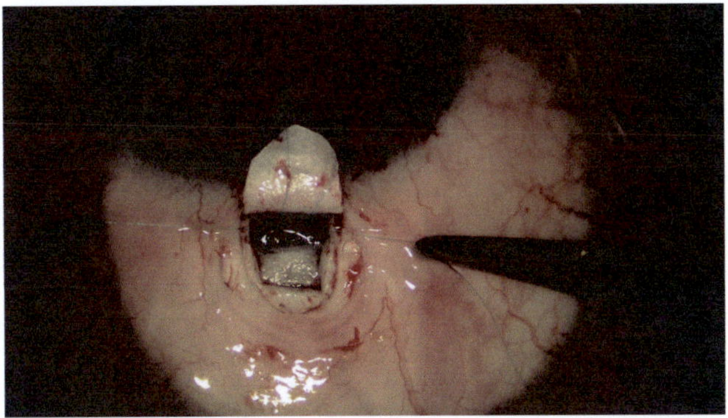

**Fig. 14.24** The corresponding ends of the Prolene sutures are tied with a slip knot that allows adjustment of tension

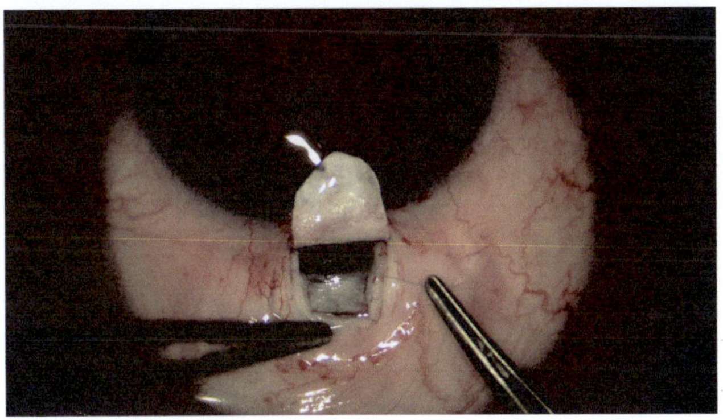

**Fig. 14.25** The desired tension is reached when the knot can barely reach the scleral spur while the sutures are being pulled posteriorly. Slight indentation of the trabeculo-Descemet's window by the suture knot can also be seen

the suture would result in more distention of SC, thus theoretically more IOP reduction (Fig. 14.26) [13]. Once satisfactory suture tension is achieved, the knots are locked and trimmed with Vannas scissors (Fig. 14.27).

Watertight closure of the superficial scleral flap is achieved with about five 10-0 nylon sutures placed in simple interrupted fashion. A cohesive high viscosity viscoelastic, such as Healon GV, may be placed under the flap to maintain the scleral lake (Fig. 14.28). It has been suggested that viscoelastics may limit fibrinogen migration [18], thereby minimizing scar formation which may obliterate scleral lake over time. Aqueous will percolate through the TDW and accumulate in this "reservoir" before being absorbed by the episcleral, scleral, and choroidal veins.

Finally, the conjunctiva is closed in a watertight fashion using 10-0 or 9-0 Vicryl suture in a running horizontal mattress fashion (Fig. 14.29) as in the case of trabeculectomy. The paracentesis and conjunctiva are checked for leaks with a Weck-cel.

## Adjunctive Measures or Alternative Techniques

If cataract surgery is planned as a combined procedure with CP, it should be performed first. After cataract extraction and intraocular lens implantation, the AC should be adequately pressurized with viscoelastic to facilitate scleral flap dissection later. The viscoelastic should be removed after the excision of the deep flap with a 27 gauge cannula on a syringe with balanced saline solution (BSS) manually, rather than with automated irrigation-aspiration, in which case the irrigation part may raise the IOP abruptly causing the TDW to rupture.

Given that the most challenging step in CP is likely the creation of a good deep scleral flap without inadvertent entry into the AC, various alternative approaches to fashion the scleral flap have been described. For deep sclerectomy, Abdelrahman reported the use of a trabeculotome to intubate

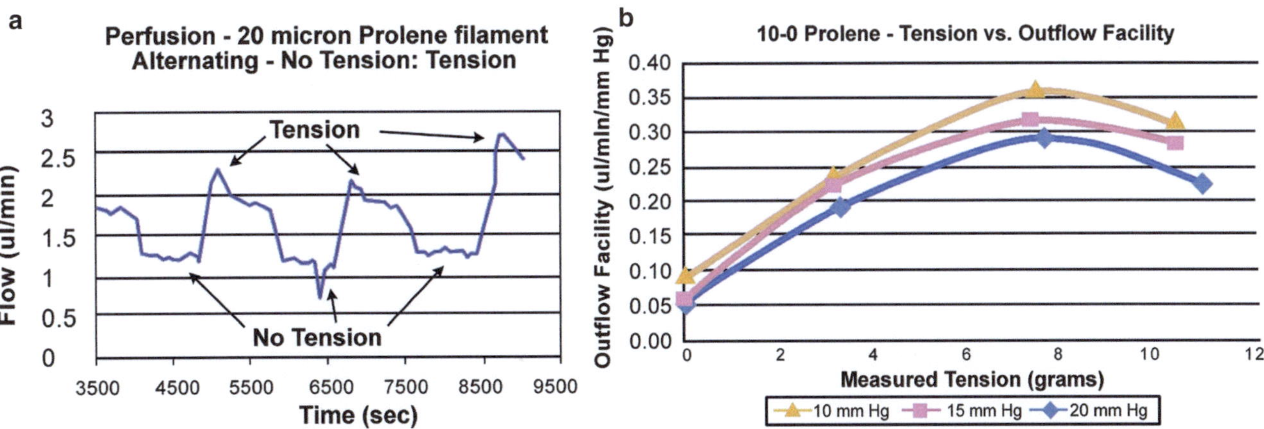


**Fig. 14.26** Outflow facility can be seen as a function of suture tension (**a**, **b**) in an ex vivo model. 10, 15 and 20 mmHg correspond to designated levels of IOP. Data from iScience Interventional Inc.

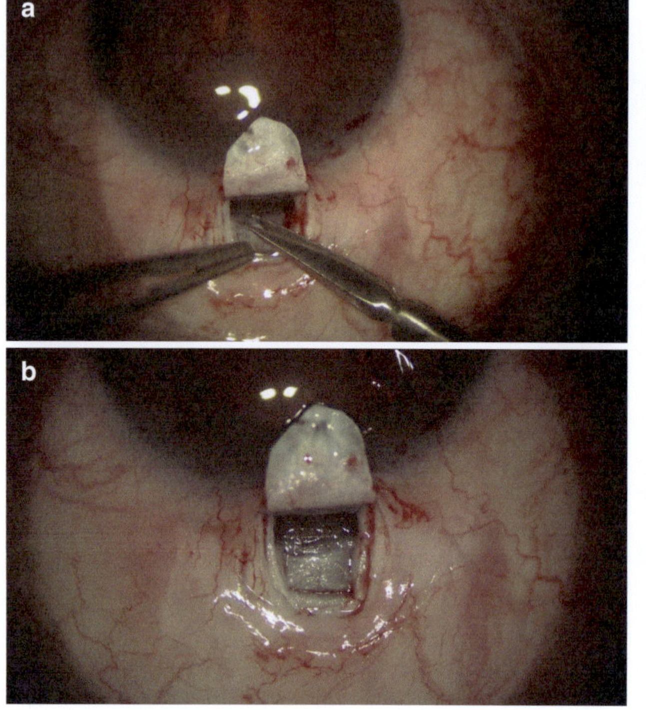

**Fig. 14.27** Vannas scissors are used to trim the knots (**a**). Slight indentation of the trabeculo-Descemet's window can be seen due to tension from the suture (**b**)

a segment of SC such that it can be well delineated prior to its unroofing [19]. Others have described using excimer laser [20], erbium:yttrium-aluminum-garnet (Er:YAG) laser [21], $CO_2$ laser [22], and the Fugo blade (Medisurg Ltd., Norristown, Pennsylvania; unpublished data by authors).

Antimetabolites such as mitomycin C (MMC) is typically not used intraoperatively in CP as bleb formation is not a planned outcome. However, it has been reported as an adjunctive agent to prevent collapse of the intrascleral lake [23, 24]. MMC (in 0.25–0.30 mg/cc) can be applied in precut soaked sponges under the superficial scleral flap prior to creation of the deep flap. The conjunctiva is lifted with non-toothed forceps to avoid its contact with antimetabolites (Fig. 14.30), which may increase risk of wound leakage.

## Intraoperative Complications

Flap or conjunctiva-related complications (e.g., partial amputation of superficial flap, buttonhole of conjunctiva) can be managed similar to the case in trabeculectomy. Inadvertent perforation of the TDW is likely the most common intraoperative complication during CP. Occult microperforations may result in trace localized leakage of aqueous with no AC

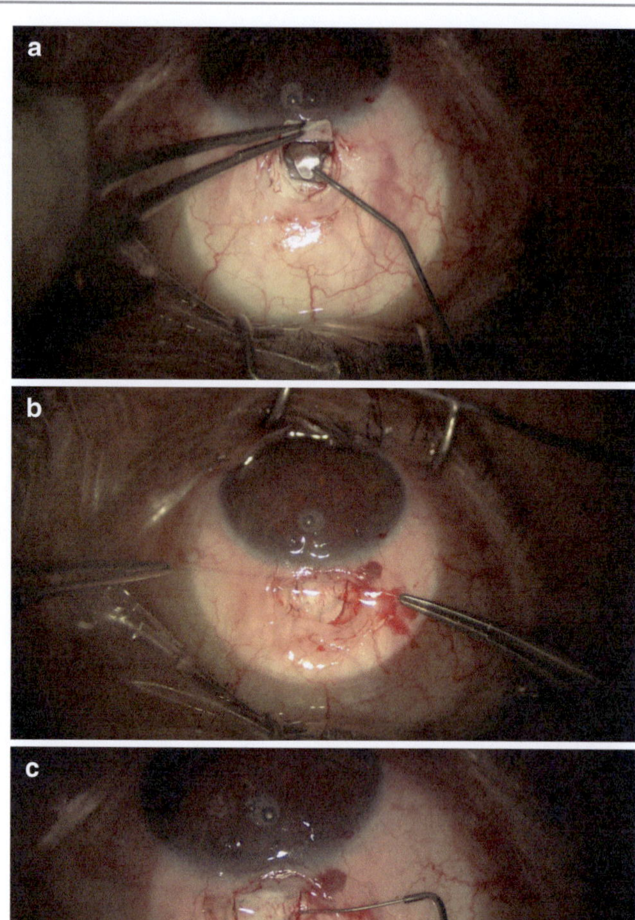

**Fig. 14.28** Cohesive viscoelastic is applied beneath the scleral flap to maintain the space for the intrascleral lake (**a, c**). 10-0 nylon sutures were placed to close the flap (**b**)

depth compromise and thus may be left alone and potentially even be beneficial to IOP lowering. On the other hand, macroperforations evident with gush of aqueous coming out with concurrent AC shallowing would indicate that CP should be aborted and essentially be converted to a penetrating procedure such as a trabeculectomy.

## Postoperative Management

The early postoperative management of CP is quite similar to that of trabeculectomy. A topical antibiotic is used, and steroid drops are administered with a frequent dosing regimen early on (e.g., every 2 h while awake) to minimize risk of

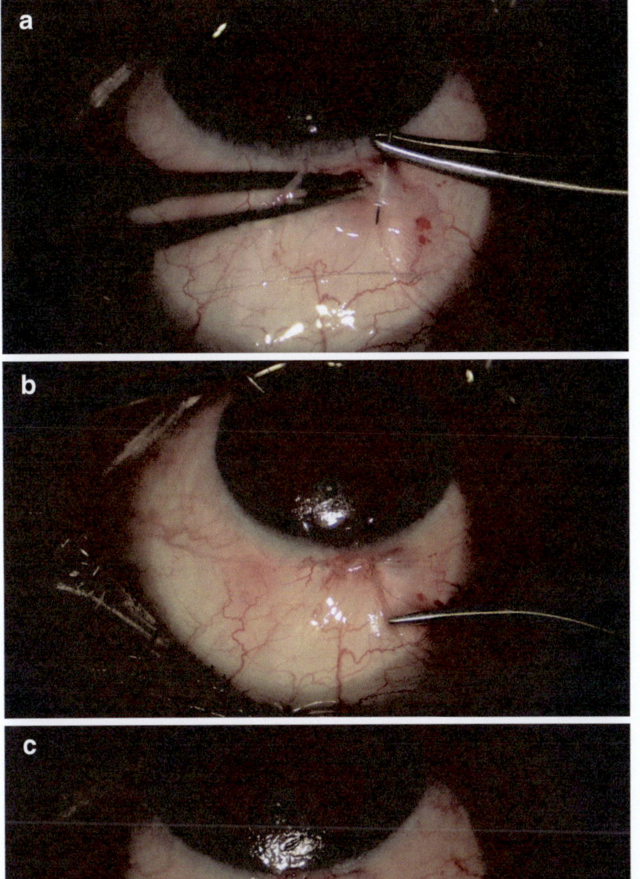

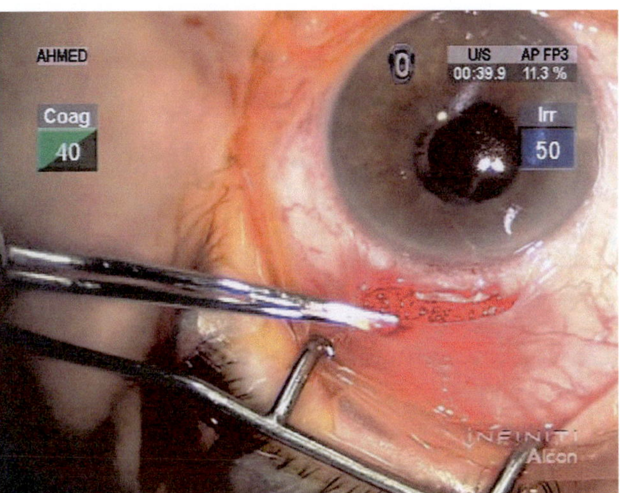

**Fig. 14.30** Sponge soaked with mitomycin C is placed under the scleral flap. The conjunctiva is lifted up with non-toothed forceps to avoid contact with antimetabolite

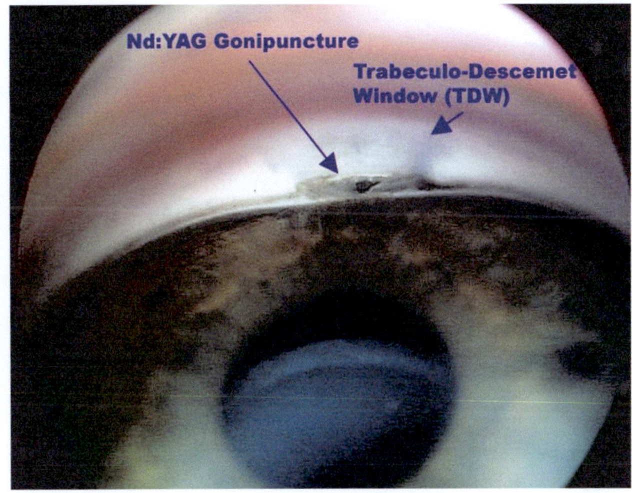


**Fig. 14.29** 10-0 Vicryl suture is placed in a running horizontal mattress fashion to close the conjunctiva (**a–c**)

**Fig. 14.31** Gonioscopic view of the angle after laser goniopuncture. A patent hole from the laser can be seen within the trabeculo-Descemet's window

scleral lake fibrosis. A miotic agent such as pilocarpine may be prescribed at a low-dosing regimen for the first month after surgery to prevent iris apposition or peripheral anterior synechiae formation against the TDW. However, one has to be careful of its use particularly in phakic patients as it may also move the lens-iris diaphragm forward. Though relatively uncommon (see below), complications such as hyphema, hypotony, and choroidal effusion should be managed as in the case of penetrating procedures. Descemet's membrane detachment may occur as a complication from ophthalmic viscoelastic device (OVD) injection into SC. In most cases these can be monitored and would resolve spontaneously. However, if it is large enough to compromise vision, it can be drained with a small needle, or neodymium-doped yttrium aluminum garnet (Nd:YAG) laser can be applied to open the descemetocele, with or without air descemetopexy [25, 26]. On the other hand, microhyphema on the first postoperative day had been suggested as a potential positive prognostic factor [27]. In contrast to trabeculectomy, ocular massage is often not recommended as it may result in inadvertent rupture of the TDW.

Late rise in IOP is usually due to fibrosis of the microperforations at the TDW and/or fibrosis of the intrascleral lake and episclera. The first approach if IOP rises above target would be laser goniopuncture (GPC), which is required in up to about 20 % of cases (Fig. 14.31) [28–30]. Even though this essentially converts CP into a penetrating procedure, because it is done after some degree of fibrosis has already occurred in the absence of antimetabolite use, the risk of hypotony is lower. GPC is performed with a YAG laser set to free-running Q-switch mode. Starting low at an energy level of around 4 mJ (which can be titrated gradually up to approximately 8 mJ as needed), about 4–8 shots are delivered to create 1–2 holes within the anterior part of the TDW under gonioscopic view. It can be done at any time after about 2 weeks postoperatively and may be repeated as needed. Nonetheless, a prerequisite for the effectiveness of giant papillary conjunctivitis (GPC), is that the TDW must be sufficiently thin and anteriorly dissected (thus further highlighting the importance of accurate dissection during surgery).

Despite the pulsed application of a miotic agent, sometimes the iris can adhere or incarcerate at the TDW early on postoperatively or after GPC (especially if the opening from GPC is too wide or placed too posteriorly), resulting in acute IOP rise. For this reason, patients should be followed closely in the first few weeks after CP, as well as shortly after GPC. Iris adherence or incarceration can be managed first with Nd:YAG laser synechialysis or argon laser iridoplasty. If the adhesion persists, a small needle (e.g., 27 or 30 gauge) can be inserted into the AC at the limbus to sweep the iris away from the TDW, with gonioscopic confirmation of release of iris after the procedure.

If IOP remains high despite goniopuncture and in the absence of iris adhesions to the TDW, it would suggest that fibrosis may have occurred within the scleral lake. One may consider a needling procedure with a 27 or 30 gauge needle to lift or dissect under the scleral flap, which can be done in the presence of a subconjunctival antimetabolite such as MMC if bleb formation is desired. Any bleb-related complications should be managed as seen in trabeculectomy.

## Literature Review

Major studies evaluating CP on its efficacy and safety are summarized in Tables 14.1 and 14.2. In general, CP demonstrates better safety profile when compared to traditional penetrating surgeries. This is because without a full-thickness sclerostomy, the semipermeable TDW provides some degree of resistance to aqueous outflow, which safeguards against large fluctuation of IOP particularly in the early postoperative period. Moreover, without a persistent patent ostium into the AC and without the need for an iridectomy, postoperative inflammation, hyphema, and endophthalmitis are less likely. Bleb-related complications are also rare because of the following: (1) flap closure is tight in CP, resulting in lower

likelihood of bleb formation; (2) in most cases antimetabolites are not used; and (3) if a bleb is formed, it tends to be more diffuse and low-lying rather than cystic and avascular, for the above reasons.

Of note are the 3-year results from a prospective multicenter international study reported by Lewis et al. in 2011, which provides the longest follow-up data with the largest number of CP subjects to date. In agreement with previous and subsequent studies [31–34], CP was shown to achieve a reduction of IOP from mid-twenties level (or at times higher) to around mid-teens while maintaining on 0–2 topical medications after surgery. Comparable efficacy is seen when CP is combined with phacoemulsification, though the cumulative failure rate is lower with the combined procedure. This may be due to the TM being put on more tension with removal of the crystalline lens in conjunction with placement of the suture in CP, thereby increasing outflow. Complications if present tend to occur early on (≤90 days), including hyphema, hypotony with AC shallowing, IOP spike, Descemet's membrane detachment, suture extrusion through the TM, and hypotony. Late postoperative complications (>90 days) include cataract formation, high IOP despite surgery, and suture extrusion [29]. The incidence and severity of these adverse outcomes are generally lower when compared to those reported for trabeculectomy and tube shunt [7, 35]. This study provides data supporting the long-term safety and efficacy of CP; however, the staging of glaucoma was not specified.

Adjunctive use of MMC had shown comparable levels of IOP reduction, though the incidence of postoperative hypotony appear to be higher than previous non-MMC studies (Table 14.2) [24]. In a retrospective case series, Ayyala et al. examined the outcome of patients who underwent CP ($n = 33$) versus trabeculectomy ($n = 46$). There was no significant difference in the percentage of IOP reduction and surgical failure rates between groups. More percentage of patients in the CP group required postoperative medications for IOP control than in the trabeculectomy group, though again the difference was not statistically significant [36].

In a recent study comparing the outcome of CP in one eye and viscocanalostomy in the opposite eye, both procedures had similar safety profiles, but CP achieved higher percentage of IOP reduction than VC at both 12- and 18-month time points [37].

Given the evidence available to date, it is still debatable if CP can consistently achieve sufficiently low IOP for patients with advanced stage of glaucoma who require more aggressive IOP targets. Nonetheless, modest IOP reduction is attainable with CP, which is thus certainly a considerable surgical option for patients with mild to moderate level of glaucomatous damage (see below).

**Table 14.1** Summary of efficacy of canaloplasty from previous studies

| Authors | Year | Design | Surgery | Adjunctive antimetabolite | GP (% required) | n (eyes) | Follow-up | Mean pre-op IOP | Mean post-op IOP | Mean # pre-op medications | Mean # post-op medications | % Complete success (qualified) | Definition of success |
|---|---|---|---|---|---|---|---|---|---|---|---|---|---|
| Shingleton et al. [31] | 2008 | Prospective non-randomized | CP + phaco | No | No | 54 | 12 | 24.4±6.1 | 13.7±4.4 | 1.5±1.0 | 0.2±0.4 | NR | NR |
| Grieshaber et al. [32] | 2010 | Prospective randomized | CP (6–0 Prolene) | No | NR | 45 | 15 | 42.7±12.5 | 19.2±6.4 | NR | NR | 51 (NR) | ≤21 |
|  |  |  | CP (10–0 Prolene) |  |  | 45 | 15 | 45.0±12.1 | 16.4±4.9 | NR | NR | 76.9 (NR) |  |
| Grieshaber et al. [33] | 2010 | Prospective non-randomized | CP | No | 0 | 60 | 30.6±8.4 | 45.0±12.1 | 13.3±1.7 | NR | NR | 77.5 (81.6) | ≤21 |
| Bull et al. [28] | 2011 | Prospective non-randomized | CP alone | No | Yes (8.3) | 82 | 36 | 23.0±4.3 | 15.1±3.1 | 1.9±0.7 | 0.9±0.9 | 40.5 (98.6) | ≤21 |
|  |  |  | CP + phaco |  | Yes (12.5) | 16 | 36 | 24.3±6.0 | 13.8±3.2 | 1.5±1.2 | 0.5±0.7 | 61.5 (100) |  |
| Lewis et al. [29] | 2011 | Prospective non-randomized | CP alone | No | Yes (8.9) | 103 | 36 | 23.5±4.5 | 15.5±3.5 | 1.9±0.8 | 0.9±0.9 | 40.4 (95.5) | ≤21 |
|  |  |  | CP + phaco |  |  | 30 | 36 | 23.5±5.2 | 13.6±3.6 | 1.5±1.0 | 0.3±0.5 | 77.8 (100) |  |
| Ayyala et al. [36] | 2011 | Retrospective | CP | No | No | 33 | 12 | 21.2±6.6 | 13.8±4.9 | 2.5±0.8 | 0.6±0.9 | NR | NR |
|  |  |  | Trab | Yes |  | 46 | 12 | 23.4±10.4 | 11.6±4.0 | 2.6±0.6 | 0.3±0.7 |  |  |
| Fujita et al. [34] | 2011 | Retrospective | CP | No | No | 3 | 12 | 23.4±5.5 | 15.0±4.1 | 2.8±0.6 | 1.2±0.8 | 81.8 (NR) | ≤21 |
|  |  |  | CP + phaco |  |  | 8 | 12 |  |  |  |  |  |  |
| Grieshaber et al. [30] | 2011 | Prospective non-randomized | CP | No | Yes (18.8) | 32 | 14.6±4.2 | 27.3±5.6 | 20.6±4.2 | 2.7±0.5 | 0.1±0.3 | 93.8 (100) | ≤21 |
| Koerber [37] | 2012 | Prospective non-randomized | CP | No | No | 15 | 18 | 26.5±2.7 | 14.5±2.6 | 2.1±1.0 | 0.3±0.5 | 60 (86.7) | ≤18 |
|  |  |  | VC | No | No | 15 | 18 | 24.3±2.8 | 16.1±3.9 | 1.9±0.8 | 0.4±0.5 | 35.7 (50) |  |
| Barnebey [24] | 2013 | Retrospective | CP | Yes | No | 20 | 12 | 23.4±4.3 | 13.4±4.3 | 2.2±1.2 | 0 | NR | NR |

*CP* canaloplasty, *Phaco* phacoemulsification, *Trab* trabeculectomy, *VC* viscocanalostomy, *NR* not reported

**Table 14.2** Summary of postoperative complications from studies on canaloplasty

| Authors | Year | Design | Surgery | $n$ (eyes) | Hyphema % | Hypotony % | Flat/shallow AC % | Choroidal detachment % | Bleb fibrosis or encapsulation % | Descemet's membrane detachment % | Induced cataract % | Late cataract progression % |
|---|---|---|---|---|---|---|---|---|---|---|---|---|
| Shingleton et al. [31] | 2008 | Prospective non-randomized | CP + phaco | 54 | 5.6 | 0 | NR | NR | NR | 1.9 | NA | NA |
| Grieshaber et al. [32] | 2010 | Prospective randomized | CP (6–0 Prolene) | 45 | 22 | 0 | 0 | 0 | 0 | 2.2 | 0 | NR |
| | | | CP (10–0 Prolene) | 45 | 33 | 0 | 0 | 0 | 0 | 2.2 | 0 | NR |
| Grieshaber et al. [33] | 2010 | Prospective non-randomized | CP | 60 | 70 (micro) | NR | 0 | 0 | 0 | 3.3 | 0 | 0 |
| Bull et al. [28] | 2011 | Prospective non-randomized | CP ± phaco | 109 | 5.5 | 0 | 0 | 0 | 0 | 3.7 | NR | 9.1 (of phakic patients) |
| Lewis et al. [29] | 2011 | Prospective non-randomized | CP ± phaco | 157 | 10.2 | 0.6 | 0 | 0 | NR | 3.2 | NR | 12.7 |
| Ayyala et al. [36] | 2011 | Retrospective | CP | 33 | 21 | 0 | NR | 0 | NR | 3 | NR | NR |
| | | | Trab | 46 | 2 | 4 | | 17 | | 0 | | |
| Fujita et al. [34] | 2011 | Retrospective | CP | 3 | 45.5 | NR | NR | NR | NR | 9 | NR | NR |
| | | | CP + phaco | 8 | | | | | | | | |
| Grieshaber et al. [30] | 2011 | Prospective non-randomized | CP | 33 | 6.1 | NR | 0 | 0 | NR | 6.1 | 0 | NR |
| Koerber [37] | 2012 | Prospective non-randomized | CP | 15 | 0 | 0 | 0 | 0 | NR | 0 | NR | NR |
| | | | VC | 15 | 0 | 0 | 0 | 0 | | 0 | | |
| Barnebey [24] | 2013 | Retrospective | CP | 20 | 5 | 15 | 0 | 0 | NR | 10 | NR | NR |

*CP* canaloplasty, *Phaco* phacoemulsification, *Trab* trabeculectomy, *VC* viscocanalostomy, *NR* not reported, *NA* not applicable

## Surgical Candidates

As supported by the available literature on the procedure, CP is indicated in patients with open-angle glaucoma who are also candidates for trabeculectomy or glaucoma drainage devices, but particularly in those with the following features:

1. When early surgical intervention is desired:

    The use of multiple topical medications is associated with low grade conjunctival inflammation and scarring, which can be a factor of failure for procedures where efficacy depends on formation of a good bleb [38]. CP is less dependent on the state of the conjunctiva than these procedures.

    Also, in conditions where large IOP fluctuations are seen (e.g., pigment dispersion glaucoma, pseudoexfoliative glaucoma), early surgery may be superior to medical therapy alone in limiting IOP fluctuation [39, 40], which is a risk factor for glaucoma progression [41]. Therefore, in light of its safety profile, CP can be a reasonable early surgery option prior to exhausting all medical options.

2. High risk for intra- and/or postoperative morbidities:

    In patients who have high risk for choroidal effusion (e.g., nanophthalmic eye) or suprachoroidal hemorrhage (e.g., those on systemic anticoagulation medications), even a brief duration of intra- or postoperative hypotony is certainly not desirable. With CP, as sudden decompression of the eye can be avoided intraoperatively, and outflow is somewhat restricted by a TDW instead of having an open ostium, it is a favorable option for these cases. Moreover, with less manipulation in the anterior segment and without the need to perform an iridectomy (both of which may incite inflammation and hypotony from hyposecretion of aqueous) [42], CP may be more favored than trabeculectomy in uveitic cases. However, the scleral lake may be prone to fibrosis in these cases; thus, frequent steroid use perioperatively would be crucial.

3. Monocular patients:

    Given their relatively higher safety profile, CP should be considered in patients who require surgery in their only functioning eye. Also, because of their non-penetrating nature and less risk for bleb-related issues, CP patients would likely have faster visual recovery than those who have penetrating procedures [43].

4. Younger patients:

    With theoretically less risk for cataract formation than penetrating procedures, CP is advantageous for younger patients who are expected to still have years of significant accommodative amplitudes ahead with their own natural crystalline lens.

5. Contact lens users:

    As no or very low blebs are present with CP, risk of blebitis is minimized.

CP is contraindicated if the TM is anatomically obstructed or damaged, such as in primary or secondary angle closure, peripheral anterior synechiae, or neovascular glaucoma, or if structural abnormality is present in the limbal or perilimbal regions such as from previous trauma or surgery. For eyes with very thin sclera, creation of scleral flaps would be challenging; thus, CP is less favored in these cases. The presence of normal angle anatomy is a prerequisite for the success of CP both intra- and postoperatively. Previous laser trabeculoplasty is not a contraindication and should not preclude the effect of non-penetrating procedures such as CP [44].

## Summary

Canaloplasty has shown to be a good (and potentially superior in selected cases) alternative to traditional penetrating surgeries for glaucoma. With the goal of improving the conventional outflow pathway, the ab externo non-penetrating nature of CP allowed a better safety profile than trabeculectomy. Adjunctive measures such as antimetabolite use and laser goniopuncture allow augmented efficacy in lowering IOP. CP can therefore be an effective option for patients with mild to moderate stage of glaucoma damage, with the benefit of lower risks than penetrating procedures. On the other hand, CP does have a steep learning curve and can be technically challenging especially for the beginning glaucoma surgeon. For this reason, as well as cost issues, CP has yet to gain widespread adoption by glaucoma surgeons in North America. The high degree of surgical precision required for CP has however provided us with greater understanding of the outflow anatomy, which has added to the foundation for the development of other innovative glaucoma procedures. Further studies are required to investigate the long-term efficacy, optimal suture tension, and prolonged effect of nonabsorbable suture in the canal in CP.

## References

1. Cairns JE. Trabeculectomy. Preliminary report of a new method. Am J Ophthalmol. 1968;66(4):673–9.
2. Molteno AC. New implant for drainage in glaucoma. Clinical trial. Br J Ophthalmol. 1969;53(9):606–15.
3. Krupin T, Podos SM, Becker B, Newkirk JB. Valve implants in filtering surgery. Am J Ophthalmol. 1976;81(2):232–5.
4. Lloyd MA, Baerveldt G, Heuer DK, Minckler DS, Martone JF. Initial clinical experience with the baerveldt implant in complicated glaucomas. Ophthalmology. 1994;101(4):640–50.
5. Coleman AL, Hill R, Wilson MR, et al. Initial clinical experience with the Ahmed Glaucoma Valve implant. Am J Ophthalmol. 1995;120(1):23–31.
6. Borisuth NS, Phillips B, Krupin T. The risk profile of glaucoma filtration surgery. Curr Opin Ophthalmol. 1999;10(2):112–6.

7. Gedde SJ, Herndon LW, Brandt JD, et al. Postoperative complications in the Tube Versus Trabeculectomy (TVT) study during five years of follow-up. Am J Ophthalmol. 2012;153(5):804–14.e1.

8. Epstein E. Fibrosing response to aqueous. Its relation to glaucoma. Br J Ophthalmol. 1959;43:641–7.

9. Krasnov MM. Externalization of Schlemm's canal (sinusotomy) in glaucoma. Br J Ophthalmol. 1968;52(2):157–61.

10. Hara T. Deep sclerectomy with Nd:YAG laser trabeculotomy ab interno: two-stage procedure. Ophthalmic Surg. 1988;19(2):101–6.

11. Sanchez E, Schnyder CC, Sickenberg M, Chiou AG, Hediguer SE, Mermoud A. Deep sclerectomy: results with and without collagen implant. Int Ophthalmol. 1996;20(1–3):157–62.

12. Stegmann R, Pienaar A, Miller D. Viscocanalostomy for open-angle glaucoma in black African patients. J Cataract Refract Surg. 1999;25(3):316–22.

13. Lewis RA, von Wolff K, Tetz M, et al. Canaloplasty: circumferential viscodilation and tensioning of Schlemm's canal using a flexible microcatheter for the treatment of open-angle glaucoma in adults: interim clinical study analysis. J Cataract Refract Surg. 2007;33(7):1217–26.

14. Moses RA, Grodzki Jr WJ, Etheridge EL, Wilson CD. Schlemm's canal: the effect of intraocular pressure. Invest Ophthalmol Vis Sci. 1981;20(1):61–8.

15. Goldsmith JA, Ahmed IK, Crandall AS. Nonpenetrating glaucoma surgery. Ophthalmol Clin North Am. 2005;18(3):443–60, vii.

16. Smit BA, Johnstone MA. Effects of viscoelastic injection into Schlemm's canal in primate and human eyes: potential relevance to viscocanalostomy. Ophthalmology. 2002;109(4):786–92.

17. Marchini G, Marraffa M, Brunelli C, Morbio R, Bonomi L. Ultrasound biomicroscopy and intraocular-pressure-lowering mechanisms of deep sclerectomy with reticulated hyaluronic acid implant. J Cataract Refract Surg. 2001;27(4):507–17.

18. Balazs EA, Denlinger JL. Clinical uses of hyaluronan. Ciba Found Symp. 1989;143:265–75; discussion 75–80, 81–5.

19. Abdelrahman AM. Trabeculotome-guided deep sclerectomy. A pilot study. Am J Ophthalmol. 2005;140(1):152–4.

20. Argento C, Sanseau AC, Badoza D, Casiraghi J. Deep sclerectomy with a collagen implant using the excimer laser. J Cataract Refract Surg. 2001;27(4):504–6.

21. Verges C, Llevat E, Bardavio J. Laser-assisted deep sclerectomy. J Cataract Refract Surg. 2002;28(5):758–65.

22. Geffen N, Ton Y, Degani J, Assia EI. CO2 laser-assisted sclerectomy surgery, part II: multicenter clinical preliminary study. J Glaucoma. 2012;21(3):193–8.

23. Choudhary A, Wishart PK. Non-penetrating glaucoma surgery augmented with mitomycin C or 5-fluorouracil in eyes at high risk of failure of filtration surgery: long-term results. Clin Experiment Ophthalmol. 2007;35(4):340–7.

24. Barnebey HS. Canaloplasty with intraoperative low dosage mitomycin C: a retrospective case series. J Glaucoma. 2013;22(3):201–4.

25. Robert MC, Harasymowycz P. Hemorrhagic descemet detachment after combined canaloplasty and cataract surgery. Cornea. 2013;32(5):712–3.

26. Jaramillo A, Foreman J, Ayyala RS. Descemet membrane detachment after canaloplasty: incidence and management. J Glaucoma. 2012. Epub ahead of print.

27. Grieshaber MC, Schoetzau A, Flammer J, Orgul S. Postoperative microhyphema as a positive prognostic indicator in canaloplasty. Acta Ophthalmol. 2013;91(2):151–6.

28. Bull H, von Wolff K, Korber N, Tetz M. Three-year canaloplasty outcomes for the treatment of open-angle glaucoma: European study results. Graefes Arch Clin Exp Ophthalmol. 2011;249(10):1537–45.

29. Lewis RA, von Wolff K, Tetz M, et al. Canaloplasty: three-year results of circumferential viscodilation and tensioning of Schlemm canal using a microcatheter to treat open-angle glaucoma. J Cataract Refract Surg. 2011;37(4):682–90.

30. Grieshaber MC, Fraenkl S, Schoetzau A, Flammer J, Orgul S. Circumferential viscocanalostomy and suture canal distension (canaloplasty) for whites with open-angle glaucoma. J Glaucoma. 2011;20(5):298–302.

31. Shingleton B, Tetz M, Korber N. Circumferential viscodilation and tensioning of Schlemm canal (canaloplasty) with temporal clear corneal phacoemulsification cataract surgery for open-angle glaucoma and visually significant cataract: one-year results. J Cataract Refract Surg. 2008;34(3):433–40.

32. Grieshaber MC, Pienaar A, Olivier J, Stegmann R. Comparing two tensioning suture sizes for 360 degrees viscocanalostomy (canaloplasty): a randomised controlled trial. Eye (Lond). 2010;24(7):1220–6.

33. Grieshaber MC, Pienaar A, Olivier J, Stegmann R. Canaloplasty for primary open-angle glaucoma: long-term outcome. Br J Ophthalmol. 2010;94(11):1478–82.

34. Fujita K, Kitagawa K, Ueta Y, Nakamura T, Miyakoshi A, Hayashi A. Short-term results of canaloplasty surgery for primary open-angle glaucoma in Japanese patients. Case Rep Ophthalmol. 2011;2(1):65–8.

35. Bindlish R, Condon GP, Schlosser JD, D'Antonio J, Lauer KB, Lehrer R. Efficacy and safety of mitomycin-C in primary trabeculectomy: five-year follow-up. Ophthalmology. 2002;109(7):1336–41; discussion 41–2.

36. Ayyala RS, Chaudhry AL, Okogbaa CB, Zurakowski D. Comparison of surgical outcomes between canaloplasty and trabeculectomy at 12 months' follow-up. Ophthalmology. 2011;118(12):2427–33.

37. Koerber NJ. Canaloplasty in one eye compared with viscocanalostomy in the contralateral eye in patients with bilateral open-angle glaucoma. J Glaucoma. 2012;21(2):129–34.

38. Lavin MJ, Wormald RP, Migdal CS, Hitchings RA. The influence of prior therapy on the success of trabeculectomy. Arch Ophthalmol. 1990;108(11):1543–8.

39. Migdal C, Gregory W, Hitchings R. Long-term functional outcome after early surgery compared with laser and medicine in open-angle glaucoma. Ophthalmology. 1994;101(10):1651–6; discussion 7.

40. Shaarawy T, Flammer J, Haefliger IO. Reducing intraocular pressure: is surgery better than drugs? Eye (Lond). 2004;18(12):1215–24.

41. Nouri-Mahdavi K, Hoffman D, Coleman AL, et al. Predictive factors for glaucomatous visual field progression in the Advanced Glaucoma Intervention Study. Ophthalmology. 2004;111(9):1627–35.

42. Chiou AG, Mermoud A, Jewelewicz DA. Post-operative inflammation following deep sclerectomy with collagen implant versus standard trabeculectomy. Graefes Arch Clin Exp Ophthalmol. 1998;236(8):593–6.

43. Egrilmez S, Ates H, Nalcaci S, Andac K, Yagci A. Surgically induced corneal refractive change following glaucoma surgery: nonpenetrating trabecular surgeries versus trabeculectomy. J Cataract Refract Surg. 2004;30(6):1232–9.

44. Ahmed II, Khan BU. Non-penetrating glaucoma surgery. In: Yanoff M, Duker JS, editors. Ophthalmology. 3rd ed. Philadelphia: Mosby Elsevier; 2009. p. 1247–60.

# The Hydrus Micro-stent

15

Shakeel Shareef, Antonio Fea, and Iqbal Ike K. Ahmed

The Hydrus micro-stent (Ivantis, Irvine CA) is a novel Schlemm's canal microinvasive glaucoma surgery (MIGS) device designed to enhance aqueous outflow into Schlemm's canal and into the distal outflow veins. Made of flexible nitinol, an elastic nickel-titanium alloy, the device is designed to conform to the arc of Schlemm's canal (Fig. 15.1). The proximal end is designed to provide a bypass inlet into the canal, with the main body of the implant designed to act as an intracanalicular scaffold which dilates the canal nine times its cross-sectional area for a length of 8mm or 3 clock hours in the eye. It has a non-luminal design to provide unimpeded access of aqueous to the collector channels and aqueous veins along the back wall of the canal, and three windows face the inner wall to stretch and increase the effective filtration area. The Hydrus thus is designed to address the underlying pathology in open-angle glaucoma – increased resistance in the inner wall and collapse of Schlemm's canal – by creating a bypass through the inner wall and stretching the inner wall as well as scaffolding open the canal and preventing collapse (Figs. 15.2 and 15.3). The device is implanted using a handheld injector through a sub 2.0 mm clear cornea incision using a specially designed cannula to incise the inner wall to permit deployment of the device using a roller wheel (Fig. 15.4). Although the device may be implanted in any clock hour in the canal, it is most readily performed in the nasal quadrant using a temporal corneal incision. The device is currently an investigational device and an FDA pivotal trial is underway. There already have been a number of basic science and early clinical studies on the Hydrus device.

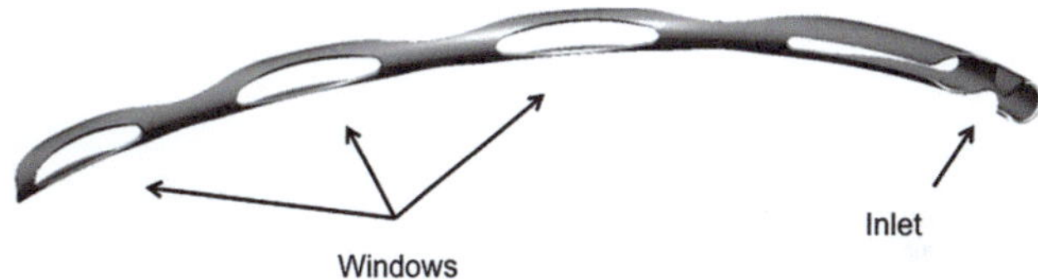


**Fig. 15.1** The Hydrus micro-stent consists of a curved implant with an inlet, three windows, and an open lumen designed to scaffold open Schlemm's canal

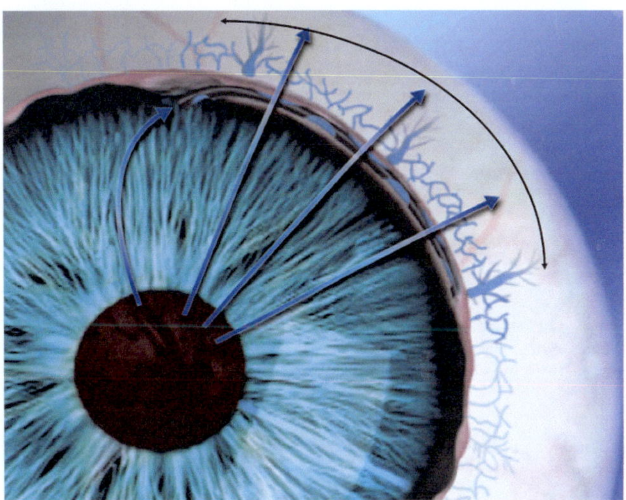

**Fig. 15.2** The Hydrus micro-stent with anterior chamber inlet providing direct aqueous access to the canal, and three windows to permit aqueous flow through the inner wall and scaffolded Schlemm's canal into collector channels and aqueous veins

S. Shareef, MD
Flaum Eye Institute, University of Rochester Medical Center, School of Medicine and Dentistry, Rochester, NY, USA
e-mail: shakeel_shareef@urmc.rochester.edu

A. Fea, MD, PhD
Clinica Oculistica-Universita' di Torino, Ospedale Oftalmico, C.so Montevecchio 62, Torino 10129, Italy
e-mail: antoniofea@interfree.it

I.I.K. Ahmed, MD, FRCSC (⊠)
Department of Ophthalmology and Vision Sciences, University of Toronto, Toronto, ON, Canada
e-mail: ike.ahmed@utoronto.ca

**Electronic supplementary material** Supplementary material is available in the online version of this chapter at http://dx.doi.org/10.1007/978-1-4614-8348-9_15. Videos can also be accessed at http://www.springerimages.com/videos/978-1-4614-8347-2

J.R. Samples, I.I.K. Ahmed (eds.), *Surgical Innovations in Glaucoma*, DOI 10.1007/978-1-4614-8348-9_15, © Springer Science+Business Media New York 2014

**Fig. 15.3** Postoperative
gonioscopic photos of the Hydrus
micro-stent in position

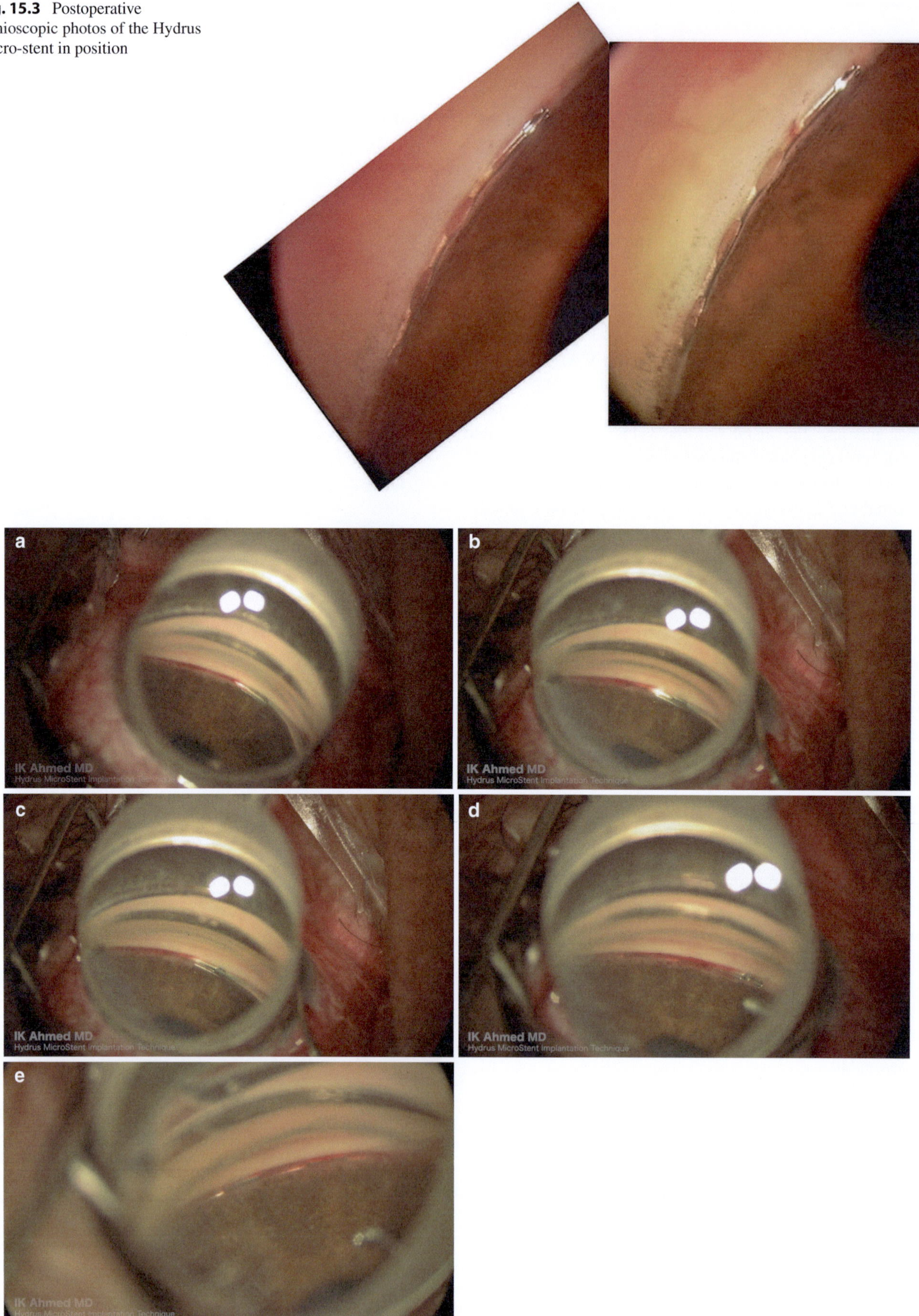

**Fig. 15.4** Surgical technique. The beveled cannula is used to incise the inner wall (**a**). The Hydrus implant is advanced into Schlemm's canal (**b**, **c**). Once implanted, the inlet is visible in the anterior chamber angle (**d**). The three windows are visible in the canal (**e**)

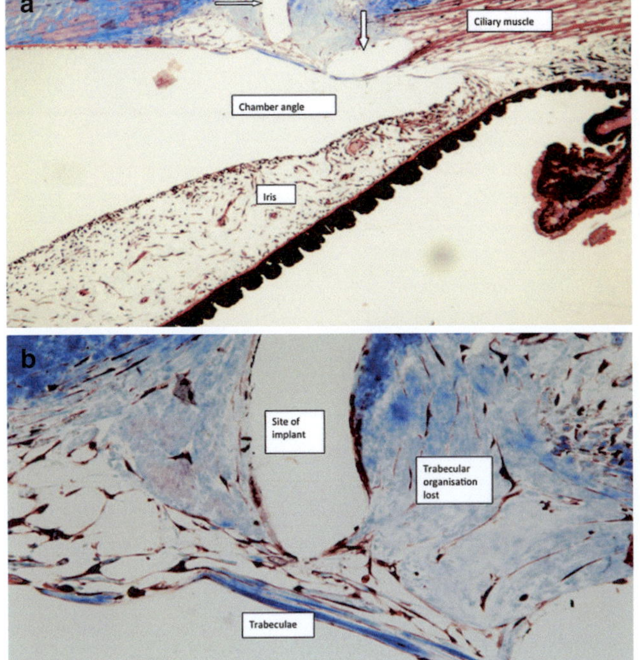



**Fig. 15.5** (**a**) Histopathology section in nonhuman primate shows two segments of the Hydrus scaffold in white (*arrows*) with no evidence of chronic inflammatory reaction in the outflow system or in adjacent tissues. (**b**) At higher magnification shows a segment of the Hydrus scaffold in white with distortion to the TM but no chronic inflammation

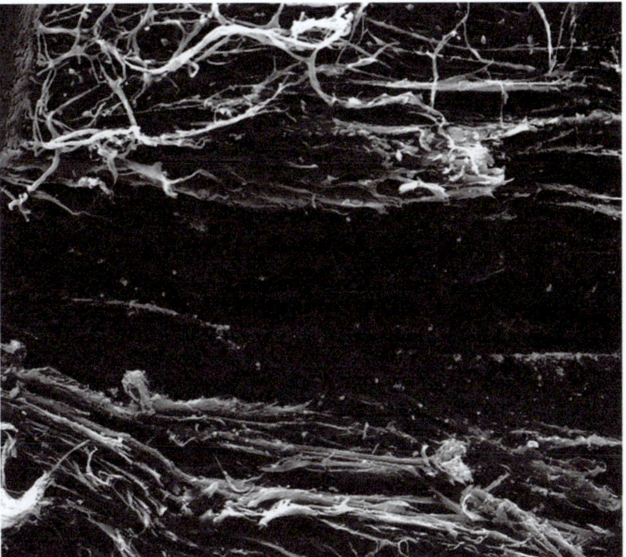

**Fig. 15.6** Scanning electron microscopy of outer wall of Schlemm's canal after implantation of Hydrus micro-stent showing minimal disruption of normal anatomy, patent collector channel ostia, and the presence of nuclear bulges in SC endothelium, a marker of cellular integrity was retained

Biocompatibility of the device has been studied histologically in both rabbit and nonhuman primates (Fig. 15.5) [1]. At 6 months, the device showed minimal inflammation in implanted New Zealand rabbits. In an analysis 13 weeks after implantation in nonhuman primates, there was no evidence of an inflammatory, foreign body response or fibrosis around the device when placed in the canal region. Based on these findings, the Hydrus micro-stent appears to be biocompatible in the eye.

A cadaveric injury study was performed to assess the impact of placement of the Hydrus into the canal using scanning electron microscopy (SEM) (Fig. 15.6) [2]. Using fresh human cadaveric anterior segments, SEM analysis showed patency of the canal, and collector channels were maintained with minimal alteration of normal Schlemm's canal anatomy. The low profile device appears to be inserted with minimal disruption of normal canal architecture.

To assess flow rates of the device, a human anterior segment perfusion model was used using perfusion pressures of 10, 20, 30, and 40 mmHg before and after the Hydrus 15 mm device was implanted into Schlemm's canal, and compared to control sham procedure eyes [3]. The mean outflow facility with the Hydrus increased from a baseline of 0.19±0.2 to 0.39±0.07 uL/min/mmHg ($p<0.01$), a 105 % increase, versus no significant change in sham procedure eyes, 0.20±0.03 to 0.23±0.03 uL/min/mmHg (15 % increase). After the Hydrus was removed from the tissue, the outflow facility returned to baseline indicating the increase was primarily from the device.

In a similar study using 24 paired human cadaveric anterior segments, the 8 mm Hydrus device was found to significantly increase outflow facility from 0.33±0.17 to 0.52 ± 0.19 uL/min/mmHg ($p<0.001$) versus sham procedure (0.39±0.21 to 0.38±0.19 uL/min/mmHg ($p=0.82$)) [4]. Using similar perfusion models and fluorescent microspheres, there was an increased amount of tracer flow into episcleral veins in implanted eyes versus controls [5]. Based on these studies, the Hydrus appears to substantially reduce the resistance and increase flow out of the conventional outflow system.

A prospective consecutive series of 29 patients with mild to moderate open-angle glaucoma who received the Hydrus implant in combination with cataract surgery was performed in Canada [6]. One-year results showed significant mean IOP reduction from medicated IOP of 17.2±4.2 mmHg on 2.5 medications and washed out IOP of 26.5±5.0 to 16.5±2.9 mmHg on 0.6 medications postoperatively (Fig. 15.7). There were no major adverse events.

A prospective multicenter case series (Video 15.1) with 1-year follow-up reported on the use of the Hydrus in either combined or solo procedures for open-angle glaucoma [7]. In the combined phaco and Hydrus cohort, mean IOP preoperatively was 21.3±5.6 mmHg with mean medication use of 2.2. Twenty-four patients were washed out preoperatively and 12 months postoperatively, and were found to have a mean washed out reduction of IOP of 8.7±4.3 mmHg (25.5–16.8 mmHg). The main adverse event was transient mild hyphema in 22 %, which resolved in all patients at 1 week. In another cohort, 40 patients who underwent solo Hydrus implant only resulted in a 69 % medication reduction (mean of 1.4 reduced to 0.5 meds) and a median IOP reduction of 4.5 mmHg (21.6–17.7 mmHg) at 1 year [8].

**Fig. 15.7** One-year results of combined phaco and Hydrus micro-stent for patients with mild–moderate glaucoma shows reduction of washed out intraocular pressure and preoperative medication use

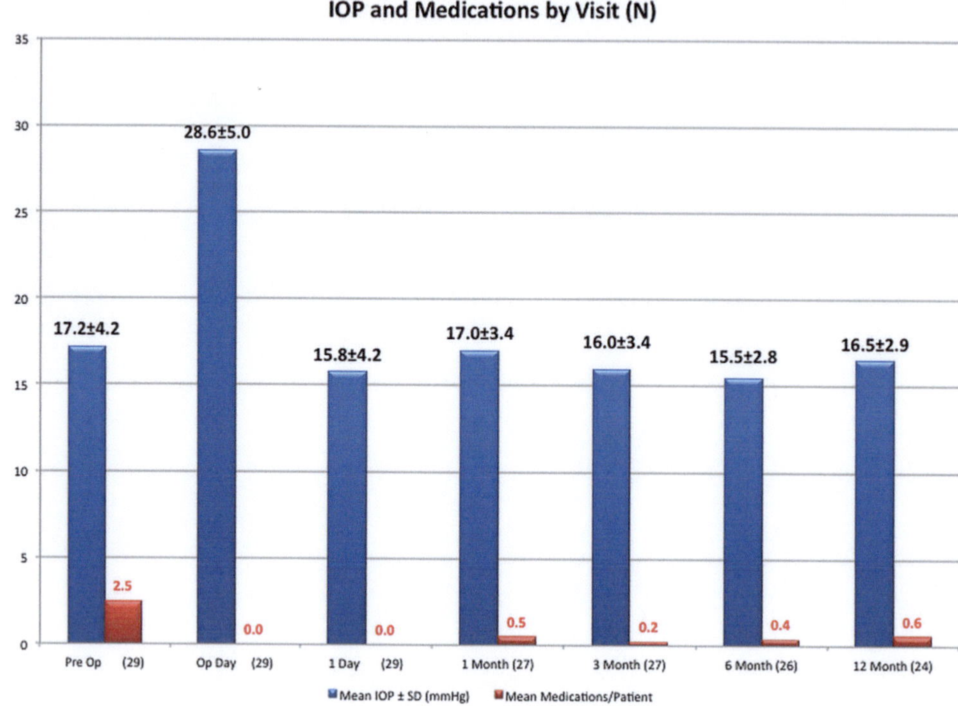


Adverse events included transient hyphema found in 17.3 % of patients, and peripheral anterior synechiae formed in 9.5 %.

The Hydrus implant, an ab interno micro-stent device designed to bypass the resistance and enhance flow through the inner wall of Schlemm's canal, and scaffold a 3 clock-hour region of the canal to prevent collapse, is designed to enhance aqueous outflow to aqueous veins. Major pivotal randomized control trials are underway, comparing phaco-emulsificaiton and Hydrus versus phacoemulsification alone. Based on early basic science and clinical studies, the Hydrus micro-stent has been shown to enhance outflow facility and reduce intraocular pressure when combined with phacoemulsification or implanted on its own. These IOP reductions are achieved with minimal mild adverse events, achieving physiological IOP control with a minimally invasive technique.

## References

1. Grierson I. In vivo biocompatibility evaluation of a novel nickel-titanium Schlemm's canal scaffold. Presented at the American Glaucoma Society annual meeting. New York City; Mar 2012.

2. Saheb H. A novel Schlemm's canal scaffold maintains patency of collector cannel Ostia in human anterior segments. Presented at the American Glaucoma Society annual meeting. New York City; Mar 2012.

3. Camras LJ, Yuan F, Fan S, Samuelson TW, Ahmed IK, Schieber AT, Toris CB. A novel Schlemm's canal scaffold increases outflow facility in a human anterior segment perfusion model. Invest Ophthalmol Vis Sci. 2012;53:6115–21.

4. Gulati V, Fan S, Hays CL, Samuelson TW, Ahmed IIK, Toris CB. A novel 8-mm Schlemm's canal scaffold reduces outflow resistance in a human anterior segment perfusion model. Invest Ophthalmol Vis Sci. 2013;54:1698–704.

5. Gong H. Characterization of aqueous outflow through a novel Schlemm's canal scaffold – a tracer study. Presented at the American Glaucoma Society annual meeting. New York City; Mar 2012.

6. Saheb H, Jampel H, Ahmed IK. One year outcomes of a Schlemm's canal microstent for IOP reduction after cataract surgery in mild to moderate open angle glaucoma. Presented at the American Glaucoma Society annual meeting. San Francisco; Mar 2013.

7. Tetz M. 12 month results from a prospective, multicenter study of a nickel-titanium Schlemm's canal microstent for IOP reduction after cataract surgery in open angle glaucoma. Presented at European Society of Cataract and Refractive Surgeons annual meeting. Milan; Sep 2012.

8. Samuelson T. One-year results of a Schlemm's canal microstent for IOP reduction in open angle glaucoma. Presented at American Academy of Ophthalmology annual meeting. Chicago; Nov 2012.

# Minimally Invasive Glaucoma Surgery: Trabeculectomy Ab Interno

Kevin Kaplowitz and Nils A. Loewen

## Introduction

Trabeculectomy ab interno with the trabectome (Neomedix, Tustin, CA) was FDA approved in 2004 [1]. It was originally described as using electrocautery to ablate trabecular meshwork (TM), unroofing the nasal Schlemm's canal over 30–60°. A first series of 37 patients was highly successful demonstrating a mean 42 % decrease in intraocular pressure (IOP) from a baseline of 28 mmHg after 1 year [1]. There were no cases of postoperative flat anterior chambers, hypotony, infection, wound leak, bleb formation, choroidal effusion, or loss of two lines of Snellen visual acuity.

The introduction of ab interno trabeculectomy with the trabectome at a time when trabeculectomy was considered the gold standard evokes memories of when cataract surgeons started to realize the benefits of phacoemulsification over extracapsular cataract extraction (ECCE). Trabectome surgery is similar to phacoemulsification in that it requires advanced equipment, is standardized, uses a small incision, and is very safe. In contrast, both ECCE and trabeculectomy require only simple instruments, feature a large incision, cannot be standardized, and produce a wide range of outcomes and complications, both early and late ones.

The aim of this chapter is to discuss the indications, to detail the techniques that the authors have adopted, and to review the results and complications of trabectome surgery.

K. Kaplowitz, MD (✉)
Department of Ophthalmology, Health Sciences Center,
Stony Brook University, Level 2, Room 152,
Stony Brook, NY 11794, USA
e-mail: kevin.kaplowitz@gmail.com

N.A. Loewen, MD, PhD
Department of Ophthalmology,
University of Pittsburgh School of Medicine, 203 Lothrop Street,
Eye and Ear Institute, Suite 819, Pittsburgh, PA 15213, USA
e-mail: loewenna@upmc.edu

## Indications

Trabectome was first described for use in glaucomas with an angle open by at least 20° or grade 2 on the Shaffer scale and an IOP level likely causing progression while on maximally tolerated medical therapy [1]. Exclusion criteria were angles with poor visibility of the trabecular meshwork and neovascular glaucoma. In our experience with more than 500 trabectome surgeries, we have found that a wide range of glaucoma types and stages can be operated on using a modified surgical technique described below. We find that only active neovascular glaucoma, elevated episcleral venous pressure, moderately active uveitis, and angle dysgenesis represent true contraindications. The patient has to be able to rotate the neck by more than 30°, or a microscope is available with a large tilt angle to compensate for the limitation. The cornea must be sufficiently free of opacities in the form of peripheral scars, deposits, vascular pannus, or arcus lipoides.

## Surgical Technique

Glaucoma surgeons do not typically learn trabectome surgery as their first glaucoma surgery but often begin with drainage device implantations and trabeculectomies. As a result, it is not surprising that more delicate microsurgery of the angle initially seems overwhelming with its requirement for higher magnification and excellent depth perception to strictly avoid structures that are only a few 100 μm apart from each other: distal to ablation, the outer wall of Schlemm's canal with collector channel intakes, posteriorly the more vascularized scleral spur, iris and ciliary body, and anteriorly the corneal endothelium.

While the beginning surgeon becomes comfortable with the goniolens relatively quickly, a considerable learning curve follows before great results can be achieved. We find that indications can be broadened, and lower target pressures, higher success rates, and earlier visual recovery

J.R. Samples, I.I.K. Ahmed (eds.), *Surgical Innovations in Glaucoma*,
DOI 10.1007/978-1-4614-8348-9_16, © Springer Science+Business Media New York 2014

can be achieved when careful attention is paid to six key elements:

1. Excellent visualization using a xenon light microscope with large tilt capabilities
2. No viscoelastic injection before or during ablation
3. Creation of a corneal incision that is 2 mm anterior to the limbus and flared on the inside
4. Avoidance of outward push applied during ablation
5. Ablation of a long, near 180° ablation arc
6. Swift tamponade of the unroofed canal with viscoelastic before and after cataract extraction

We will discuss these key elements in detail in the following.

## Angle Visualization: Xenon Light and Large Tilt Angle

The impact of an outstanding microscope with excellent optics and blue-white illumination using xenon light (e.g., Zeiss Lumera, Carl Zeiss Meditec, Jena, Germany) cannot be overestimated to visualize the target of ablation, the lacy, delicate, 50-µm-thick trabecular meshwork.

Preoperative considerations pertaining to anesthesia are minimal. Adequate anesthesia can be achieved with intracameral 1 % preservative-free lidocaine [1]. The surgeon sits temporally. For patients who will face significant difficulty rotating the neck, the microscope tilt can be increased. If the

patient is unable to rotate the neck, then the superior axial core may be rotated by placing blankets underneath the half of the patient's back and shoulder on the side closest to the surgeon. Preoperative pilocarpine is not necessary, and when trabectome surgery is combined with phacoemulsification, routine dilation can be used. The intact lens of a young patient should be protected by preoperative pilocarpine or intracameral carbachol.

## No Viscoelastic Prior to or During Trabectome Ablation

The paracentesis is fashioned as for phacoemulsification. As is common practice for goniotomy for pediatric glaucoma, no viscoelastic should be used because it interferes with optimal visualization from different optical densities and interfaces, traps ablation gas bubbles, and can bake into the tip during ablation.

## Incision 2 mm Anterior to Limbus, Slight Flare of Innermost Aspect

The main incision is positioned at the standard clock hour position as for phacoemulsification. The size is only 1.6 mm wide, and the incision should be made 2 mm anterior to the limbus and parallel to the iris (Fig. 16.1). The more anterior

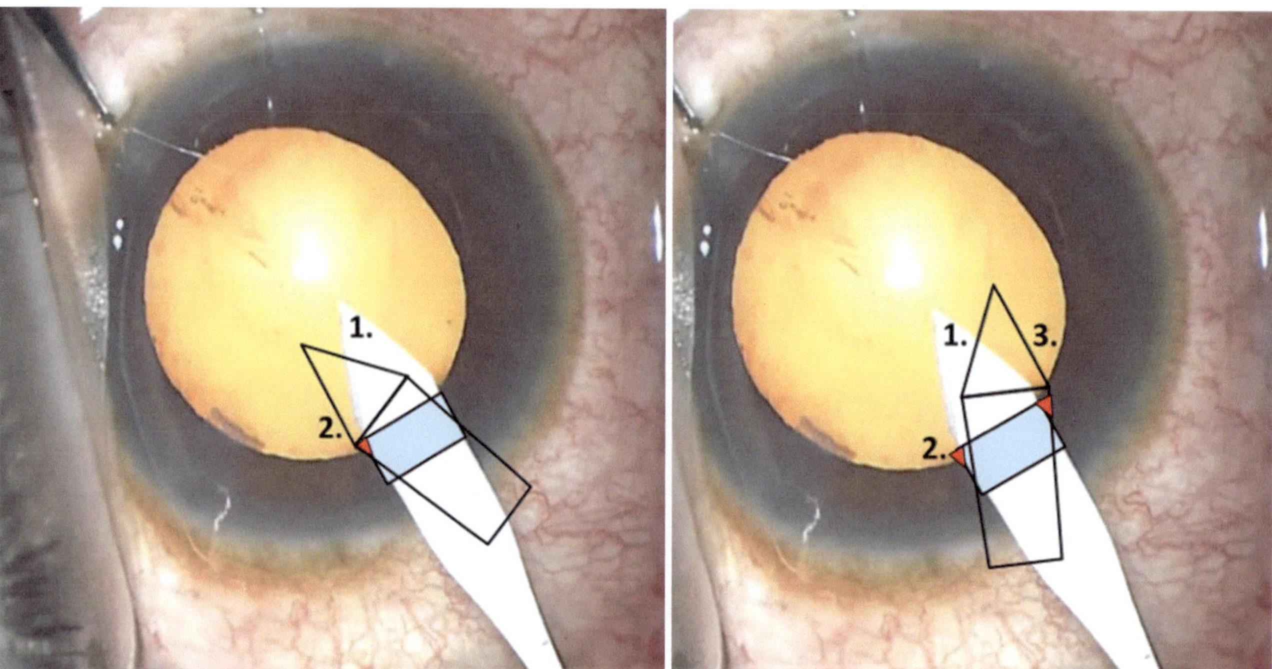


**Fig. 16.1** Main incision for trabectome surgery into the anterior chamber filled with 1 % lidocaine solution. (*1*) Entry is made 2 mm anterior to limbus and parallel to the iris in the left and right photos. Line diagrams showing how to position the blade for internal enlargement to the left (*2*) and to the right (*3*), allowing for better trabectome range without striae can be achieved by nicking Descemet's membrane and slightly flaring the incision

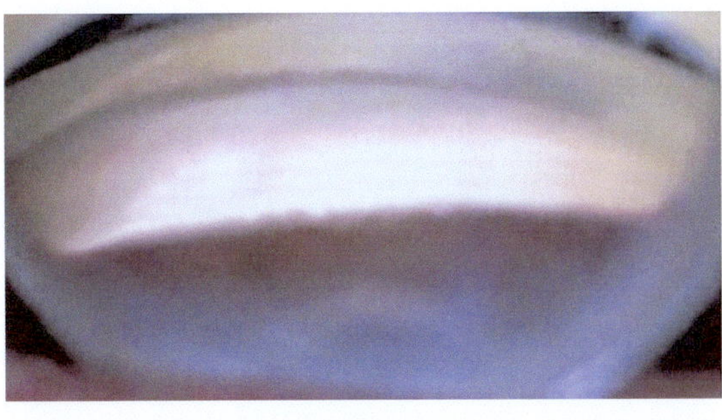
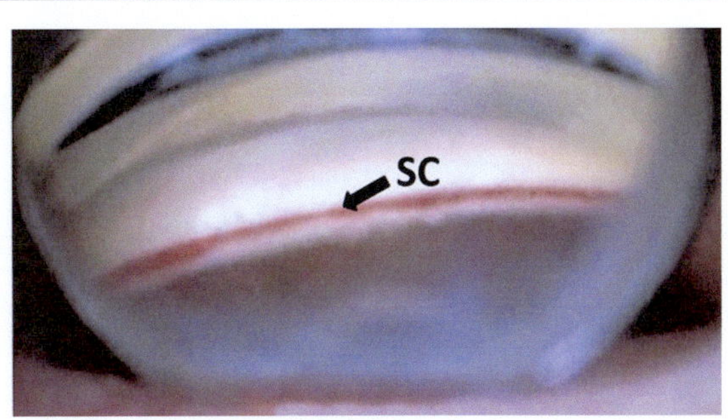


**Fig. 16.2** Schlemm's canal (SC, *right*) can be easily identified by gaping the main incision to induce hypotony and blood reflux from the collector channels. This is useful in nonpigmented TM but more generally to differentiate angle landmarks that may look similar (e.g., Sampaolesi's line, TM, ciliary body band)

incision and planar orientation – compared with a regular incision for phacoemulsification – will greatly reduce striae during manipulation of the handpiece and prevent iris prolapse. Following full entry, after only partially retracting the blade in the initial incision, a slight forward cut is made to the left and to the right, pointing toward the anticipated end of the ablation arc, flaring the incision. Only the innermost 25 % of the wound needs to be flared for the first-generation handpiece. This prevents the metal irrigation sleeve from getting caught at the level of Descemet's membrane and reduces corneal striae that can reduce visibility when the incision is torqued at the end of large ablation arcs. The redesigned second-generation tip has a sloped irrigation sleeve and allows for a much smoother insertion.

The anterior chamber will not collapse as long as the keratome is kept parallel to the incision plane and no viscoelastic is needed for insertion. A small amount of fluid egress can induce temporary hypotony. This will allow blood to reflux into Schlemm's canal and clearly outline the target structure (Fig. 16.2). Oftentimes the trabecular meshwork may not be pigmented or other pigmented structures are confusing. Misidentification and ablation of the wrong structure by beginning surgeons is the primary reason for arterial bleeding. Since the correct structure was not unroofed, the hyphema cannot exit the anterior chamber and the high persistent IOP will ensue.

Following the main incision, the patient's head is rotated about 30° away from the surgeon, while the microscope headpiece is tilted approximately 45° toward the surgeon. A direct Swan-Jacobs gonioscopy lens with proper handedness (Ocular Instruments, Bellingham, Washington) is placed to assure an adequate view of the trabecular meshwork after adjusting zoom and focus. The trabectome handpiece is then inspected under the microscope to assure the integrity of the tip. Continuous irrigation should be activated on the foot pedal but without activating electroablation which can damage the tip.

The irrigation bottle should be raised to near maximum height to deepen the angle and improve the view. The impact on visibility is manifold: surge is prevented, the iris root and peripheral iris are maximally displaced posteriorly resulting in an immediately apparent angle opening, and the cornea is forced into a stable spherical shape without striae. This also prevents reflux from the collector channels, while any pigment or bubbles are swiftly washed out through the main incision. The trabectome handpiece is inserted through the main wound. If the shoulder of the handpiece (19 gauge) cannot be inserted easily through the wound, a twisting motion with rotation along the long axis can be used as gentle but increasing pressure is applied at the wound. If this is inadequate, the upper lip of the corneal wound can be grasped and pulled anteriorly with forceps to offer less resistance to insertion. The insertion should be done quickly to avoid excess aqueous egress and anterior chamber collapse. The handpiece tip should be advanced to the center of the pupil before the goniolens is placed back onto the cornea. With the modified Swan-Jacobs lens, no coupling fluid is needed other than balanced salt solution (BSS). The goniolens should only gently touch the cornea: if striae are noted (first seen at the most superior aspect of the view), then too much downward pressure is being applied.

## Identifying and Engaging Schlemm's Canal, No Outward Pressure During Ablation

Without certain identification of Schlemm's canal, this procedure can produce either no IOP effect when ablation occurs in the cornea or create arterial bleeding with large hyphemas and dangerous postoperative IOP. If the TM is nonpigmented, then induction of hypotony by wound gape is an effective means to visualize the TM (Fig. 16.2).

Under gonioscopic view, the trabectome tip is moved toward the trabecular meshwork (TM). It is easier to initiate ablation at a point that is more toward the left than exactly at the opposite site of the chamber. This offers a better angle of engagement because the tip is now pointed toward, and not parallel to, the TM (Fig. 16.3).

The TM is approached with the tip at a 45° angle aimed upward (Fig. 16.4), from just inferior to the TM at the scleral

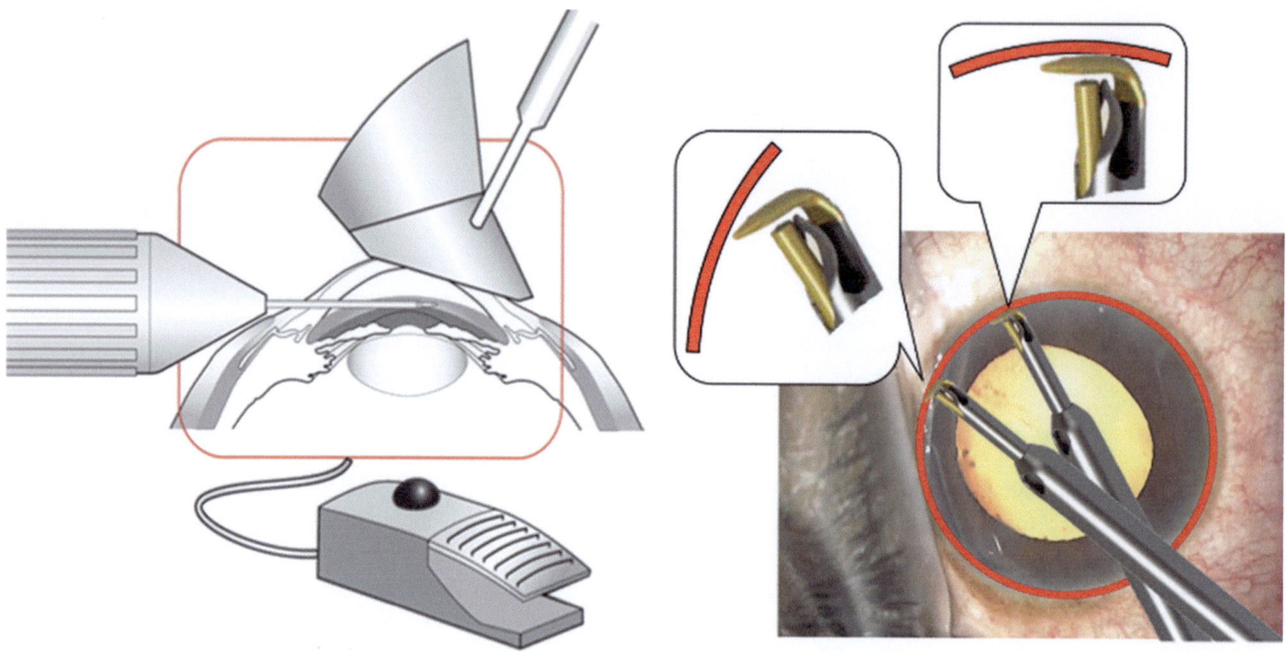

**Fig. 16.3** *Left*: Sketch of trabectome, lens and eye. *Right*: If entry of Schlemm's canal opposite of the main incision is difficult, the tip should be moved toward the left to allow a more pointed encounter

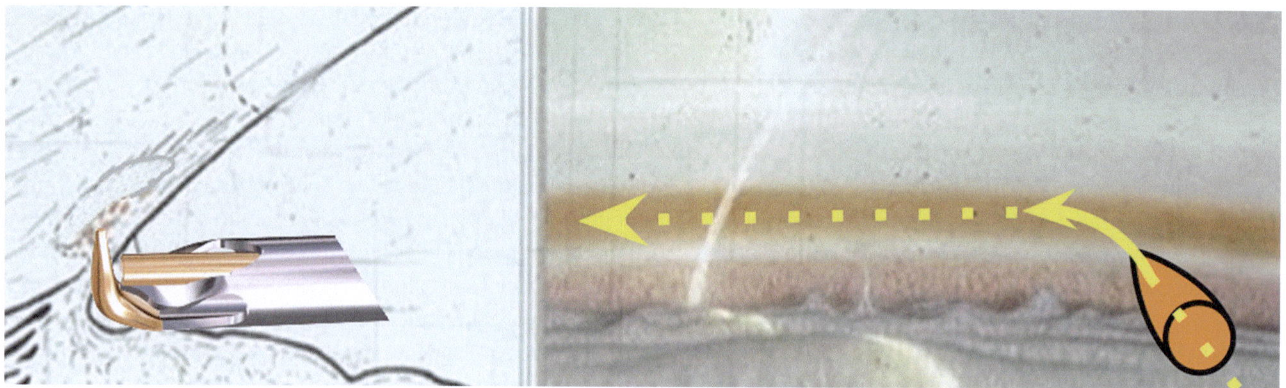

**Fig. 16.4** Entry of Schlemm's canal with the trabectome is easiest directly anterior to the scleral spur in a 45° angle because the space is maintained by it. If the trabectome is held parallel to the trabecular meshwork, Schlemm's canal collapses

spur. The spur will keep the space open and resist collapse of Schlemm's canal which occurs when the trabectome tip is held parallel and pushed outward when engagement is attempted directly across from the incision. Once the footplate is behind the TM, a slight inward pull should be exerted to counteract the tendency to push outward. This tenting of the TM changes the visibility of the ablation tip and confirms proper insertion. Ablation is started toward the surgeon's nondominant hand.

Ablation can be carried out starting at 0.8 mW and titrated up. Power should be decreased if visible blackening of the upper and lower edges of the TM occurs. This is possible although heat transfer through the footplate to the outer wall is only 1.2 °C. As discussed, the bottle height should be at maximum. The trabectome foot pedal can be tapped (black ball switch) for continuous, gravity-fed irrigation, then depressed to position 1 for continuous, nonlinear aspiration and position 2 for continuous and constant ablation power. Aspiration has a maximum flow rate of 10 ml/min [2].

During ablation, it is pertinent to avoid any outward pressure, ideally preventing touching the outer wall entirely. The outer wall of Schlemm's canal is lined with 50-μm orifices of the collector system that easily scar over when the lining endothelium is damaged (Fig. 16.5). Yet because beginning surgeons are focused on trying to enter Schlemm's canal and engaging the TM, this mistake is extremely common leading to disappointing pressure results either early on or after several weeks as a response to endothelial damage.

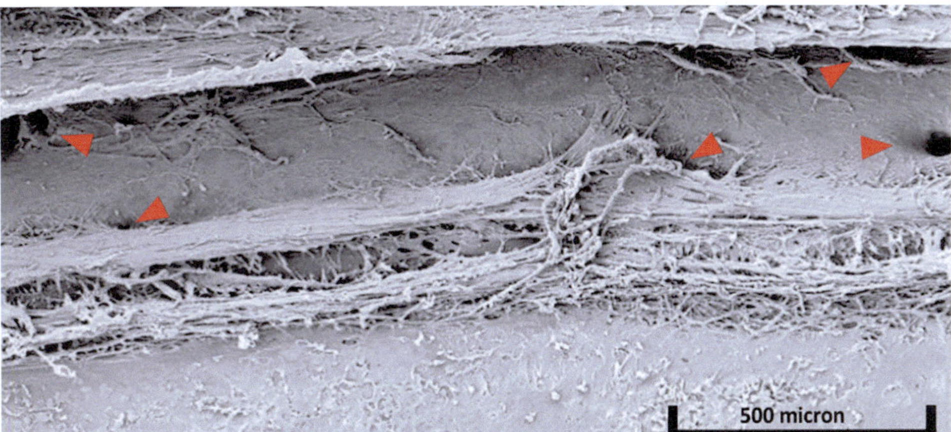

**Fig. 16.5** Location of collector channel orifices. Many intakes are close to the upper (anatomic anterior) and lower (anatomic posterior) portion of Schlemm's canal, providing a possible explanation why removal of TM with the trabectome might be superior to goniotomy which merely incises the TM allowing the remaining lips to roll inward and occlude those

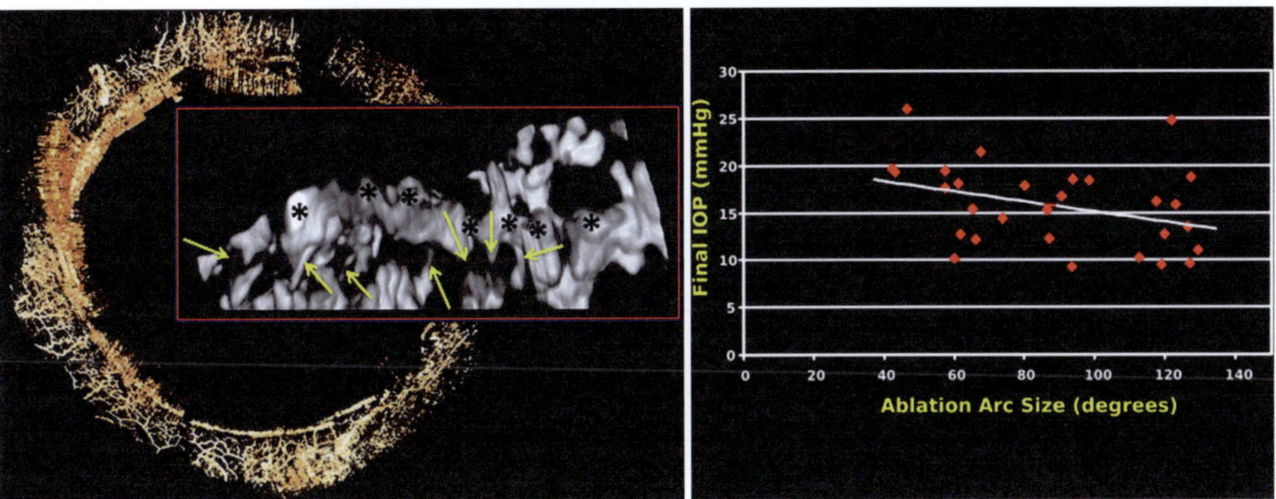


**Fig. 16.6** *Left*: In vivo, Schlemm's canal is often not contiguous and may have duplications (After Kagemann et al. [3]; *asterisks*: Schlemm's canal, *yellow arrows*: collector channels). *Right*: ablation arc length correlates with final IOP (After Sit et al. [4])

## Achieve 180° of Ablation

Aiming to ablate 180° of trabecular meshwork increases the chance of obtaining successful access to viable collector channels. Contrary to common belief, aqueous flow is not circumferential (Fig. 16.6). Studies ranging from injecting intracameral tracer [5] to anterior segment optical coherence tomography (OCT) [6] have shown that aqueous outflow through Schlemm's canal is segmental, increasing near collector channels. For instance, Schlemm's canal was shown to be 33 % wider nasally than temporally [7], and actual septae have been imaged in 2-μm resolution 3d micro-computerized tomography scans [8]. Adequate ablation can be confirmed by the white appearance of the outer wall of Schlemm's canal. The first 60° can usually be ablated continuously without many adjustments. As visualization is turned to the remaining 30°, the goniolens is rotated in the same direction the ablation is occurring, and the eye is tilted closer to the endpoints to increase visibility (Fig. 16.7).

Although the goal should be to ablate a full 90°, the final 10–15° cannot always be visualized for ablation. Once the full extent of visualization is reached, the tip is retracted from Schlemm's canal by pulling inward. It is rotated with one hand and under continuous gonioscopic view, tip down, by a full 180° and reinserted into Schlemm's canal where the original ablation was started.

The handpiece is rotated between the index finger, ring finger, and thumb while the wrist is increasingly pronated during the ablation of the remaining 90° (Fig. 16.8). The metal sleeve of the trabectome can be rested firmly against the proximal, straight edge of the goniolens during the 180° rotation into the opposite direction. Visualization of the wall of Schlemm's canal is confirmed as ablation continues. It is advisable not to force the tip ahead but instead stop and retract the tip. This will unwrinkle the TM or retract the tip from the outer wall and collector openings, and then ablation can be continued. After ablation is complete, the handpiece is withdrawn completely from the TM. The handpiece can then be removed from the eye.

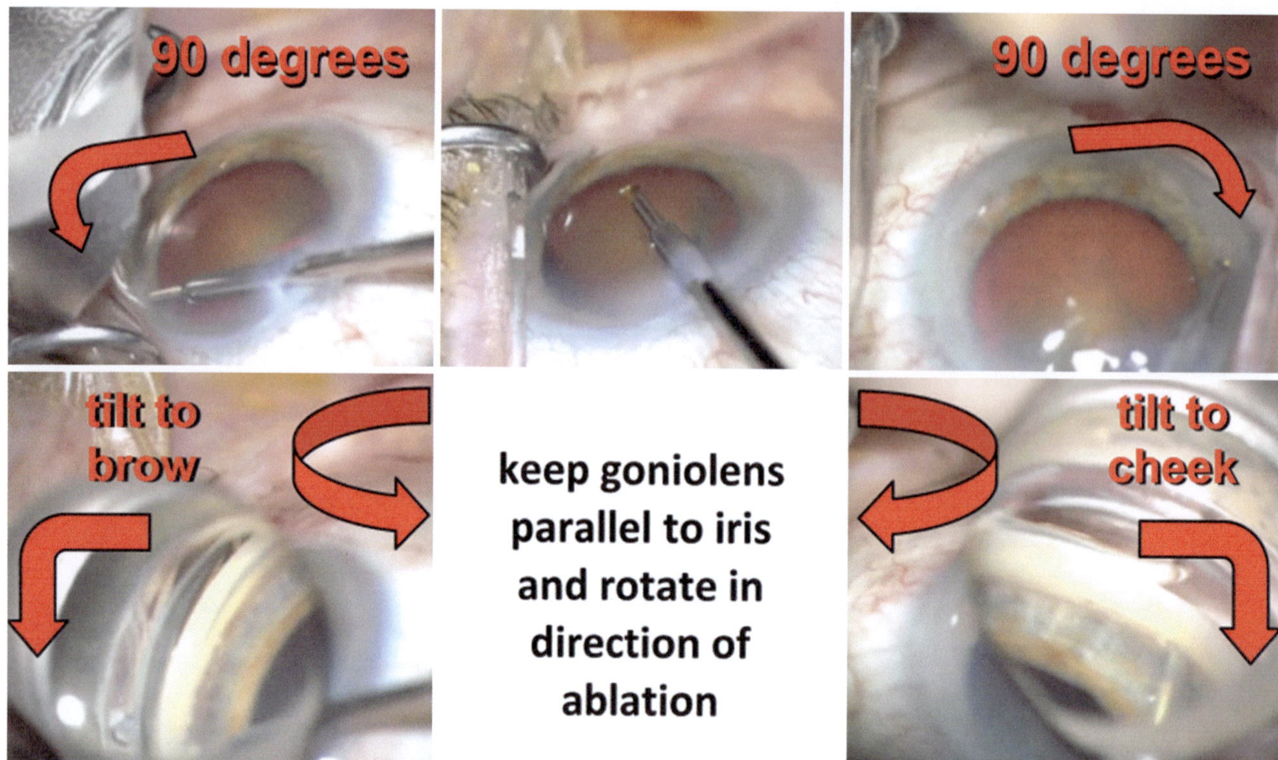


**Fig. 16.7** A modified Swan-Jacob goniolens designed for trabectome surgery is placed on the cornea without compressing it. It is held parallel to the iris and rotated into the direction of ablation. The eye can be tilted upward or downward by lifting the trabectome up in the incision to increase visibility of the superior and inferior chamber angle and maximize the ablation arc to achieve near 180°. Gonioscopic prism power and angle view at these ablation endpoints is increased by lifting the distal part of the lens off the cornea to float in the pool of saline that forms during the procedure (*lower left* and *right*)

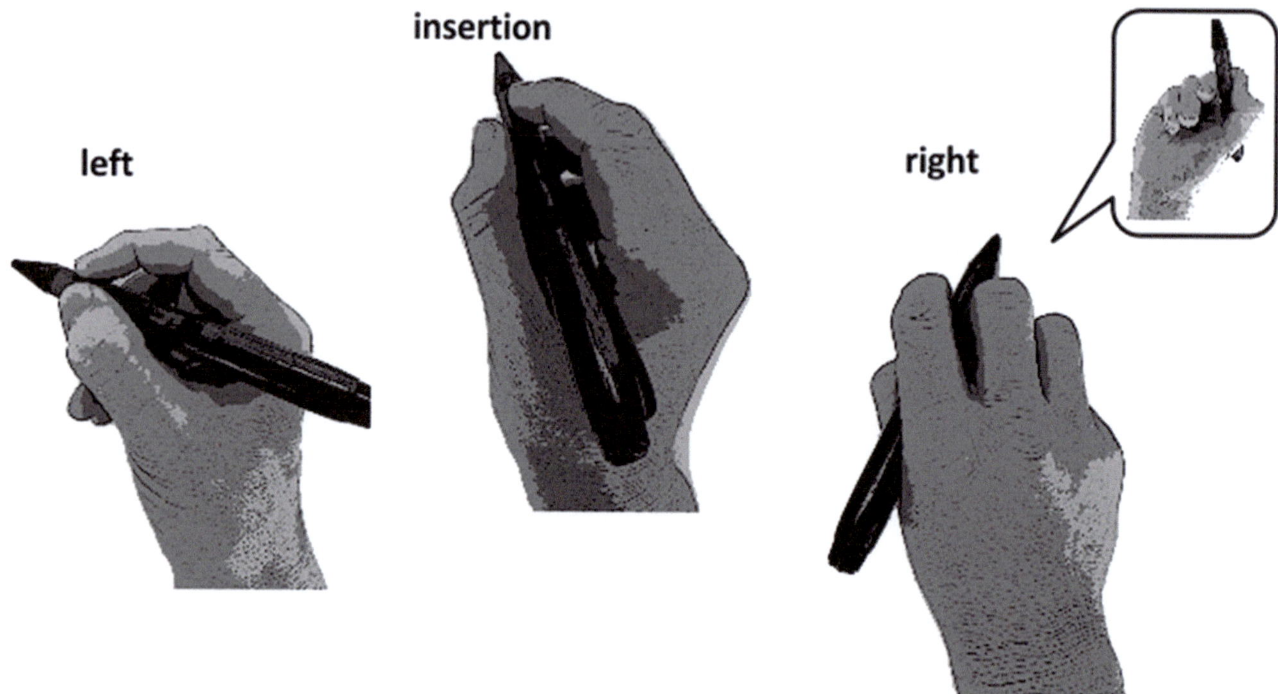


**Fig. 16.8** Hand position during trabectome surgery. The trabectome handpiece is held like with phacoemulsification during insertion with the tip pointing toward the left (*middle*). As ablation continues toward the nondominant hand, the hand is increasingly supinated and more held like a pen (*left*). The handpiece is then rotated 180° under gonioscopic view and ablation continued toward the right while the hand is increasingly pronated (*right*; *inset*: finger position from *below*). The tip is rolled between the thumb, index finger, and ring finger to keep it parallel to Schlemm's canal

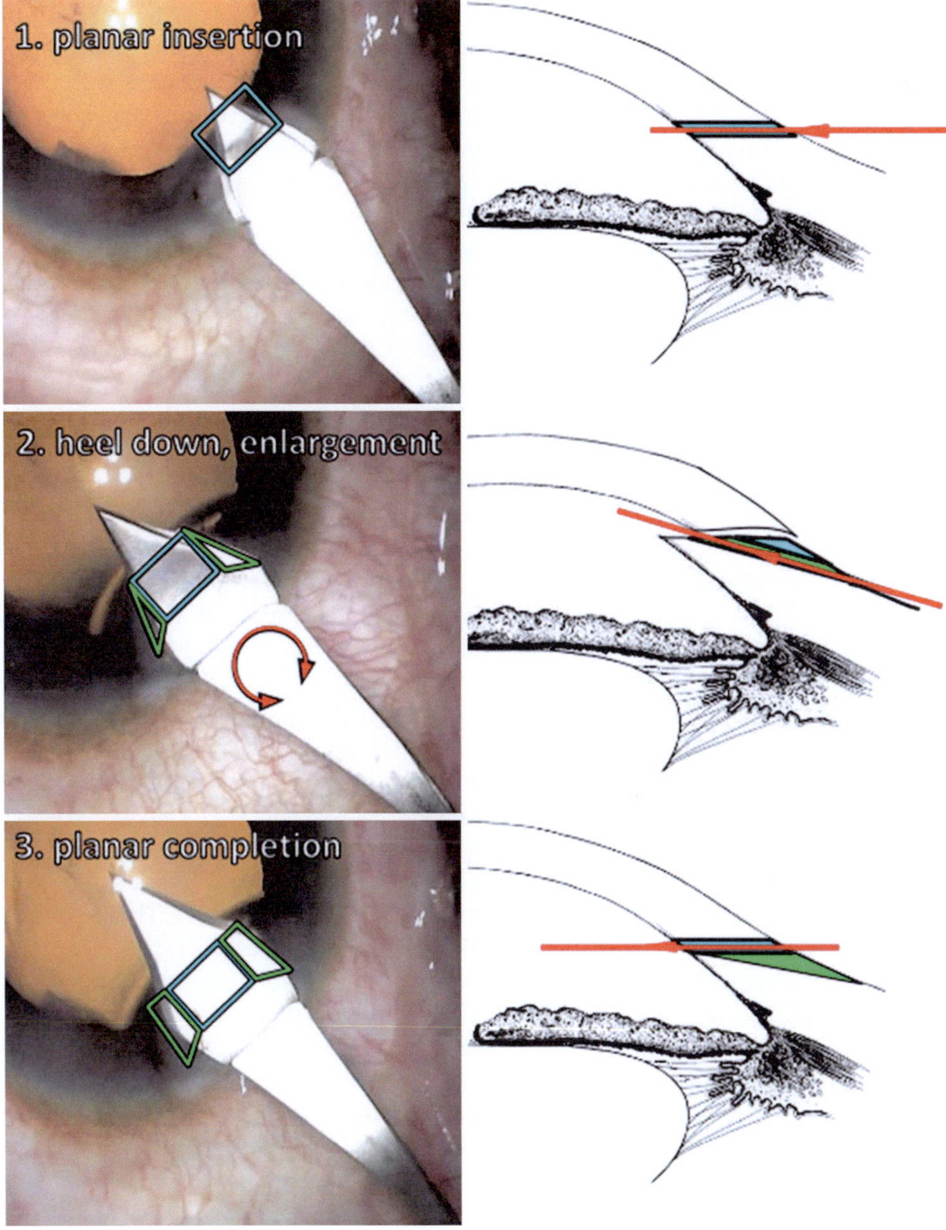


**Fig. 16.9** Enlargement of the main incision (*blue*) to prepare for cataract surgery; tri-planar wings (*green*) are fashioned that allow a single self-sealing incision. This requires that in step 2 the heel of the keratome be almost flush on the conjunctiva while the keratome is gradually advanced with careful rotations. The *red arrow* in the drawing on the right represents the base of the keratome's triangular blade

## Immediate Viscoelastic Tamponade of Ablated Canal, Chamber Pressurization

Once the ablation is complete, viscoelastic is injected directly along the ablation arc at the root of the iris. This will displace non-coagulated as well as coagulated blood and tamponade Schlemm's canal and collector channels. We compared five different viscoelastic substances for this purpose and recommend a premixed viscoelastic with both cohesive and dispersive agents in one syringe (e.g., DiscoVisc, Alcon, Fort Worth, TX). The dispersive properties allow the viscoelastic to flow easily into the chamber angle including the orifices of the collector channels, while the cohesive properties allow to maintain the space and prevent displacement. The entire anterior chamber can be pressurized while the patient's head

is still rotated, or the head can be rotated back and the chamber then fully filled and pressurized with the remaining viscoelastic. The patient and microscope are now rotated back until they are again perpendicular to the floor.

To continue with cataract surgery, a standard keratome is partially inserted planar to the iris into the main incision (Fig. 16.9), the tip is carefully advanced past the inner lip of Descemet's membrane, and then the heel is moved all the way down against the conjunctiva before the keratome is carefully inserted further, aided by small rotating movements around the axis of the handle if necessary. This will create a partial tri-planar incision that has a slight inverted U-shape like a scleral tunnel in ECCE and provide self-sealing features on the left and right aspects of the smaller, initial trabectome keratome incision. To conclude the enlargement of the incision, the blade is now held parallel to the iris again and the keratome moved forward to complete the incision.

Capsulorrhexis and the remaining phacoemulsification steps are done in standard fashion. Just before lens insertion, viscoelastic is injected again to prepare the capsule for implantation, and a second viscoelastic crescent is injected directly along the root of the iris again with the goal to tamponade and displace refluxing blood. Following lens implantation, viscoelastic can be partially removed and the incision is hydrated. We recommend retaining at least 30 % of viscoelastic in the eye to create a positive pressure gradient from the anterior chamber to the outflow system. This will avoid postoperative hypotony and hyphema with better vision early on, and may also provide better early pressures by reducing the phacocytotic load on the remaining trabecular meshwork from red blood cells while minimizing blood clotting along the unroofed canal. It is especially important to maintain postoperative IOP because evidence suggests that fluctuations in IOP, even the brief hypotony induced following a blink, can lead to flow from the ocular surface through the clear corneal incision and into the anterior chamber [9, 10]. OCT has shown full-thickness gaping of a clear corneal wound when the IOP was at 5 mmHg [11]. The wound is hydrated but a suture is not needed and may in fact cause gaping hypotony and instant hyphema. Although the viscoelastic mentioned above has a tendency to cause considerable postoperative hypertension after regular cataract surgery if not carefully removed, the unroofing of Schlemm's canal in trabectome surgery will allow for improved evacuation similar to glaucoma drainage device surgery.

The patient is seen the following day, at 1 week, at 1 month, and finally at 3 months. All glaucoma medications are discontinued the day of surgery. The postoperative regimen for the first week consists of a fourth-generation fluoroquinolone, prednisolone acetate 1 %, and pilocarpine 1 or 2 %, all of which are started four times daily on the day of surgery. The fluoroquinolone is continued for 7 days. The prednisolone is tapered weekly by one drop for a 4-week course. Pilocarpine is usually maintained at 4 times daily for about 4 weeks, then three times per day 4 more weeks. Flattening the iris out using pilocarpine is thought to reduce the chance of forming peripheral anterior synechiae [12]. If trabectome surgery is combined with phacoemulsification, then a proper refraction cannot be obtained until pilocarpine is stopped.

## Results

The steps described above are designed to maximize visibility, facilitate identification of the correct structure, maximize the area that gains access to the outflow system, and reduce or eliminate hyphema. Our own results with this evolved technique in 192 trabectome surgeries that consisted of open-angle glaucomas and approximately one third of patients with uveitic, traumatic, angle-closure, or low-pressure glaucomas suggest that a 30 % IOP drop can be achieved from a relatively low preoperative IOP of $20 \pm 8$ to $14 \pm 4$ mmHg at year 1. The incision technique described above produces predictable astigmatism as any standard cataract incision which allows to implant toric lenses in the same session and deliver high quality of vision and satisfaction to glaucoma patients undergoing combined procedures.

The first retrospective series of 37 patients by Minckler et al., which were stand-alone trabectome cases, demonstrated a 42 % decrease in mean IOP, lowering the baseline IOP from 28 to 16 mmHg at 12 months. The series was later extended to 101 patients [1]. The larger series still demonstrated a 40 % IOP decrease. Eleven of those patients had follow-up for 30 months, and that group sustained a 33 % mean IOP decrease. A further report revealed a mean IOP decrease of 42 % after 36 months, although only five patients were still available at that time [13]. A series of 1,127 patients was composed of 738 patients who underwent stand-alone trabectome in addition to 366 cases combined with phacoemulsification [14]. This study retrospectively followed patients for up to 5 years and defined failure as either final IOP over 21 mmHg or demonstrating less than a 20 % decrease from baseline IOP and found a 55 % failure rate after 4 years. The published results of trabectome surgery are divided into stand-alone trabectome cases below in Table 16.1 and combined trabectome-phacoemulsification in Table 16.2. There are no published randomized trials involving trabectome. Longer follow-up is needed to elucidate the long-term success rates. The largest case series dating back to the first trabectome cases had 1,878 trabectome cases (alone or with phacoemulsification) recorded as of 2010 [20]. There was data on five patients who had been evaluated a full 6 years after the procedure and still maintained a 38 % mean IOP decrease.

Only a few studies have identified risk factors for failure. Studies that stratified their results by baseline IOP suggest that trabectome lowers the IOP significantly more starting from a higher baseline IOP. In one study, when the baseline IOP was below 20 mmHg, the IOP reduction at 1 year was only 0.2 % versus a 28 % decrease when baseline IOP was 20–25 mmHg, and a 45 % decrease when baseline IOP was over 25 mmHg (absolute values were not reported, only percentages) [2]. A prospective study of 1,401 cases came to similar conclusions [21]. From a baseline IOP below 17 mmHg, the decrease in IOP was only 7 % versus a 33 % decrease from a baseline IOP between 23 and 29. One study reported on risk factor analysis and found that younger age and lower baseline IOP were significant risk factors after multivariate analysis [16].

**Table 16.1**  Review of published results with trabectome-only cases

| Authors | Type of study | Number of patients | Mean baseline IOP | Mean or final % decrease IOP | Mean # decrease in medication | Length of study |
|---|---|---|---|---|---|---|
| Minckler et al. [1] | Prospective | 37 | 28 | 40 | 0.9 | 13 months |
| Minckler et al. [1] | Prospective | 101 | 28 | 40 | Not reported | 30 months |
| Minckler et al. [14] | Retrospective | 738 | 26 | 35 | 1.1 | 5 years |
| Ting et al. (POAG patients only) [15] | Prospective | 450 | 26 | 34 | 0.6 | 12 months |
| Ting et al. (PXG patients only) [15] | Prospective | 67 | 29 | 44 | 0.9 | 12 months |
| Jea et al. [16] | Retrospective | 115 | 28 | 41 | 1 | 30 months |
| Minckler et al. [17] | Retrospective | 1,151 | 26 | 36 | 1.7 | 60 months |
| Mosaed et al. [18] | Retrospective | 538 | 26 | 31 | 0.8 | 12 months |

*PDG* pigmentary dispersion glaucoma, *POAG* primary open-angle glaucoma, *PXG* pseudoexfoliation glaucoma

**Table 16.2**  Review of published results with combined phacoemulsification and trabectome cases

| Authors | Type of study | Number of patients | Mean baseline IOP | Mean or final % decrease IOP | Mean # decrease in medication | Length of study |
|---|---|---|---|---|---|---|
| Minckler et al. [14] | Retrospective | 366 | 20 | 20 | 1.2 | 5 years |
| Francis et al. [2] | Prospective | 304 | 20 | 25 | 1.2 | 21 months |
| Francis and Winarko [19] | Prospective | 89 | 22 | 27 | 1 | 12 months |
| Ting et al. (POAG patients only) [15] | Prospective | 263 | 20 | 22 | 0.7 | 12 months |
| Ting et al. (PXG patients only) [15] | Prospective | 45 | 22 | 35 | 0.9 | 12 months |
| Minckler et al. [14] | Retrospective | 681 | 20 | 21 | 0.9 | 36 months |
| Mosaed et al. [18] | Retrospective | 290 | 20 | 18 | 0.8 | 12 months |

*JRA* juvenile rheumatoid arthritis, *PDG* pigmentary dispersion glaucoma, *POAG* primary open-angle glaucoma, *PXG* pseudoexfoliation glaucoma

**Table 16.3**  Reported failure rate defined as IOP >21 or less than 20 % IOP decrease

| Study | Length of time analyzed | Failure rate for trabectome only | Failure rate for combined phaco/trabectome |
|---|---|---|---|
| Minckler et al. [14] | 4 years | 45 % (only one value reported for both stand-alone and combined cases) | 45 % (only one value reported for both stand-alone and combined cases) |
| Francis and Winarko [19] | 1 year | Not studied | 5 % |
| Ting et al. [15] | 1 year | 27 % for POAG, 21 % for PXG | 9 % for POAG, 13 % for PXG |
| Jea et al. [16] | 2 years | 78 % | Not studied |

*POAG* primary open-angle glaucoma, *PXG* pseudoexfoliation glaucoma

There was some concern that damage to the outflow pathway by laser trabeculoplasty could lead to downstream scarring which would lower the efficacy of the trabectome procedure [22]. The issue was examined in a retrospective review of 1,345 trabectome patients, 493 of whom had previous laser trabeculoplasty (there was no differentiation between micropulse diode, Nd:YAG or argon laser). Despite starting from a very similar baseline IOP, there was actually a larger mean decrease in IOP at 36 months in the group who had previously undergone laser trabeculoplasty (39 % decrease versus 32 %), though the difference was not statistically significant. There was also no statistically significant difference in the complication rate between the two groups.

The various studies reporting on the success of the trabectome procedure have used different definitions of success, from a multitude of absolute and relative change in IOP to just demonstrating a decrease in medication [2]. The wide range of definitions makes it difficult to compare the results. Using a less stringent definition of a decrease in medications (all patients in this group had a baseline IOP ≤21 mmHg) yielded a success rate just over 70 % at 18 months. There were four studies [14–16, 19] which reported a similar definition of failure being IOP >21 or demonstrating less than a 20 % IOP decrease from baseline (see Table 16.3). For stand-alone trabectome cases, the failure rate using this definition ranged from 21 to 78 %. For cases combined with phacoemulsification, the failure rate ranged from 5 to 45 %. The longest study to analyze failure rates reported on 1,415 patients and followed them for as long as 6 years [23]. The main definition of failure used was needing any further glaucoma surgery. The failure rate (given for all cases, stand alone and combined) with this definition was 10 % at 5 years. Using another less stringent definition of failure being IOP >21 and less than 20 % IOP decrease, the failure rate was about 5 % for combined cases (reported out to 3 years) and about 48 % for the stand-alone trabectome cases after 6 years.

Since combined cataract surgery and trabectome has not been compared with trabectome as a stand-alone procedure in a randomized controlled fashion, it is not possible to conclude that cataract surgery added to trabectome surgery increases the success rate as outcomes might simply be a consequence of eyes with different disease status. However, it is possible that reduced incidence of peripheral anterior synechiae (PAS) does improve the success rate [24]. Cataract surgery might have an IOP-lowering effect from ultrasound-mediated trabeculoplasty of the remaining trabecular meshwork [25], but there was no regression of the success rate toward trabectome alone over time in a single-surgeon prospective study [2]. The average IOP decrease after 2 years was 7 mmHg in the stand-alone trabectome group versus only 2 mmHg in the stand-alone phacoemulsification group.

## Surgical Failure

A study examining the timing of 100 failed trabectome procedures [14] found that only 12 occurred by 2 weeks but 76 by 6 months, and 95 by 18 months. This could suggest that the majority of failures will be seen by the 6-month visit. This was corroborated in a study on failed trabectome surgeries which went on to need a trabeculectomy [26]. The range of time to trabeculectomy was 3 days to 18 months, with an average of 4.9 months. Possible reasons for failure to reach the target IOP following an apparently successful procedure may be inferred from a preclinical study of the trabectome handpiece on donor corneoscleral rims [27]. One specimen still had an intact TM after the procedure, and the authors suggest that the footplate never entered into Schlemm's canal. Another specimen revealed damage only to the superficial TM, suggesting that although the footplate may have come into contact with the TM, it was not properly positioned entirely in Schlemm's canal with the TM engaged between the footplate and the electrodes. At least two specimens did show successful ablation of TM, but the edges had re-approximated. Long-term studies are needed to evaluate the time course and rate of possible re-approximation of the ablated edges. One study reports on neodymium-doped yttrium aluminum garnet (Nd:YAG) goniopuncture intervention for eight patients with post-trabectome IOP elevation 33 % above baseline [12]. Four of the eight patients had visible peripheral anterior synechiae (PAS) lysis during the laser, while the other four were seen to have cleft closure which was considered reopened upon blood reflux into the AC. An average of 10.5 months following goniopuncture, the IOP had been lowered again to 21 % below baseline. The settings used were 0.2–0.6 mJ for 3–15 shots. Supporting the use of postoperative pilocarpine to reduce formation of synechiae, none of the patients in that study received any pilocarpine.

If trabectome surgery does not lower pressure sufficiently, every conventional treatment can be attempted, including SLT, trabeculectomy ab externo, Express shunts, aqueous shunts, endocyclophotocoagulation,and external cyclophotocoagulation [21]. Outcomes of subsequent glaucoma procedures involving the conjunctiva such as glaucoma drainage devices are not affected by trabectome that uses a clear corneal incision. One study examined the effect of trabectome on subsequent trabeculectomy [26]. A retrospective review of 34 patients who failed trabectome surgery was compared to 42 patients who underwent primary trabeculectomy. Starting from a baseline IOP of 28 mmHg in the failed trabectome group and 29 in the primary trabeculectomy group, the mean IOP was 11 in both groups after 24 months, with no statistically significant difference in IOP between the two groups at any time point. Kaplan-Meier survival curve analysis also confirmed no statistically significant difference in success rates, indicating that a failed trabectome does not increase the risk of failure of a subsequent trabeculectomy. There was also no statistically significant difference in rates of complication between the two groups, with 6 % of the primary trabectome group and 7 % of the primary trabeculectomy group going on to need further surgery. The benefit of repeating trabectome, for instance, by operating across the nose and unroofing the temporal Schlemm's canal, remains unclear at this time. Although it has certainly been reported [20], there is no subgroup analysis or any specific reports on the efficacy.

## Results with Various Subtypes of Glaucoma

Although many secondary open-angle glaucomas have been reported to be treated with trabectome, the results often do not detail subgroup success rates. Out of the 1,127 cases reviewed by Minckler, the second largest group (after POAG) was pseudoexfoliation with 109 cases [14]. Only one study analyzed glaucoma subtypes: the study by Ting et al. compared a group of patients with POAG to those with PXG [15]. With both stand-alone trabectome and trabectome-phacoemulsification combined procedures, the PXG group started with a higher mean baseline IOP and showed a greater IOP decrease as compared to POAG. There was a 5 mmHg further decrease in IOP for PXG patients versus POAG patients with trabectome only and a 3 mmHg further decrease from the combined procedure. Other types of glaucoma reported to be treated with trabectome but without subgroup success rate analysis include: pigmentary, uveitic, steroid-induced, and chronic angle-closure glaucoma (that still offered a view of nasal TM with or without goniosynechialysis).

## Complications

Table 16.4 summarizes the complications reported following trabectome surgery. The most common complication is hyphema, occurring in up to 100 % of cases, depending on

**Table 16.4** Complications reported after trabectome

| Hyphema |
| --- |
| PAS |
| Corneal injury |
| Transient IOP spike |
| Cyclodialysis cleft [16] |
| Transient hypotony (it has not been reported past 30 days) |
| Iris injury |
| Lens injury |
| Aqueous misdirection [20] |
| Choroidal hemorrhage [20] |

the definition of hyphema versus microhyphema [16]. In our experience, visual acuities of 20/30 can be expected if the anterior chamber is properly pressurized and maintained as described above. Given that blood refluxes into Schlemm's canal when episcleral pressure exceeds IOP, and Schlemm's canal is unroofed during this procedure, this can be an expected occurrence. There is only one published case detailing surgical intervention for hyphema associated with an IOP spike [28]. The vast majority are cleared by 1 week. As described in the technique section above, using a crescent of viscoelastic to tamponade the unroofed area limits the extent of postoperative hyphema. It is especially important to forewarn patients about this common occurrence.

A case series of 12 patients who complained of transient decrease in vision between 2 and 31 months following trabectome demonstrated a spontaneous rebleed associated with a mean IOP 12 mmHg higher than the preceding visit [28]. Six of them reported the episode occurring four or more times, and ten of them awoke with the blurring. Only three of them had a visible hyphema. Knape and Smith reported on a patient with an intraoperative hyphema during a trabeculectomy done 11 months after a failed trabectome surgery [29]. When the sclerostomy was made, the authors noted reflux bleeding from the nasal angle. This led the authors to suggest using viscoelastic and releasable sutures to avoid hypotony during second surgeries following a trabectome, a practice that we employ already during primary trabectome surgery for the same reason. In the study by Jea et al. comparing trabeculectomy after failed trabectome to primary trabeculectomy, there was a higher incidence of postoperative hyphema in the group who had a previous trabectome surgery (20 % versus 7 %), but this difference was not statistically significant ($p=0.1$) [26].

In one study, the second-most common complication was PAS, which was found in 24 % of patients [1]. Transient postoperative IOP spikes of at least 10 mmHg may be seen in 4 [19]–10 % [15]. It occurred in 6 % of a series with 1,127 cases [14]. One study examined the time course of these postoperative IOP spikes and found that while 9 % had an IOP spike over 10 mmHg on post-op day 1, only 2 % still had an IOP spike at post-op day 7 [2]. Liu et al. found that IOP

spikes after post-op day 7 resolved after stopping or switching to a less potent steroid [30].

## Comparison to Other Glaucoma Surgeries

One of the main benefits of performing trabectome is that there is no bleb formation with the perpetual increased risk of infection nor is there any hardware left in the eye to erode or become infected. The conjunctiva is spared in case further surgery is needed. The main disadvantage is that trabectome should not be relied upon when the target IOP is in the low teens. The success rate of trabectome performed alone however, without same session or prior phacoemulsification, is lower. Even after failed trabeculectomy or tube shunt surgery, trabectome surgery can have a success rate of 70 % at year one ($n=107$, success definition = IOP less than 21 mmHg and 20 % decrease and no need for another surgery; Loewen et al., unpublished data).

Two studies compared the trabectome to trabeculectomy with mitomycin C but neither was randomized. The first was a prospective study that showed at 1-year trabeculectomy lowered the IOP by 52 % versus a 30 % decrease following trabectome [19]. Using the stringent success criteria (like the Tube versus Trabeculectomy Study) [31] of final IOP <21 mmHg and maintaining a 20 % IOP decrease while avoiding persistent hypotony and reoperation, the 12-month success rates were statistically similar at 95 % for trabectome and 83 % for trabeculectomy, $p=0.1$. The second, retrospective study followed 217 patients for 2.5 years [16]. The final IOP decrease was 41 % with stand-alone trabectome and 62 % for trabeculectomy. Despite a 41 % mean decrease in IOP, the reported success rate of trabectome after 2 years ranged from 10 to 43 % versus 66–76 % with trabeculectomy, depending on which IOP cutoff was chosen. Excluding hyphema (none of which required treatment), the complication rate was only 4 % with trabectome versus 35 % with trabeculectomy.

As suggested by the American Academy of Ophthalmology report on Novel Glaucoma Procedures [32], trabectome is meant to augment conventional outflow rather than offer an alternative route such as with an aqueous shunt. The report points out that at this time, the goal with minimally invasive glaucoma surgery may be more to reduce the amount of glaucoma medications needed while maintaining a lower risk of devastating complications as compared to traditional, incisional glaucoma surgery. Given the improved side effect profile (as in the study by Jea et al. with a 4 % complication rate with trabectome versus 35 % with trabeculectomy), trabectome may be offered earlier in the course of glaucomatous nerve damage. One of the goals of this minimally invasive glaucoma surgery is to avoid devastating complications. As of October 2012, there are no published cases of postoperative flat anterior chambers, hypotony past 1 month, wound leak, bleb formation, or choroidal effusion.

## Conclusion

Trabeculectomy ab interno with the trabectome is a mature surgery that was first reported in 2004. By maximizing visibility, identifying and ablating the correct structures, enlarging the ablation, and reducing hyphema through generous use of viscoelastic, the range of indications can be extended and outcomes can be improved. The average IOP reduction is 30–40 %. Longer-term studies indicate a failure rate that may be favorable to trabeculectomy. It is a fast procedure that can easily be combined with phacoemulsification, thus making it an excellent option to provide improved quality of life in glaucoma patients. No randomized controlled trials currently exist comparing trabectome surgery with trabeculectomy or glaucoma drainage devices. IOP reductions in the low teens are uncommon. No long-term complications occur.

## References


1. Minckler D, Baerveldt G, Ramirez MA, Mosaed S, Wilson R, Shaarawy T, et al. Clinical results with the Trabectome, a novel surgical device for treatment of open-angle glaucoma. Trans Am Ophthalmol Soc. 2006;104:40.
2. Francis BA, Minckler D, Dustin L, Kawji S, Yeh J, Sit A, et al. Combined cataract extraction and trabeculotomy by the internal approach for coexisting cataract and open-angle glaucoma: initial results. J Cataract Refract Surg. 2008;34(7):1096–103.
3. Kagemann L, Wollstein G, Ishikawa H, Nadler Z, Sigal IA, Folio LS, et al. Visualization of the conventional outflow pathway in the living human eye. Ophthalmology. 2012;119(8):1563–8.
4. Khaja HA Hodge D, Sit A. Poster 4191. ARVO Annual Meeting. Fort Lauderdale, Florida, 2008. Epub 27 Apr 2008.
5. Battista SA, Lu Z, Hofmann S, Freddo T, Overby DR, Gong H. Reduction of the available area for aqueous humor outflow and increase in meshwork herniations into collector channels following acute IOP elevation in bovine eyes. Invest Ophthalmol Vis Sci. 2008;49(12):5346–52.
6. Kagemann L, Wollstein G, Ishikawa H, Sigal IA, Folio LS, Xu J, et al. 3D visualization of aqueous humor outflow structures in-situ in humans. Exp Eye Res. 2011;93(3):308–15.
7. Kagemann L, Wollstein G, Ishikawa H, Bilonick RA, Brennen PM, Folio LS, et al. Identification and assessment of Schlemm's canal by spectral-domain optical coherence tomography. Invest Ophthalmol Vis Sci. 2010;51(8):4054–9.
8. Hann CR, Bentley MD, Vercnocke A, Ritman EL, Fautsch MP. Imaging the aqueous humor outflow pathway in human eyes by three-dimensional micro-computed tomography (3D micro-CT). Exp Eye Res. 2011;92(2):104–11.
9. Chawdhary S, Anand A. Early post-phacoemulsification hypotony as a risk factor for intraocular contamination: in vivo model. J Cataract Refract Surg. 2006;32(4):609–13.
10. Shingleton BJ, Wadhwani RA, O'Donoghue MW, Baylus S, Hoey H. Evaluation of intraocular pressure in the immediate period after phacoemulsification. J Cataract Refract Surg. 2001;27(4):524–7.
11. McDonnell PJ, Taban M, Sarayba M, Rao B, Zhang J, Schiffman R, et al. Dynamic morphology of clear corneal cataract incisions. Ophthalmology. 2003;110(12):2342–8.
12. Wang Q, Harasymowycz P. Goniopuncture in the treatment of short-term post-trabectome intraocular pressure elevation: a retrospective case series study. J Glaucoma. 2013;22(8):e17–20.
13. Mosaed S. Ab interno trabeculotomy with the trabectome surgical device. Tech Ophthalmol. 2007;5(2):63–6.
14. Minckler D, Mosaed S, Dustin L, Francis B. Trabectome (trabeculectomy—internal approach): additional experience and extended follow-up. Trans Am Ophthalmol Soc. 2008;106:149.
15. Ting JLM, Damji KF, Stiles MC. Ab interno trabeculectomy: outcomes in exfoliation versus primary open-angle glaucoma. J Cataract Refract Surg. 2012;38(2):315–23.
16. Jea SY, Francis BA, Vakili G, Filippopoulos T, Rhee DJ. Ab interno trabeculectomy versus trabeculectomy for open-angle glaucoma. Ophthalmology. 2012;119(1):36–42.
17. Minckler D, Dustin L, Mosaed S. Trabectome UPdate: 2004–2010. Poster. American Glaucoma Society, Naples, 2001.
18. Mosaed S, Rhee D, Filippopoulos T. Trabectome outcomes in adult open-angle glaucoma patients: one-year follow-up. Clin Surg Ophthalmol. 2010;28(8):5–9.
19. Francis BA, Winarko J. Ab interno Schlemm's canal surgery: trabectome and i-stent. Dev Ophthalmol. 2012;50:125.
20. Vold SD. Ab interno trabeculotomy with the trabectome system: what does the data tell us? Int Ophthalmol Clin. 2011;51(3):65–81.
21. Vold S. Impact of preoperative intraocular pressure on trabectome outcomes: a prospective, non-randomized, observational, comparative cohort outcome study. Clin Surg Ophthalmol. 2010;28:11.
22. Vold SD, Dustin L. Impact of laser trabeculoplasty on trabectome® outcomes. Ophthalmic Surg Lasers Imaging. 2010;41(4):443–51.
23. Mosaed S, Dustin L, Minckler DS. Comparative outcomes between newer and older surgeries for glaucoma. Trans Am Ophthalmol Soc. 2009;107:127.
24. Vizzeri G, Weinreb RN. Cataract surgery and glaucoma. Curr Opin Ophthalmol. 2010;21(1):20.
25. Heijl A, Leske MC, Bengtsson B, Hyman L, Bengtsson B, Hussein M. Reduction of intraocular pressure and glaucoma progression: results from the Early Manifest Glaucoma Trial. Arch Ophthalmol. 2002;120(10):1268.
26. Jea SY, Mosaed S, Vold SD, Rhee DJ. Effect of a failed trabectome on subsequent trabeculectomy. J Glaucoma. 2012;21(2):71.
27. Francis BA, See RF, Rao NA, Minckler DS, Baerveldt G. Ab interno trabeculectomy: development of a novel device (Trabectome (TM)) and surgery for open-angle glaucoma. J Glaucoma. 2006;15(1):68–73.
28. Ahuja Y, Malihi M, Sit AJ. Delayed-onset symptomatic hyphema after Ab interno trabeculotomy surgery. Am J Ophthalmol. 2012;154(3):476–80.e2.
29. Knape RM, Smith MF. Anterior chamber blood reflux during trabeculectomy in an eye with previous trabectome surgery. J Glaucoma. 2010;19(7):499–500.
30. Liu J, Jung J, Francis BA. Ab interno trabeculotomy: trabectome™ surgical treatment for open-angle glaucoma. Expert Rev Ophthalmol. 2009;4(2):119–28.
31. Gedde SJ, Schiffman JC, Feuer WJ, Herndon LW, Brandt JD, Budenz DL. Treatment outcomes in the Tube Versus Trabeculectomy (TVT) Study after five years of follow-up. Am J Ophthalmol. 2012;153(5):789–803.e2.
32. Francis BA, Singh K, Lin SC, Hodapp E, Jampel HD, Samples JR, et al. Novel Glaucoma Procedures: a report by the American academy of ophthalmology. Ophthalmology. 2011;118(7):1466–80.

# XEN Gel Stent: The Solution Designed by AqueSys®

Vanessa I. Vera and Christopher Horvath

## History

At the University of Western Australia Lions Eye Institute, Professor Dao-Yi Yu conducted studies and research programs for 6 years to evaluate the feasibility of implanting a microfistula in the eye for the treatment of open-angle glaucoma in animals.

A gelatin-based implant material was chosen with the initial idea to cross-link the material so that it would bioabsorb in the eye over the course of a few months or years. There was an expectation that the disappearing gelatin tube would leave a cell-lined scleral channel behind that functions a microfistula, maintaining outflow. Very early, this approach was changed to use a permanently cross-linked version of the gelatin tube. Preclinical testing was performed to assess safety, feasibility, device performance, and functionality using both bench testing and animal experiments. Several studies were done on animals (rabbits and primates) with hundreds of microfistulas implanted (Yu DY, 2005, Biological microfistula implantation for the surgical management of glaucoma, unpublished data recorded). Cross-linked times and inflammatory reaction were evaluated to achieve the best biocompatibility possible. First, an ab externo approach was evaluated, resulting in cell proliferation and scaring from the surgical trauma created to the conjunctiva. However, an ab interno approach showed excellent biocompatibility and functional drainage, with a longer persistence of drainage when compared to trabeculectomy in rabbits. In primates, a study demonstrated a similar biologic response to that which was observed in rabbits, with a conjunctival bleb that formed immediately, a natural cell-lined channel formed in the sclera, and drainage vessels formed in the conjunctiva. The safety of this procedure was also demonstrated with no complications such as hypotony, endophthalmitis, flat anterior chamber, macular edema, choroidal detachment, or erosion observed during the study. The safety and feasibility of the microfistula implant for the treatment of open-angle glaucoma was successfully accomplished.

## Scientific Rationale

Trabeculectomy and glaucoma drainage devices (GDD) are currently the most commonly used and established surgical procedures, but in both cases, complications are still a major problem [1–7].

The inadequacy of safe surgical treatments for uncontrolled intraocular pressure (IOP) has led the search into new technologies that may surpass the efficacy and safety of the currently considered gold standard surgical approaches (trabeculectomy and glaucoma drainage device (GDD)) with the goal to achieve lower complication rates. A variety of new techniques are emerging and have been referred to as minimally invasive glaucoma surgery (MIGS). Most of these new technologies take advantage of an ab interno approach, which eliminates external manipulation of the eye and may be inserted into the same incision and at the same time as cataract surgery. These procedures are less invasive and much safer.

The superiority of external filtration surgery in terms of intraocular pressure lowering is unquestionable. All other drainage spaces (Schlemm's canal and suprachoroidal) have a limitation since aqueous humor outflow critically depends in the venous system; therefore, most devices are unable to reduce IOP below the pressure of the distal outflow system when performed as a stand-alone procedure.

V.I. Vera, MD (✉)
Unidad Oftalmologica De Caracas,
Caracas, Venezuela
e-mail: vera_vane@hotmail.com

C. Horvath, PhD
AqueSys, Inc, 26970 Aliso Viejo Parkway,
Suite 200, Aliso Viejo, CA 92656, USA
e-mail: chorvath@aquesys.com

**Electronic supplementary material** Supplementary material is available in the online version of this chapter at http://dx.doi.org/10.1007/978-1-4614-8348-9_17. Videos can also be accessed at http://www.springerimages.com/videos/978-1-4614-8347-2



J.R. Samples, I.I.K. Ahmed (eds.), *Surgical Innovations in Glaucoma*,
DOI 10.1007/978-1-4614-8348-9_17, © Springer Science+Business Media New York 2014

From the subconjunctival space, the aqueous humor has numerous potential drainage pathways including diffusion through the conjunctiva, diffusion into the venous system of the sclera and conjunctiva, as well as potential lymphatic pathways [8–11].

Taking the best of both worlds, proven outflow mechanism of action in the subconjunctival space with a minimally invasive approach (MIME: Minimally Invasive Maximum Efficacy), using all the learned lessons from preclinical and early clinical studies, AqueSys, Inc. developed the XEN Gel Stent.

The XEN Gel Stent is a hydrophilic tube composed of a porcine gelatin and cross-linked with glutaraldehyde to provide a more physiologic approach to the treatment of glaucoma and avoid the limitation of other technologies. It decreases intraocular pressure by creating a permanent patent outflow pathway from the anterior chamber to the subconjunctival space through which the aqueous humor can flow to numerous potential drainage pathways.

The implant is derived from collagen and made of gelatin. The material has an extensive track record for medical use in a variety of geographic regions including the European Union, USA, Japan, and Canada. The implant has been successfully developed and used in two material versions: bovine derived or porcine derived. Both versions are crosslinked to become permanent gelatin implants. The XEN Gel Stent is made with gelatin that meets the compendial requirements of the European Pharmacopeia. The biocompatibility properties of gelatin are well established as proven in early clinical trials, and a remarkable lack of foreign body reaction has been shown in the human eye.

Complete verification and validation of all product specifications, sterilization validation and biocompatibility testing to confirm the safety and biocompatibility of the XEN Gel Stent has been performed.

Using the fact from initial animal studies that concluded that a scleral channel of 2–4 mm was optimal to create a bleb, a 6 mm length implant was created to be positioned with approximately 2.0 mm in the subconjunctival space, 3 mm in the sclera, and 1.0 mm in the anterior chamber. During later stages of studies, it was observed that achieving these suggested placement dimension parameters was not critical as long as a 2–4 mm scleral channel was achieved, which made the surgical procedure very simple and forgiving (Yu DY, 2009, Surgical procedure for microfistula tube implantation, unpublished data recorded).

The placement of the implant could be achieved through an ab externo or an ab interno procedure. The ab externo approach required the dissection and pullback of conjunctival and Tenon tissue to allow access to the sclera for implant placement. After implant placement, the conjunctival flap was sutured on

$$\phi \;=\; \frac{dV}{dt} \;=\; \upsilon \pi R^2 = \frac{\pi R^4}{8\eta}\left(\frac{-\Delta P}{\Delta \chi}\right) = \frac{\pi R^4}{8\eta}\frac{|\Delta P|}{L}$$

**Fig. 17.1** Hagen–Poiseuille equation

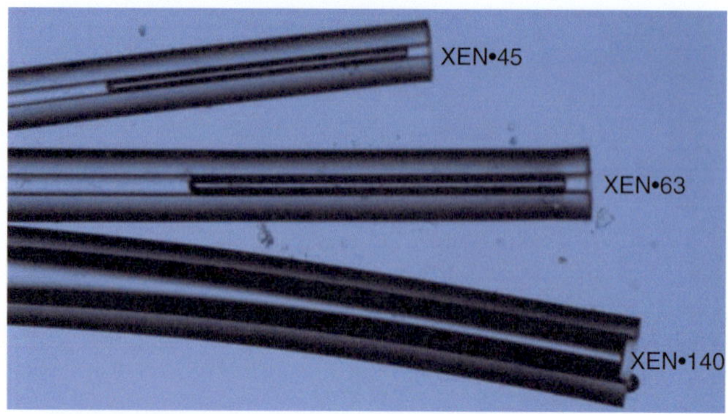


**Fig. 17.2** Microscopic pictures (side view) of the three different implant versions (water column present at inner lumen)

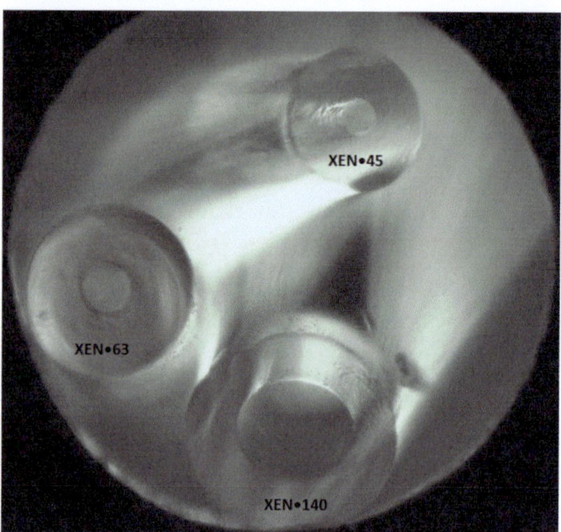


**Fig. 17.3** Microscopic picture from a transectional view of the three different implant versions

a watertight fashion. Similar to the first and last steps of a trabeculectomy, this ab externo approach requires a more traumatic and complex procedure than the ab interno approach, where the conjunctival space remains virtually untouched. AqueSys, Inc. early on decided to focus on perfecting the ab interno approach giving all the advantages of this technique, and since then, all animal studies and human patients have been so far treated with the ab interno method.

To reach the best IOP-lowering outcome possible, the laminar flow through the implant was calculated using the Hagen–Poiseuille equation (Fig. 17.1).

From these calculations, three different versions of implants (Figs. 17.2 and 17.3) were designed to accommodate the needs of different glaucoma stages. The XEN•140 Stent has an inner diameter of ~140 μm. At that size and typical aqueous production rates of 2.5 μl/min, it does not provide any significant outflow restriction. It is designed to rely on physiologic outflow resistances only. XEN•63 with a smaller lumen of ~63 μm creates some outflow resistance in the order of 2–4 mmHg and is designed for patients with moderate glaucoma, and the smallest inner lumen in XEN•45 with ~45 μm provides around 6–8 mmHg flow resistance and was created for patients with less advanced disease or OHT where very minimum risks should be taken at time of surgery.

The MIME approach of the XEN Gel Stent was designed as a solution to provide several key advantages over conventional and other new glaucoma technologies:

- Minimum invasive procedure that reduces surgical risks to the patient and minimizes damage from the surgery
- Ab interno approach that eliminates incisions in the conjunctiva and the need to perform a scleral flap, therefore reducing postoperative inflammation and scarring
- Minimal damage to conjunctiva and tissues which allows multiple and repeatable implantations over the lifetime of the patient, if necessary
- Bypassing the trabecular meshwork, Schlemm's canal, and the collector channels entirely, thus eliminating the risk of reducing the efficacy of the implant due to any other outflow obstruction in the eye
- Low and diffuse outflow into intact tissue anatomy and intact drainage pathways in the conjunctiva, giving maximum efficacy pressure reduction

## Surgical Method

As mentioned before, a mayor difference from conventional glaucoma surgeries is the ab interno approach. As we all know, this approach is less invasive and preserves the integrity of the patient's conjunctiva which means that the patient's natural drainage pathways are intact and the risks of fibrosis and scarring are reduced.

To achieve this ab interno with a minimally invasive approach, the injector system ends up in a small needle (25G or 27G depending on the implant used) which holds inside the gelatin implant. The inserter is designed to protect the XEN Gel Stent and to accurately place the implant into the correct anatomical location (Figs. 17.4a, b).

An overview of the main suggested surgical steps is as follows:

1. Standard ophthalmic care preoperative preparation.
2. Intended landing zone in the superonasal quadrant of the conjunctiva is visualized and marked as shown in

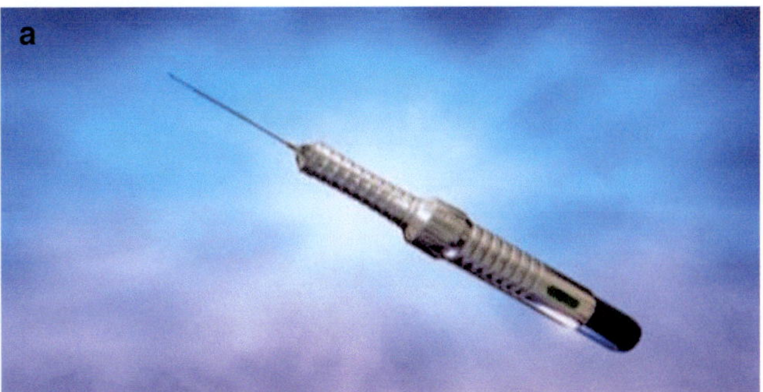
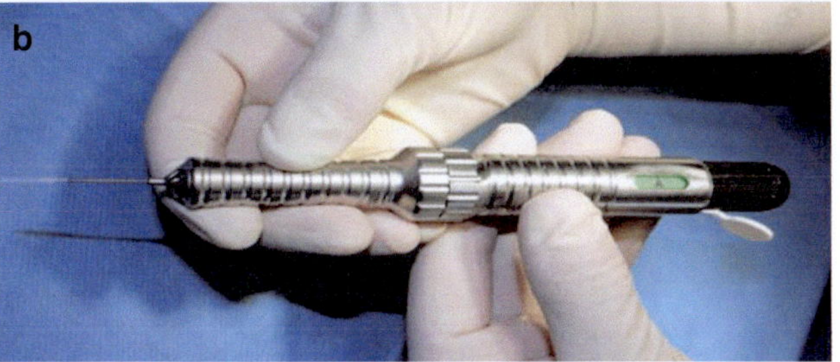

**Fig. 17.4** (a) Animation image of XEN injector. (b) Picture of XEN injector

Fig. 17.5 (blue arrow showing 3 mm marks in the conjunctiva).
3. Corneal incisions (main and side port) are created.
4. A preloaded/single-use injector is provided to the physician, which comes individually packaged and sterile.
5. Enter main incision at peripheral cornea and direct the needle across the anterior chamber to the angle (Fig. 17.6).
6. Optional goniolens use for angle visualization. The entry zone in the angle is a broad and forgiving area (anywhere from the Schwalbe's line to the Scleral spur), not a specific target which gives flexibility to use gonioscopy or not during the procedure.
7. The needle is pushed to go through the sclera and into the subconjunctival space. As the needle bevel exits the sclera, an ideal 3 mm intrascleral channel is usually achieved (Fig. 17.7).

   With this approach, the needle bevel angle at the exit site is close to parallel to the conjunctiva tissue. This leads to the Tenon and conjunctiva layers above the needle bevel to be rather pushed up versus being engaged in a penetrating fashion. As a result of this, perforating the conjunctiva with the needle bevel when coming out of the sclera can be avoided.
8. Once the needle is out at the subconjunctival space, direct visualization of the entire needle's bevel through the surgical microscope is possible and confirms correct location (Fig. 17.8).

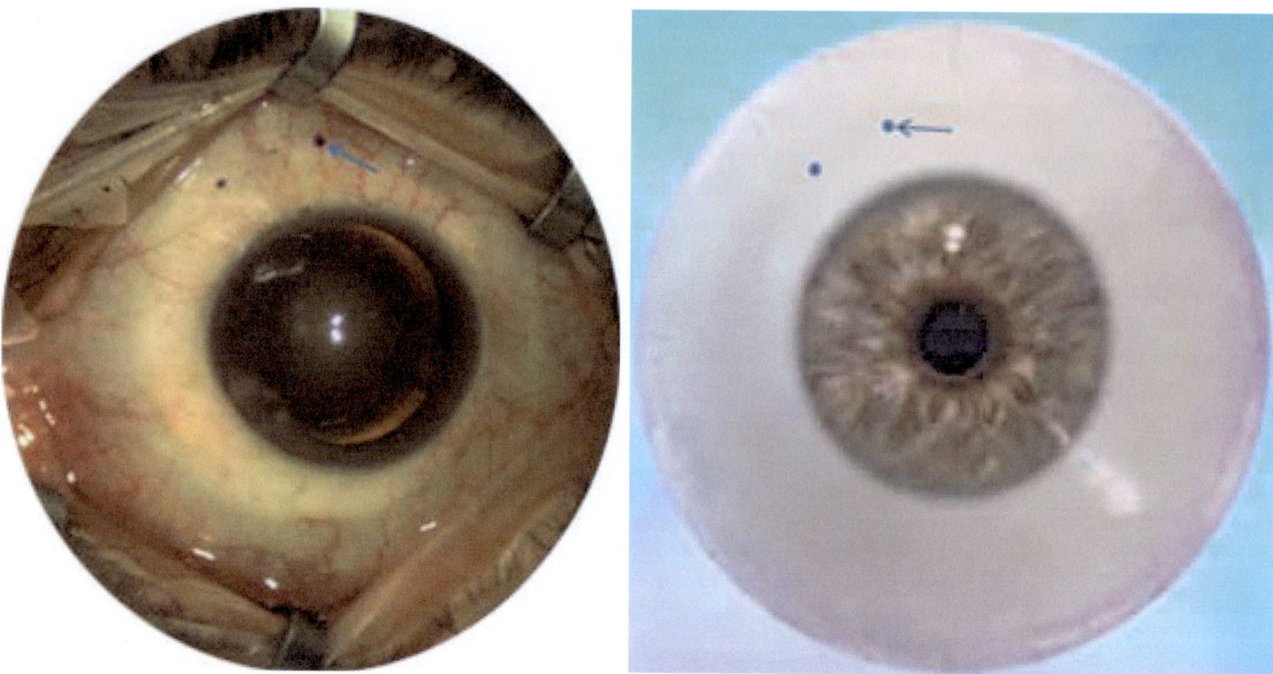

**Fig. 17.5** *Left side* shows a picture from the surgical microscope view. *Right side* shows an animation image

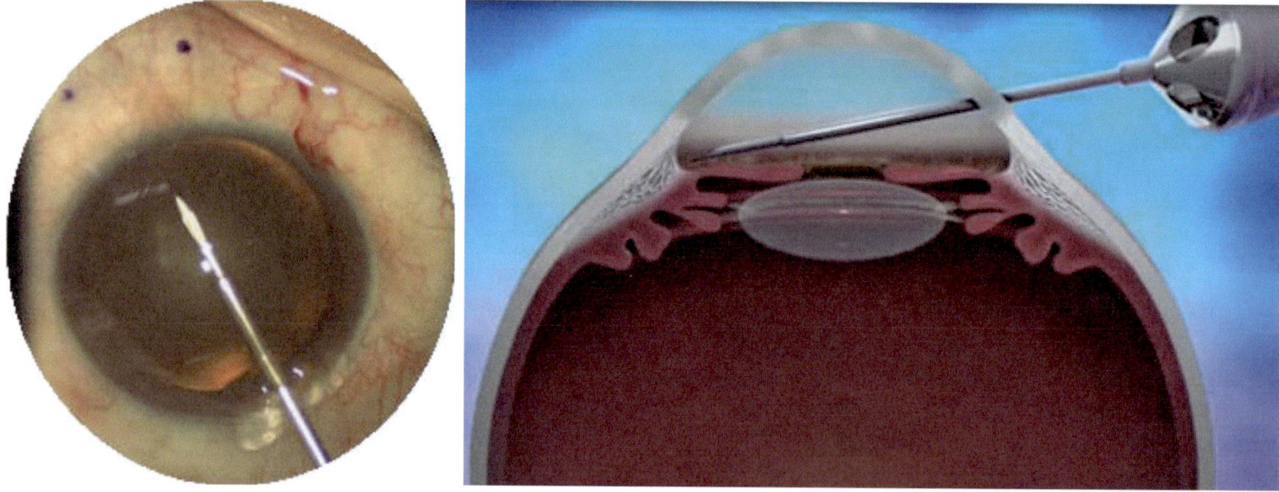

**Fig. 17.6** *Left side* shows a picture from the surgical microscope view. *Right side* shows an animation image (sagittal view) of needle passing across the anterior chamber

9. The XEN Gel Stent is then deployed by turning a wheel on the inserter (similar procedure to a two-hand IOL insertion) until the wheel has been fully turned (Fig. 17.9).

   During this step, the implant is being slowly deployed forward into position by the internal mechanism, and the needle is being fully withdrawn into the sleeve of the injector.

10. The procedure is then complete, and the surgeon simply removes this blunt sleeve from the patient's eye. The implant immediately begins shunting fluid from the anterior chamber to the subconjunctival space (Fig. 17.10).

   During the implantation procedure, the implant hydrates and swells in place to become a soft non-migrating drainage channel that is tissue conforming. The cross-linked gelatin material gives a fixed inner diameter wall that does not change after swelling, allowing more predictable IOP value and hypotony protection.

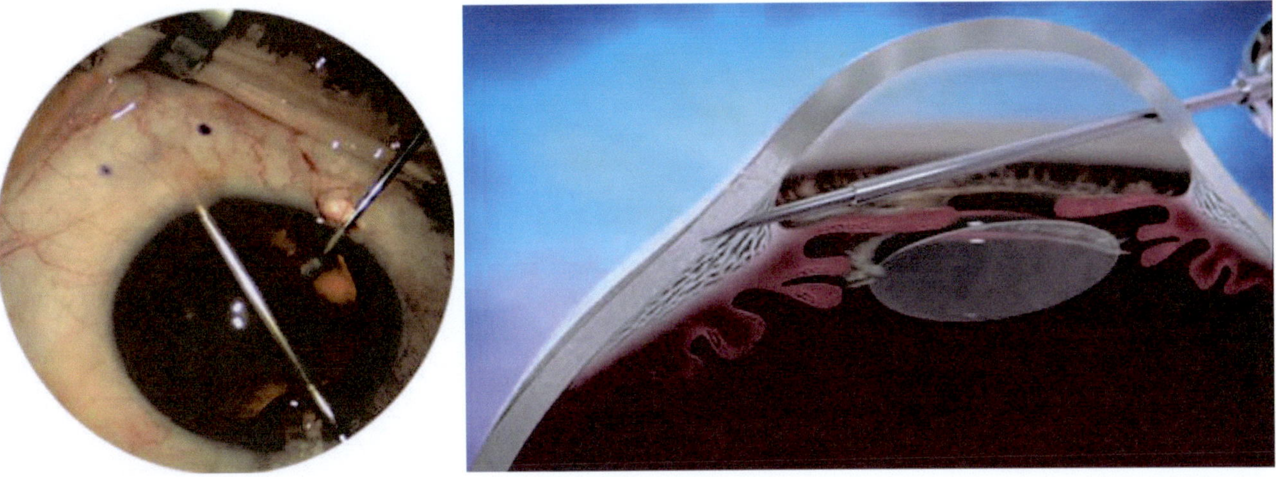

**Fig. 17.7** *Left side* shows a picture from the surgical microscope view. *Right side* shows an animation image (sagittal view) of scleral tunnel being created by the needle

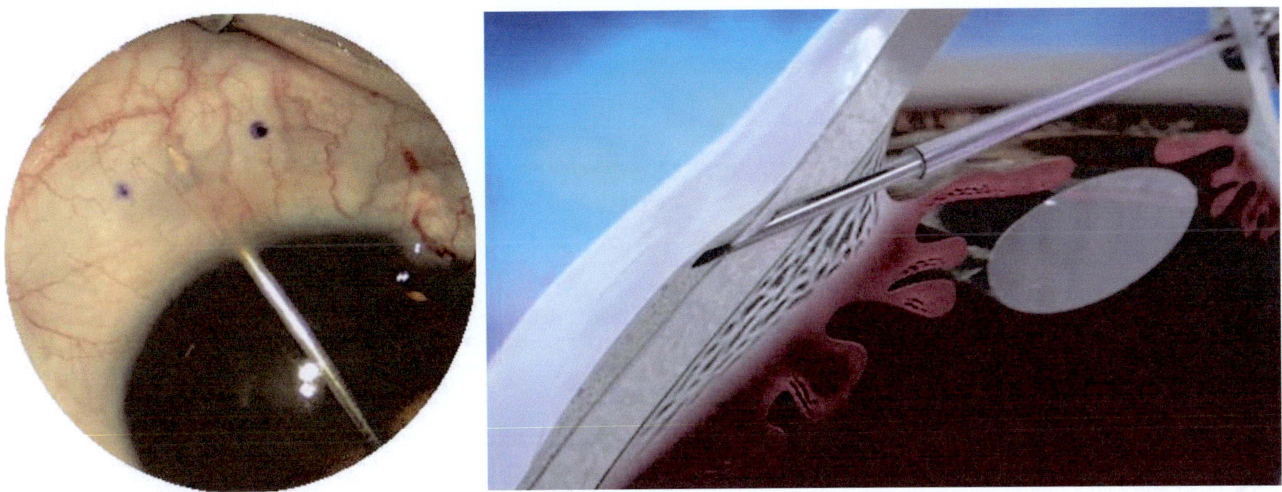

**Fig. 17.8** *Left side* shows a picture from the surgical microscope view. *Right side* shows an animation image (sagittal view) of needle's bevel exiting at subconjunctival space

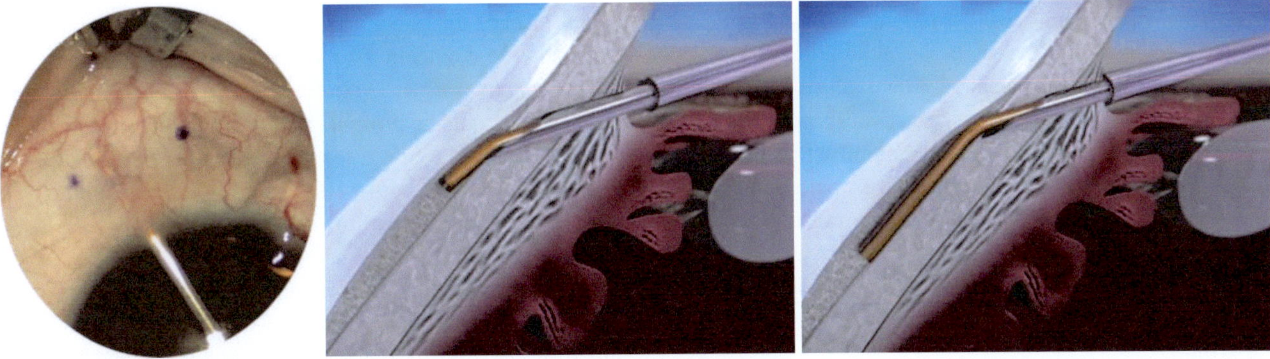

**Fig. 17.9** *Left side* shows a picture from the surgical microscope view. *Middle* and *right side* images show an animation image (sagittal view) of XEN Gel Stent being deployed in position

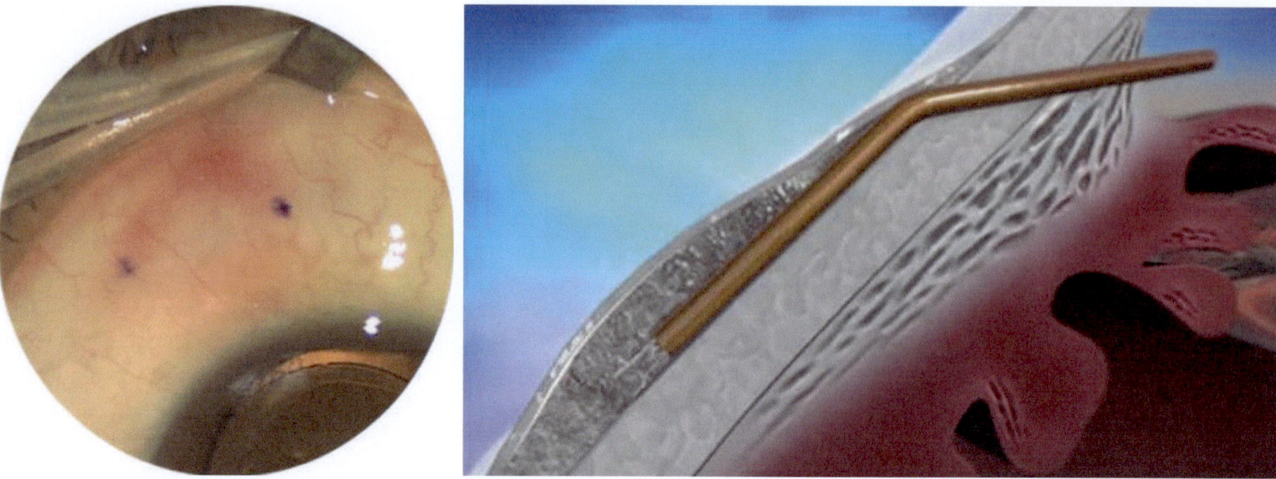

**Fig. 17.10** *Left side* shows a picture from the surgical microscope view. *Right side* shows an animation image (sagittal view) of fluid present at subconjunctival space

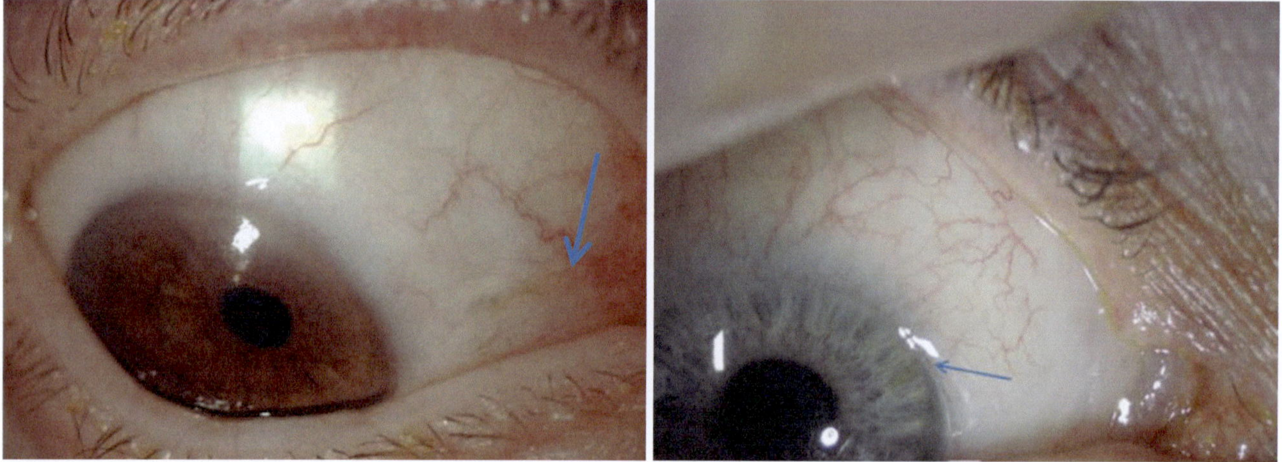

**Figs. 17.11 and 17.12**   Slit lamp picture of XEN Gel Stent (*blue arrow*) at 12 months postoperative

The mechanism of action is fundamentally consistent with other full-thickness surgical treatments for glaucoma, bypassing all potential outflow obstructions and mitigating several of the limitations of those technologies. The XEN Gel Stent maintains a patent outflow pathway between the anterior chamber and the subconjunctival space while the tissues surrounding the implant heal naturally. By allowing the tissue to heal naturally around it, there is no need to create an iridotomy, and with the minimum amount of trauma, subsequent inflammation and fibrosis is minimized and many of the complications associated with more invasive procedures such as trabeculectomy, and aqueous shunt implantation can be avoided.

Another advantage of this procedure is the very simple and easy to perform surgical technique that does not requires long training, extraordinary surgical skills, or long learning curves.

## Drainage Path

The presence of subconjunctival fluid upon implantation confirms the connection between the anterior chamber and subconjunctival space. An initial medium or high bleb appearance could be present during immediate postoperative stages. During the first week, this bleb gradually reduces in volume as drainage pathways form from the subconjunctival space to the various outflow channels (see Videos 17.1 and 17.2) [10].

At later stages, due to the gentle and diffuse dispersion of aqueous humor into the non-dissected Tenon's and subconjunctival space, the morphology of an established and functioning bleb differs from the blebs seen after traditional filtering surgeries (i.e., trabeculectomy with antifibrotic agents). Subconjunctival fluid disperses over wide areas giving a low-lying and diffuse appearance (Figs. 17.11 and 17.12).

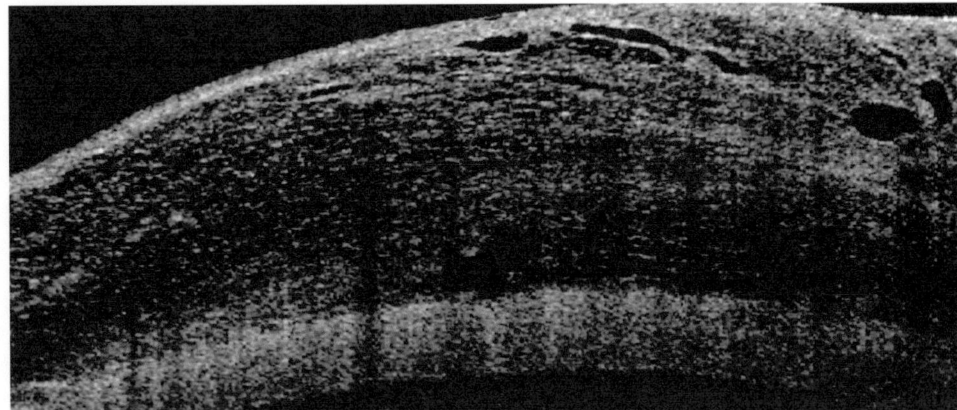

**Fig. 17.13** AS-OCT image (radial high resolution) of bleb at 1 day postoperative after XEN implantation. Non-dissected conjunctiva shows presence of microcysts, stripping and shading phenomenon

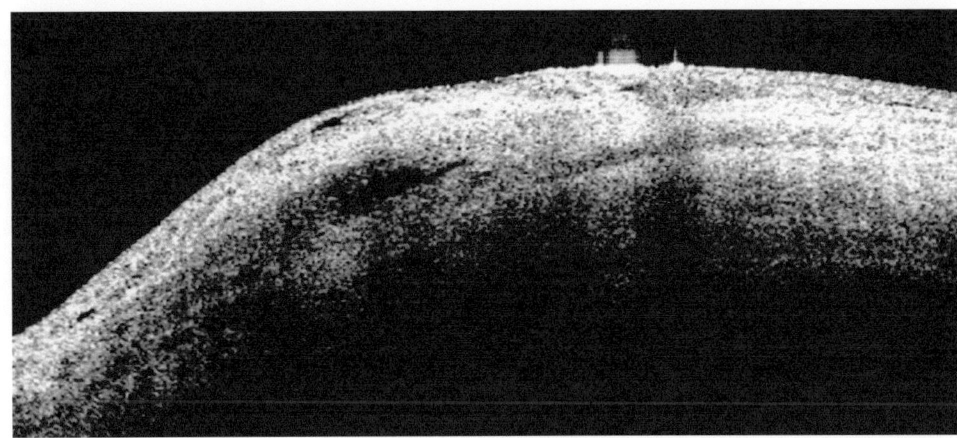

**Fig. 17.14** AS-OCT image (radial high resolution) of bleb at 1 month postoperative. Intrableb cysts, few subepithelial cysts, and initial thickening of the conjunctiva

Previous studies have shown that anterior segment optical coherence tomography (AS-OCT) is able to objectively quantify bleb morphology after trabeculectomy [12]. Theelen et al. [13] demonstrated poor visualization of the sclera below the bleb calling it shading phenomenon and multi-hyporeflective layers within Tenon's capsule described as striping phenomenon in successful blebs in the first operative week using slit lamp-adapted OCT. Studies using imaging of blebs and histological results of filtering blebs showed that striping phenomenon represents collections of aqueous humor with loosely arranged subepithelial connective tissue [14–18]. Shading phenomenon seems to represent the absorption profile of water that significantly worsens tissue transparency and limits light backscatter of deeper structures. Early studies had been done using Visante AS-OCT images to analyze morphology and qualitative changes in the bleb structure after XEN implantation (Shoham–Hazon N, 2012, Aquesys anterior segment optical coherence tomography (OCT) (Visante), unpublished data recorded).

The early and late changes in the bleb morphology appearance mentioned before were also present and documented during the AS-OCT study. Presence of microcysts throughout the epithelium during initial postoperative stages (Fig. 17.13) adds further anatomic evidence to the fact that the aqueous humor moves transconjunctivally after filtration surgery [19–21].

Gradually, several outflow p channels [10] take over the incoming fluid, which makes a reduction in volume of the bleb appearance (Fig. 17.14). This morphology changes correlate with AS-OCT images showing fewer subepithelial cysts and an initial thickening of the conjunctiva.

These findings might indicate that a more diffuse and controlled manner of outflow through the XEN Gel Stent could produce lower-lying and diffuse appearance blebs compared to the blebs observed after traditional trabeculectomy or an ExPRESS device (Fig. 17.15).

At later postoperative stages, in the majority of the eyes, a hyporeflective space between the conjunctiva and the sclera indicated good filtration. In those cases, bleb appearances were low lying and diffuse, and good IOP control was also noted. Conjunctival thickening was also associated with reduction in IOP (Figs. 17.16, 17.17, and 17.18).

In the majority of cases, the implant has been shown to create a long-term, effective IOP lowering without the use of antimetabolites such as mitomycin C (MMC) at the time of surgery. In some cases, patients with high-risk factors, such as previous history of fibrosis (i.e., refractory cases), race, and age, a postoperative needling procedure using antimetabolites is suggested to improve the long-term performance of the gelatin implant. This ability to tune the implant performance in the postoperative phase is another benefit of the

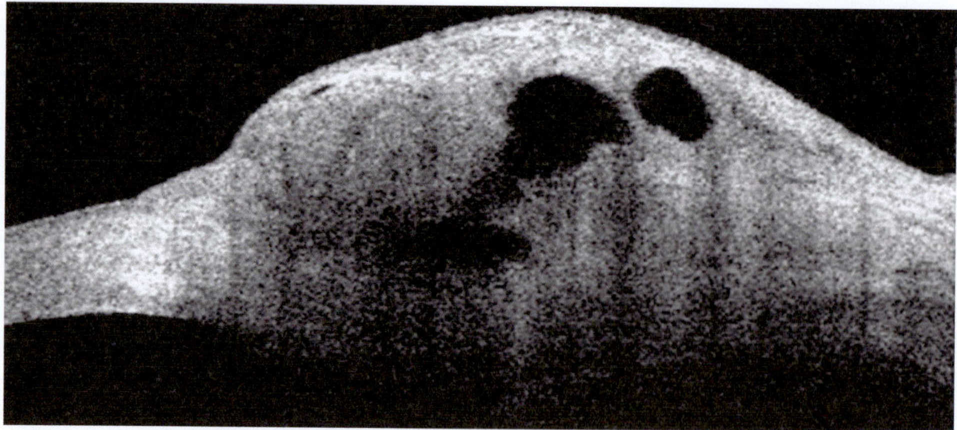

**Fig. 17.15** AS-OCT image (radial high resolution) of bleb at 1 month after ExPRESS surgery

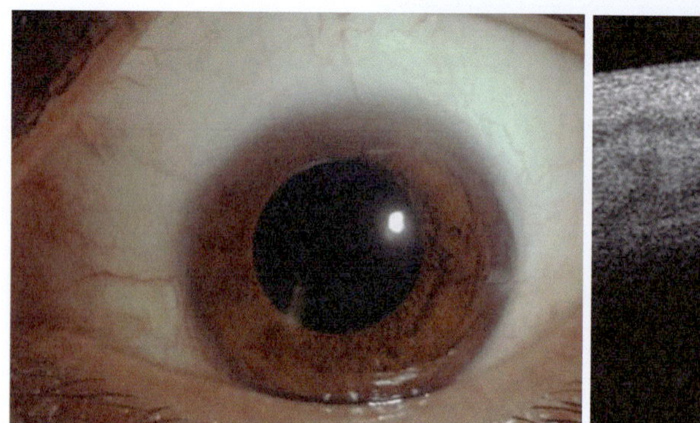

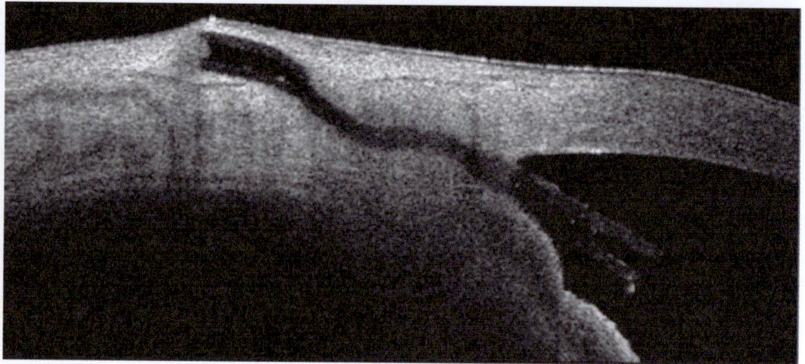

**Fig. 17.16** On the *left*, an SL picture at 12 months postoperative OS showing low-lying and diffuse superonasal bleb. On the *right*, an AS-OCT image (radial high resolution) of bleb with thickened and hyperreflective bleb wall

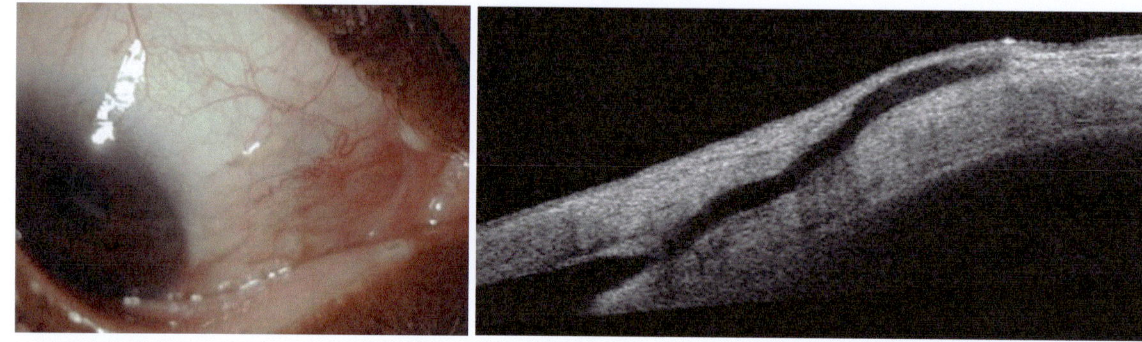

**Fig. 17.17** On the *left*, an SL picture at 12 months postoperative OD with low-lying and diffuse superonasal bleb. On the *right*, an AS-OCT image (radial high resolution) of bleb with thick and hyperreflective wall bleb

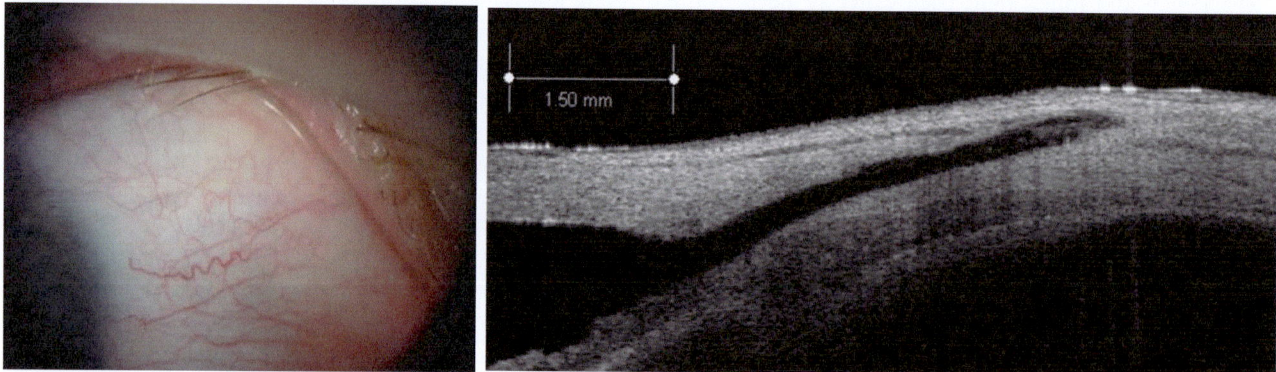


**Fig. 17.18** On the *left*, an SL picture at 12 months postoperative OD with low-lying and diffuse superonasal bleb. On the *right*, an AS-OCT image (radial high resolution) hyperreflective wall bleb

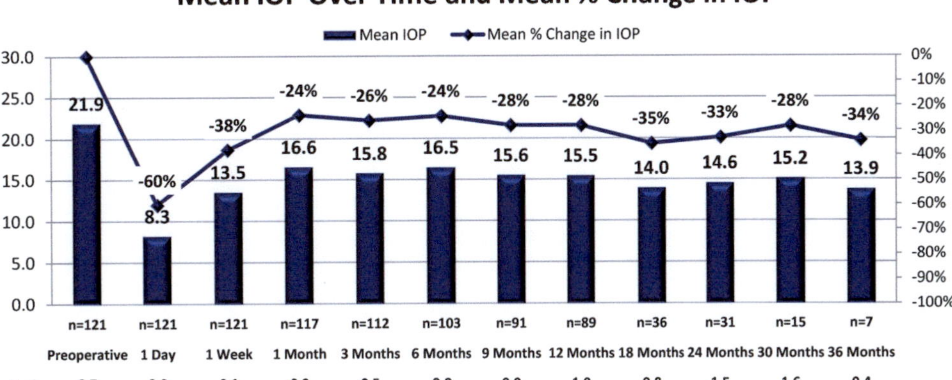



**Fig. 17.19** Current international clinical study results. *Mean preoperative IOP is best medicated. Patients were not washed out prior to surgery

XEN procedure. Early glaucoma patients without a long history of glaucoma drug usage showed remarkable low fibrosis rates and great long-term performances without any use of antimetabolites.

## Clinical Results

International studies are being held with the purpose of establishing the safety and effectiveness of the Aquecentesis procedure in reducing IOP in patients with primary open-angle glaucoma. In this multicentric, prospective, nonrandomized, open-label study, 121 patients undergoing either primary or secondary surgery were followed for up to 36 months, and their outcomes for mean IOP, IOP change, and reduction of medications were recorded.

Effectiveness was determined by comparing the baseline IOP and number of glaucoma medication taken with the postoperative values during a period of 36 months. Safety parameters were evaluated using IOP, frequency of patients with loss of visual acuity, and assessment of any adverse events.

The study enrollment and follow-up is still ongoing in Canada, Europe, Asia, Australia, and South America. Partial results were collected during product development and learning curve phases. Clinical ophthalmic examinations were performed at the preoperative visit and on postoperative day 1, weeks 1 and 2, and months 3, 6, 9, 12, 18, and 24. The exams included applanation tonometry, anterior chamber OCT imaging, visual acuity, visual field, and assessment of any complications. Effectiveness was evaluated by comparing the baseline and postoperative IOPs and reduction in glaucomatous medications.

Mean preoperative IOP was 21.9 mmHg (±3.4) on 2.7 medications (patients were not washed out prior to surgery). Mean postoperative IOPs were 15.5 mmHg (±4.4) on 1.0 medication at 12 months, 14.6 mmHg (±3.4) on 1.5 medications at 24 months, and 13.9 mmHg (±4.0) on 0.4 medications at 36 months. The mean decrease in IOP (mmHg) from best medicated IOP was −6.4 mmHg (−28 % reduction) at 12 months, −7.8 mmHg (−33 % reduction) at 24 months, and −7.5 mmHg (−34 % reduction) at 36 months. At 24 months, anti-glaucomatous medications were reduced by 49 % from the preoperative median of 3 (Fig. 17.19).

## Summary

The Aquecentesis procedure is a MIME procedure where a hollow 27GA or 25GA needle penetrates the sclera from an ab interno approach. A twist of the handle withdraws the needle as it deposits a trans-scleral aqueous drainage tube which connects the anterior chamber to the subconjunctival space. The XEN Gel Stent is manufactured from a soft, flexible, permanent gelatin. XEN Gel Stent is an effective surgical approach for controlling intraocular pressure in early, moderate, advanced, or refractory patients who have primary open-angle glaucoma. The Aquecentesis procedure bypasses all of the trabecular and scleral resistance to create outflow, but unlike other full-thickness procedures, it provides sufficient resistance flow through the tube to avoid flat chambers or clinically significant hypotony, and obviates the need to do any conjunctival dissection. This conjunctiva-sparing ab interno approach allows an additional benefit where future XEN Gel Stents could be placed later on during the patient's lifetime, giving the ophthalmologists a tool to adjust over the course of the patient's disease to different target IOP needs (XEN•45, XEN•63, and XEN•140).

## References


1. Watson PG, Jakeman C, Ozturk M, Barnett MF, Barnett F, Khaw KT. Complications of trabeculectomy (a 20-year follow-up). Eye (Lond). 1990;4:425–38.
2. Nouri-Mahdavi K, Brigatti L, Weitzman M, Caprioli J. Outcomes of trabeculectomy for primary open-angle glaucoma. Ophthalmology. 1995;102:1760–9.
3. Ticho U, Ophir A. Late complications after glaucoma filtering surgery with adjunctive 5-fluorouracil. Am J Ophthalmol. 1993;115:506–10.
4. Costa VP, Wilson RP, Moster M, Schmidt CM, Gandham S. Hypotony maculopathy following the use of topical mitomycin C in glaucoma filtration surgery. Ophthalmic Surg. 1993;24:389–94.

5. Topouzis F, Coleman AL, Choplin N, Bethlem MM, Hill R, Yu F, Panek WC, Wilson MR. Follow-up of the original cohort with the Ahmed glaucoma valve implant. Am J Ophthalmol. 1999;128:198–204.

6. Smith SL, Starita RJ, Fellman RL, Lynn JR. Early clinical experience with the Baerveldt 350-mm glaucoma implant and associated extraocular muscle imbalance. Ophthalmology. 1993;100: 914–8.

7. Topouzis F, Yu F, Coleman AL. Factors associated with elevated rates of adverse outcome after cyclodestructive procedures versus drainage device procedures. Ophthalmology. 1998;105: 2276–81.

8. Singh D. Conjunctiva lymphatic system. J Cataract Refract Surg. 2003;29:632–3.

9. Yucel YH, Johnston MG, Ly T, et al. Identification of lymphatics in the ciliary body of the human eye: a novel "uveolymphatic" outflow pathway. Exp Eye Res. 2009;89:810–9.

10. Yu D-Y, et al. The critical role of the conjunctiva in glaucoma filtration surgery. Prog Retin Eye Res. 2009;28:303–28.

11. Schmid-Schonbein GW. Microlymphatics and lymph flow. Physiol Rev. 1990;70:987–1028.

12. Singh M, Aung T, Tun TA, et al. Quantitative analysis of the change in bleb morphology over time after successful trabeculectomy [abstract]. Invest Ophthalmol Vis Sci. 2009;50:E-abstract 3370.

13. Theelen T, et al. A pilot study on slit lamp-adapted optical coherence tomography imaging of trabeculectomy filtering blebs. Graefes Arch Clin Exp Ophthalmol. 2007;245:877–82.

14. Addicks EM, Quigley HA, Green WR, et al. Histologic characteristics of filtering blebs in glaucomatous eyes. Arch Ophthalmol. 1983;101:795–8.

15. Labbé A, Dupas B, Hamard P, Baudouin C. In vivo confocal microscopy study of blebs after filtering surgery. Ophthalmology. 2005;112:1979–86.

16. Guthoff R, Klink T, Schlunck G, Grehn F. In vivo confocal microscopy of failing and functioning filtering blebs: results and clinical correlations. J Glaucoma. 2006;15:552–8.

17. Messer EM, Zapp DM, Mackert MJ, et al. In vivo confocal microscopy of filtering blebs after trabeculectomy. Arch Ophthalmol. 2006;124:1095–103.

18. Schmitt JM, Knüttel K, Yadlowsky M, Eckhaus MA. Optical-coherence tomography of a dense tissue: statistics of attenuation and backscattering. Phys Med Biol. 1994;39:1705–20.

19. Picht G, Grehn F. Sickekissenentwicklung nach trabekulektomien. Ophthalmologe. 1998;95:380–7.

20. Singh M, Chew PTK, Friedman DS, et al. Imaging of trabeculectomy blebs using anterior segment optical coherence tomography. Ophthalmology. 2007;114:47–53.

21. Teng CC, Chi HH, Katzin HM. Histology and mechanism of filtering operations. Am J Ophthalmol. 1959;47:16–33.

Lindsay A. McGrath, Graham A. Lee, and Ivan Goldberg

## Introduction

Since the introduction of trabeculectomy in 1968, the technique of glaucoma filtration surgery has evolved progressively. Use of adjuvants such as mitomycin C (MMC), 5-fluorouracil, and β-radiation as well as non-penetrating approaches and small-incision trabeculectomy has attempted to improve the procedure's outcomes and safety [1, 2]. Devices such as the Ex-Press mini glaucoma shunt (Alcon Laboratories, Fort Worth, TX) try to improve predictability of aqueous flow through the sclerostomy and thus control one factor that influences the resulting intraocular pressure (IOP).

The Ex-Press glaucoma filtration device is a small stainless steel, non-valved flow-restricting device. This shunt is implanted under a partial-thickness scleral flap to drain aqueous from the anterior chamber to the intrascleral and then subconjunctival spaces, to form a filtration bleb as seen in traditional trabeculectomy [3, 4]. The pilot Ex-Press model (R-50) has a 2.96-mm long tube, 2.5 mm of which is intraocular, with a 400-μm (27 gauge) external diameter and 50-μm internal diameter. There are two other commercially available models which differ in length and lumen diameter. The R model has a beveled tip and a uniform back plate, but the T model's tip is round and short with a split back plate [5]. Initially, two models (R and T) were produced; however, the T model has recently been replaced by the P model (Fig. 18.1). The P-50 and P-200 models are 2.64 mm in length and have internal diameters of 50 and

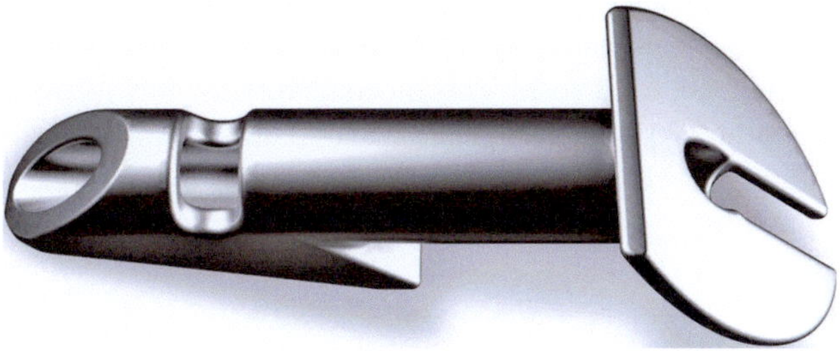

**Fig.18.1** Ex-Press glaucoma shunt (P model)

200 μm respectively [6]. The P models also have a beveled tip for controlled device insertion and a vertical channel in the faceplate posteriorly, to facilitate flow in this direction [7, 8]. Neither the manufacturer nor the literature has provided guidelines for the clinical use of the different models. All models have been shown to create a relatively constant resistance to flow, and the tube diameter is the only parameter to control fluid drainage in vitro [6].

The Ex-Press device is made of implantable stainless steel similar to that used in cardiac stenting and is considered non-ferromagnetic [9, 10]. The device features an outer disc-like flange to stabilize depth of implantation and a spur-like inner projection to prevent extrusion after implantation [10, 11]. The flange and spur are designed and angled to conform to the anatomy of the peri-limbal sclera to stabilize the device [10]. There are three holes in the device near the distal tip providing an alternate conduit for aqueous humor flow, should blood, fibrin, or the iris block the main orifice [12]. The Ex-Press glaucoma filtration device was first described in 1998 in Israel and received the Food and Drug Administration approval in 2002. Approximately 75,000 devices have been implanted since that time [13].

L.A. McGrath, MBBS

G.A. Lee, MBBS (Qld), MD, FRANZCO (✉)
Department of Ophthalmology,
City Eye Center, University of Queensland,
10/135 Wickham Terrace, Brisbane, QLD 4000, Australia
e-mail: lindsay.mcgrath@uqconnect.edu.au; eye@cityeye.com.au

I. Goldberg, AM, MBBS, FRANZCO, FRACS
Department of Ophthalmology, Sydney Eye Hospital, Level 4,
Park House, 187 Macquarie Street, Sydney, NSW 2000, Australia
e-mail: eyegoldberg@gmail.com

**Electronic supplementary material** Supplementary material is available in the online version of this chapter at http://dx.doi.org/10.1007/978-1-4614-8348-9_18. Videos can also be accessed at http://www.springerimages.com/videos/978-1-4614-8347-2

J.R. Samples, I.I.K. Ahmed (eds.), *Surgical Innovations in Glaucoma*,
DOI 10.1007/978-1-4614-8348-9_18, © Springer Science+Business Media New York 2014

## Biocompatibility

In 2003, Nyska et al. found no evidence of active inflammatory reaction or tissue irritation at 3 and 6 months post-Ex-Press implantation in 8 rabbit eyes [10]. They reported a fibrotic capsule of variable thickness (up to 0.04 mm) surrounding the implants, devoid of inflammatory cells. Granulomatous inflammation and fibroblastic proliferation around foreign implants can be a major complication for glaucoma devices [14]. Aziz and colleagues described a histopathologic specimen of human ocular tissue surrounding an Ex-Press shunt [14]. They found minimal cellular reaction surrounding the implant and a thin fibrocellular tissue present deep to the implant. There was no granulomatous nor cellular inflammation identified around a shunt that had been in situ for 2 years. This biocompatibility may relate to the minimal tissue manipulation and trauma during implantation, as well as reduced cautery and absence of an iridectomy [10].

## Indications

The general indications for implantation of an Ex-Press glaucoma shunt are similar to those for standard trabeculectomy and include failure to control IOP with maximal tolerable medical and/or laser therapy, nonadherence to medication (financial or physical restrictions), and intolerance of medical therapy (reactive or allergic) [12]. The Ex-Press shunt can be placed either nasally or temporally as long as there are 2–3 clock hours of viable conjunctiva available. This renders Ex-Press implantation a possible alternative in cases of failed glaucoma surgery where there is a small, non-scarred area of the remaining conjunctiva [15, 16]. Lankaranian and coworkers reported an IOP of 15 mmHg or lower 3 months after Ex-Press implantation in 65.3 % of patients who had previously undergone unsuccessful trabeculectomy [17].

The device is approved for use in open-angle glaucoma in phakic, pseudophakic, or aphakic eyes [18]. The use of an Ex-Press device has also been described in uveitic, pigmentary, traumatic, and neovascular glaucoma if there is no conjunctival scarring, inflammation, or uncontrolled bleeding [16, 19, 20]. There is, however, a potential risk of postoperative hyphema in neovascular glaucoma which may occlude the stent [1]. Dahan and Carmichael reported the use of Ex-Press devices in neovascular glaucoma secondary both to retinal vein occlusion and proliferative diabetic retinopathy [21]. After good initial lowering of IOP, 6 of the 12 cases failed owing to bleb fibrosis or uncontrolled rubeosis and 5 eyes had hyphema. Further reports of Ex-Press device use in chronic angle-closure and pseudoexfoliation glaucoma show good intermediate [17] (27 ± 13.2 months) and longer-term [22] (up to 5 years) success [1, 16, 19, 22]. Lankaranian and colleagues showed

that the Ex-Press shunt lowered IOP to 5–21 mmHg with no medications in 55.4 % (83.7 %, with medications) of patients with primary open-angle, angle-closure, or pseudoexfoliative glaucoma over a mean follow-up period of 27 ± 13.2 months [17]. A single case report in 2007 described the efficacy of the Ex-Press glaucoma implant in an 11-year-old male with Sturge-Weber syndrome [23].

The Ex-Press device has shown short-term efficacy in the IOP reduction in vitrectomized eyes [24]. Ocular hypertension induced by pars plana vitrectomy is often resistant to medical therapy, and in cases where emulsified silicone oil blocks the trabecular meshwork, filtering surgery is a valid strategy. Vetrugno and colleagues reported four vitrectomized eyes with persistent ocular hypertension that following Ex-Press shunt insertion had IOP lower than 18 mmHg with no severe adverse effects [24]. There are no larger series or follow-up longer than 6 months published on this indication for Ex-Press implantation.

Ex-Press mini glaucoma shunt implantation in post-penetrating keratoplasty glaucoma has been reported since 2010 [25, 26]. In contrast to other glaucoma drainage devices, Ates and colleagues had relative success with the implantation of the Ex-Press device in patients with corneal grafts [25]. They reported a 93.3 % rate of glaucoma control (IOP <21 mmHg with or without medications) with a mean follow-up of 12.2 months. During this period of follow-up, there were no graft failures in their 15 eyes, with no observed endothelial damage related to the Ex-Press shunt, compared with that seen with other implantable devices [25, 27]. A potential advantage of a rigid metal shunt, if positioned correctly, is that it may be less likely than a flexible silicone tube to damage the endothelium.

## Contraindications

In their discussion of Ex-Press shunt insertion, Sarkisian and colleagues discouraged implantation in patients with a narrow angle, owing to angle crowding and risks of endothelial and/or iris trauma [28]. In general, concurrent cataract extraction with Ex-Press insertion for IOP regulation has been recommended for cases of angle closure [12]. Congenital glaucoma and glaucoma associated with anterior segment dysgenesis (aniridia, Axenfeld-Rieger, or microphthalmia) are also relative contraindications for Ex-Press implantation. Such eyes often have thin sclera and altered angle anatomy, either of which may compromise successful and stable placement of an Ex-Press [29].

Another relative contraindication for Ex-Press implantation might be the presence of an anterior chamber intraocular lens [18]. Such a lens may increase risk of corneal endothelial damage should there be postsurgical hypotony with anterior chamber collapse.

## Preoperative Considerations

At the preoperative review, the surgeon should determine the status and mobility of the conjunctiva and the health of the sclera in the anticipated surgical site, along with careful gonioscopy to determine angle depth and configuration. Peripheral anterior synechiae should be excluded near the planned insertion site. Lenticular status determines any need for combined cataract and glaucoma surgery [12]. If safe to do so, discontinuation of blood "thinners" may reduce the risk of intraoperative hemorrhage.

## Anesthesia

Choice of anesthetic used for intraocular surgery depends on the patient, surgeon, and anesthetist [12]. Ex-Press shunt insertion is similar to trabeculectomy and can usually be performed under local or regional anesthesia (Video 18.1) [2, 7]. General anesthesia is required only in young, uncooperative, or disorientated patients.

Peribulbar, retrobulbar, and sub-Tenon injections are commonly used [12, 30]. Subconjunctival or topical anesthetic has been successful in cooperative patients, using tetracaine, lidocaine, or lignocaine jelly. Intracameral preservative-free lidocaine 1 % can be combined with topical anesthetic. Although no difference in pain has been reported when topical anesthesia is compared with peribulbar, the inability of the former to provide akinesia may compromise anterior chamber stability [31].

## Surgical Technique

As originally conceived, the Ex-Press device was placed subconjunctivally [10]. This was associated with significant incidence of device erosion and overfiltration; in late 2005, implantation was reported to be safer under a scleral flap [11, 32]. This closely resembles trabeculectomy, requiring a conjunctival flap, scleral trapdoor, antimetabolite augmentation if indicated, and meticulous conjunctival closure [16, 33].

Optimal exposure of the surgical site can be attained with a corneal traction suture of 6/0–7/0 polyglactin or silk to infraduct the eye [12]. A standard fornix or limbal conjunctival incision in an upper quadrant allows access to the scleral bed, which is gently cauterized for hemostasis. The scleral flap can be shaped to the surgeon's preference (square, rectangular, triangular, or trapezoidal), although shape is not as important as extension anteriorly to clear cornea. The flap should be at least 2.5×2.5 mm to cover the implant well by at least 1 mm around the plate [34]. Alternatively, a 5×5 mm limbus-based scleral flap of 50–60 % depth can be fashioned, with the dissection plane forward into clear cornea. At the surgeon's discretion, an anti-fibrotic agent can be applied to the scleral flap and sub-Tenon's tissue. The type, concentration, and exposure time of an anti-fibrotic agent will vary according to the patient's individual needs.

A 26–27-gauge needle is used to create an ostium into the anterior chamber under the scleral flap. This incision should be placed in the center of the blue-grey transition zone between the sclera and cornea, approximately 1–2 mm from the surgical limbus to allow scleral reinforcement for the implanted device. The needle should be passed parallel to the iris plane and aimed at the center of the pupil. This avoids the device touching the iris or corneal endothelium in a normal depth anterior chamber. Any lateral movement as the needle perforates should be avoided to minimize the risk of aqueous leak around the implant [2]. A temporal limbal paracentesis facilitates ophthalmic visco-surgical insertion into the anterior chamber and/or the placement of an anterior chamber maintainer [33].

The Ex-Press glaucoma shunt, mounted on its introducer (Fig. 18.2), is inserted tip first, on its side, into the anterior chamber, radial to the limbus and parallel to the iris, through the perforation site. The shunt should be inserted all the way into the wound until the plate is flush with the scleral bed and then rotated through 90° so the plate lies flush with the scleral bed beneath the trapdoor (Fig. 18.3). The injector is depressed to retract the wire introducer, separate the inserter from the

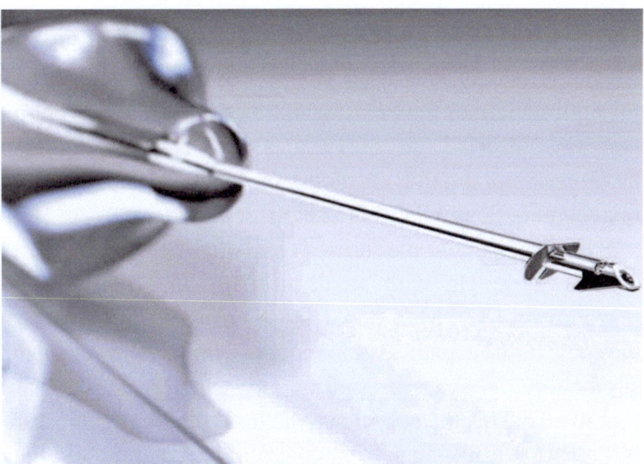

**Fig. 18.2** Ex-Press shunt mounted on wire introducer

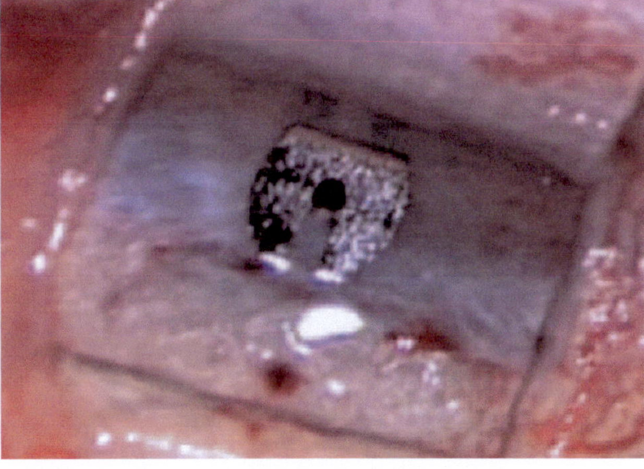

**Fig. 18.3** Appearance of Ex-Press plate flush with the scleral bed, under the trapdoor

shunt, leaving the shunt in situ [35]. The scleral flap is sutured securely with 10/0 nylon sutures to cover the flange on the Ex-Press device. As in a trabeculectomy, sutures are placed in the scleral flap according to the surgeon's preferred technique. The conjunctiva is replaced and sutured to prevent wound edge leakage.

## Modifications to Surgical Technique

Some authors have modified implantation techniques to enhance IOP reduction with the Ex-Press shunt. Mermoud described the use of a deep sclerectomy to simplify the difficult dissection of Schlemm's canal and trabeculo-Descemet's membrane [36]. He found that by performing a partial posterior deep sclerectomy and inserting an Ex-Press implant into the anterior portion under the superficial scleral flap, there were fewer postoperative complications.

In 2010 in 27 eyes, Bissig and colleagues [19] described a $4 \times 5$ mm limbus-based superficial scleral flap of 300-$\mu$m thickness and then removal of a rectangle of deep sclera ($4 \times 2 \times 0.5$ mm) in the posterior part of the scleral bed behind Schlemm's canal, taking care not to open it [19]. A 21-gauge needle was used to enter the anterior chamber, through which an Ex-Press device of 200-$\mu$m lumen diameter was inserted. At $40.1 \pm 10.8$ months post-combined Ex-Press implantation in modified deep sclerectomy with phacoemulsification, Gindroz et al. reported complete (IOP <18 mmHg without medication) and qualified success rates (IOP <18 mmHg with medication) of 45.6 and 85.2 % respectively [37]. Modified deep sclerectomy possibly creates new outflow pathways for aqueous drainage through the suprachoroidal space as well as intrasclerally and subconjunctively. This technique may be less technically demanding than the traditional non-penetrating procedure and may protect against device erosion, obstruction, or dislocation [19, 36, 37].

An Ex-Press shunt can be implanted at the same time as phacoemulsification surgery. Rivier and coworkers found a cumulative qualified success rate (IOP 6–18 mmHg with or without medication) of 53.7 % at 48 months ($p < 0.05$) [35]. Kanner and colleagues examined a further 114 eyes treated with Ex-Press implant under a scleral flap combined with phacoemulsification [38]. Their findings showed slightly worse long-term IOP control than trabeculectomy alone [38]. Three years after surgery, the authors found a surgical success (IOP 5–21 mmHg) of 95.6 % (with or without medications), with the most common device-related complication reported as tube obstruction by inflammatory matter.

## Postoperative Management

Similar to trabeculectomy, postoperative topical treatment consists of frequent steroids and a prophylactic antibiotic. Most studies advocate these drops for at least 4 weeks, with or without tapering [24, 35, 39]. Cycloplegics can also be used for anterior chamber maintenance, especially in phakic eyes [7]. On the first postoperative day, the IOP can vary widely. There have been reports of increased IOP at 2–4 weeks postimplantation [3, 4, 33, 39]. This is usually self-limiting; however, interventions such as cessation of topical steroidal agents, suture lysis, suture release, or bleb needling can be performed as required. When an Ex-Press shunt bleb is needled, the anterior chamber cannot be entered and the needle should never be passed under the scleral flap radially as there is a risk of dislodging the shunt into the anterior chamber. Instead, the needle should be passed parallel to the limbus to elevate the scleral flap, and tactile feedback permits navigation over the base of the device [40].

## Outcomes

The success rates of Ex-Press implantation in studies of greater than 20 subjects have been summarized in Table 18.1. The first publication detailing the short-term results of the Ex-Press glaucoma shunt, implanted subconjunctivally, reported a mean IOP reduction of 36 % from baseline with a 67 % probability of maintaining an IOP of 16 mmHg without medication [47]. Dahan and Carmichael pioneered the subscleral placement of the Ex-Press shunt in 2005, reporting significant reduction in IOP from $27.2 \pm 7.1$ mmHg preoperatively to $14.2 \pm 4.2$ mmHg after 24 months [11]. They found this technique of implantation to be safe with minimal side effects compared with previous reports of subconjunctival placement. Coupin and colleagues reported a short-term surgical success in 87 % of 99 eyes with an Ex-Press shunt placed under a scleral flap [48]. A longer-term study (follow-up $25.7 \pm 11.1$ months) of subscleral shunt placement found surgical success (IOP 5–21 mmHg) of 94.8 %, with a decrease in glaucoma medications from $3.7 \pm 1.0$ to $1.0 \pm 1.4$ at 42 months post-surgery [38].

De Feo and colleagues used Kaplan-Meier calculations to describe the efficacy of an Ex-Press device implanted under a scleral flap, reporting that the device maintained IOP <18 mmHg in 72.6 % of eyes and <15 mmHg in 47.9 % at 1 year, without medications [39]. Only 6 of 37 eyes (16.2 %) required glaucoma medications, a better rate than that commonly reported for trabeculectomy [39]. Ex-Press shunt implantation may transiently affect posterior corneal astigmatism, anterior chamber depth, and anterior chamber volume; however, these changes normalize by 3 months postoperatively [20].

**Table 18.1**  The success rates of Ex-Press implantation in published studies of greater than 20 subjects

| Investigator | No. eyes | Study design | Type shunt | Definition of IOP reduction success | Types of glaucoma | % success | Follow-up (months) | Significant complications |
| --- | --- | --- | --- | --- | --- | --- | --- | --- |
| Dahan Carmichael [11, 21] | 24 | Prospective | Prototype | ≥50 % | POAG (22), PXFG (2) | 41 % 1 year, 45 % 2 years | 17.8 (6.5–26) | Iris touch (1) |
| Traverso et al. [5] | 26 | Prospective multicenter | R50 | ≤21 mmHg with or without medication | POAG | 76.9 % | 23.9±10.4 | Rotation (2) Erosion (3) |
| Rivier et al. [35] | 35 | Prospective | R50 | Complete: 6–18 mmHg with no medications. Qualified: IOP 6–18 mmHG with or without medication | POAG (22), PXFG (13) | Complete: 32.7 % Qualified: 53.7 % | 36.9±18.2 | Erosion (4) |
| Maris et al. [16] | 50 | Retrospective | R50 | 5–21 mmHg with or without medication | POAG (37), PXFG (2), other (11) | 85.6 % | 10.8 (3.5–18) | Endophthalmitis (1) |
| Gallego-Pinazo et al. [41] | 20 | Prospective | R50 | 5–21 mmHg without medication | POAG (14), PXFG (6) | 90 % | 9.7 (4.5–15) | N/K |
| Kanner et al. [38] | 231 | Retrospective | T-50, R-50, X-50 | 5–21 mmHg with or without medication | POAG (157), PXFG (4), NVG (6), uveitic (11), CACG (7), other (46) | 94.8 % | 25.7±11.1 (1–46.2) | Erosion (1) Dislocation (1) |
| De Feo et al. [39] | 37 | Prospective | X-200 | <18 mmHg without medications | POAG | 78.4 % | 18 (12–24) | N/K |
| De Jong et al. [43] | 40 | Prospective Randomized | Not stated | 4–18 mmHg without medication | POAG (38), PXFG (1), other (1) | 84.6 % | 12.4±2.7 (0.3–13) | Iris touch (1) |
| Bissig et al. [19] | 26 | Prospective | X-200 | Complete: 6–18 mmHg without medication Qualified: 6–18 mmHg with or without medication | POAG (8), PXFG (7), uveitic (2), CACG (1), other (8) | Complete: 69 % Qualified: 85 % | 18.6±2.4 | N/K |
| Good and Kahook [3] | 35 | Retrospective case control series | P-50 | Complete: 5–18 mmHg and 30 % decrease without medication Qualified: 5–18 mmHg and 30 % decrease with or without medication | POAG (21), CACG (5), PXFG (5), other (4) | Unqualified: 77.14 % Qualified: 82.85 % | 28±3.2 | N/K |
| Seider et al. [44] | 36 | Retrospective | R-50 (22), X-50 (11), not stated (3) | Complete: 6–21 mmHg with no medication Qualified: 6–21 mmHg with or without medication | POAG (28), PXFG (1), CACG (1), other (6) | Complete: 48 % Qualified: 91 % | 6–12 | Hypotony (1) |
| Lankaranian et al. [17] | 100 | Retrospective | R-50, T-50 | Complete: 5–21 mmHg without medications Qualified: 5–21 mmHg with or without medications | POAG (67), CACG (13), PXFG (20) | Complete: 60 % Qualified: 24 % | 27±13.2 (12–66) | Wound leak (1) Choroidal effusion (1) |
| Marzette and Herndon [45] | 76 | Retrospective | Not stated | Complete: 5–21 mmHg without medications Qualified: 5–21 mmHg with or without medications | POAG (62), PXFG (3), other (11) | Complete: 69 % Qualified: 12 % | 9.1±3.5 | Further glaucoma surgery (8) |
| De Jong et al. [22] | 39 | Prospective Randomized | Not stated | Complete: ≤15 mmHg without medication Qualified: ≤15 mmHg with or without medication | POAG (37), PXFG (1), other (1) | Complete: 59.0 % Qualified: 92.1 % | 65.6±1.0 (62.8–78.5) | N/K |
| Gindroz et al. [37] | 24 | Prospective | LR-50 | Complete: 6–18 mmHg without medication Qualified: 6–18 mmHg with or without medication | PXFG (12), POAG (5), other (5) | Complete: 45.6 % Qualified: 85.2 % | 40.1±10.8 | Endophthalmitis (1) Macular edema (1) Late obstruction (1) |
| Dahan et al. [33] | 35 | Prospective Randomized | X-200 | Complete: 5–18 mmHg without medications Qualified: 5–18 mmHg with or without medications | POAG | Complete: 63 % Qualified: 76 % | 23.6±6.9 | N/K |
| Salim et al. [46] | 43 | Retrospective | P-50 | 5–18 mmHg without medications | POAG (26), PXFG (2), other (15) | 83.3 % | 31.9±9.8 (14.6–47) | Hypotony maculopathy (1) |

Sugiyama and colleagues published the first report on intermediate-term outcome of Ex-Press device implantation, compared with trabeculectomy in Japanese patients [4]. They found a low incidence of early postoperative complications: overall, there was no significant difference between the two procedures, although they noted a tendency for fewer postoperative glaucoma medications in the Ex-Press group [4, 16, 43]. Salim and coworkers reported a comparative case series of 36 eyes of African-Americans and 43 eyes of white Americans with the Ex-Press shunt [46]. They found similar IOP-lowering effects and complications across the two groups and concluded that the insertion of the Ex-Press glaucoma filtration device, augmented by antimetabolite use, may be a better surgical option for African-American patients than traditional trabeculectomy. This conclusion was based on the potential advantages associated with Ex-Press insertion, with reduced tissue removal, more predictable outcomes related to consistent shunt lumen size, and controlled flow that may reduce postoperative complications and overall failure rates [46].

## Comparative Outcomes

The first direct comparison of Ex-Press shunt implantation with traditional trabeculectomy was published 5 years after the release of the device [16]. Maris and coworkers retrospectively compared 100 eyes over 10.8 months post-glaucoma-filtering surgery. They found a similar reduction in IOP in both groups after 3 months with no significant difference in the number of glaucoma medications between the groups nor overall success [16]. There was a significant difference in the incidence of choroidal effusions, however, totaling 18 eyes in the trabeculectomy group versus 4 in the Ex-Press group [16]. A further retrospective comparison of the two procedures found that final IOP measurements were slightly lower after trabeculectomy compared with Ex-Press, although there were no significant differences over longer follow-up (28±3.23 months) [3].

Gallego-Pinazo and colleagues compared trabeculectomy with Ex-Press shunt implantation, with 20 eyes in each group [41]. While the mean IOP was significantly higher in the 50-μm Ex-Press group in the immediate postoperative period, complications were not significantly different. De Jong and coauthors published a prospective randomized study of 80 eyes comparing the two procedures: the Ex-Press device produced better results than trabeculectomy in all efficacy parameters, with superior IOP control maintained up to 12 months postoperatively with fewer fluctuations [43]. These results were extended over 5 years; patients with Ex-Press devices continued to require less IOP medication and fewer surgical interventions over the follow-up period [22]. Ex-Press device insertion resulted in a more significant IOP reduction over the first 3 postoperative years; however, after 4–5 years, the IOP effect of trabeculectomy matched that of Ex-Press implantation [22].

Marzette and coworkers retrospectively compared trabeculectomy and Ex-Press shunt implantation in 153 eyes: Ex-Press device use was at least as effective as standard trabeculectomy in the treatment of glaucoma [45]. Comparisons of IOP and complications were not significantly different. The first direct comparison of trabeculectomy and Ex-Press implantation in fellow eyes of the same 15 patients was published in 2012 [33]. Trabeculectomy eyes had a higher rate of postoperative complications (33 %) than did Ex-Press implants (20 %); the latter also showed a higher qualified success rate (hazard ratio 0.21, IOP 5–18 mmHg) after 30 months of follow-up [33].

## Complications

### Technique Specific

The manufacturer recommends anterior chamber filling with ophthalmic viscoelastic after insertion of an Ex-Press shunt [13]. Overfilling of the anterior chamber is the most common cause for early raised IOP. Dahan suggests that only one-third of the anterior chamber should be filled with ophthalmic viscoelastic when the R50 model is used and two-thirds for other models (P50/P200) [18]. The entire anterior chamber should be filled, however, in eyes post-vitreoretinal surgery, especially if they are aphakic [24]. In the case of IOP spike on the first day postoperatively, the anterior chamber can be decompressed manually through the limbal paracentesis.

As with any glaucoma-filtering surgery, there is a risk of subconjunctival scar formation after implantation of an Ex-Press device. Stewart and colleagues described two cases of failed implantation due to fibrosis [49]. In both cases, the implant was not removed; instead, a trabeculectomy or insertion of an alternative device was carried out with success. This complication can be minimized by the use of intraoperative MMC [30, 39]. In particular, MMC should be used in cases where filtration surgery has previously failed or in patients who have been treated long-term with maximal medical therapy [11, 39, 43].

In addition to fibrotic changes, other complications that are associated with traditional filtration surgery can occur after Ex-Press shunt implantation. These include immediate postoperative hypotony, shallow anterior chamber, hyphema, and choroidal effusions or detachment [45, 50]. They have been shown to occur at a lower rate in patients post-Ex-Press insertion, likely due to the small drainage orifice and a more controlled flow of aqueous humor [12]. Additionally, bleb-related complications such as bleb leaks, blebitis, endophthalmitis,

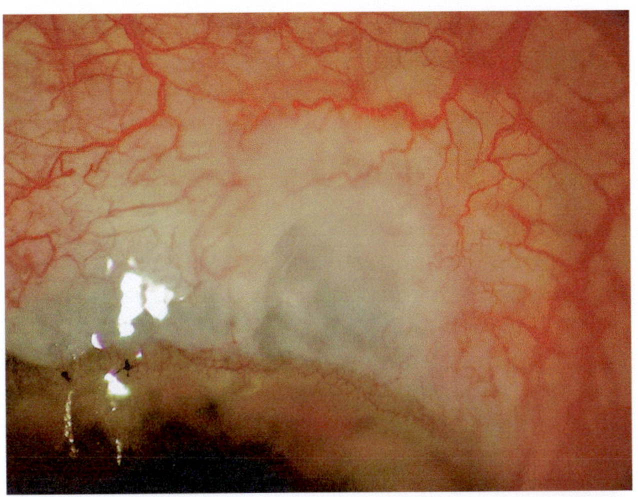

**Fig. 18.4** Failed Ex-Press shunt bleb due to conjunctival scarring

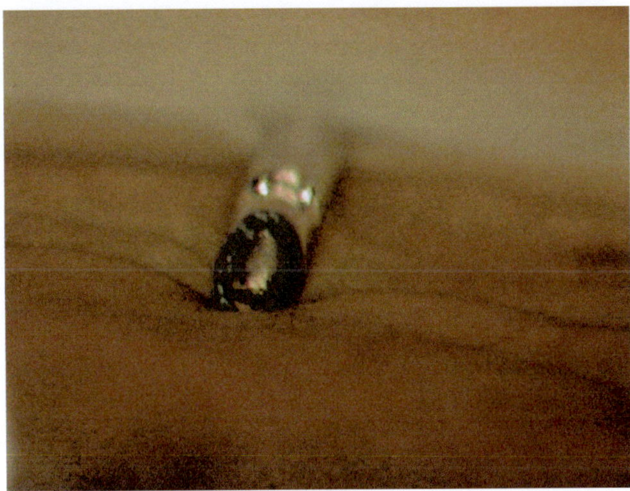

**Fig. 18.5** Gonioscopic view of Ex-Press device with implant-iris touch

bleb encapsulation, and scarring (Fig. 18.4) are not avoided [12, 37]. In general, techniques used to treat and prevent these complications in trabeculectomy can be applied to glaucoma surgery with the Ex-Press device.

Implant-iris touch can result from an insertion incision which is not parallel to the iris (Fig. 18.5). In phakic eyes, if there is a risk of iris trauma, repositioning may be necessary. In some cases, iris touch seen in the immediate postoperative period can resolve with subsequent deepening of the anterior chamber [43].

## Device Specific

The first report of Ex-Press shunt dislocation was in 2005 [51]. This followed blunt trauma to the eye: the shunt protruded through the superior limbal sclera and conjunctiva.

The authors were able to remove the device through a limbus-based conjunctival flap. The previous implantation of an Ex-Press shunt should therefore alert the clinician to confirm normal device position after ocular trauma.

A small case series highlighted the association of conjunctival erosion of an Ex-Press device and endophthalmitis, seen in one patient [49]. The manufacturer lists the prevalence of device exposure as 5.31 % for all devices and that of partial exposure as 0.88 % [13]. The prevalence of endophthalmitis is not listed in these guidelines. Several authors have suggested that spontaneous device erosion may also follow incorrect placement where the flange is not aligned completely flat against the sclera [11, 52]. The incidence of conjunctival erosion has significantly decreased with the adoption of implantation under a scleral flap, rather than beneath conjunctiva alone [11, 35]. Despite this, Ex-Press glaucoma device exposure continues to be reported, and care should be taken to ensure that the scleral flap is of adequate thickness [52, 53].

Anterior Ex-Press shunt dislocation has also been reported [54]. Teng and colleagues presented the first case report of this phenomenon and attributed the dislocation to the use of a 25-gauge needle to perforate the anterior chamber beneath the scleral flap [54]. This opening was slightly wider than the suggested 26–27-gauge tunnel, which may have allowed device migration. In addition, early bleb manipulation was required postoperatively which may have contributed to the anterior dislocation. Saricaoglu and coworkers reported a further malpositioned Ex-Press device in 2008 [55]. They found severe fibrosis at the site of implantation, which they believe led to the anterior dislocation of the device 6 months postoperatively [55].

Ex-Press tube obstruction can affect outcomes [5, 16, 35, 38]. Rivier and colleagues noted an 11.4 % rate of tube obstruction over 18 months postimplantation (in 35 eyes) [35]. A large consecutive case series of 345 implants published by Kanner in 2009 described Ex-Press luminal blockage as the most common adverse effect (1.74 % prevalence) [38]. Blockage was hypothesized to be caused by inflammatory deposits or debris; it manifested as increased IOP and a flat bleb which did not respond to laser suture lysis [38]. Kanner et al. used the neodymium:yttrium-aluminum-garnet (Nd:YAG) laser to clear material from the tip of the device in the anterior chamber [38]. This was successful in all six cases and has been reported elsewhere with similar success [38, 56].

Over time, an Ex-Press shunt may dislocate anteriorly into the corneal limbus causing device obstruction. This phenomenon was reported by Vetrugno and colleagues in 2011, and they described a technique to reposition the device [57]. The initial scleral flap is reopened by removing the sutures and searching for the previous cleavage plane. The corneal tissue covering the flange is then dissected using Vannas scissors, with the shunt manipulated and repositioned using forceps. In this case, the flange was sutured to the scleral bed with polypropylene suture. Repositioning can restore device function and preserve adjacent conjunctiva for future surgery if required [57].

## Removal of the Device

Stein and colleagues retrospectively reported eight eyes with exposed Ex-Press devices [53]. The average time to shunt exposure from time of implantation was 8.5 months (range 3–16 months). The authors describe a technique for Ex-Press shunt removal. Care must be taken to release the sharp spur and remove it through the sclera to avoid damage to surrounding tissues. The external plate should first be blunt dissected with a sharp blade. The device can then be rotated through 90° along its axis to facilitate removal. A trephine or 15° blade can be used to incise around the sclerostomy to create a narrow tract through which the miniature shunt can be removed, using anterior pressure to dislodge the spur. A scleral patch graft is overlaid and sutured with 8–0 polygalactin [53]. Grafting is important to help avoid complications such as wound leakage, hypotony, infection, and epithelial downgrowth [53]. A pre-placed paracentesis permits control of the anterior chamber volume.

If the Ex-Press device is placed too anteriorly, it may erode through the scleral flap over time or may angulate posteriorly toward the iris root due to lack of tissue support [7, 58]. The removal of an anteriorly dislocated device was described by Saricaoglu and coworkers [55]. They incised the fibrous capsule at the site of implantation and were able to view the external plate. A Y-shaped manipulator was applied under ophthalmic visco-surgical device support through a side port to the anterior chamber. The implant was then pushed toward the spur. Ophthalmic visco-surgical device was applied under the spur portion, and, with pressure at the base of the incision, the Ex-Press implant was removed [55]. A nylon suture was used to close the incision, and a traditional trabeculectomy was carried out in adjacent sclera.

## Ex-Press Shunt Imaging

Given the size and implantation location of the Ex-Press shunt, it can be difficult to visualize clinically. Verbraak and colleagues described the use of optical coherence tomography (OCT) to help localization [59]. High-resolution anterior segment OCT was able to show the exact position of the device relative to the surrounding tissues in ex vivo porcine eyes. The authors suggest that this imaging modality could be used to identify parameters or structures contributing to device failure [59].

With the increasing popularity of the Ex-Press device and thousands of implantations worldwide, there has been interest in the magnetic properties of the implant during magnetic resonance imaging (MRI) [9, 42, 60]. The initial report of MRI testing of the Ex-Press device's magnetic properties was commissioned by the original manufacturer (Optonol Ltd.); the device was suggested not to present an additional hazard or risk to a patient undergoing an MRI with a static 3 T magnetic field or less. Patients were advised to avoid MRI scanning for 2 weeks after device insertion.

De Feo and colleagues evaluated MRI images taken in patients with Ex-Press implants in situ [42]. Despite an absence of safety concerns, they did find that imaging artifacts generated by the device could potentially compromise diagnostic evaluation, particularly of the optic nerves [42]. Geffen and coauthors demonstrated movement of the Ex-Press shunt under 1.5 and 3.0 T conditions ex vivo [60]. These results were not demonstrated in vivo, where the devices showed no movement. Similarly, Seibold et al. found Ex-Press only minimal movement in the 3.0 T MRI but extreme angular deflection in the 4.7 T environment [9]. They found no evidence of temperature changes or radiofrequency heating under any MRI environment. The literature suggests that the Ex-Press glaucoma drainage device can be considered MRI safe up to 3.0 T and is weakly ferromagnetic [9, 60]. There is concern that micromovements during the early postoperative period could induce inflammation and may decrease the success of filtration surgery; therefore, MRI should be avoided in this early period [9].

## Ex-Press Use in Training

Several publications have addressed teaching Ex-Press shunt implantation, rather than trabeculectomy, to ophthalmology residents in training [40, 44, 61]. Possibly, the surgical efficacy and low rate of complications seen in comparative studies of the Ex-Press shunt may be limited to insertion by experienced practitioners [44]. Although there is no evidence of superiority of the Ex-Press shunt over trabeculectomy, it has been argued that device implantation is less technically demanding which may favor implantation by a trainee or comprehensive ophthalmologist [61]. Seider and colleagues compared the outcomes of patients undergoing Ex-Press shunt and trabeculectomy surgery performed by supervised ophthalmology residents in their third year of training [44]. In the hands of these residents, Ex-Press shunt implantation and trabeculectomy procedures performed comparably in terms of postoperative IOP control and risk of complications.

For a new procedure to replace trabeculectomy in residency training, the newer procedure must have a significant advantage in terms of success rates and/or reduction in complications [61]. If these features are equivocal, other considerations include a technically easier procedure, reduced surgical time, lower cost, or improved accessibility. While several authors have concluded that Ex-Press implantation is less technically challenging, the evidence to date does not support routine Ex-Press use by trainees [40, 61].

## Summary

Glaucoma-filtering surgery with the Ex-Press device shows potential for safe and predictable control of IOP with a side effect profile similar to that of trabeculectomy. Placed under a scleral flap, with or without concomitant phacoemulsification, this shunt has been shown to be effective for the longer-term management of open-angle glaucoma.

To date, most studies that have reported the success and efficacy of the Ex-Press shunt have been retrospective, either Ex-Press alone or combined with cataract surgery. Comparative studies are limited to only two prospective cohort studies and two prospective randomized trial comparing Ex-Press with trabeculectomy. Generally, the Ex-Press shunt at 1-year follow-up has been shown to achieve an IOP of up to 21 mmHg for 73–100 % of eyes with or without medications. Given the significant cost difference between Ex-Press implantation and standard trabeculectomy, surgeons need to weigh the perceived benefits of the device against the cost [40].

In conclusion, the Ex-Press glaucoma drainage device offers a modification of the traditional trabeculectomy technique. Most steps in the procedure are similar with the advantage of a more controlled sclerostomy and avoidance of a peripheral iridectomy. Postoperative management is similar to that of trabeculectomy; however theoretically the more controlled flow of aqueous through the shunt may provide more predictable IOP control in the immediate postoperative period. Longer-term IOP outcomes appear to be similar. The Ex-Press shunt involves initial extra cost of the device, and the cost-benefit ratio of this technology has yet to be determined. Long-term complications of dislodgement and extrusion of the prosthesis, as well as the potential effects of MRI are also concerns. Long-term studies regarding the safety and efficacy of this device will elucidate the role of these shunts in glaucoma surgery. Evolution of the device design may lead to improved clinical outcomes.

## References

1. Dahan E, de Smedt S, Garcia Feijoo J, et al. Minimally penetrating glaucoma surgery with the Ex-PRESS miniature shunt. In: Fine IH, Mojon D, editors. Minimally invasive ophthalmic surgery. Berlin: Springer; 2009. p. 172–82.
2. Sarkisian SR. The ex-press mini glaucoma shunt: technique and experience. Middle East Afr J Ophthalmol. 2009;16(3):134–7.
3. Good TJ, Kahook MY. Assessment of bleb morphologic features and postoperative outcomes after Ex-PRESS drainage device implantation versus trabeculectomy. Am J Ophthalmol. 2011;151(3):507–13.e1.
4. Sugiyama T, Shibata M, Kojima S, et al. The first report on intermediate-term outcome of Ex-PRESS glaucoma filtration device implanted under scleral flap in Japanese patients. Clin Ophthalmol. 2011;5:1063–6.
5. Traverso CE, De Feo F, Messas-Kaplan A, et al. Long term effect on IOP of a stainless steel glaucoma drainage implant (Ex-PRESS) in combined surgery with phacoemulsification. Br J Ophthalmol. 2005;89(4):425–9.
6. Estermann S, Yuttitham K, Chen JA, et al. Comparative in vitro flow study of 3 different Ex-PRESS miniature glaucoma device models. J Glaucoma. 2013;22(3):209–14.
7. Hendrick AM, Kahook MY. Ex-PRESS mini glaucoma shunt: surgical technique and review of clinical experience. Expert Rev Med Devices. 2008;5(6):673–7.
8. Francis BA, Singh K, Lin SC, et al. Novel glaucoma procedures: a report by the American Academy of Ophthalmology. Ophthalmology. 2011;118(7):1466–80.
9. Seibold LK, Rorrer RA, Kahook MY. MRI of the Ex-PRESS stainless steel glaucoma drainage device. Br J Ophthalmol. 2011;95(2):251–4.
10. Nyska A, Glovinsky Y, Belkin M, Epstein Y. Biocompatibility of the Ex-PRESS miniature glaucoma drainage implant. J Glaucoma. 2003;12(3):275–80.
11. Dahan E, Carmichael TR. Implantation of a miniature glaucoma device under a scleral flap. J Glaucoma. 2005;14(2):98–102.
12. Salim S. Ex-PRESS glaucoma filtration device-surgical technique and outcomes. Int Ophthalmol Clin. 2011;51(3):83–94.
13. Ex-press glaucoma filtration device: directions for use. Fort Worth: Alcon Laboratories, Inc. Manufacturer's instructions (unpublished).
14. Aziz H, Fantes F, Dubovy S. Histopathology of the Ex-PRESS shunt. Ophthalmic Surg Lasers Imaging. 2011;42 Online:e94–6.
15. Wamsley S, Moster MR, Rai S, et al. Results of the use of the Ex-PRESS miniature glaucoma implant in technically challenging, advanced glaucoma cases: a clinical pilot study. Am J Ophthalmol. 2004;138(6):1049–51.
16. Maris Jr PJ, Ishida K, Netland PA. Comparison of trabeculectomy with Ex-PRESS miniature glaucoma device implanted under scleral flap. J Glaucoma. 2007;16(1):14–9.
17. Lankaranian D, Razeghinejad MR, Prasad A, et al. Intermediate-term results of the Ex-PRESS miniature glaucoma implant under a scleral flap in previously operated eyes. Clin Experiment Ophthalmol. 2011;39(5):421–8.
18. Dahan E. Ex-Press miniature glaucoma implant. Expert Rev Ophthalmol. 2007;2(6):899–909.
19. Bissig A, Feusier M, Mermoud A, Roy S. Deep sclerectomy with the Ex-PRESS X-200 implant for the surgical treatment of glaucoma. Int Ophthalmol. 2010;30(6):661–8.
20. Hammel N, Lusky M, Kaiserman I, et al. Changes in anterior segment parameters after insertion of Ex-PRESS miniature glaucoma implant. J Glaucoma. 2013;22(7):565–8.
21. Dahan E, Carmichael TR. The surgical treatment of neovascular glaucoma with a 200 micron miniature glaucoma shunt. In: The association for research in vision and ophthalmology. Fort Lauderdale: Invest Ophthalmol Vis Sci; 2005. p. 77.
22. de Jong L, Lafuma A, Aguade AS, Berdeaux G. Five-year extension of a clinical trial comparing the EX-PRESS glaucoma filtration device and trabeculectomy in primary open-angle glaucoma. Clin Ophthalmol. 2011;5:527–33.
23. Elgin U, Simsek T, Batman A. Use of the ex-press miniature glaucoma implant in a child with Sturge-Weber syndrome. J Pediatr Ophthalmol Strabismus. 2007;44(4):248–50.
24. Vetrugno M, Ferreri P, Sborgia C. Ex-PRESS miniature glaucoma device in vitrectomized eyes. Eur J Ophthalmol. 2010;20(5):945–7.
25. Ates H, Palamar M, Yagci A, Egrilmez S. Evaluation of Ex-PRESS mini glaucoma shunt implantation in refractory postpenetrating keratoplasty glaucoma. J Glaucoma. 2010;19(8):556–60.
26. Yildirim N, Gursoy H, Sahin A, et al. Glaucoma after penetrating keratoplasty: incidence, risk factors, and management. J Ophthalmol. 2011;2011:951294.
27. Freedman J. What is new after 40 years of glaucoma implants. J Glaucoma. 2010;19(8):504–8.
28. Sarkisian Jr SR. Use of an injector for the Ex-PRESS mini glaucoma shunt. Ophthalmic Surg Lasers Imaging. 2007;38(5):434–6.

29. Li JY, Lim MC, Mannis MJ. Traumatic cataract associated with mini glaucoma shunt. J Cataract Refract Surg. 2011;37(7):1360–2.

30. Salim S. Current variations of glaucoma filtration surgery. Curr Opin Ophthalmol. 2012;23(2):89–95.

31. Pablo LE, Perez-Olivan S, Ferreras A, et al. Contact versus peribulbar anaesthesia in trabeculectomy: a prospective randomized clinical study. Acta Ophthalmol Scand. 2003;81(5):486–90.

32. Dahan E. Subconjunctival insertion of Ex-PRESS R-50 miniature glaucoma implant. J Cataract Refract Surg. 2008;34(5):716; author reply −7.

33. Dahan E, Ben Simon GJ, Lafuma A. Comparison of trabeculectomy and Ex-PRESS implantation in fellow eyes of the same patient: a prospective, randomised study. Eye (Lond). 2012;26(5):703–10.

34. Rouse JM, Sarkisian Jr SR. Mini-drainage devices: the Ex-PRESS mini-glaucoma device. Dev Ophthalmol. 2012;50:90–5.

35. Rivier D, Roy S, Mermoud A. Ex-PRESS R-50 miniature glaucoma implant insertion under the conjunctiva combined with cataract extraction. J Cataract Refract Surg. 2007;33(11):1946–52.

36. Mermoud A. Ex-PRESS implant. Br J Ophthalmol. 2005;89(4):396–7.

37. Gindroz F, Roy S, Mermoud A, Schnyder CC. Combined Ex-PRESS LR-50/IOL implantation in modified deep sclerectomy plus phacoemulsification for glaucoma associated with cataract. Eur J Ophthalmol. 2011;21(1):12–9.

38. Kanner EM, Netland PA, Sarkisian Jr SR, Du H. Ex-PRESS miniature glaucoma device implanted under a scleral flap alone or combined with phacoemulsification cataract surgery. J Glaucoma. 2009;18(6):488–91.

39. De Feo F, Bagnis A, Bricola G, et al. Efficacy and safety of a steel drainage device implanted under a scleral flap. Can J Ophthalmol. 2009;44(4):457–62.

40. Freidl KB, Moster MR. Express shunt surgery: preferred glaucoma surgery in residency training? Surv Ophthalmol. 2012;57(4):372–5.

41. Gallego-Pinazo R, Lopez-Sanchez E, Marin-Montiel J. Postoperative outcomes after combined glaucoma surgery. Comparison of ex-press miniature implant with standard trabeculectomy. Arch Soc Esp Oftalmol. 2009;84(6):293–7.

42. De Feo F, Roccatagliata L, Bonzano L, et al. Magnetic resonance imaging in patients implanted with Ex-PRESS stainless steel glaucoma drainage microdevice. Am J Ophthalmol. 2009;147(5):907–11. 11.e1.

43. de Jong LA. The Ex-PRESS glaucoma shunt versus trabeculectomy in open-angle glaucoma: a prospective randomized study. Adv Ther. 2009;26(3):336–45.

44. Seider MI, Rofagha S, Lin SC, Stamper RL. Resident-performed Ex-PRESS shunt implantation versus trabeculectomy. J Glaucoma. 2012;21(7):469–74.

45. Marzette L, Herndon LW. A comparison of the Ex-PRESS mini glaucoma shunt with standard trabeculectomy in the surgical treatment of glaucoma. Ophthalmic Surg Lasers Imaging. 2011;42(6):453–9.

46. Salim S, Du H, Boonyaleephan S, Wan J. Surgical outcomes of the Ex-PRESS glaucoma filtration device in African American and white glaucoma patients. Clin Ophthalmol. 2012;6:955–62.

47. Gandolfi S, Traverso CF, Bron A, et al. Short-term results of a miniature draining implant for glaucoma in combined surgery with phacoemulsification. Acta Ophthalmol Scand Suppl. 2002;236:66.

48. Coupin A, Li Q, Riss I. Ex-PRESS miniature glaucoma implant inserted under a scleral flap in open-angle glaucoma surgery: a retrospective study. J Fr Ophtalmol. 2007;30(1):18–23.

49. Stewart RM, Diamond JG, Ashmore ED, Ayyala RS. Complications following ex-press glaucoma shunt implantation. Am J Ophthalmol. 2005;140(2):340–1.

50. Mosaed S, Minckler DS. Aqueous shunts in the treatment of glaucoma. Expert Rev Med Devices. 2010;7(5):661–6.

51. Garg SJ, Kanitkar K, Weichel E, Fischer D. Trauma-induced extrusion of an Ex-PRESS glaucoma shunt presenting as an intraocular foreign body. Arch Ophthalmol. 2005;123(9):1270–2.

52. Tavolato M, Babighian S, Galan A. Spontaneous extrusion of a stainless steel glaucoma drainage implant (Ex-PRESS). Eur J Ophthalmol. 2006;16(5):753–5.

53. Stein JD, Herndon LW, Brent Bond J, Challa P. Exposure of Ex-PRESS miniature glaucoma devices: case series and technique for tube shunt removal. J Glaucoma. 2007;16(8):704–6.

54. Teng CC, Radcliffe N, Huang JE, Farris E. Ex-PRESS glaucoma shunt dislocation into the anterior chamber. J Glaucoma. 2008;17(8):687–9.

55. Saricaoglu MS, Karakurt A, Recep OF, Hasiripi H. Retrieval of a mispositioned Ex-PRESS glaucoma device. Ophthalmic Surg Lasers Imaging. 2008;39(5):404–6.

56. Bagnis A, Papadia M, Scotto R, Traverso CE. Obstruction of the Ex-PRESS miniature glaucoma device: Nd: YAG laser as a therapeutic option. J Glaucoma. 2011;20(4):271.

57. Vetrugno M, Ferreri P, Cardascia N, Sborgia C. Surgical reposition of a dislocated Ex-PRESS miniature device. Eur J Ophthalmol. 2011;21(2):212–4.

58. Gregory L, Khouri AS, Lari HB, Fechtner RD. Technique for intraoperative reuse of Ex-PRESS delivery system. J Glaucoma. 2013;22(4):e5–6.

59. Verbraak FD, de Bruin DM, Sulak M, et al. Optical coherence tomography of the Ex-PRESS miniature glaucoma implant. Lasers Med Sci. 2005;20(1):41–4.

60. Geffen N, Trope GE, Alasbali T, et al. Is the Ex-PRESS glaucoma shunt magnetic resonance imaging safe? J Glaucoma. 2010;19(2):116–8.

61. Buys YM. Trabeculectomy versus Ex-PRESS shunt surgery: preferred glaucoma surgery in residency training. Surv Ophthalmol. 2012;57(4):375–8.

Jeffrey Freedman

## The Development of the Molteno Implant

The precipitating factor for the development of the implant was an observation by Molteno, some 45 years ago, who as a resident in ophthalmology was perturbed by the poor results of traditional glaucoma procedures, at that time full-thickness thermal sclerostomies (Scheie procedures), despite a meticulous surgical technique. Furthermore when comparing the results in white and black patients, it was found that the black patients failed earlier and to a greater extent [1]. Epstein expressed a similar finding 9 years earlier, when he noted that in black patients "the results of drainage operations are strangled by the relatively rapid fibrosis that occurs." Epstein further suggested that surgical trauma condemns the operation to failure. As a result of these observations, Epstein devised an operation whereby thin polyethylene tubing was inserted from the anterior chamber to the subconjunctival space by means of a trocar both eliminating a surgical procedure and possible fibrosis of the bleb. Drainage did occur in all the patients; however, the blebs all failed within a few months due to a fibrous cap seen over the subconjunctival ends of the tubing. Epstein concluded that something in the aqueous had induced the fibrosis; the report by him in the literature was called "Fibrosing response to aqueous its relation to glaucoma" [2]. Epstein was correct in his assessment of his finding, but did not know what this substance was calling it the "Epstein factor." As will be discussed this factor(s) was destined to play a major role in the future effectiveness of glaucoma implants. Taking into account Epstein's observation, Molteno began to search for a means whereby the longevity of the bleb could be facilitated. He concluded that this "might be achieved by the use of a plastic implant designed to fit the scleral surface over a large area to prevent

shrinkage of the bleb from fibrosis" [1]. A device that would dilute the "Epstein factor", by spreading it over a large area, is a so-called "Bleb spreading device".

## Anterior Molteno Implants

The first Molteno implant was adapted for human use after testing the implant in rabbit eyes [3].

The first Molteno implants were placed anteriorly beneath the upper eyelid. The implant was made of methyl methacrylate, from a mold. The implant consisted of a translimbal tube with a length from 0.75 to 1 mm. The internal diameter was 0.75 mm. This tube was attached to a plate approximately circular in shape 8.5 mm long and wide. The anterior two thirds of the plate was facetted; thus the plate thickness varied from 0.15 mm anteriorly to 1 mm posteriorly. The plate had two suture holes placed anteriorly (Fig. 19.1). The initial implant was used mainly in cases of buphthalmos that had failed conventional therapy, aphakic glaucoma, and uveitic glaucoma [4]. A few implants were placed into patients with primary open-angle glaucoma. With the use of the initial implant, Molteno noted a constant course characterized by:

1. A stage of hypotony, lasting 10 days.
2. The hypertensive stage lasting 6–10 weeks.
3. The stable stage in which the intraocular pressure remained steady or fell slowly. This began after 8–12 weeks.

The hypertensive stage coincided with the formation of a thick-walled hyperemic bleb. Thus the early implants produced bleb pathophysiology, which has continued in all the upgraded implants that have developed over the years. The unchanged factors over the years have been the tissue and the aqueous, and thus the "Epstein factor(s)" continues to play a major role in bleb function related to implant use.

Systemic steroids were used in some of these initial implants. Prednisone 30 mg was given daily beginning 1 week after operation and was maintained in gradually diminishing dosage until the eye was completely quiet after 6–12 weeks.

J. Freedman, MBBCh, FRCS (Edin), FCS (SA)
Ophthalmology, SUNY, Downstate University Hospital,
161 Atlantic Ave, Brooklyn 11201, NY, USA
e-mail: jfreedman50@hotmail.com

J.R. Samples, I.I.K. Ahmed (eds.), *Surgical Innovations in Glaucoma*,
DOI 10.1007/978-1-4614-8348-9_19, © Springer Science+Business Media New York 2014

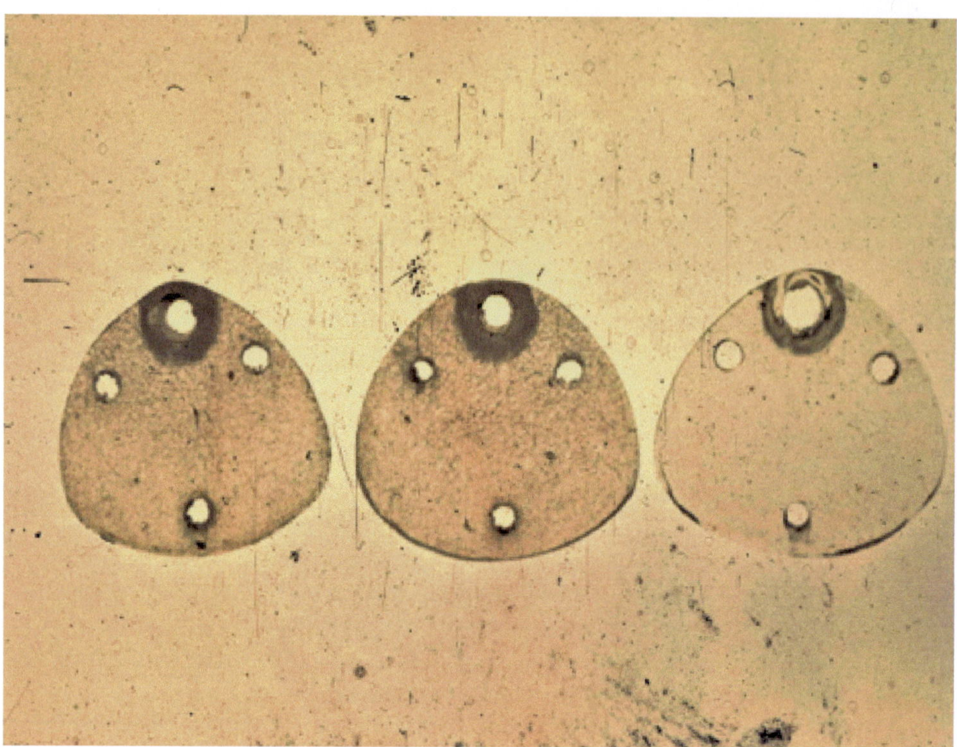

**Fig. 19.1** Original single-plate Molteno implant, 1967

Systemic steroids had a marked effect in every case giving a shorter hypertensive phase, thinner bleb, and stable intraocular pressure of between 10 and 23 mm. This observation of the use of anti-inflammatory medication was to play a much more significant role in the yet to be redesigned Molteno device. Complications of the initial implant included corneal dystrophy due to the tube as well as uveitis and discomfort from the large anteriorly situated bleb. In older patients the implant was removed usually at 3 months, or later, when the bleb was well established, to avoid the complications listed. Removal was not done in young patients as this resulted in a tendency for the bleb to fibrose. The initial implant had made headway in the treatment of refractory cases of glaucoma, and when the results obtained with the implant were compared to those of the Scheie procedure as an initial procedure, only a small difference in favor of the implant was noted. However, a marked difference in the success obtained with the implant over the Scheie was seen in secondary glaucomas, previously failed glaucoma procedures, and buphthalmic cases. The anterior implant was technically difficult to implant, had to be removed at a later date, and combined with the complications of corneal dystrophy, uveitis, and bleb dysesthesia encouraged Molteno to modify the implant. The availability of medical grade silicon and polypropylene allowed Molteno to develop the long-tube implant, which became the prototype of all the long-tube implants available today.

## Long-Tube Implants

The long-tube implant was developed because more suitable materials, polypropylene and silicone, became available. This allowed the delivery system from plate to anterior chamber to become more flexible, which in turn provided the opportunity to move the plate away from the limbal area to a more posterior location [5]. The long-tube implant plate now had a larger plate surface 13.5 mm, resulting in a larger bleb and more drainage. The polypropylene plate and the silicone delivery systems were easy to handle surgically and, more importantly, afforded the opportunity of placement in a quadrant of the eye where paralimbal surgery may not have been possible. Indeed this new design would stand the test of time and become the prototype for a new generation of long-tube implants. The development of the long-tube implant resulted in the introduction of a bleb different from those seen with standard glaucoma surgeries. The function of the tube was to deliver aqueous from the anterior chamber to the surface of the plate, situated away from the locations that had been prevalent with standard glaucoma procedures. The function of the plate was to initiate the presence of a bleb, generally as large or larger than the plate surface. This bleb would then regulate the flow of aqueous to the surrounding conjunctiva, and this in turn would be regulated by the final permeability of the fibrovascular lining of the bleb wall. The implant thus now became simply a conduit for delivering aqueous from the anterior chamber to the subconjunctival space, and the process of bleb formation, as well as surgical aspects related to the implant itself, would become the important aspects which would drive the search for mechanisms to improve the function of these new glaucoma implants. Molteno predominantly, and other researchers to a lesser extent, would become involved in the further evolution of Molteno's discovery.

Molteno made the observation that the bleb formed around the implant depended on the age of the patient and to some degree on the severity of the glaucoma, in particular to the level of the intraocular pressure immediately prior to inserting the implant [6]. Infants and elderly patients form thin-walled blebs, which function well. Older children and fit young adults were found to produce a series of changes in the blebs after implant surgery, which often led to the formation of a fibrosed bleb. Based on these observations Molteno began extensive research on the pathophysiology of the blebs and discovered that the changes that accompany formation of a bleb over an implant can be named according to the intraocular pressure within the eye, at that particular stage of bleb formation [6].

The initial stage of bleb formation is the hypotensive stage, lasting approximately 7–10 days, and is characterized by vascular congestion and edema of the tissues over the plate. This is followed by a period of steadily rising pressure, disappearance of the edema, and the formation of the bleb itself. About 4–6 weeks after implant insertion, the blood vessels over the bleb become congested, and the intraocular pressure rises to usher in the hypertensive phase. This phase lasts from 2 to 4 weeks after which time the bleb becomes less congested; the pressure falls until a stable plateau is reached about 3–6 months after implant insertion. This results in the stable stage, hopefully remaining for the rest of the patient's life.

Two major problems associated with the use of the long-tube implants were immediate postoperative hypotony and the development of bleb fibrosis as mentioned in some patients. Methods for dealing with these two problems therefore required solutions.

of the conjunctiva in the area of the plate, consisting of decreasing the size of the dissection in the area of plate deposition, by inserting a single Weck-Cel sponge into the area to accomplish the dissection, rather than utilizing scissors to dissect a much larger space [7]. This technique did help to limit postoperative flow into the surrounding tissue, thereby decreasing the potential for shallow or flat anterior chambers but was by no means ideal.

Molteno developed a two-stage procedure for use in those patients where medical control of intraocular pressure was sufficient to allow the eye to tolerate a delay of 5 weeks prior to allowing aqueous to reach the plate surface [8]. This technique consisted of inserting the implant rather than connecting the tube to the anterior chamber, to place it beneath a rectus muscle but to connect it to the anterior chamber at a second operation 5–6 weeks later when a sufficient capsule had developed over the plate, thereby preventing postoperative hypotony. This procedure, although effective, required two surgeries and was replaced by the "vicryl tie" procedure [9]. Herein the tube was constricted by placing a 5-0 vicryl suture tightly around the tube prior to inserting it into the anterior chamber at the time of implant insertion. This resulted in delaying aqueous access to the plate surface for 3–5 weeks, the usual time taken for dissolution of the suture, at which time a sufficient capsule had developed over the plate, once again preventing excessive hypotony.

The ability to control postoperative hypotony allowed Molteno to increase the drainage area by introducing a multiple plate system. The concept being if one plate lowers pressure, then surely two or more plates will multiply the pressure-lowering effect. Molteno tried using as many as four plates, one in each eye quadrant, but found that one or two were sufficient. The introduction of the double-plate implant would usher in a phase of glaucoma implant development which would change the thinking related to glaucoma implants, resulting in the development of different implants, a process that is still continuing, and revert to the all important pathophysiology of bleb formation and its importance [10].

## Control of Hypotony in the Immediate Postoperative Period

In the beginning the single-plate implant was used without restricting flow to the surface of the plate. Shallow to flat anterior chambers were the norm in the postoperative period. Homeostasis of aqueous flow usually took 10–14 days, after which, due to early capsule development over the plate, the anterior chamber began to reform. The earliest attempt at restricting aqueous flow was a modification of the dissection

## The Influence of the Double-Plate Molteno Implant on Glaucoma Implant Research and Development

The double-plate implant consisted of two single plates joined together by a silicone tube. Aqueous would therefore pass from the surface of one plate to the other plate, and this flow could be restricted by placing a vicryl suture around the connecting tube, thereby restricting flow until a sufficient capsule had formed over the second plate. A major problem

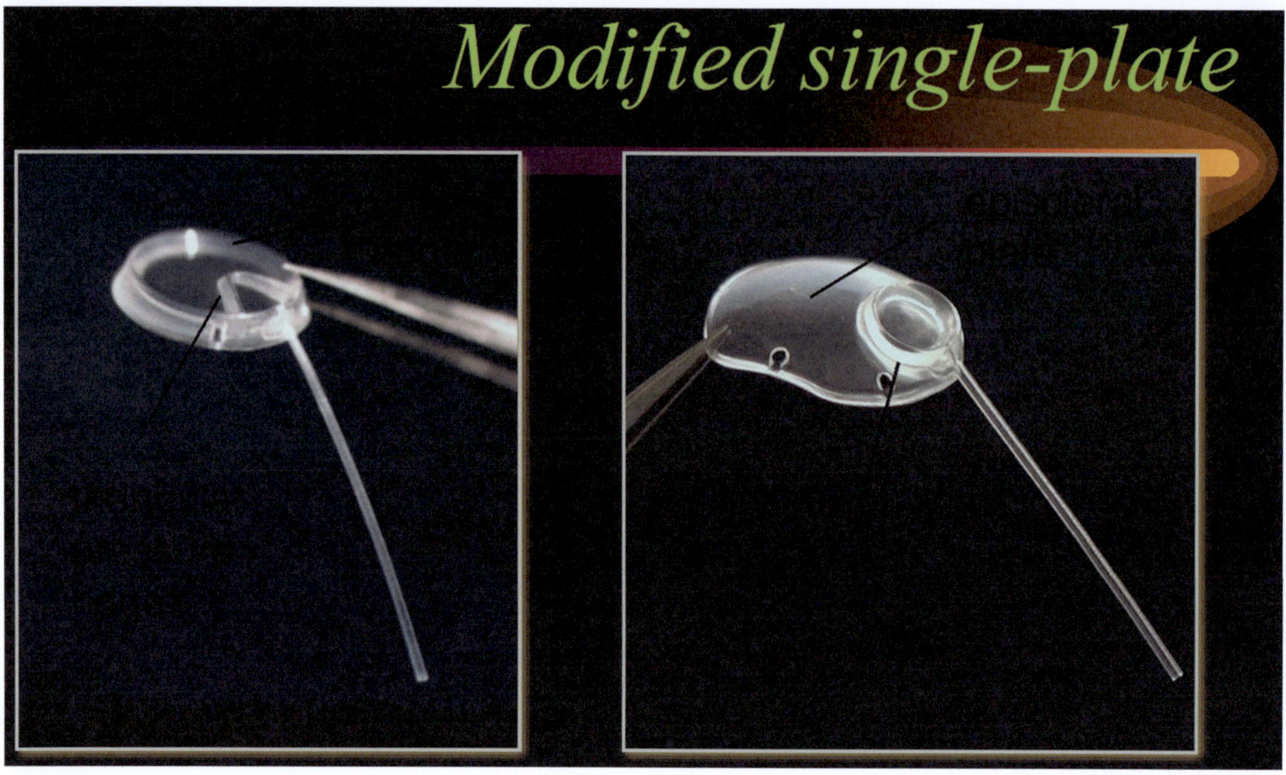


**Fig. 19.2** Dual chamber Molteno3 implant

with the double-plate implant was the need to isolate the superior rectus muscle, allowing placement of the second plate beneath the muscle into the adjacent eye quadrant. This technique was that used by Molteno and by most surgeons using double-plate implants. This procedure was complicated and time consuming. Placement over the muscle, which was much easier and just as effective, was suggested, but most surgeons continued to use the standard "under" the muscle technique. The first Molteno implant was inserted into an eye in the USA by the author who was a resident with Molteno. Molteno mailed this implant to the author, with instructions on its use. The author subsequently mailed an implant to Baerveldt, also with instructions on its use. A study published by the doctors working with Baerveldt concluded that the two-plate implant was better in intraocular pressure control than the single plate, and therefore this implant became the implant of choice when glaucoma implants were chosen [11]. The surgical difficulty of placing the second implant persisted. Baerveldt concluded that a single-plate implant, with at least the surface area of the double plate or larger, would be more practical and could be placed into a single quadrant. Thus the Baerveldt implant came into being. The single-plate implant would subsequently become the future of all glaucoma implants, including the Molteno implant.

The problem of hypotony with the introduction of larger single-plate implants became more important. Control of hypotony resulted in further developmental advances in design of implants as well as in surgical innovations.

Molteno developed the dual chamber implant, prior to the introduction of the Baerveldt implant [12, 13] (Fig. 19.2). This implant was available in both a single- and double-plate model.

The dual chamber implant is placed with the anterior edge of its plate in line with the insertion of the rectus muscles. This allows Tenon's capsule to be pulled tightly over the anterior situated chamber, which has a posterior pressure ridge. This pressure ridge when covered by Tenon's capsule acts as a pressure-sensitive valve which regulates the flow of fluid into the main bleb cavity. The intraocular pressure at which aqueous flows into the main chamber depends on the tension of the Tenon's capsule over the anterior chamber as well as the swelling of covering tissue in the postoperative period. The pressure ridge needs to be of sufficient height to produce this valve action. The swelling of the tissue decreases allowing a bleb to form over the anterior chamber, as a capsule has developed enclosing the space. This prevents flow into the second chamber and prevents hypotony. As the intraocular pressure increases, the aqueous will flow over the ridge into the main chamber maintaining a low intraocular pressure. The dual chamber implant will not function as a valve unless it is used as Molteno suggested, which is by pulling Tenon's tightly over the ridge and suturing it to the muscle insertion. Without this technique the dual ridge implant acts as a non-dual chamber device. The pressure at which aqueous flows across the pressure ridge depends on the turgor and elasticity of the overlying tissue. Molteno has found that irrespective of variation in tissue over the chamber, that pressure during the first postoperative week is maintained at 6–22 mmHg.

The advantage of the dual ridge valve is that it can clear itself rapidly after blockage by inflammatory exudate or solid blood clot. Unfortunately the dual ridge implant had not been used as proposed by Molteno, resulting in the search for a different valve mechanism leading to the development of the Ahmed implant, with its pressure-sensitive valve. The Ahmed implant differed from the Molteno implants in that it was a single-quadrant larger single plate with a valve mechanism [14]. Double-plate Ahmed implants were introduced at a later date.

The Baerveldt implant required a mechanism to prevent postoperative hypotony, as did all the Molteno implants including the dual chamber implant, the latter due to the failure in adopting the correct means of insertion of the implant. Use of intraluminal stents and tubal occlusion with circumferential sutures became the usual means of hypotony control. The tying off of tubes required a mechanism to relieve postoperative increases in pressure, prior to tube opening. Sherwood suggested making a relieving slit in the tube anterior to the area of occlusion, allowing aqueous to escape into the tissue surrounding the tube, lowering the intraocular pressure [15] (Fig. 19.3). This slit needs to be made on the lateral side of the tube to prevent occlusion of the overlying patch material. As a result of the restriction of aqueous flow to the plate surface until pressure had normalized in the eye, it became apparent that the hypertensive phase, as described previously, became less marked and often did not occur at all. This phenomenon appeared to be due to a decrease in the

release of proinflammatory substances to the plate surface, as will be explained later in the chapter. The discovery that double plates had a better pressure-lowering potential than single-plate implants, as pointed out earlier, led to the concept that bigger is better. This in turn resulted in the development of large single-plate implants, with different sizes available in the Molteno and Baerveldt groups. However with further studies relating to the efficacy of size, it became apparent that beyond a size equivalent to the 300 mm Baerveldt, that additional pressure lowering was minimal if at all present [16]. The single-plate implants used most frequently at the present time include the single-plate Molteno3 implants 175 and 230 mm$^2$, the Baerveldt implant 250 and 350 mm$^2$, and the Ahmed and Krupin implants both 184 mm$^2$. A newer single-plate Molteno implant, a modified Molteno3, will be described later (Fig. 19.4). Very little additional pressure lowering is obtained with implants larger than 175 mm$^2$. The introduction of the single-plate larger-size implants has made the surgical procedure easier, as well as freeing up an additional superior quadrant should an additional implant be required.

The introduction of delayed release of aqueous to the plate surface was observed to result in a less intensive tissue reaction over the plate, especially if the intraocular pressure was elevated. Molteno made the observation that the intensity of the inflammation depended on the patient's age and the intensity of the glaucoma. The immediate release of aqueous onto the plate surface in the presence of high IOP resulted in a more fibrosed and less efficient bleb. This reaction occurs as a result of the passage of proinflammatory cytokines present in glaucomatous aqueous. In infants and the elderly, without severe glaucoma, the tube opening is followed by low-normal IOP and 3–4 weeks later moderately elevated IOP. In severe glaucoma and young healthy patients, the pressure rises sooner and is higher with a more marked inflammatory reaction over the plate. Molteno found that in these patients, this reaction and the hypertensive phase could be modified with the use of anti-fibrosis systemic medication.

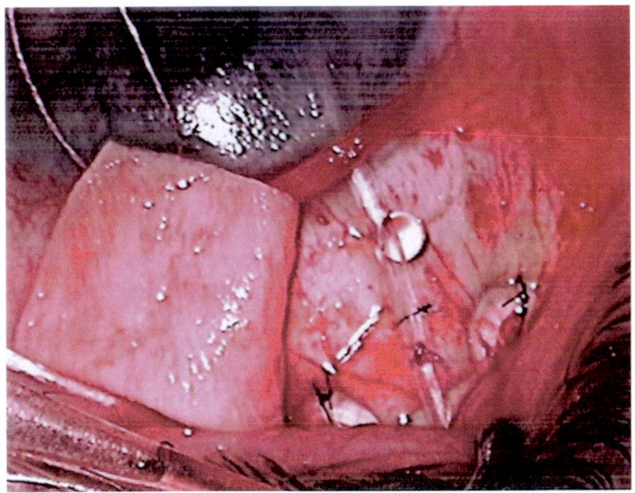

**Fig. 19.3** Aqueous bubble exiting anterior chamber via Sherwood slit in silicone tube

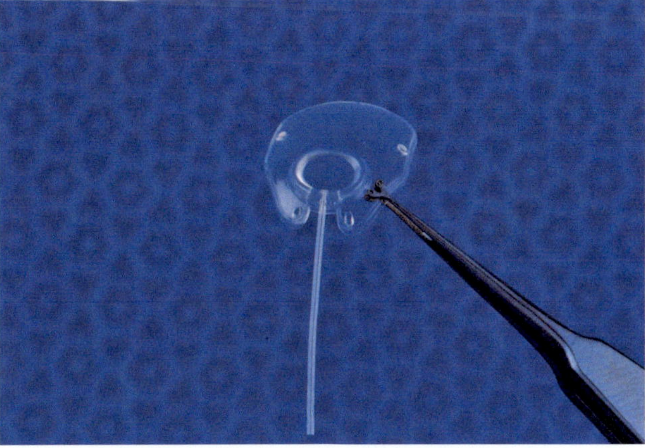

**Fig. 19.4** Molteno3 with low ridge and anteriorly placed suture holes

## The Control of Postoperative Inflammation and the Hypertensive Phase of the Bleb

Molteno found that the use of a systemic combination of drugs, comprising steroids, nonsteroidal anti-inflammatories, and colchicine, given in combination, reduced postoperative inflammation [6]. Furthermore the additional use of topically applied epinephrine and atropine had an additive effect. According to Molteno the medication should not be given prior to the flow of aqueous onto the plate surface as this will prevent the formation of a preformed bleb lining, resulting in increased hypotony after the tube opens. The use of Molteno's anti-fibrosis drug regimen, albeit effective, has not been adopted universally. The reason for this is that the drugs need to be taken within 4–5 days after the operation and continued usually for a period of 6 weeks. There are multiple side effects related to their use, and often the patients need to be hospitalized in order to be monitored, an impractical situation in many countries.

Maintaining a low IOP after the tube opens will result in a more functional bleb. This can be achieved with the use of hypotensive medications used from the time of implant insertion for 12 weeks, a period that will include the hypertensive phase. An alternative method has been introduced to treat the hypertensive phase, consisting of removing aqueous from the bleb, using a 30-gauge needle, a procedure that can be done in the office and which can be repeated weekly or less frequently until the stable stage of the bleb is reached [17]. The use of this technique has resulted in the development of thinner and more functional blebs. Aqueous removed from blebs during the hypertensive phase has been shown to contain cytokines, namely, TGFβ (transforming growth factor beta) and PGE2 (prostaglandin E2) [18]. Recent research has discovered additional cytokines in glaucomatous aqueous, the most consistent being interleukin-8 and monocyte chemotactic protein (MCP-1 and MCP-2), all of which are proinflammatory (current research to be published). Therefore tapping the bleb not only lowers the IOP but also at the same time removes these proinflammatory products resulting in less postoperative inflammation and subsequently thinner and more functional blebs.

Clinical observation, relating to the effect of the hypertensive phase of the bleb, has indicated that a hypertensive phase in which the pressure is very high and prolonged will result in a final bleb with a thicker lining rendering it less effective. Another observation made is that the hypertensive phase is more marked if the aqueous is allowed to reach the plate surface at the time of surgery [19]. As previously stated, "glaucomatous aqueous" has been shown to contain proinflammatory cytokines, which will result in an early intense inflammatory reaction over the plate producing an inflamed bleb wall, which in turn results in a more intense hypertensive phase. Preventing aqueous from reaching the plate surface, until the IOP has been lowered and thereby containing less cytokines, has proven to decrease the intensity of the inflammatory reaction over the plate as well as a less intense hypertensive phase.

## Development of Ancillary Methods for Bleb Fibrosis Control

The understanding of bleb physiology has resulted in the development of ancillary methods for bleb fibrosis control. The implant per se only really acts as a conduit for transporting aqueous from the anterior chamber to the subconjunctival space as has been previously mentioned. The main factors involved in bleb formation are the aqueous and the tissue over the plate. The initial aqueous is proinflammatory due to its contents of cytokines, and the tissue, most specifically Tenon's capsule, contains the messenger RNA (mRNA) for tumor necrosis factor-beta (TGFβ), a proinflammatory cytokine [20]. Controlling aqueous flow to the plate and manipulating Tenon's capsule or a combination of both was thought to offer promise in the control of bleb fibrosis.

Preventing aqueous from reaching the plate surface in non-valved implants is accomplished by tubal occlusion as has been described. Prior to this technique Molteno utilized a two-stage procedure to prevent aqueous flow to the plate. Following placement of the implant, the tube was not introduced into the eye, but only done so 6 weeks later when a thin fibrous capsule had developed over the plate. This technique was associated with actively lowering the IOP as much as possible with medications, so that when the tube was finally introduced into the eye, the IOP was lower than the IOP at the original surgery, thereby lowering cytokine levels and thus the fibrotic potential of the aqueous. Because the two-stage procedure was originally designed to prevent postoperative hypotony, with the advent of the vicryl tie method, this technique was abandoned by Molteno. However it also led to the development of the dual chamber implant. Although developed to control hypotony as previously explained, the dual chamber implant also prevented the flow of aqueous to the second chamber, and this occurred usually after the IOP had been lowered by its isolation in the anterior chamber and subsequent formation of a draining bleb over this chamber, before allowing flow to the main plate surface. This resulted in a different type of aqueous flowing onto the plate, one with less cytokines, resulting in the formation of a thinner and more efficient bleb. Molteno has demonstrated this occurrence with histology gleaned from a postmortem eye (Fig. 19.5).

Removal of Tenon's capsule has been described associated with standard glaucoma procedures with good results regarding improvement of bleb function [21]. The manipulation of Tenon's capsule with glaucoma implant surgery was introduced some 20 years ago. This method consists of the fashioning of a pocket between the conjunctiva and Tenon's

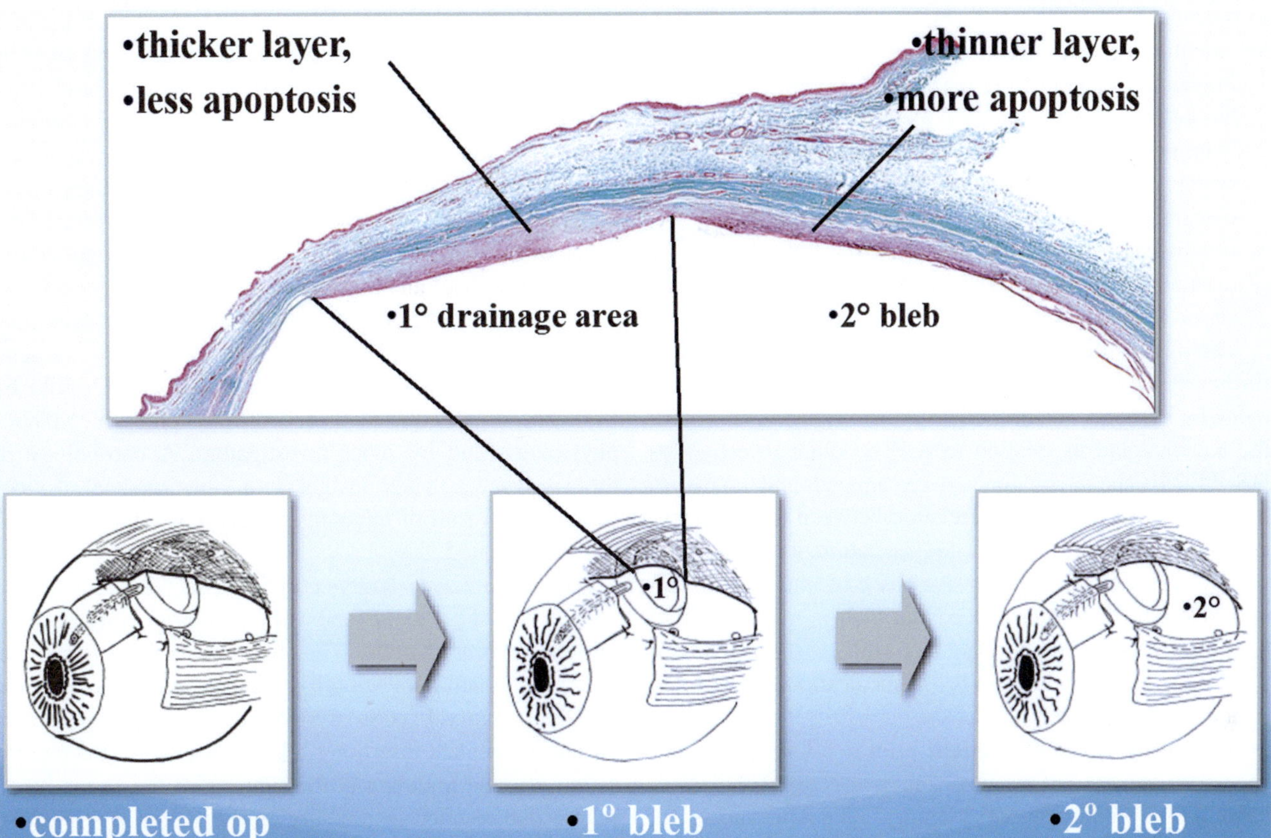



**Fig. 19.5** Histology of bleb over dual chamber Molteno implant, showing thick bleb reacting to initial cytokine aqueous over anterior plate chamber and thin bleb over plate when IOP is lower and cytokine content has decreased

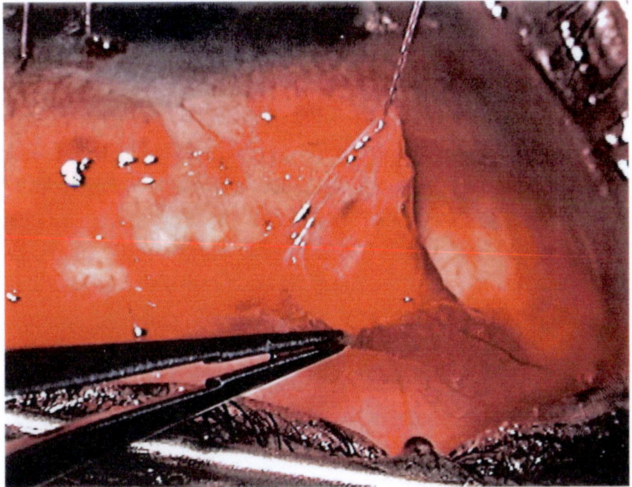

**Fig. 19.6** Pocket between Tenon's capsule anteriorly and conjunctiva posteriorly for insertion of supra-Tenon implant

capsule into which the implant was placed (Fig. 19.6). The technique has been described. The thought behind this procedure was twofold: firstly to decrease the thickness of the tissue forming the bleb capsule, comprised mainly of Tenon's capsule, and secondly to remove a potent source for the pro-inflammatory cytokine TGFβ, whose mRNA has been shown to reside in Tenon's capsule. Clinically this method has proven to be effective in refractory glaucoma case [22, 23]. The procedure was initially done with the original single-plate Molteno implant and subsequently with the larger Molteno3 implant which also has an anterior ridge forming a dual chamber. This ridge became a problem when used for supra-Tenon placement of the implant, as the thinning of the covering tissue led to erosions over the ridge necessitating removal of the implant. At the request of the author, Molteno agreed to lower the ridge and as an adjunct to this modification also moved the suture holes anteriorly, resulting in the development of a modified Molteno3 implant. Although specifically designed for supra-Tenon placement, the modified Molteno3 has become popularized for use in standard implant procedures as well.

The understanding of bleb physiology, as well as techniques described to assist in decreasing bleb fibrosis, suggests a template for managing bleb fibrosis which can be summarized in the following paragraphs.

Raised IOP results in the production of proinflammatory substances consisting predominantly of cytokines. Methods to prevent these cytokines from reaching the plate surface include the following:

1. Preventing aqueous from reaching plate surface until IOP has been lowered by medical therapy.
2. If immediate IOP lowering cannot be accomplished, use systemic anti-fibrosis medical regime as soon as aqueous reaches plate surface.
3. If fibrosis still occurs with the above methodology, the tissue may be manipulated by placing the implant into a supra-Tenon pocket.

The interaction between aqueous and the tissue has been further defined by the histological findings of bleb development, by Molteno, and the defining of the cytokine content of the aqueous and its relation to IOP, by other investigators [18, 24, 25]. The interaction between aqueous and the tissues has shown that there is a correlation between the hypertensive phase of bleb physiology and the nature of the final bleb function. Should the hypertensive phase be intense, not well controlled, and prolonged, the final bleb is more likely to have a thick poorly functioning bleb wall.

The use of systemic anti-fibrosis medication will result in a more successful bleb.

The ability to control the IOP, prior to allowing aqueous access to the plate surface, results in an aqueous with a lower content of proinflammatory cytokines and a more successful bleb. A further observation has been that prolonged normalization of the IOP in the postoperative period will enhance the success of the bleb. Elevation of IOP in the bleb has been shown to be associated with higher levels of proinflammatory cytokines, which in turn increases inflammation in the bleb resulting in bleb wall fibrosis.

Molteno has explained bleb behavior of bleb tissue around implants. He suggests that in cases of severe glaucoma, there is impairment of blood supply, resulting in the production within the eye of "metabolites" which are shed into the aqueous. These "metabolites" have been identified as proinflammatory cytokines, the main one being TFGβ. The cytokines cause marked inflammation in the episcleral tissue overlying the implant plate. The levels of cytokines are proportional to the severity of the glaucoma, more specifically to the height of the IOP. Higher IOP results in increased cytokine levels [18]. This would account for the observations that control of IOP prior to allowing aqueous to reach the plate surface results in less fibrotic blebs, as does control of the hypertensive phase of bleb development. The inflammatory response varies with individual patients; nonetheless there does appear to be a decrease of both the inflammatory response and fibrous tissue deposition with increasing age, that is elderly patients, as well as with infants in the first few years of life. The stable bleb that occurs with normalization of IOP shows a loss of fibroblasts with

degeneration and fragmentation and disappearance of collagen fibrils, as reported by Teng Chi and Katzin [26]. These changes are largely confined to approximately the inner half of the bleb wall and may reflect the fact that aqueous is being removed by a network of small vessels in the inner bleb wall. These changes may be occurring due to the loss of the effect of the cytokines in the aqueous.

Based on Molteno's original implants, changes have evolved, leading to physical changes in implant design and the application of additional surgical techniques utilized in present-day glaucoma implants.

Many of the aspects relating to present-day long-tube glaucoma implants have evolved directly from the Molteno implant and have done so as a result of research both by Molteno, in particular his excellent research on bleb pathophysiology, and by other investigators. A chronology of these advances lends insight into how medical devices change as a result of ongoing research once the initial seed has been planted.

Molteno utilized a lamellar scleral dissection to form a flap under which the silicone tube was placed prior to its insertion into the anterior chamber. The elimination of this technique, by the introduction of the full-thickness donor scleral patch, was the first modification of Molteno's original surgical procedure for implant insertion [27]. The reason for the modification was the finding that the suturing of the fornix-based scleral flap resulted in pressure on the posterior end of the tube pushing the intraocular distal end close to the cornea. Furthermore as the original scleral flap was lamellar, it was thin and led at times to erosion of the tube. Based on these observations it made sense to try and cover the tube with full-thickness sclera as this would allow the anterior part of the tube to follow the contour of the globe and therefore on insertion into the eye actually be deflected away from the cornea. The full-thickness sclera would also be less likely to erode. Molteno continued to use his lamellar technique, but at times would place a full scleral patch over the lamellar technique. Interestingly at the present time the use of the combined technique has been adopted by other surgeons and may be the best way to avoid later tube erosion. The subsequent use of different materials to cover the tube has been introduced to include the dura [28], pericardium, artificial collagen, and cornea. A technique has been described for handling the tube without a lamellar scleral dissection, nor the use of a covering patch. This technique consists of the use of a long episcleral 23-gauge needle track for introducing the tube into the eye [29]. The reason given for using this technique is that the tight fit around the tube, by preventing lateral movements around the tube, decreases the supposed trauma which may be the reason for the erosion seen with the patch and lamellar dissection. Nonetheless erosion has also been reported associated with this track method of tube coverage.

The problem of hypotony, as described, resulted in the development of the valved implant and the process of tubal occlusion by internal and external suture techniques.

The pressure ridge Molteno implant, although at present utilized in routine implant surgery, was to a large extent developed for use in neovascular glaucoma. Neovascular glaucoma commonly presents with very high IOP, requiring immediate pressure lowering. A "valve" of sorts needed to be developed. The subsidiary ridge of the pressure ridge implant acts as a pressure-sensitive valve limiting postoperative hypotony, but only when inserted according to the method described by Molteno as previously indicated.

Although there is still limited use of double-plate implants today, the present trend is for the use of single-plate implants. This has led to the development of larger-size single-plate implants as seen in all of the implants in use today. Clinical studies regarding the effect of plate size has led to the change from double-plate to larger single-plate use. These studies have shown that although larger-sized plates do have a pressure-lowering advantage, this increase in plate size is not exponential, and the ideal plate size lies probably between 175 and 250 mm. Experiments have shown that by increasing the internal radius of the bleb, the surface tension increases, Laplace's law, causing bleb fibrosis and capsule thickening, thereby decreasing the efficiency of the bleb [30]. Additionally the surgical advantages of single-plate use, which include ease of insertion, and single-quadrant use have also contributed to the change from double-plate use.

## The Changes in Glaucoma Implant Use

Molteno originally suggested a template for the use of Molteno implants, and this template affords a review of changes that have taken place in implant use.

The Molteno template concerns use of single- and double-plate implants. The decision as to which model to use was based on the area of bleb required for long-term control of IOP. This decision has largely been eliminated now by the introduction of large single-plate implants. However, the following concept elucidated by Molteno may still be in effect with very large models of single-plate implants. Molteno suggested that the ciliary body function was of importance in deciding single or double plates and therefore by inference, smaller or larger single-plate implants. Where ciliary body function is impaired, the template suggests use of a single plate as excessive drainage in these eyes, by double plates or very large single plates, could result in excessive hypotony. The following have been suggested as possible causes for decreased aqueous production: older and frail patients, previous cyclodestructive

procedures, intraocular inflammation, and advanced vascular disease. Clinical signs suggestive of poor aqueous production include advanced glaucomatous changes in the absence of raised IOP, the presence of iris neovascularization, and evidence of carotid stenosis. Much of this part of the template can be ignored today as even the smallest size single plate is usually sufficient to obtain the necessary lowering of IOP, and if not, a second plate can be inserted into the unused quadrant of the eye.

The template suggested a two-stage procedure, where medical control was good enough to tolerate a delay of up to 5 weeks, before drainage is established. This technique had the advantage of reducing the amount of fibrous tissue in the bleb wall. This also has been eliminated by the stent and vicryl occlusion method. However, the introduction of the valved implant negates the advantage obtained by utilizing this method of delayed bleb formation. The template suggested the use of the pressure ridge implant for treating neovascular glaucoma. The larger Molteno implants, apart from the newest modified Molteno3, can still be used for this purpose. For the treatment of neovascular glaucoma, a valved implant does have an advantage. Non-valved implants may be used, even in the presence of a dual chamber, by ignoring the dual chamber and using an occlusive technique on the tube, with the addition of the relieving slit technique.

The template advocated by Molteno was specifically for the use of Molteno implants. With the subsequent introduction of different glaucoma implants, has the template remained the same, have there been changes, and what influence has the template had on our current use of glaucoma implants today? The template for present-day glaucoma implants incorporates many of the features introduced by Molteno, with, perhaps, one very significant change, that being the question of which implant is the most efficient in reducing IOP. Comparative studies involving the three most commonly used implants, Molteno, Baerveldt, and Ahmed, in different computations and performed by independent investigators, as well as in multicenter, randomized clinical trials, have in general indicated that no implant demonstrates a marked superiority in IOP control. The original concept of plate size being important has largely been negated by the use of large single-plate implants, available in all three implants.

The use of the different implants depends mainly on factors that have to do with ease of surgical implantation, postoperative management, and lack of complications, with the assumption that all lower the IOP similarly. However, studies comparing valved to non-valved implants have shown that the pressure-lowering ability of non-valved implants does have a better IOP-lowering ability in the long term, albeit minimal.

The newer implants are all based on the original long-tube implant of Molteno. The modifications incorporated into the Ahmed and Baerveldt implants were done predominantly to facilitate surgical implantation.

## Changes Incorporated to Facilitate Surgical Implantation

The introduction of a large single-plate Baerveldt implant, and later the large single-plate Ahmed implant, essentially improved on the difficulty associated with inserting the double-plate implant requiring two-quadrant placement. Molteno has subsequently followed this change by introducing large single-plate Molteno implants. The placement of the anterior suture holes in the original small and subsequently larger Molteno3 implant was specifically situated in a posterior position, to facilitate the suturing of the implant adjacent to the insertions of the recti muscles, which placed the bulk of the implant plate at the equator. With the introduction of the dual ridge implant, the placement of these suture holes became even more important, allowing Tenon's capsule to be pulled tightly over the ridge, thereby isolating the anterior small chamber. This was accomplished by suturing Tenon's to the muscle insertions. The difficulty presented by these posterior suture hole placements resulted in many surgeons changing to either Baerveldt or Ahmed implants with their anterior suture hole placement. The recently introduced modified Molteno3 has anteriorly placed suture holes for the previously described reasons. Thus the placement of the suture holes in an anterior position, in all commonly used implants, has been a modification that has significantly improved the ease of insertion.

The original Molteno implant plates consist of polypropylene, a hard and relatively inflexible material. The Baerveldt and some Ahmed implants are made of silicone, a slightly more flexible and therefore easier material to handle surgically. An additional modification of the Baerveldt implant is the low profile, again facilitating ease of insertion. Modified Molteno3 implants now also are more flexible, being thinner, more curved to follow the contour of the globe, and made of a different polypropylene.

The introduction of a valve system in the Ahmed implant resulted in the ability to avoid postoperative hypotony, a major problem previously confronted with implant use. Other methods for preventing postoperative hypotony have also been instituted as mentioned, consisting of tubal occlusion and the use of the dual chamber Molteno implants in a manner described by Molteno. Although most of the modifications associated with further developments in long-tube implants have been advantageous, there also have been some deleterious effects.

## Adverse Effects Associated with Long-Tube Glaucoma Implant Modifications

The utilization of the muscles for implantation of the Baerveldt implant, as well as the increase in size and thereby the height of the bleb, has been associated with diplopia [31]. Further modification, being introduction of holes into the plate, was instituted to decrease this complication. The holes allowed the plate to be more firmly attached to the underlying sclera by fibrous tissue growth through them, thus lowering the plate profile.

The use of a valved implant resulted in early access of "glaucomatous" aqueous to the plate surface, which resulted in a more severe hypertensive phase and consequently a more fibrosed and less efficient bleb.

The introduction of an external material to cover the external portion of the silicone tube has not proven to be fail-safe in preventing erosion and tube exposure. The cure for these tubal exposures has proven to be challenging. Reverting to a combination of a lamellar scleral flap, in addition to a superimposed patch, may be an option to preventing tubal exposure. The nature of the silicone tubing has remained unchanged since the inception of long-tube implants, apart from the final location within the eye. Tubes are now placed into the anterior chamber, the sulcus, retrolenticular in pseudophakia, and the vitreous chamber, after total vitrectomy. The effect of anterior chamber tubes on endothelial health has been a concern, but no prospective, comparative study has been done to confirm the deleterious effect of tubes on the endothelium. Localized endothelial tube touch may result in local corneal decompensation, but whether this will routinely produce diffuse corneal decompensation has not been determined.

## What Is the Status of Glaucoma Implant Use at the Present Time?

Glaucoma implant use has increased exponentially since the introduction of the Molteno long-tube implant 40 years ago. A report on the use of various glaucoma surgeries specifically on Medicare patients in the USA indicated a 184 % increase in the number of tube-shunt procedures and a concurrent 43 % decrease in trabeculectomies performed between 1995 and 2004 [32]. Practice patterns in glaucoma surgery reported by the American Glaucoma Society, gleaned from a survey of its members, indicated that the selection of tube implants as the preferred surgical approach increased from 17.5 % in 1966 to 50.8 % in 2008 [33].

Numerous studies reporting results obtained with the different implants either individually or comparatively are available. The majority of the studies are retrospective reports, involving individual implants. Characteristically comparative reports have been done between two different types of implant, comparing the effect of size and the presence or absence of a valve [34–37]. There are also prospective studies comparing two different types of implant [38], but of these there is only one multicentral, randomized study that has been done [39]. This study compared Ahmed and Baerveldt implants. The conclusions derived from this study indicated that the pressure-lowering effect of the Baerveldt was minimally better. A prospective study comparing single-plate Ahmed implants to single-plate Molteno implants found that the Molteno group had a greater percentage drop in IOP from baseline at 2 years than did the Ahmed group.

In a literature review, Hong et al. reported that the overall success rate of four individual long-tube implants, namely, Molteno, Krupin, Baerveldt, and Ahmed implants, averaged between 72 and 79 % [40]. A study comparing the efficacy of single- and double-plate Molteno implants indicated that the double plate had a better IOP-lowering potential than the single plate. This report together with Molteno's earlier observation suggested that the double-plate implant was more efficient in lowering IOP. This observation was retracted by Molteno based on the results of a long-term later study, by him, which indicated that there was no statistical difference in pressure lowering between the original single-plate and double-plate Molteno implants [41]. Studies comparing double-plate Molteno implants to the single-plate larger implants, Ahmed and Baerveldt, have shown that the double-plate Molteno and the 350 mm$^2$-Baerveldt implant had relatively similar reduction in IOP [36]. The double-plate Molteno implant produced a statistically lower IOP than the single-plate Ahmed implant [37]. The newer large-size single-plate Molteno implants have, as of yet, not been compared in a prospective or retrospective study to any of the other non-Molteno long-tube single-plate implants.

Based on the present reports available regarding pressure-lowering ability of the various implants, there appears to be no clear advantage ascribed to any of the available implants mainly used at the present time. Non-valved implants do, however, seem to have a minimal advantage in IOP lowering in the long term, as seen in direct comparative studies. The individual choices of implant use would appear to depend on the implant used during fellowship training, the ease of surgical implantation, and to a lesser extent the belief in possible fewer complications associated with the chosen implant. This observation would suggest that no single implant in the eyes of the surgeon has a more likely pressure-lowering ability than any other implant. The implants have therefore become predominantly conduits for the transportation of aqueous from the eye to the subconjunctival space. Results obtained with the individual implant will therefore depend predominantly on the pathophysiology of bleb formation in the individual patient.

The factors mainly concerned in bleb physiology are the aqueous and the tissue reaction over the plate.

## The Future Direction of Glaucoma Implants

In the last 40 years, glaucoma implants have progressed from paralimbal large inflexible implants to the present-day variety of single-plate long-tube implants. Changes over the years have involved mainly the plate portion of the implant, the tube remaining essentially as introduced originally. The size of the plate appears to have reached a size that is able to produce a standard pressure-reducing effect, with little advantage obtained by utilizing single plates any larger than 175 mm$^2$. Studies comparing the different plate materials available in the same variety of implant, namely, silicone and polypropylene, arrived at various conclusions. One study suggested improved intraocular pressure control with silicone implants, whereas a second study suggested that the silicone implants were only more effective in the first 3 months after implantation, but the complication rate with the polypropylene implants was higher than the silicone group. A third study suggested better pressure lowering in the silicone group and once again more complications with the polypropylene group [42–44]. The more flexible silicone material did result in ease of implantation of the device. There are many grades of polypropylene, some more inert and more flexible than others, and unless the grade of polypropylene is indicated, the comparative studies to silicone are flawed. The thickness of the plate will also affect the flexibility. The development of a more suitable material for the implant plate is an area for future research.

Future possible modifications relating to the silicone tube do appear to be necessary. The two main problems related to the tube are the methods available for covering the tube in its path from plate to anterior chamber. Erosions in the tissue covering the tube present one of the most common and frustrating problems seen in implant use. The present methods utilized for covering the tube have proven to be anything but fail-safe. Various tissues have been tried as coverings for the tube, with or without an associated lamellar scleral flap, but none has shown any marked superiority in preventing tube erosion. A possible solution to this problem may be to shorten the external exposure of the tube, as well as changing the direction of the tube to a more posterior situation, thus avoiding pressure of the tube on the overlying covering tissue. Both of these modifications would be achieved by placing the tube into the vitreous, rather than the anterior chamber. This modification would also eliminate the possible effect the tube has on the vitality of the corneal endothelium, another unwanted complication of glaucoma implant use. This modification would necessitate a total vitrectomy, which has become a safer and simpler procedure with the introduction of small-bore needle vitrectomy.

The glaucoma implants are presently used mainly following failure of previous glaucoma filtering procedures, as well as primarily in eyes with complicated glaucoma, such as uveitic and neovascular glaucoma. A prospective study comparing tubes to trabeculectomy in patients with previous ocular surgery resulted in a higher success rate in IOP control in the tube group after 5 years of follow-up [45]. The study comparing trabeculectomy to tubes in patients without previous glaucoma surgery has not as yet published results. Individual reports comparing tubes and trabeculectomy have been published [46]. The results of these studies indicated that the cumulative probability of success was similar between the two treatment groups after 1 year follow-up. There may be a trend in the future to use tubes as the primary surgical procedure for all types of glaucoma requiring glaucoma surgery.

The mechanism involved in bleb physiology remains the key for the future research relating to the improvement of results with glaucoma implant use. The choice of implant use at the present time depends primarily on the implant that the glaucoma specialist was using during fellowship training, and this trend is adhered to as the variety of implants available today, differ minimally from each other.

Many reports have appeared in the literature over the years discussing the pros and cons of the various long-tube implants available today. The reports all tend to focus on which implant is better, what changes in implant materials are needed, which is easiest to insert, and which has the least complications. The findings are mostly inconclusive regarding all of the parameters mentioned. What is consistent in most of the studies relating to long-tube glaucoma implants is that almost all the reports concentrate on the device. Large, small, polypropylene, silicone, and surgical-related problems. As previously mentioned all devices in the end are simply conduits transporting fluid from the anterior chamber to the chosen place, most commonly the subconjunctival space. The true mechanism which determines the IOP is the bleb, and this depends on the physiology of its formation and the chemical contents of the aqueous. The shunt itself plays only a small role in determining the effectivity of the bleb. The patient's inflammatory reaction, the nature of the tissue, and the aqueous contents will determine the effectivity of the bleb. Molteno has shown over the past 40 years that the bleb is a viable and changing structure. This is the reason that different results are obtained in different patients using the same devices very often by the same surgeon. Finally the choice of device more often than not has more to do with the ease of insertion, lack of complications, and postoperative ease of care, which often has little to do with the final outcome of pressure control.

This suggests that in order to improve results in IOP lowering, research should be directed into the better understanding of the mechanisms involved in bleb formation and methods that might be employed to improve bleb filtration.

## References


1. Molteno ACB, Luntz MH. Proceedings of the first South African international ophthalmological symposium, Butterworths; 1969. p. 1215–31.
2. Epstein E. Fibrosing response to aqueous. Its relation to glaucoma. Br J Ophthalmol. 1959;43:641–7.
3. Molteno ACB. New implant for drainage in glaucoma. Animal trial. Br J Ophthalmol. 1969;53:161–8.
4. Molteno ACB. New implant for drainage in glaucoma. Clinical trial. Br J Ophthalmol. 1969;53:606–15.
5. Molteno ACB, Straughan JL, Ancker E. Long tube implants in the management of glaucoma. SA Med J. 1976;50:1062–6.
6. Molteno ACB, Dempster AG. Methods of controlling bleb fibrosis around draining implants. Glaucoma. Proceedings of the fourth international symposium of the Northern Eye Institute. Manchester: Pergamon Press; 1988. p. 192–211.
7. Freedman J, Trope GE. Drainage implants. In: Yanoff M, Ducker JS, editors. Ophthalmology. 3rd ed. Boca Raton, FL: Taylor & Francis Group; 2005. p. 1277–82.
8. Molteno ACB, BiljonVan G, Ancker E. Two-stage insertion of glaucoma drainage implants. Trans Ophthalmol Soc N Z. 1979;31:17–26.
9. Molteno ACB, Polkinhorne PJ, Bowbyes JA. The vicryl tie technique for inserting a drainage implant in the treatment of secondary glaucoma. Aust N Z J Ophthalmol. 1986;14:343–54.
10. Molteno ACB. The optimal design of drainage implants for glaucoma. Trans Ophthalmol Soc N Z. 1981;33:39–41.
11. Heuer DK, Lloyd MA, Abrams DA, et al. Which is better? One or two? A randomized clinical trial of single-plate versus double-plate Molteno implantation for glaucomas in aphakia and pseudophakia. Ophthalmology. 1992;99:1512–9.
12. Molteno ACB. The dual chamber single plate implant its use in neovascular glaucoma. Aust N Z J Glaucoma. 1990;18:431–6.
13. Freedman J. Clinical experience with the Molteno dual chamber single plate implant. Ophthalmic Surg. 1992;38:241–3.
14. Barton K, Heuer DK. Chapter 97. Aqueous shunts: choice of implant. In: Sharawy TK, Sherwood MB, Hitchings RA, Crowston JG, editors. Glaucoma surgical management. Saunders Elsevier: www.elsevierhealth.com; 2009. p. 395–401.
15. Sherwood MB, Smith MF. Prevention of early hypotony associated with Molteno implants by a new occluding stent technique. Ophthalmology. 1993;100:85–90.
16. Lloyd MA, Baerveldt G, Fellenbaum PS, et al. Intermediate term results of a randomized clinical trial of the 350-versus the 500 mm² Baerveldt implant. Ophthalmology. 1994;101:1456–63.
17. Freedman J. Aqueous tube shunts. In: Spaeth GL, Danish-Meyer H, Goldberg I, Kampic A, editors. Ophthalmic surgery. Principles and practice. 4th ed. Edinburgh: Elsevier Saunders; 2012. p. 264–73.
18. Freedman J, Goddard D. Elevated levels of transforming growth factor b and prostaglandin $E_2$ in aqueous humor from patients undergoing filtration surgery for glaucoma. Can J Ophthalmol. 2008;43:370.
19. Nour-Mahdavi K, Caprioli J. Evaluation of the hypertensive phase after insertion of the Ahmed glaucoma valve. Am J Ophthalmol. 2003;136:1001–8.
20. Tripathi RC, Tripathi BJ, Chan WFA. Expression of growth factor mRNA's by human Tenon's capsule fibroblasts. Invest Ophthalmol Vis Sci. 1994;35(Suppl):1432.
21. Sira B, Ticho U. Excision of Tenon's capsule in fistulizing operations on Africans. Am J Ophthalmol. 1969;68:336–40.
22. Freedman J, Chamnongvonse P. Supra-Tenon's placement of a single-plate Molteno implant. Br J Ophthalmol. 2008;92:669–72.

23. Freedman J, Bhandari R. Supra-tenon capsule placement of original Molteno vs Molteno 3 tube implants in black patients with refractory glaucoma. Arch Ophthalmol. 2011;129:993–7.

24. Jampel HD, Roche N, Stark WJ, Roberts AB. Transforming growth factor beta in human aqueous humor. Curr Eye Res. 1990;9:963–9.

25. Tripathi RC, Tripathi BJ, Borisuth NSC. Growth factors in the aqueous humor and their clinical significance. J Glaucoma. 1994;3:248.

26. Teng CC, Chi h, Katzin HM. Histology and mechanism of filtering operations. Am J Ophthalmol. 1959;47:16–34.

27. Freedman J. Scleral patch grafts with Molteno setons. Ophthalmic Surg. 1987;18:532–4.

28. Brandt JD. Patch grafts of dehydrated cadaveric dura mater for tube shunt glaucoma surgery. Arch Ophthalmol. 1993;111:1436–9.

29. Albis-Donado O. The Ahmed valve. In: Sharaawy T, Mermoud A, editors. Atlas of glaucoma surgery. New Delhi: Jaypee Brothers; 2008. p. 58–76.

30. Wilcox MJ, Barad JP, Wilcox CC, et al. Performance of a new low-volume, high-surface aqueous shunt in normal rabbit eyes. J Glaucoma. 2000;9:74–82.

31. Smith SL, Starita RJ, Fellman RL, et al. Early clinical experience with the Baerveldt 350 mm$^2$ glaucoma implant and associated extraocular muscle imbalance. Ophthalmology. 1993;1001:914–8.

32. Ramulu PY, Corcoran SL, Robin AL. Utilization of various glaucoma surgeries and procedures in Medicare beneficiaries from 1995 to 2004. Ophthalmology. 2007;114:2265–70.

33. Desai MA, Gedde SJ, Feuer WJ, et al. Practice preferences for glaucoma surgery: a survey of The American Glaucoma Society in 2008. Ophthalmic Surg Lasers Imaging. 2011;42:202–8.

34. Tsai JC, Johnson CC, Dietrich MS. The Ahmed shunt versus the Baerveldt shunt for refractory glaucoma: a single-surgeon comparison of outcome. Ophthalmology. 2003;110:1814–21.

35. Syed HM, Law SK, Nam SH, et al. Baerveldt −350 implant versus Ahmed valve for refractory glaucoma. A case-controlled comparison. J Glaucoma. 2004;13:38–45.

36. Smith MF, Doyle JW, Sherwood MB. Comparison of the Baerveldt glaucoma implant with the double-plate Molteno drainage implant. Arch Ophthalmol. 1995;113:444–7.

37. Ayyala RS, Zurakowski D, Monshizadeh R, et al. Comparison of double-plate Molteno and Ahmed glaucoma valve in patients with advanced uncontrolled glaucoma. Ophthalmic Surg Lasers. 2002;33:94–101.

38. Nassiri N, Khamali G, Rahanavardi M, et al. Ahmed glaucoma valve and single – plate Molteno implants in treatment of refractory glaucoma: a comparative study. Am J Ophthalmol. 2010;149:893–902.

39. Budenz DL, Barton K, Feuer WJ, et al. Treatment outcomes in the Ahmed Baerveldt Comparison Study after one year of follow up. Ophthalmology. 2011;118:443–52.

40. Hong CH, Arosemena A, Zurakowski D, et al. Glaucoma drainage devices: a systematic literature review and current controversies. Surv Ophthalmol. 2005;40:48–60.

41. Molteno ACB, Bevin TH, Herbison P, Houliston MJ. Otago glaucoma surgery outcome study. Long-term follow-up of primary glaucoma with additional risk factors drained by Molteno implants. Ophthalmology. 2001;108:2193–200.

42. Law SK, Nguyen BS, Coleman AL, et al. Comparison of safety and efficacy between silicone and polypropylene Ahmed glaucoma valves in refractory glaucoma. Ophthalmology. 2005;112:1514–20.

43. Ishihada K, Netland PA, Costa VP, et al. Comparison of polypropylene and silicone Ahmed glaucoma valves. Ophthalmology. 2006;113:1320–6.

44. Mackenzie PJ, Schertzer R, Ibister CM. Comparison of silicone and polypropylene Ahmed glaucoma valves. Can J Ophthalmol. 2007;42:227–32.

45. Gedde SJ, Schiffman JC, Feuer WJ, et al. Treatment outcomes in the Tube Versus Trabeculectomy Study after five years of follow-up. Am J Ophthalmol. 2012;153:787–1012.

46. Wilson MR, Mendis U, Smith SD, Paliwal A. Ahmed glaucoma valve implant vs. trabeculectomy in the surgical treatment of glaucoma: a randomized clinical trial. Am J Ophthalmol. 2000;130:267–73.

Peter A. Netland

## Introduction

Glaucoma drainage devices are helpful in the management of intractable glaucoma, which does not respond well to conventional medical and surgical therapies. Surgeons also may choose to use glaucoma drainage devices for primary surgery for glaucoma [1]. The Ahmed Glaucoma Valve is a glaucoma drainage device that has a flow-resistive valve mechanism [1]. This valve is helpful in minimizing postoperative hypotony and complications associated with hypotony, including flat anterior chamber, choroidal effusions, and suprachoroidal hemorrhage [2, 3].

After Ahmed Glaucoma Valve implantation, patients may require adjunctive antiglaucoma medications for adequate control of intraocular pressure (IOP) [2–4]. With smaller glaucoma valve implants, such as the Molteno implant, increasing the device surface area may lead to lower mean IOP and fewer adjunctive glaucoma medications [5, 6]. However, additional surface area does not dramatically improve the results with larger implants, such as the Ahmed Valve and the Baerveldt implant [7–10]. In contrast with trabeculectomy, use of adjunctive mitomycin C does not appear to improve the results with the Ahmed Glaucoma Valve [11].

In experimental studies, different glaucoma drainage implant plate materials may influence capsule formation and influence the results of glaucoma drainage implants [12, 13]. In clinical comparisons, different plate materials have been associated with significant difference of mean postoperative intraocular pressure in some [14–16] but not in all studies [17, 18]. In a randomized prospective trial, transient elevation of IOP during the early postoperative period, known as a "hypertensive phase," was less frequent after silicone plate compared with polypropylene plate Ahmed Glaucoma Valve implantation [14]. In addition to implant plate size and material, other variables influencing success of glaucoma drainage implant surgery have been identified, including race, treatment with silicone oil endotamponade, and neovascular glaucoma [19].

A silicone plate Ahmed Glaucoma Valve has demonstrated efficacy and safety in clinical studies [14–18]. An Ahmed Glaucoma Valve plate constructed with porous material has been developed and is Food and Drug Administration (FDA) approved. This new plate material may offer advantages in reducing encapsulation of the implant, thereby potentially improving postoperative IOP control.

## Device Description

The Ahmed Glaucoma Valve (New World Medical, Inc., Rancho Cucamonga, CA) Model FP7 has a silicone plate, which has 184 mm² surface area. The Model M4 (Fig. 20.1) has a porous polyethylene plate, which has 160 mm² surface area not including the surface area of the pores. The M4 plate length is 14 mm, the plate width is 10.5 mm, and the thickness is 2 mm. Both the Model FP7 and Model M4 are Food and Drug Administration approved for implantation in humans with intractable glaucoma.

The Model M4 plate is approximately the same size as the Model FP7 plate (191 and 160 mm² surface area, respectively). However, the theoretical surface area of the M4 is much higher because of the porous nature of the material. The porous polyethylene material is a biocompatible alloplastic material, which is formed by a proprietary process (Porex Corporation, Fairburn, GA). The porous plate material is high-density polyethylene with a long history of use in surgical implants (MEDPOR Biomaterial implants). The

P.A. Netland, MD, PhD
Department of Ophthalmology,
University of Virginia School of Medicine,
1300 Jefferson Park Avenue, 800715, Charlottesville,
VA 22908-0715, USA
e-mail: pnetland@virginia.edu, pnetland@gmail.com

**Electronic supplementary material** Supplementary material is available in the online version of this chapter at http://dx.doi.org/10.1007/978-1-4614-8348-9_20. Videos can also be accessed at http://www.springerimages.com/videos/978-1-4614-8347-2

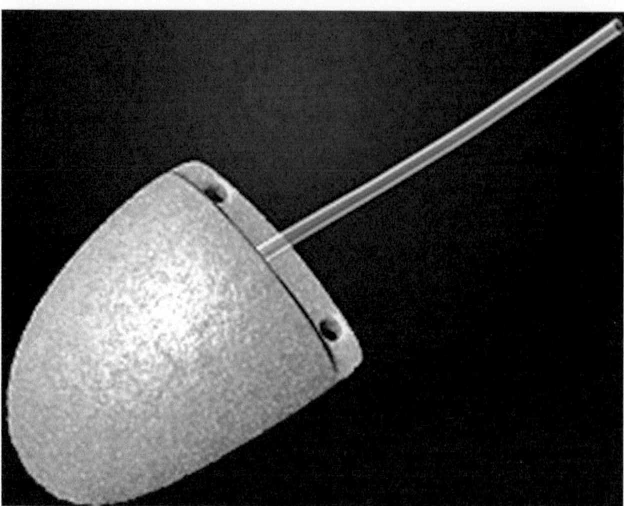

**Fig. 20.1** Ahmed Glaucoma Valve M4 (porous plate). The device has a porous polyethylene shell, which allows soft tissue growth into pores and integration with surrounding tissue (Photograph courtesy New World Medical, Inc., Rancho Cucamonga, California)

pores allow collagen and mature blood vessels to grow into the material [20]. Tissue integration and vascular ingrowth into the pores improve resistance to infection, exposure, and extrusion [21, 22]. In the Model M4, average pore sizes are greater than 100 μm and pore volume is in the 50 % range, with an interconnecting open pore structure that allows for tissue ingrowth.

In experimental models, the Ahmed Glaucoma Valve with a surrounding porous membrane of expanded polytetrafluoroethylene (ePTFE) has thinner and more vascular capsules compared with the unmodified implant [23]. Implants with a ePTFE membrane showed higher resistance at low flow rates and lower resistance at high flow rates [24]. The porous polyethylene used in the Model M4 Ahmed Glaucoma Valve is stiffer and less deformable compared with porous ePTFE, which provided better fluid pressure distribution in the implant approved for human use.

## Surgical Procedure

The surgical procedure is similar for the Model FP7 (silicone plate) and the Model M4 (porous plate) Ahmed Glaucoma Valves (Video 20.1). The implant should be examined and primed prior to implantation. Priming is accomplished by injecting balanced salt solution (BSS) through the drainage tube and valve, using a blunt cannula. Because the valve is encased in the porous material, streaming of BSS is not observed during priming. Flow is verified by visualizing oozing of BSS through the porous material.

An incision is made at or near the limbus, through the conjunctiva and Tenon's capsule. A pocket is formed at the superior quadrant between the medial and lateral rectus muscles by blunt dissection of Tenon's capsule from the episclera. The valve body is inserted into the pocket between the rectus muscles and sutured to the episclera. The leading edge of the device should be at least 8–10 mm from the limbus. The "rough" surface of the Model M4 helps to hold the implant in position while anchoring the plate to the sclera.

The drainage tube is trimmed to permit 2–3 mm insertion of the tube into the anterior chamber. The tube is cut bevel up to an anterior angle of approximately 30° to facilitate insertion and avoid occlusion by the iris. A paracentesis is performed and the anterior chamber is entered at the limbus with a sharp 23-gauge needle, parallel to the iris. The drainage tube is inserted approximately 2–3 mm into the anterior chamber, through the needle track and parallel to the iris. The leading edge of the device should be 8–10 mm from the limbus.

The exposed drainage tube is covered with a small piece of preserved donor cornea, sclera, or pericardium, which is sutured into place and the conjunctiva is closed. As an alternative, a partial-thickness limbal-based scleral flap may be made. The tube is inserted into the anterior chamber through a 23-gauge needle puncture made under the flap. Postoperatively, the patient is treated with topical corticosteroids and antibiotics, tapered over approximately 6 weeks. After surgery, patients are usually examined at 1 day, 1 week, 3–4 weeks, and at regular 3–4-month intervals thereafter.

## Clinical Results

In a retrospective comparative study [25], 40 eyes were implanted with the Model M4 implant with an average of 1.4-year follow-up and compared with 38 eyes treated with the Model S2 (polypropylene plate) and 76 eyes treated with the Model FP7 (silicone plate). After treatment with the Model M4 implant, the mean IOP was reduced from $27.0 \pm 12.0$ to $15.0 \pm 4.0$ mmHg at 1 year, which was not statistically significantly different, compared with the groups treated with Models S2 and FP7. The cumulative probability of success was higher, but not statistically significantly different in the M4 group (80 %) compared with the FP7 (70 %) and S2 (66 %) groups ($P = 0.99$). Blebs formed in the M4 group were low profile. In this small series, complications were similar among groups, although statistically significantly lower mean IOP at 1–3 months in the M4 group suggested less "hypertensive phase" in patients treated with the Model M4 implant. Further studies are needed to determine the long-term safety and efficacy of the Ahmed Glaucoma Valve M4 implant.

## Conclusion

The Ahmed Glaucoma Valve Model M4 has a porous plate, which allows integration of vascular tissue with the plate. Early clinical results suggest similar intraocular pressure control compared with other Ahmed Glaucoma Valve plates. Potential advantages include reduction of hypertensive phase and low-profile bleb. It is anticipated that, if needed, explantation of the device would be more difficult compared with other Ahmed Glaucoma Valve plates. The long-term safety and efficacy of this device are under evaluation at this time.

**Financial Disclosure**  The University of Virginia has received research support from New World Medical for a multicenter randomized clinical trial.

## References


1. Boyle IV JW, Netland PA. Ahmed glaucoma valve drainage implant. In: Shaarawy TM, Sherwood MB, Hitchings RA, Crowston JG, editors. Glaucoma, Surgical management, vol. 2. 1st ed. Edinburgh: Saunders Elsevier; 2009. p. 425–35.
2. Coleman AL, Hill R, Wilson MR, Choplin N, Kotas-Neumann R, Tam M, Bacharach J, Panek WC. Initial clinical experience with the Ahmed glaucoma valve implant. Am J Ophthalmol. 1995;120: 23–31.
3. Huang MC, Netland PA, Coleman AL, Siegner SW, Moster MR, Hill RA. Intermediate-term clinical experience with the Ahmed glaucoma valve implant. Am J Ophthalmol. 1999;127:27–33.
4. Ayyala RS, Zurakowski D, Smith JA, Monshizadeh R, Netland PA, Richards DW, Layden WE. A clinical study of the Ahmed glaucoma valve implant in advanced glaucoma. Ophthalmology. 1998;105:1968–76.
5. Heuer DK, Lloyd MA, Abrams DA, Baerveldt G, Minckler DS, Lee MB, Martone JF. Which is better? One or two? A randomized clinical trial of single-plate versus double-plate Molteno implantation for glaucomas in aphakia and pseudophakia. Ophthalmology. 1992;99:1512–9.
6. Broadway DC, Iester M, Schulzer M, Douglas GR. Survival analysis for success of Molteno tube implants. Br J Ophthalmol. 2001;85:689–95.
7. Smith MF, Doyle JW, Sherwood MB. Comparison of the Baerveldt glaucoma implant with the double-plate Molteno drainage implant. Arch Ophthalmol. 1995;113:444–7.
8. Siegner SW, Netland PA, Urban Jr RC, Williams AS, Richards DW, Latina MA, Brandt JD. Clinical experience with the Baerveldt glaucoma drainage implant. Ophthalmology. 1995;102:1298–307.
9. Britt MT, LaBree LD, Lloyd MA, et al. Randomized clinical trial of the 350-mm$^2$ versus the 500-mm$^2$ Baerveldt implant: longer term results. Is bigger better? Ophthalmology. 1999;106:2312–8.
10. Al-Aswad LA, Netland PA, Bellows AR, et al. Clinical experience with the double-plate Ahmed glaucoma valve. Am J Ophthalmol. 2006;141:390–1.
11. Costa VP, Azuara-Blanco A, Netland PA, Lesk MR, Arcieri ES. Efficacy and safety of adjunctive mitomycin C during Ahmed glaucoma valve implantation. A prospective randomized clinical trial. Ophthalmology. 2004;111:1071–6.
12. Ayyala RS, Harman LE, Michelini-Norris B, Ondrovic LE, Haller E, Margo CE, Stevens SX. Comparison of different biomaterials for glaucoma drainage devices. Arch Ophthalmol. 1999;117: 233–6.
13. Ayyala RS, Michelini-Norris B, Flores A, Haller E, Margo CE. Comparison of different biomaterials for glaucoma drainage devices: part 2. Arch Ophthalmol. 2000;118:1081–4.
14. Ishida K, Netland PA, Costa VP, Shiroma L, Khan B, Ahmed II. Comparison of polypropylene and silicone Ahmed glaucoma valves. Ophthalmology. 2006;113:1320–6.
15. Hinkle DM, Zurakowski D, Ayyala RS. A comparison of the polypropylene plate Ahmed glaucoma valve to the silicone plate Ahmed glaucoma flexible valve. Eur J Ophthalmol. 2007;17:696–701.
16. Mackenzie PJ, Schertzer RM, Isbister CM. Comparison of silicone and polypropylene Ahmed glaucoma valves: two-year follow-up. Can J Ophthalmol. 2007;42:227–32.
17. Law SK, Nguyen A, Coleman AL, Caprioli J. Comparison of safety and efficacy between silicone and polypropylene Ahmed glaucoma valves in refractory glaucoma. Ophthalmology. 2005;112:1514–20.
18. Brasil MV, Rockwood EJ, Smith SD. Comparison of silicone and polypropylene Ahmed glaucoma valve implants. J Glaucoma. 2007;16:36–41.
19. Netland PA. The Ahmed glaucoma valve in neovascular glaucoma. Trans Am Ophthalmol Soc. 2009;107:325–42.
20. Wellisz T. Clinical experience with the Medpor porous polyethylene implant. Aesthetic Plast Surg. 1993;17:339–44.
21. Katwitter JJ, Bagwell JG, Weinstein AM, et al. An evaluation of bone growth into porous high density polyethylene. J Biomed Mater Res. 1976;10:311–23.
22. Spector M, Harmon SL, Kreutner A. Characteristics of tissue growth into Proplast and porous polyethylene implants in bone. J Biomed Mater Res. 1979;13:677–92.
23. DeCroos FC, Ahmad S, Kondo Y, et al. Expanded polytetrafluoroethylene membrane alters tissue response to implanted Ahmed glaucoma valve. Curr Eye Res. 2009;34:562–7.
24. DeCroos FC, Kondo Y, Mordes D, et al. In vitro fluid dynamics of the Ahmed glaucoma valve modified with expanded polytetrafluoroethylene. Curr Eye Res. 2011;36:112–7.
25. Kim J, Allingham RR, Hall J, et al. Clinical experience with a novel glaucoma drainage implant. J Glaucoma. 2013. Epub ahead of print.

# The CyPass Suprachoroidal Micro-Stent



Tsontcho Ianchulev

The CyPass Micro-Stent is the first suprachoroidal micro-stent developed by Transcend Medical. At the current time, it is an investigational device under FDA IDE studies in the USA. In the EU, the micro-stent is approved to use for intraocular pressure (IOP) lowering in open-angle glaucoma under a CE mark.

The CyPass device is a fenestrated micro-stent which is implanted in the supraciliary space to provide a permanent conduit for uveoscleral outflow of aqueous from the anterior chamber. The stent is made of biocompatible, nonbiodegradable polyimide material which has demonstrated minimal inflammatory and fibrotic reaction in preclinical studies of rabbit implantations [1]. It is 6.35 mm in length and 510 μm in external diameter and is implanted through a 1.5 mm clear cornea incision. When the micro-stent is correctly inserted into the supraciliary space, the material stiffness, in conjunction with a series of retention rings at the proximal end, helps ensure the stability of the device in the angle and the supraciliary space (Fig. 21.1). The micro-stent is designed to improve aqueous outflow through the uveoscleral pathway.

Implantation technique is achieved in a blebless, minimally invasive way through a clear cornea incision, sparing the conjunctiva and the sclera. For implantation of the CyPass device, the anterior chamber is refilled with a viscoelastic agent of the surgeon's choice to maintain the chamber and expand the angle. Visualization is achieved with a surgical goniolens (Swan-Jacob, Hill or TVG lens) prior to and during implantation. The CyPass device is loaded onto a retractable guidewire of a specially designed applier. Under gonioscopy, the implant is inserted into the anterior chamber through a 1.5 mm paracentesis or the phacoemulsification incision when done in combination with phaco.

Non-incisional dissection is initiated with the tip of the guidewire below the scleral spur at the interface of the ciliary body and the sclera. The guidewire is designed to bluntly disinsert the ciliary body and create passage into the supraciliary space. The micro-stent is then implanted with all retention features engaged. The guidewire is retracted and the applier withdrawn from the eye. Viscoelastic agent is evacuated using irrigation and aspiration.

The CyPass Micro-Stent can be implanted in a goniofree technique as well (without the use of surgical intraoperative gonioscopy), as demonstrated by Ianchulev [2] and illustrated in Fig. 21.2. A specially designed tactile gonioprobe is used to measure the depth of the angle from

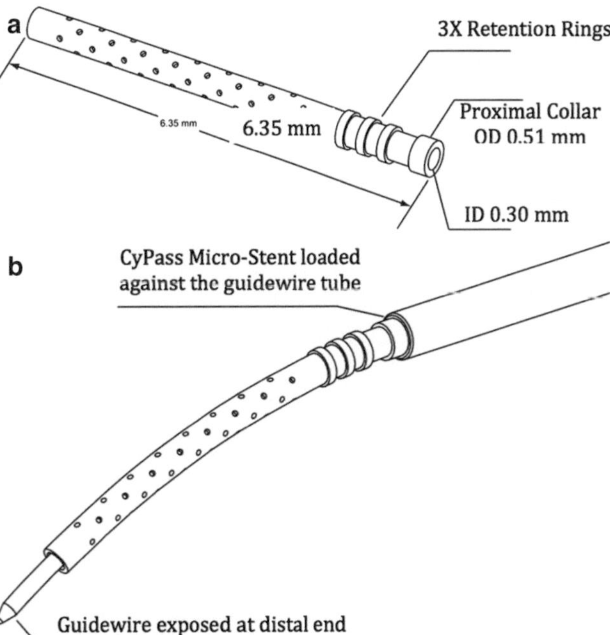


**Fig. 21.1** CyPass Micro-Stent. (**a**) Configuration and dimensions of the micro-stent. (**b**) Applicator tool, with retractable guidewire, for insertion of the micro-stent into the supraciliary space


T. Ianchulev, MD, MPH
Department of Ophthalmology,
University of California, San Francisco (UCSF),
707 Oregon Ave, San Francisco, CA 94402, USA
e-mail: sianchulev@transcendmedical.com


J.R. Samples, I.I.K. Ahmed (eds.), *Surgical Innovations in Glaucoma*,
DOI 10.1007/978-1-4614-8348-9_21, © Springer Science+Business Media New York 2014

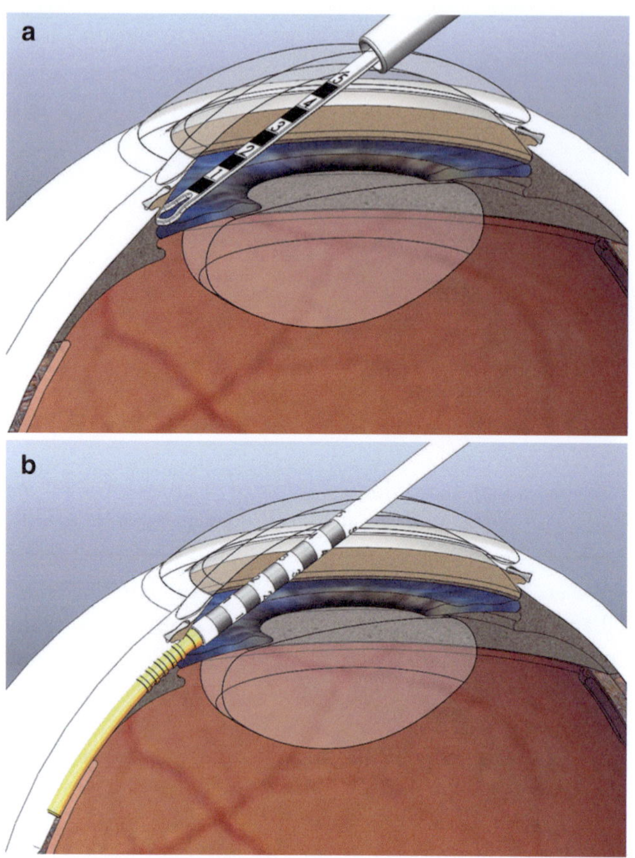

**Fig. 21.2** Implantation of the CyPass Micro-Stent with gonio-free technique. (**a**) Positioning tool with measurement scale. (**b**) Implantation using the curved guidewire

the ciliary body insertion to the limbus at the site of implantation. A measurement scale on the probe and a corresponding one on the applier allow for high-precision implantation and micro-stent positioning without need for goniovisualization (Fig. 21.2a). The tip and the curvature of the guidewire are also designed for a gonio-free approach as they allow the surgeon to find the insertion landmark and to initiate blunt dissection along the supraciliary plane by following the contour of the scleral wall without direct view of the scleral spur.

OCT Visante or Ultrasound biomicroscopy (UBM) images can be used to confirm the micro-stent position in the supraciliary space (Fig. 21.3). They allow visualization of postoperative morphological outcomes not visible by slit lamp or indirect ophthalmoscopy – not only the micro-stent position but the drainage area and the space surrounding or posterior to the stent. This is critical as proper positioning and implantation of any micro-stent are essential to drainage and function. Describing the findings of OCT images after suprachoroidal micro-stent implantation and correlating the morphological outcomes with IOP outcomes are novel and informative ways to further understand the effect of microinvasive glaucoma surgery (MIGS), specifically on the suprachoroidal space. The AS-OCT or UBM images can demonstrate areas of hypodensity surrounding the micro-stent, both posteriorly and circumferentially. These areas of hypodensity likely represent aqueous traveling through and around the micro-stent and accumulating in the suprachoroidal space. Posterior accumulation of

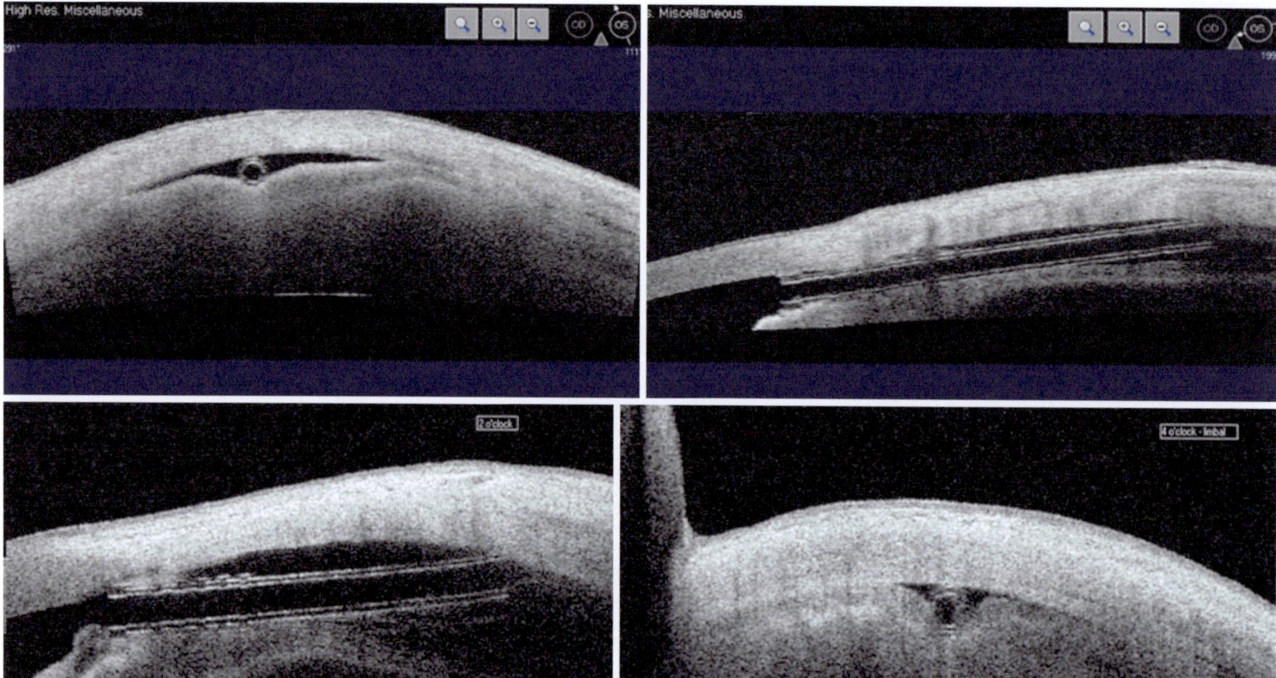

**Fig. 21.3** Visualization of CyPass Micro-Stent placement using anterior segment OCT imaging

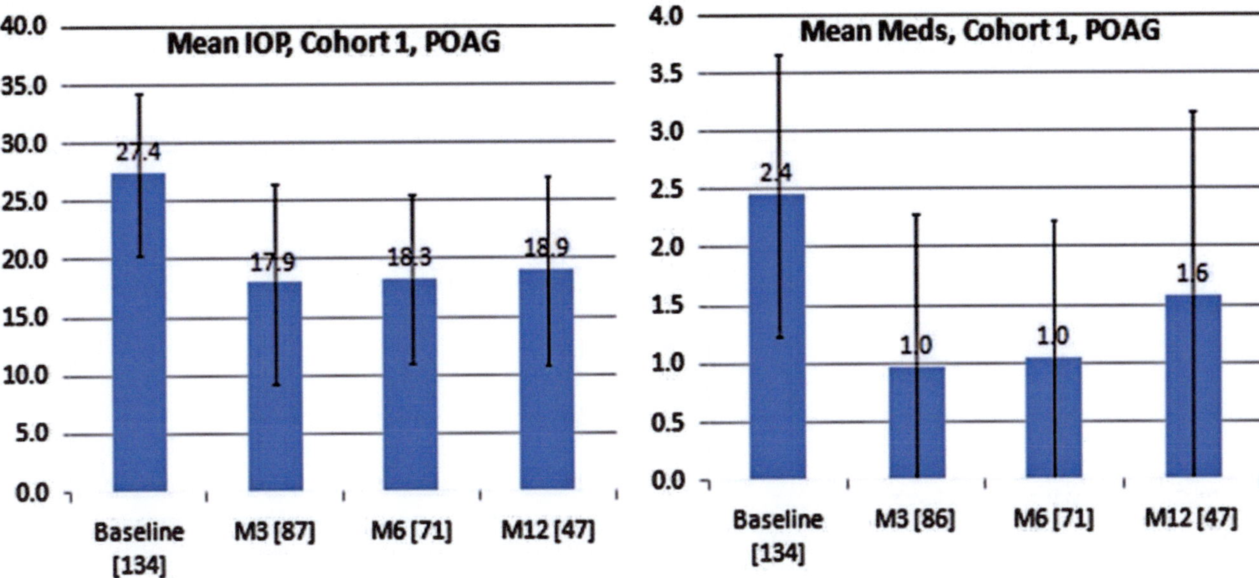


**Fig. 21.4** IOP results for Cohort 1 (uncontrolled IOP preoperatively) in the CyCLE OAG Study (From Garcia-Feijoou et al. [8]). Error bars = 1 SD

fluid is of functional significance as it may suggest fluid filtration and aqueous lake formation which are essential for suprachoroidal absorption and outflow.

## Biologic Rationale for Suprachoroidal Stenting

There is a strong biologic rationale for increasing suprachoroidal outflow as a means of lowering intraocular pressure in glaucoma. The suprachoroidal space is a target for therapeutic intervention for a number of important reasons. Experimental evidence suggests there is a negative pressure gradient between the suprachoroidal space and the anterior chamber, which provides a driving force for aqueous outflow [3]. In some areas the pressure difference can exceed 3–4 mmHg with a gradient which increases along the posterior aspect of the suprachoroidal space. Secondly, clinical experience demonstrates that traumatic or iatrogenic cyclodialysis is associated with significant IOP lowering by creating additional non-trabecular outflow through the uveoscleral route [4]. The effect is often transient and diminishes once the cyclodialysis cleft closes. Thirdly, experience from glaucoma pharmacotherapy demonstrates that some of the most effective topical therapies for IOP reduction act primarily by increasing the uveoscleral outflow [5]. While it may be secondary to the trabecular outflow, the uveoscleral outflow may have a higher capacity for therapeutic effect on IOP.

Additional discussion on suprachoroidal and uveoscleral outflow as a therapeutic target is available in Chap. 3.

## Clinical Experience

Ianchulev et al. [6] first reported on 81 glaucomatous (OAG) eyes that underwent cataract surgery (phacoemulsification) followed by CyPass implantation. At 6 months after surgery, the mean IOP had decreased to 16 mmHg from a preoperative mean value of 22.9 mmHg. The procedure was well tolerated, with postoperative complications of shallow anterior chamber and transient hyphema in one patient each. The following year, Craven et al. reported on safety outcomes of 121 eyes that underwent phacoemulsification and CyPass implantation [7]. The adverse events following the procedure were transient hyphema ($n = 8$), persistent inflammation ($n = 1$), branch retinal vein occlusion ($n = 1$), and diabetic macular edema exacerbation ($n = 1$).

More recent data presented at the 2012 European Society of Cataract and Refractive Surgeons Annual Meeting provide additional clinical experience with the micro-stent [8, 9]. The CyCLE OAG study (A Cypass open angle glaucoma study) was conducted in 460 patients, over 83 % of whom had a diagnosis of open-angle glaucoma. Of the 460 total patients, 222 patients were treated with CyPass alone and 238 received the CyPass procedure in combination with cataract removal.

Of the 222 patients treated with CyPass alone, 134 had uncontrolled IOP (Cohort 1; $\geq 21$ mmHg; mean = 25.4 mmHg) and 88 had controlled IOP (Cohort 2; <21 mmHg; mean = 17.9 mmHg) preoperatively. Approximately half of the patients (50.2 %) had received prior glaucoma interventions, and 27.2 % had received prior trabeculectomy or tube shunt implantation. Figure 21.4 shows the mean IOP and mean number of

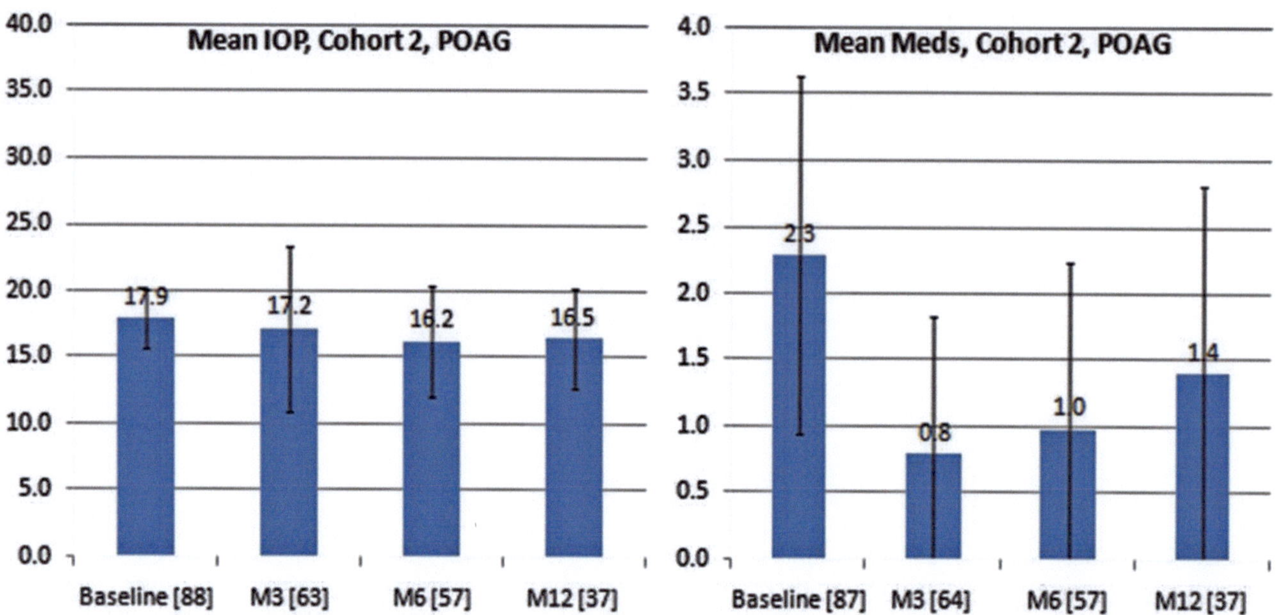


**Fig. 21.5** IOP results for Cohort 2 (controlled IOP preoperatively) in the CyCLE OAG Study (From Garcia-Feijoo et al. [8]). Error bars = 1 SD

antiglaucoma medications for Cohort 1 at preoperative baseline and at 3, 6, and 12 months after CyPass implantation. At 12 months after surgery, Cohort 1 patients experienced a 26 % reduction from baseline IOP and a greater than 33 % reduction in the number of antiglaucoma medications required.

Figure 21.5 shows the mean IOP and mean number of antiglaucoma medications for Cohort 2 at preoperative baseline and at 3, 6, and 12 months after CyPass implantation. At 12 months after surgery, IOP remained stable, but a 39 % reduction in antiglaucoma medications was achieved.

The safety profile of the CyPass micro-stent is consistent with what one would expect from a minimally invasive, clear-cornea ab interno procedure. There were no occurrences of hypotony maculopathy, suprachoroidal hemorrhage, retinal detachment, iris atrophy, or endophthalmitis. Other adverse events included the need for additional surgical intervention (10.8 %), postoperative IOP increase (7.6 %), obstruction (3.6 %), transient inflammation (1.8 %), anterior chamber shallowing (1.8 %), endothelial contact (1.8 %), transient hypotony (1.3 %), repositioning (0.4 %), explantation (0.4 %), and loss of BCVA (0.4 %) due to macular edema.

Of the 238 patients in the CyCLE study for whom CyPass implantation was combined with cataract removal surgery, 90 had uncontrolled IOP (Cohort 1; ≥21 mmHg; mean = 25.3 mmHg) and 148 had controlled IOP (Cohort 2; <21 mmHg; mean = 16.6 mmHg) preoperatively. Prior glaucoma interventions had been performed in 11.3 % of the patients, and 27.2 % had received prior trabeculectomy or tube shunt implantation. Figure 21.6 shows the mean decrease from preoperative IOP achieved at 3, 6, and 12 months after surgery in Cohort 1. The IOP reduction was clear at month 3 and remained stable at >33 % through month 12.

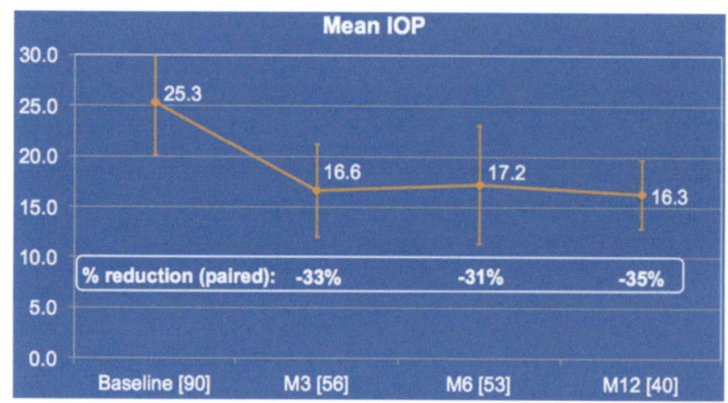


**Fig. 21.6** Effect of CyPass implantation on IOP relative to preoperative baseline in Cohort 1 (uncontrolled IOP) of patients who received CyPass in combination with cataract removal surgery (From Hoeh et al. [9]). Error bars = 1 SD

Figure 21.7 shows the mean reduction in antiglaucoma medications required in patients with uncontrolled IOP (Cohort 1) at baseline through 12 months after surgery. At 12 months, the number of medications required was decreased by 48 % in addition to the IOP reduction effect.

Figure 21.8 shows the mean IOP at 3, 6, and 12 months after surgery in controlled patients (Cohort 2) where the therapeutic objective of suprachoroidal micro-stenting was eliminating or reducing the number of IOP-lowering medications after a combined phaco-CyPass procedure. The mean IOP remained stable with patients under control on average through 12 months. However, as shown in Fig. 21.9, the mean number of antiglaucoma medications required was dramatically reduced by ≥75 % compared with baseline at months 3, 6, and 12 after surgery.

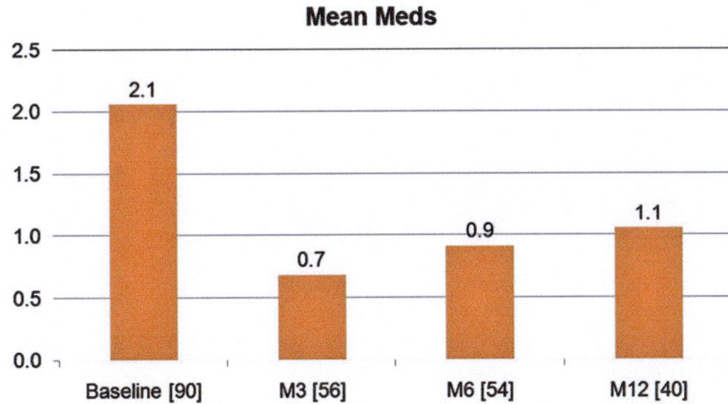

Fig. 21.7 Effect of CyPass implantation on a number of antiglaucoma medications required relative to preoperative baseline in Cohort 1 (uncontrolled IOP) of patients who received CyPass in combination with cataract removal surgery (From Hoeh et al. [9])

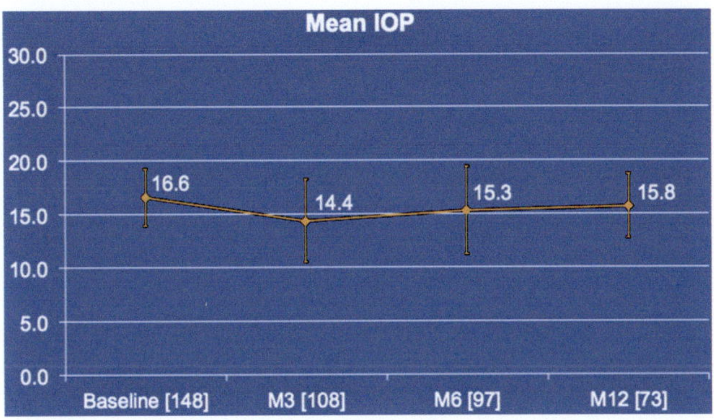

Fig. 21.8 Effect of CyPass implantation on IOP relative to preoperative baseline in Cohort 2 (controlled IOP) of patients who received CyPass in combination with cataract removal surgery (From Hoeh et al. [9]). Error bars = 1 SD

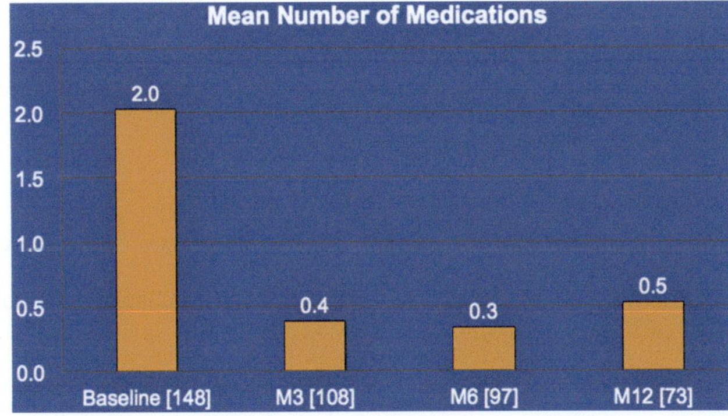

Fig. 21.9 Effect of CyPass implantation on a number of antiglaucoma medications required relative to preoperative baseline in Cohort 2 (controlled IOP) of patients who received CyPass in combination with cataract removal surgery (From Hoeh et al. [9])

Adverse events among the 238 patients treated with CyPass implantation in combination with cataract removal surgery, as with CyPass alone, were minimal – particularly in comparison to conventional glaucoma surgery (trabeculectomy or shunts).

There were no occurrences of hypotony maculopathy, suprachoroidal hemorrhage, retinal detachment, iris atrophy, or endophthalmitis. Other adverse events included obstruction (5.0 %), need for additional surgical intervention (3.3 %), postoperative IOP increase (1.7 %), transient hyphema (0.8 %), endothelial contact (0.8 %), and loss of best corrected visual acuity (BCVA; 0.4 %). In 0.4 % of patients the micro-stent had to be explanted or repositioned.

In summary, micro-stent implantation in the supraciliary space is a novel therapeutic approach which provides minimally invasive access to the suprachoroidal space for enhanced non-trabecular outflow. The procedure can be done as a stand-alone treatment in open-angle glaucoma patients or in combination with phaco surgery. Because of the clear-cornea, ab interno approach without interfering with the conjunctival and scleral tissue, this intervention is applicable earlier in the disease spectrum with mild-to-moderate glaucoma. Definitive clinical results are still pending, and the CyPass Micro-Stent is currently being evaluated in a large randomized controlled FDA trial of 505 patients which will provide Level I evidence of safety and efficacy of this therapy.

## References


1. Nguyen QH, Ahmed II, Craven ER, Anton-Lopez A, Grisante S, Ianchuler T. Biocompatibility of a polymide suprachoroidal microstent (Cypass) for intra-ocular pressure lowering in glaucoma: 6 months rabbit animal model. Association for Research in Vision and Ophthalmology annual meeting, Ft Lauderdale, FL, 6–9 may 2012.
2. Guguchkova P, Samsonova B, Topov A, Ianchulev T. Conio-free minimally invasive glaucoma suprachoroidal microstent implantation. American Society of cataract and Refractive surgery annual meeting, San Francisco, CA, 19–23 Apr 2012.
3. Emi K, Pederson JE, Toris CB. Hydrostatic pressure of the suprachoroidal space. Invest Ophthalmol Vis Sci. 1989;30(2):233–8.
4. Razeghinejad MR, Spaeth GL. A history of the surgical management of glaucoma. Optom Vis Sci. 2011;88(1):E39–47.
5. Toris CB. Pharmacotherapies for glaucoma. Curr Mol Med. 2010; 10(9):824–40.
6. Ianchulev T, Ahmed K, Hoeh HR, Rau M. Minimally invasive ab interno suprachoroidal device (CyPass) for IOP control in open-angle glaucoma. American Academy of Ophthalmology annual meeting, Chicago, 18–19 Oct 2010.
7. Craven ER, Khatana A, Hoeh H, Rau M, Ianchuler T. Safety of minimally invasive, abinterno suprachoroidal micro-stent for IOP reduction used in combination with phaco cataract surgery. American academy of Ophthalmology annual meeting, Orlando, FL, 22–25 Oct 2011.
8. Garcia-Feijoo J, Rau M, Ahmed I, Anton A, Grabner G, Ianchulev T. Safety and efficacy of CyPass Micro-Stent as a stand-alone treatment for open-angle glaucoma: worldwide clinical experience. European Society of Cataract and Refractive Surgeons annual meeting, Milan, 8–12 Sept 2012.
9. Hoeh H, Rau M, Reitshamer H, Rapisarda A, Ianchulev T, editors. Clinical outcomes of combined cataract surgery and implantation of the CyPass Micro-Stent for the treatment of open-angle glaucoma. In: European Society of Cataract and Refractive Surgeons, Milan, 10 Sept 2012.

# STARflo™: A Suprachoroidal Drainage Implant Made from STAR® Biomaterial


Sayeh Pourjavan, Nathalie J.M. Collignon, Veva De Groot, Rich A. Eiferman, Andrew J. Marshall, and Cecile J. Roy


## Introduction

Aqueous humor is produced in the posterior chamber of the eye by the ciliary body epithelium at a relatively constant rate of about 2.5 µl/min and flows into the anterior chamber, passing around the lens and through the pupillary opening in the iris. It is a complex mixture of electrolytes, organic solutes, growth factors, and other proteins that supply nutrients to the nonvascularized tissues of the anterior chamber (i.e., trabecular meshwork, lens, and corneal endothelium). Egress of aqueous humor from the anterior chamber occurs via two distinct pathways: conventional and uveoscleral. In the primary (conventional) outflow pathway, accounting for the majority of the aqueous outflow in normal individuals, aqueous humor passes through the trabecular meshwork, enters a space lined with endothelial cells (Schlemm's canal), and drains into collector channels and then into the aqueous veins. The uveoscleral outflow pathway, which may account for 10–60 % of total flow in the human eye [1–4], comprises the interstitium of the ciliary body, the suprachoroidal space, and, ultimately, the choroidal and scleral vasculature. Elevated intraocular pressure (IOP) typically results from increased resistance or compromise in either or both outflow pathway.

While research is investigating ways to protect the optic nerve and the vision from an elevated pressure, the only therapeutic approach currently available in glaucoma is to reduce the intraocular pressure. Glaucoma surgery is intended to reduce the IOP when the target IOP cannot be reached with maximal medical therapy or laser treatment. Due to complications with established surgical approaches such as trabeculectomy (early hypotony, blebitis, endophthalmitis, shallow anterior chamber, etc.) and closure by the body's natural healing process, a variety of seton devices, including aqueous shunts, are in use or being evaluated as alternative surgical treatments for patients with glaucoma. Glaucoma drainage devices (GDDs) aim at creating an alternate aqueous pathway from the anterior chamber by channeling aqueous humor out of the eye, hence reducing IOP. Traditionally, GDDs have been developed to provide an artificial conduit (small tube) for aqueous humor to travel from the anterior chamber and spread across a subconjunctivally located plate to form a filtering bleb [5, 6]. Although this filtration is nonphysiologic, the traditional tube shunts can effectively reduce IOP. However, they share similar postoperative challenges with trabeculectomy including bleb leakage, overfiltration, bleb dysesthesia, bleb encapsulation, and fibrosis. They also have their own unique set of postoperative risks, such as corneal endothelial cell death, ptosis, diplopia, tube migration, tube or plate exposure, and tube lumen occlusions. As a result,


S. Pourjavan, MD, PhD
Department of Ophthalmology, Cliniques Universitaires
St. Luc, UCL, Avenue Hippocrate 10, Brussels 1100, Belgium
e-mail: sayehpourjavan@hotmail.com

N.J.M. Collignon, MD, PhD
Division of Neuro-Ophthtalmology and Glaucoma,
Department of Ophthalmology, University Hospital of Liège,
Domaine du Sart Tilman B35 avenue de l'hôpital 1,
avenue de l'hôpital 1, Liège 4000, Belgium
e-mail: nathalie.collignon@chu.ulg.ac.be

V. De Groot, MD, PhD
Department of Ophthalmology, University
Hospital Antwerp, Edegem, Belgium
e-mail: Veva.DeGroot@uza.be

R.A. Eiferman, MD, FACS
Department of Ophthalmology, University of Louisville,
6400 Dutchmans Pkwy, Louisville, KY 40205, USA
e-mail: reiferman@cs.com

A.J. Marshall, PhD
Healionics Corporation, 2121 N 35th St,
Seattle, WA 98103, USA
e-mail: andrewm@healionics.com

C.J. Roy, PhD (✉)
iSTAR Medical SA, Rue Phocas Lejeune 25/3,
Isnes 5032, Belgium
e-mail: cecile@istarmed.com



**Electronic supplementary material** Supplementary material is available in the online version of this chapter at http://dx.doi.org/10.1007/978-1-4614-8348-9_22. Videos can also be accessed at http://www.springerimages.com/videos/978-1-4614-8347-2



J.R. Samples, I.I.K. Ahmed (eds.), *Surgical Innovations in Glaucoma*,
DOI 10.1007/978-1-4614-8348-9_22, © Springer Science+Business Media New York 2014

                                                                    

many recent efforts have been directed towards new "blebless" procedures that do not rely on conjunctival placement and are less prone to these complications.

STARflo™ is a new glaucoma drainage device designed to provide a pathway for aqueous humor to travel from the anterior chamber into the suprachoroidal space, enhancing the natural uveoscleral outflow and eliminating the need for a filtering bleb. It is comprised entirely of Healionics' proprietary silicone STAR® Biomaterial, a precision-pore structure that creates a permanent multi-porous wicking system and that enhances biointegration and reduces fibrosis [7–9].

## Background

The shape of the STARflo Glaucoma Implant is based on designs developed by Dr. Robert Nordquist in the 1990s [10, 11]. Originally based on cellulosic membrane, the material composition of the seton has evolved towards the use of a more advanced biomimetic structure and a more robust biocompatible material – the silicone STAR® Biomaterial manufactured by Healionics Corporation.

## Cellplant Device

The use of setons to permanently lower IOP has been attempted for many decades. The first seton made of horsehair was implanted in 1906 to drain fluid out of the anterior chamber [12]. Since then, devices made from numerous other materials including silk thread, nylon, hydrogels, collagen, gold, platinum, silicones, and polythene have been described in the literature [13, 14]. Over time, these devices have varied widely in size, material composition, and design. In the 1990s, a novel approach was created by Drs. Robert Nordquist and Bing Li to overcome shortcomings that limit conventional aqueous tube shunts, such as foreign body reactions, inflammation, tube obstruction, and infection. Nordquist and Li described the material, the design, and the surgical protocol for a novel method of lowering the IOP [10, 11, 15, 16]. The material should exhibit certain characteristics for seton use:

- Biocompatible to avoid foreign body reaction, inflammation, and capsule formation
- Highly resistant to cellular attachment and invasion
- Nonabsorbable and stable at body temperature
- Pliable so as to fit the contours of the eye
- Soft enough to avoid scleral erosion, corneal irritation, inducement of undesirable changes in eye curvature, or damage to adjacent vasculature and tissue, but resilient enough to maintain shape and thickness
- Strong enough to keep the surgical fistula open permanently
- Porous so as to naturally regulates the flow of aqueous humor through the seton by mimicking the trabecular meshwork

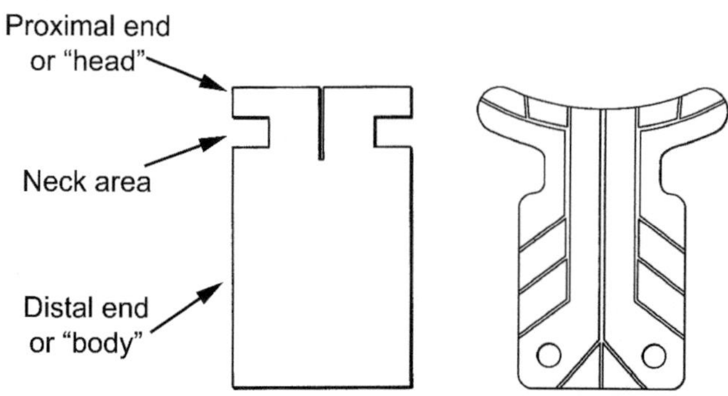


**Fig. 22.1** Norquist's designs for seton use [11, 15]. Seton is comprised of a head, a neck, and a body portions. Further versions of the seton included grooved drainage channels, curved edges and proximal end, and suture holes

The multi-porous structure should also exhibit an inherent controlled resistance to flow first to prevent postoperative hypotony and second to regulate the rate of aqueous humor outflow proportional to the intraocular pressure. The material should also inhibit closure at the surgical site without producing inflammation, obstruction, or infection.

In the initial iteration, the seton devices were formed as thin flexible sheets with bottle-shaped profiles (Fig. 22.1). The proximal end ("head") extended into the anterior chamber and reduced to a narrow neck area passed through a limbal opening at the iridocorneal angle. The neck shape regulated the flow and securely held the seton in position. The distal end ("body") was rectangular shaped and entirely placed under a conventional 50 % thickness scleral flap. Typically, these setons were designed approximately 8–10 mm long with a width of 4–6 mm and a thickness of 50 μm. Some versions further included grooved drainage channels to facilitate increased ocular fluid flow from the anterior chamber, curved proximal ends to conform with the curvature of the anterior chamber, and suture holes in the body to secure the implant to the sclera.

The resultant "CELLplant" device (Fig. 22.2) was a filtering implant of similar shape to the first model shown on the left in Fig. 22.1 and made from the cellulosic membrane material widely used for hemodialysis filtering [10, 11]. This material exhibited many of the needed characteristics.

Toxicity, safety, and efficacy of the CELLplant device were successfully demonstrated in rabbits [10, 11]. In a first short study, the average IOP dropped from 22.0 to 14.3 mmHg in the eyes treated with the CELLplant device, whereas the control eyes treated with a normal filtering surgery had an average IOP of 20.2 mmHg after 70 days ($p$-value of 0.001). A 1-year study showed similar results with an average IOP reduction more than 30 % at the end of the experiment (Fig. 22.3). None of the rabbits developed corneal decompensation, conjunctival erosion, or uveitis as a result of the implants. Scanning electron microscopy of the angle structures showed no evidence of corneal endothelial damage, iris atrophy, necrosis, or hypertrophy although there was iris touch. In all experimental eyes, except for one due to malposition of the implant, a functional filtering bleb was maintained, and the fistulas remained well open. Similar IOP results were also obtained in a cat with glaucomatous eyes.

Based on the promising preliminary animal studies devoid of complications, a human clinical trial was conducted in the Republic of China in 1994–1995 by Dr. Li [10, 11, 17]. Twenty-three patients, exhibiting uncontrolled glaucoma of various type (neovascular, open angle, closed angle, traumatic) averaging over 60 mmHg of IOP and with previous failure to respond to conventional medical treatment, underwent filtration surgery with the CELLplant seton. The average IOP was 12 mmHg by the third-day postoperative, and all remained below 18 mmHg through 180 days. During the 24-month follow-up of the study (13 cases), no postoperative hypotony; complications including hyphema, uveitis, or infection; or flat chambers were observed, and the devices still functioned at the end of the study.

The feasibility of the surgical procedure and the promising results of the CELLplant device in significantly and sustainably dropping the IOP have been reported in both animal and human trials; further bench testing and an animal study on rabbits were conducted in response to the then newly issued (1998) US FDA Guidelines for Aqueous Shunts 510(k) (later issued as ANSI Z80.27-2001 Aqueous Shunts for Glaucoma Application) with the aim of commercializing the CELLplant device. Although IOP results correlated with those earlier observed (see Fig. 22.3), this animal study revealed certain issues of long-term fibrosis and mechanical fragmenting of the cellulosic material [18, 19]. The use of a more robust, long-term stable material was therefore required to overcome the drawbacks of the cellulose and to provide a future for Norquist's design. This material was found in the STAR® Biomaterial, invented at the University of Washington in 2003.

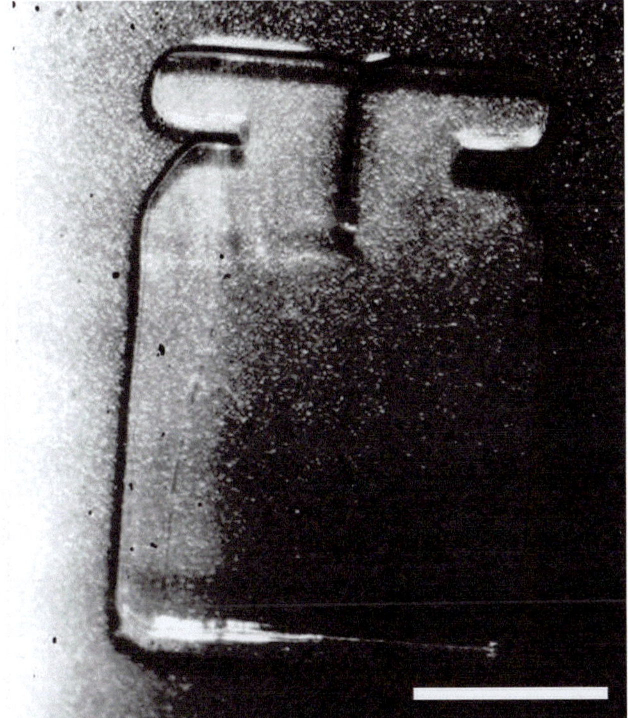

**Fig. 22.2** Image of a hydrated CELLplant device. Once hydrated, CELLplant thickness was about 75 μm. *White scale bar* represents 3 mm (Used with permission of Dr. Robert Nordquist)

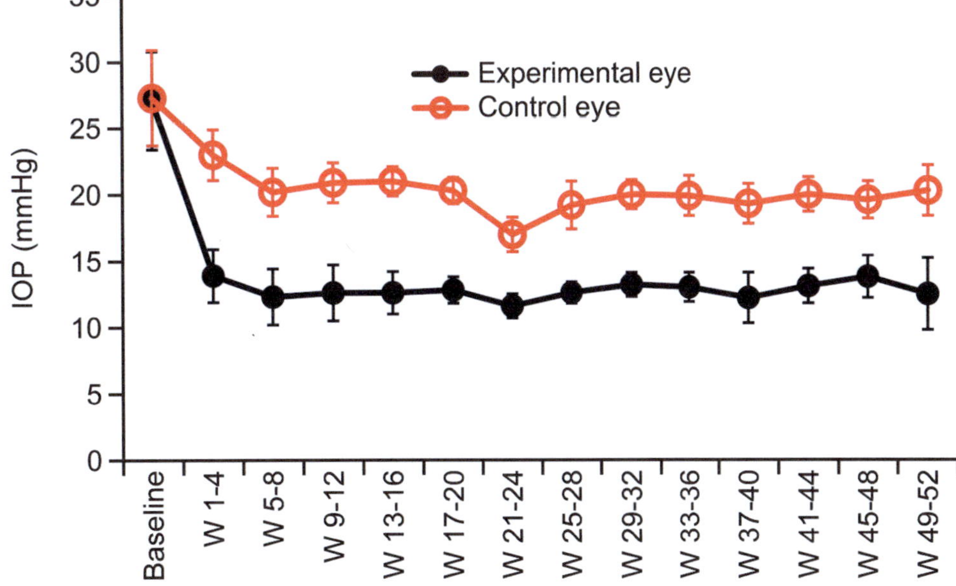



**Fig. 22.3** One-year IOP follow-up in rabbits. For each animal (12 rabbits in total), one eye was implanted with CELLplant (experimental eye – *black line*) and the contralateral eye was used as control (open markers, *red line*)

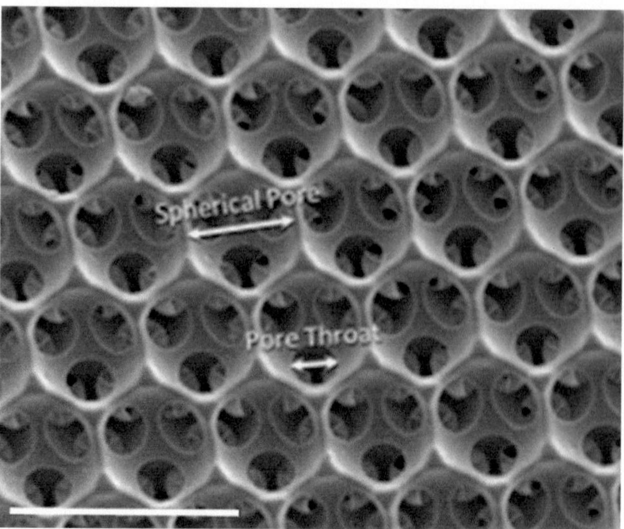


**Fig. 22.4** SEM image of STAR® Biomaterial surface showing uniform dimensions of the pores and pore throats. *White scale bar* represents 50 μm

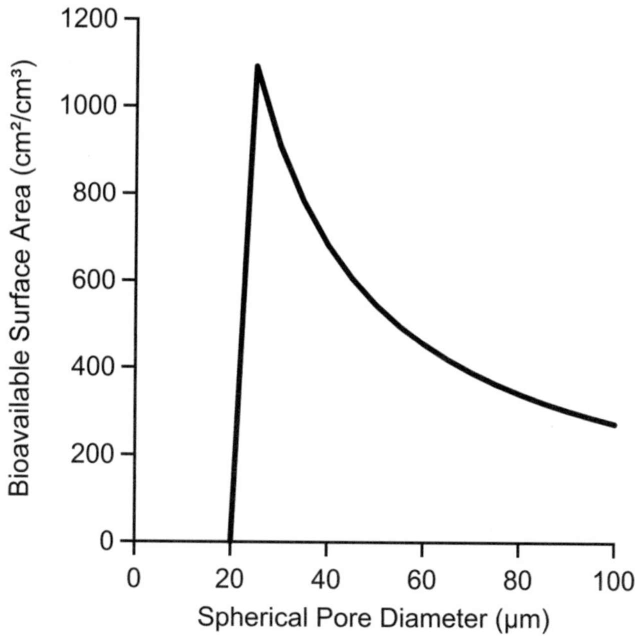


**Fig. 22.5** Calculated bioavailable surface area for sphere-templated biomaterials as a function of the pore diameter. Note: calculations assume 40 % throat-pore size ratio, porosity of 65 %, 7.5 throats per pore, and 10-μm minimum throat size for cellular access [20]

## STAR Material

Healionics' proprietary STAR® Biomaterial is a porous tissue engineering scaffold designed to promote healing of tissue around implanted medical devices with less scarring, improved vascularity, and a more stable long-term tissue-biomaterial interface.

## A Precision-Pore Structure

STAR® Biomaterial contains a precisely controlled pore geometry made with a sphere-templating process developed at the University of Washington by Andrew Marshall and Buddy Ratner. Healionics has exclusively licensed patents from the University of Washington covering porous biomaterials with the optimized pore size for promoting vascular ingrowth and the sphere-templating methods for making them [7–9].

The sphere-templating process yields a pore structure with interconnected uniformly sized spherical pores. Since the size of the necks formed during the sintering step is carefully controlled, the size of the interconnections, or "throats," between the pores of the templated biomaterial is also precisely controlled. Figure 22.4 shows a scanning electron microscopy (SEM) image of the sphere-templated STAR® pore structure, with uniform dimensions of the pores and pore throats indicated. The ordered arrangement of the pores is an outcome of the fabrication method but is not believed essential to biological function so long as overall porosity and interconnection is maintained.

The pore size and structure of the STAR® Biomaterial are optimized for several biological effects that contribute the functionality of the STARflo™ Glaucoma Implant. These effects include maximized recruitment of macrophage cells

into the pores, the subsequent vascularization of the implant with high capillary density, and the minimization of fibrotic scarring in the peri-implant tissues.

## Maximized Macrophage Concentration

Macrophages are known to play a key role in the body's response to the tissue injury created upon implantation of a foreign biomaterial; these cells arrive at the tissue-biomaterial interface and attach to any exposed biomaterial surface area.

Pore structure of the STAR® Biomaterial is optimized so as to attract a maximized concentration of host macrophages into the pore structure. This is achieved by maximizing the surface area per unit volume available for macrophage attachment. As shown in Fig. 22.5, the so-called bioavailable surface area in the sphere-templated materials exhibits a sharp peak at the pore size of ~25 μm – the smallest pore size that allows macrophages to enter the spherical pores via the circular pore throats. Figure 22.6 demonstrates the sharp spike in macrophage concentration at 35 μm pore size, hence defining a "sweet spot" pore range between 25 and 35 μm represented by STAR® Biomaterial [21].

Beside the pore size, tight control of the pore throat diameter is also a critical parameter. On one hand, this dimension is on the same size scale as the macrophage cells (a human macrophage is 10–20 μm in diameter) [22]. To facilitate cellular infiltration, pore throats must therefore be at least ~10 μm in diameter. On the other hand, the throat-pore size

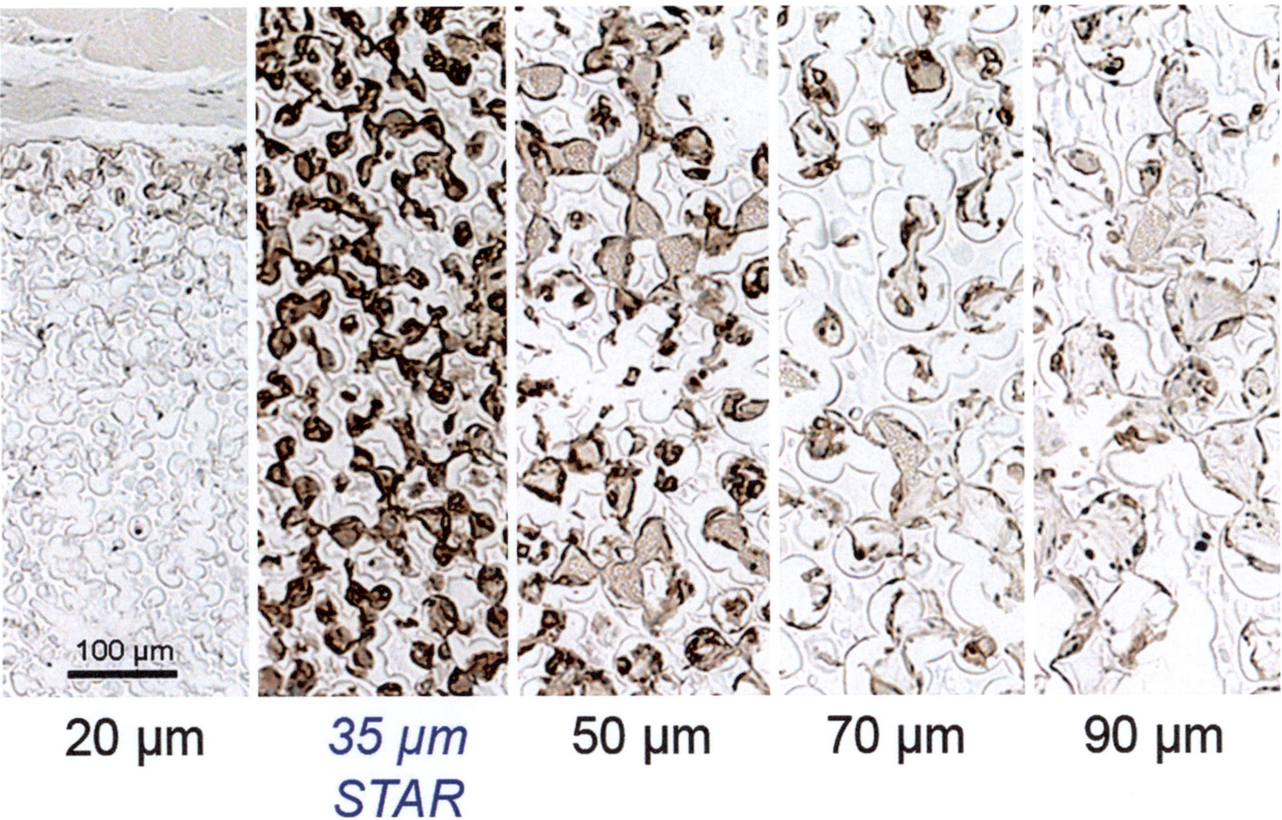



**Fig. 22.6** Tissue sections of sphere-templated scaffolds with a series of controlled pore sizes implanted subcutaneously in mice for 4 weeks, stained with F4/80 macrophage marker. The 35-µm pore size (STAR® Biomaterial) is infiltrated with the largest number of F4/80 positive cells

ratio is constrained by practical considerations of the sphere-templated geometry: if the pore throat size is increased much beyond ~40 % of the spherical pore diameter, the neighboring pore throats within each pore would nearly overlap, and mechanical strength of the templated porous structure may fall off precipitously.

### Maximized Vascularization

The STAR pore dimensions also encourage vascularization of the porous biomaterial with a robust capillary network. Figure 22.7 demonstrates that maximum blood vessel density occurs in the same "sweet spot" pore range of 25–35 µm and that the increased vascular density is observed not only within the pores but also in the capsule tissue immediately adjacent to the outer boundary of the porous implant [21]. The vascularizing effect mirroring the pore size dependent trend observed with macrophages suggests that the macrophages within the pores promote angiogenesis via the release of proangiogenic factors. The neovascularization effects of implanted porous biomaterials had been observed previously by other researchers [23, 24]. The precise dimensional control of the STAR® sphere-templating method allowed the optimum pore size for maximizing density of vascular ingrowth to be determined with greater accuracy. Since the method ensures all pores and

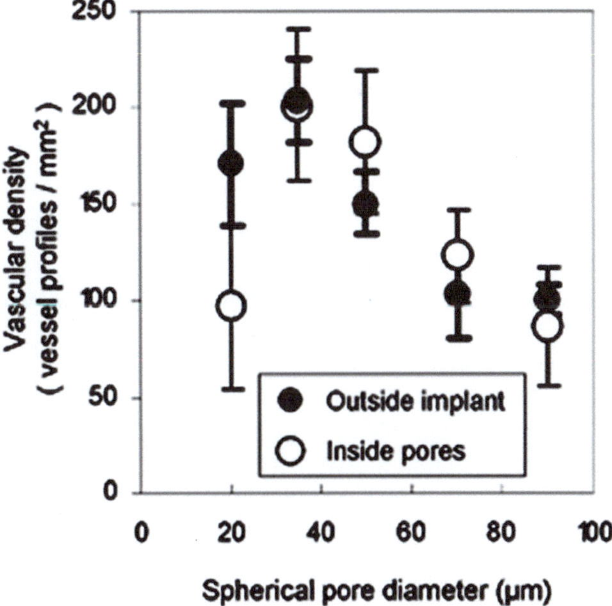



**Fig. 22.7** In the "sweet spot" pore range around ~30 µm, the density of blood vessels is maximized both inside the implant and in the adjacent tissue within 50 µm of the implant. Vessels counted from sections of 4-week subcutaneous mouse implants stained with MECA-32 endothelial cell marker

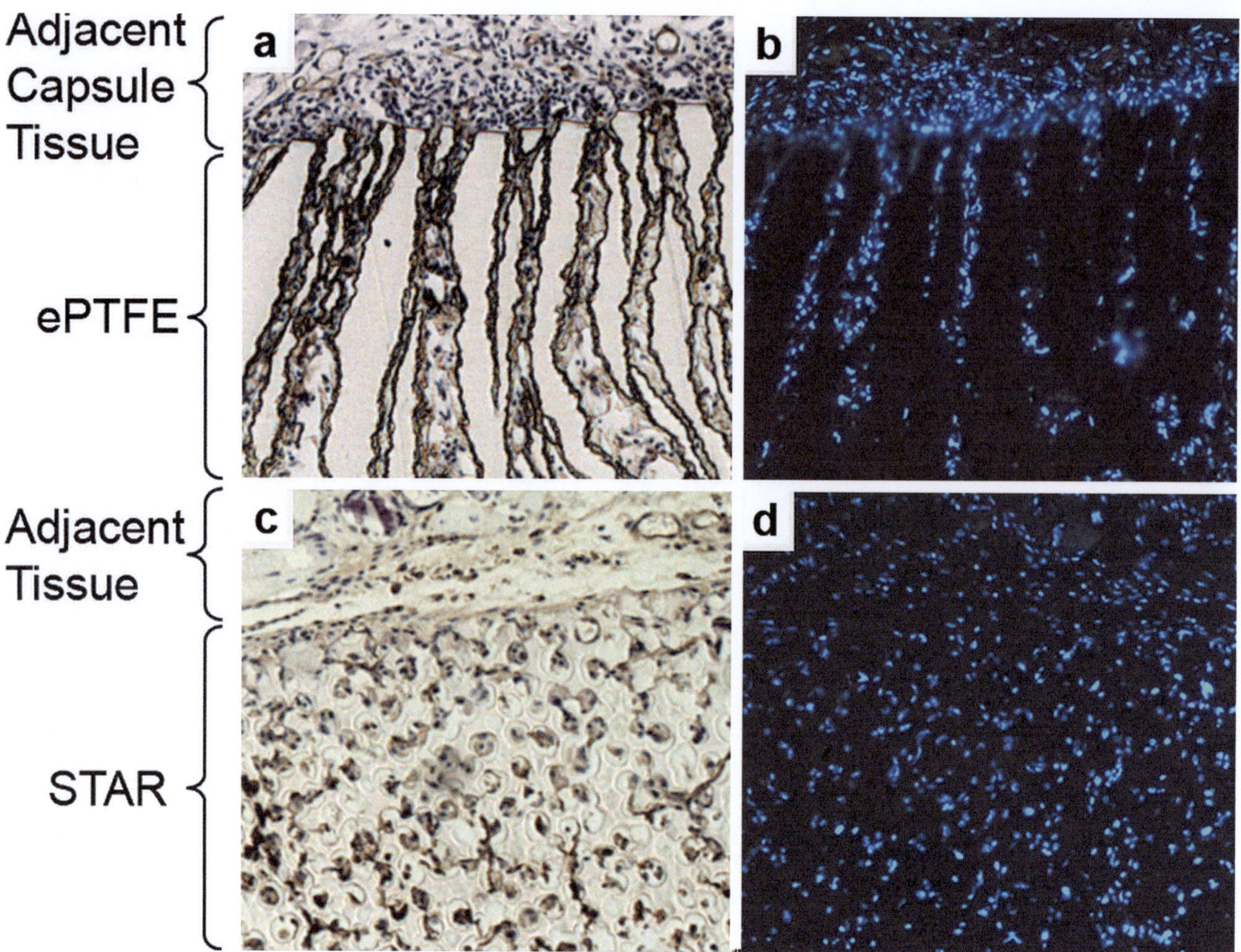



**Fig. 22.8** Comparison of cellular integration at tissue-biomaterial interface for expanded polytetrafluoroethylene (ePTFE) (panels **a** and **b**) and STAR® Biomaterial (panels **c** and **d**). Tissue sections from scaffolds implanted subcutaneously in mice for 2 weeks, stained with MECA-32 brown endothelial marker (panels **a** and **c**) and with DAPI inflammatory cell nuclei marker (panel **b** and **d**). STAR material exhibits a more integrated interface with cells equally dispersed in scaffold and adjacent tissue while inflammatory cells accumulate and concentrate in adjacent capsule tissue around ePTFE implant (Used with permission of the authors and excerpted from [26])

pore throats in the structure are optimized in size, the localized proangiogenic effect is more pronounced.

The biointegration of STAR® Biomaterial was compared to expanded polytetrafluoroethylene (ePTFE) with 60-μm internodal distance – a porous biomaterial of similar pore size that has been investigated for glaucoma implants [25]. It was found that the STAR material induced a more smoothly integrated interface. As shown in Fig. 22.8, inflammatory cells accumulate in high concentration in the capsule tissue bordering the ePTFE implant, while the interface between the STAR® Biomaterial and the surrounding capsule tissue features a smooth transition in cellular density across the capsule-biomaterial boundary. Also, Fig. 22.9 shows that the endothelial cell concentration within the pores of STAR® Biomaterial was significantly greater than for ePTFE, indicating significantly increased intrapore neovascularization. The enhanced vascularizing effect compared to other porous biomaterials provided inspiration for the "STAR" acronym for sphere-templated angiogenic regeneration.

It has been hypothesized that the increased neovascularization associated with STAR Biomaterial could be attributed in part to a shift in macrophage polarity triggered when the spatially confined macrophages within the pore structure are directed by geometric cues towards a proangiogenic phenotype [27].

## Anti-fibrotic Properties

Severalfold reductions in foreign body capsule thickness compared to nonporous controls have been observed for STAR Biomaterial in a variety of small and large animal models [21, 27, 28]. In Fig. 22.10, implant made from STAR® Biomaterial elicits remarkably thinner and looser foreign body capsule compared to nonporous control of same size and shape in a porcine subcutaneous implant model [28].

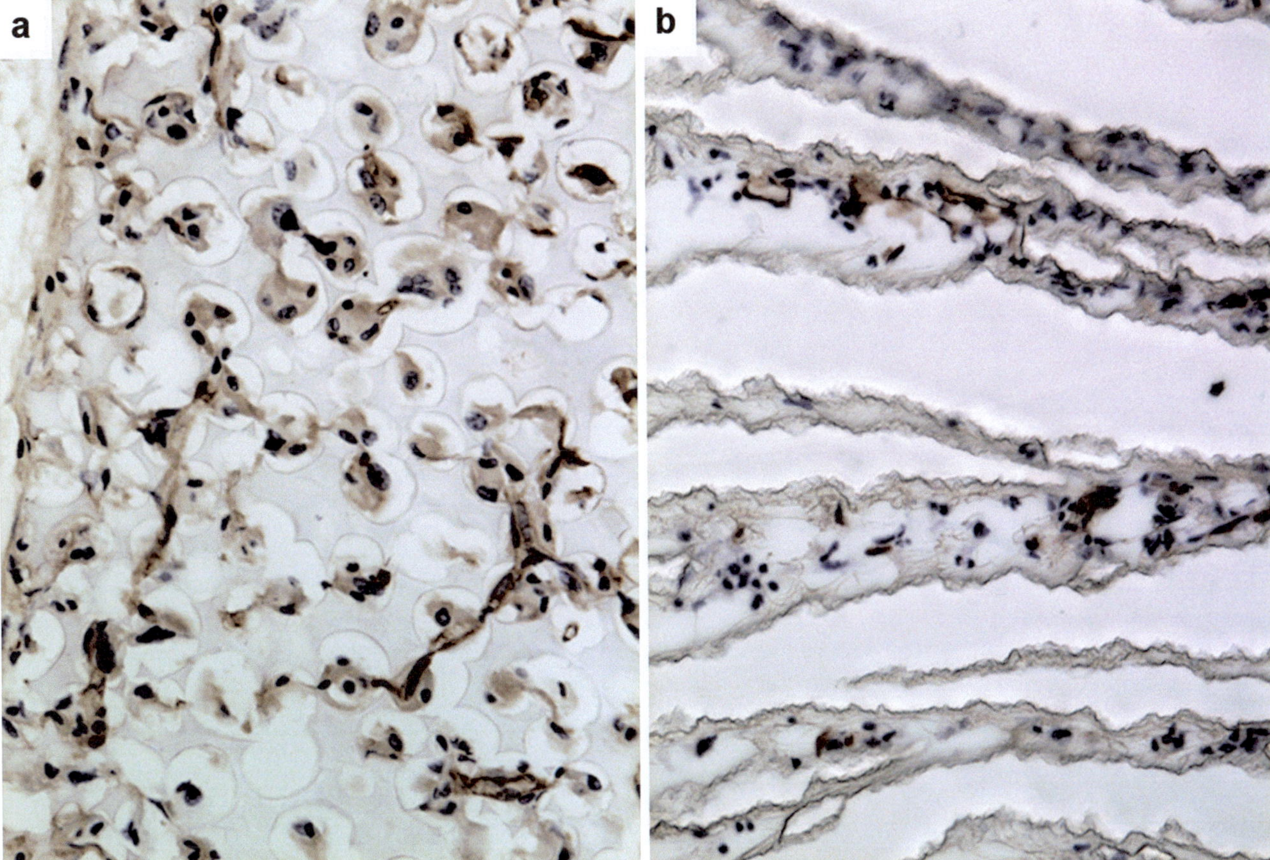

**Fig. 22.9** Comparison of level of vascularization within STAR® Biomaterial and expanded polytetrafluoroethylene (ePTFE). Tissue sections from scaffolds implanted subcutaneously in mice for 2 weeks, stained with MECA-32 brown endothelial marker. STAR scaffold (panel **a**) shows much higher level of neovascularization than ePTFE (panel **b**) (Used with permission of the authors and excerpted from [26])

Although the mechanism for the reduction of peri-implant fibrosis is not fully understood, a plausible explanation is based on the idea that the vascularized tissue-biomaterial interface disrupts collagen lattice contraction. This "lattice slack" hypothesis is supported by a study where the capsule-reducing effects of STAR® Biomaterial were amplified by combining macrotopographic features and optimized microporosity in complementary configurations [28]. In that study, the absence of a myofibroblast layer in the capsule suggested a stress-relaxed condition with minimal fibrotic scar.

STAR Biomaterial's high resistance to fibrotic scarring represents a tremendous advantage for the STARflo device over other types of GDDs where fibrosis is a recurring problem in the sustainability of IOP-lowering efficacy.

## STARflo Glaucoma Implant

Of similar shape to the CELLplant device, the STARflo™ Glaucoma Implant is entirely made from silicone STAR® Biomaterial. Besides meeting the specific physical characteristics defined by Nordquist, this biomaterial exhibits advantageous inherent properties for a glaucoma drainage device:

- The angiogenic properties are exploited by positioning the implant body in contact with the choroid, forming a well-integrated drain for the aqueous flow diffusing from the anterior chamber and minimizing the formation of a filtering bleb and its associated complication.
- The biomaterial's ability to reduce the thickness and density of the peri-implant fibrous capsule layer that forms during the course of the foreign body response may benefit longer-term pressure-lowering performance of the implant.

## Material and Design

The STARflo device design is based on the previously mentioned patents. To overcome drawbacks associated with the cellulosic material of the CELLplant (e.g., long-term fibrosis and mechanical fragmentation), the STARflo device is made entirely from a long-term, implant silicone material (Nusil Technologies LLC, Carpinteria, USA) formed into the STAR

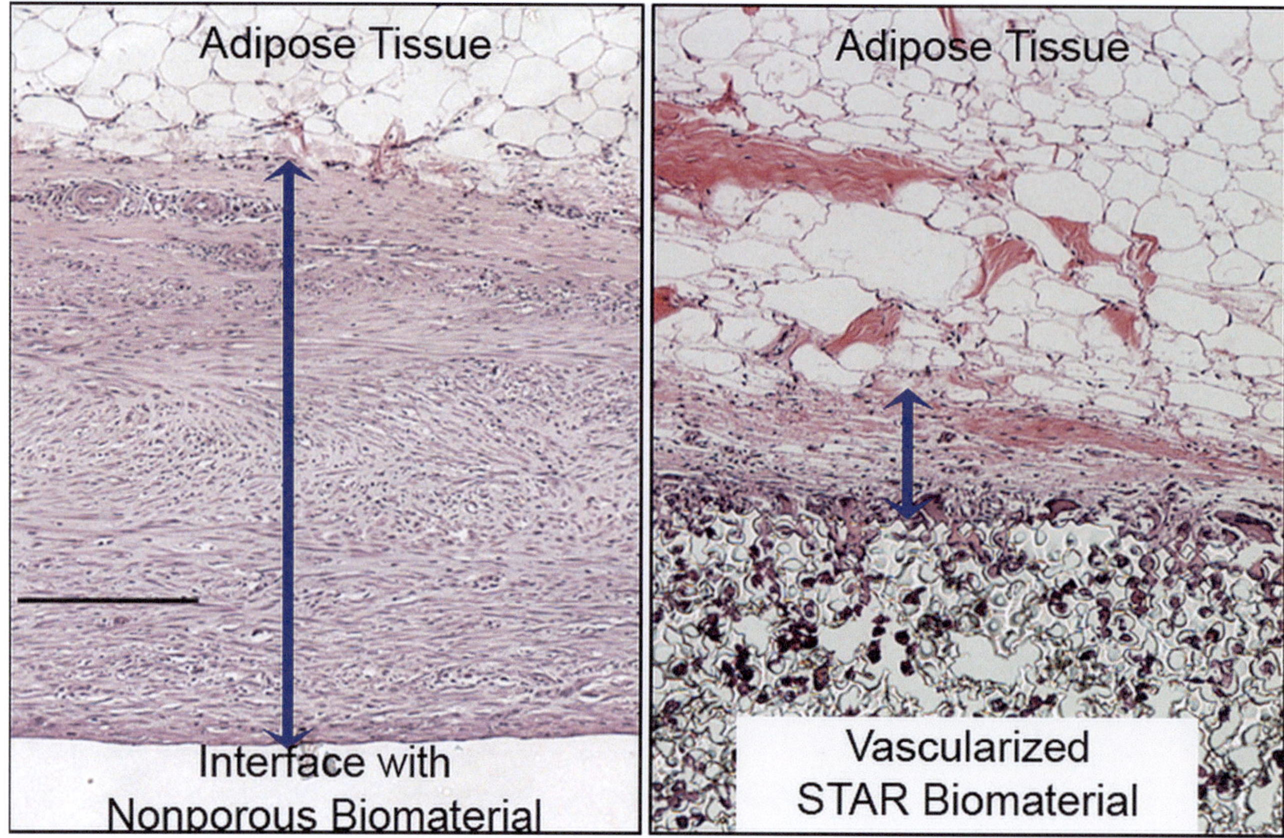


**Fig. 22.10** H&E-stained tissue sections from 6-week subcutaneous porcine implants. *Blue bands* denote capsule thickness. The average thickness of capsules surrounding nonporous control implants (panel **a**) was nearly 4-fold greater than capsules surrounding STAR implants with 27-μm pore size (panel **b**). *Black scale bar* represents 200 μm

structure. Silicones exhibit superior mechanical properties, durability, and reduced inflammation in ophthalmic implants [29]. The device is made as a single continuous sheet of porous silicone STAR scaffold free from seams, joints, coatings, metal, or degradable substances. Pore size and throat size within the material are uniformly 27 and 9 μm, respectively, through the entire volume of the device (Fig. 22.11) and comprised within the "sweet spot" pore range. The device has the same length and width, and general shape as the CELLplant predecessor, but a nominal thickness of 300 μm. In use, most of the body sits in the suprachoroidal space.

The structure and pore dimensions of the STAR material forming the STARflo closely mimic those of the trabecular meshwork and the ~10-μm-sized natural drain openings into Schlemm's canal, making the head section mimic the normal drainage path.

avoided. For ease of access and technical performance of the surgery, upper quadrants are the most commonly chosen location (1–2 o'clock (OS) or 10–11 o'clock (OD)).

Since the implant is entirely made from very soft porous silicone, the head area may be folded for ease of insertion to the anterior chamber via a small incision, just sufficient to retain the device neck. The anterior portion of the body then rests under a tight scleral flap while the posterior portion of the body is placed between the sclera and choroid (Fig. 22.12). This configuration provides a controlled fluid path for aqueous humor to drain from the anterior chamber to the suprachoroidal space of the eye. The implant bypasses the obstructed normal outflow passages and reduces the IOP without the need of a filtering conjunctival bleb prone to numerous complications. It also may spare patients wound healing issues associated with filtering surgery.

## Intended Use and Implant Location

The STARflo device is indicated for open-angle glaucoma. Implantation can be made in any location around the circumference of the globe providing that the rectus muscles are

## Surgical Procedure

The device is designed to be surgically placed in an *ab externo* fashion, under local retro- or parabulbar anesthesia. Because of its anti-fibrotic properties, STARflo implantation does not

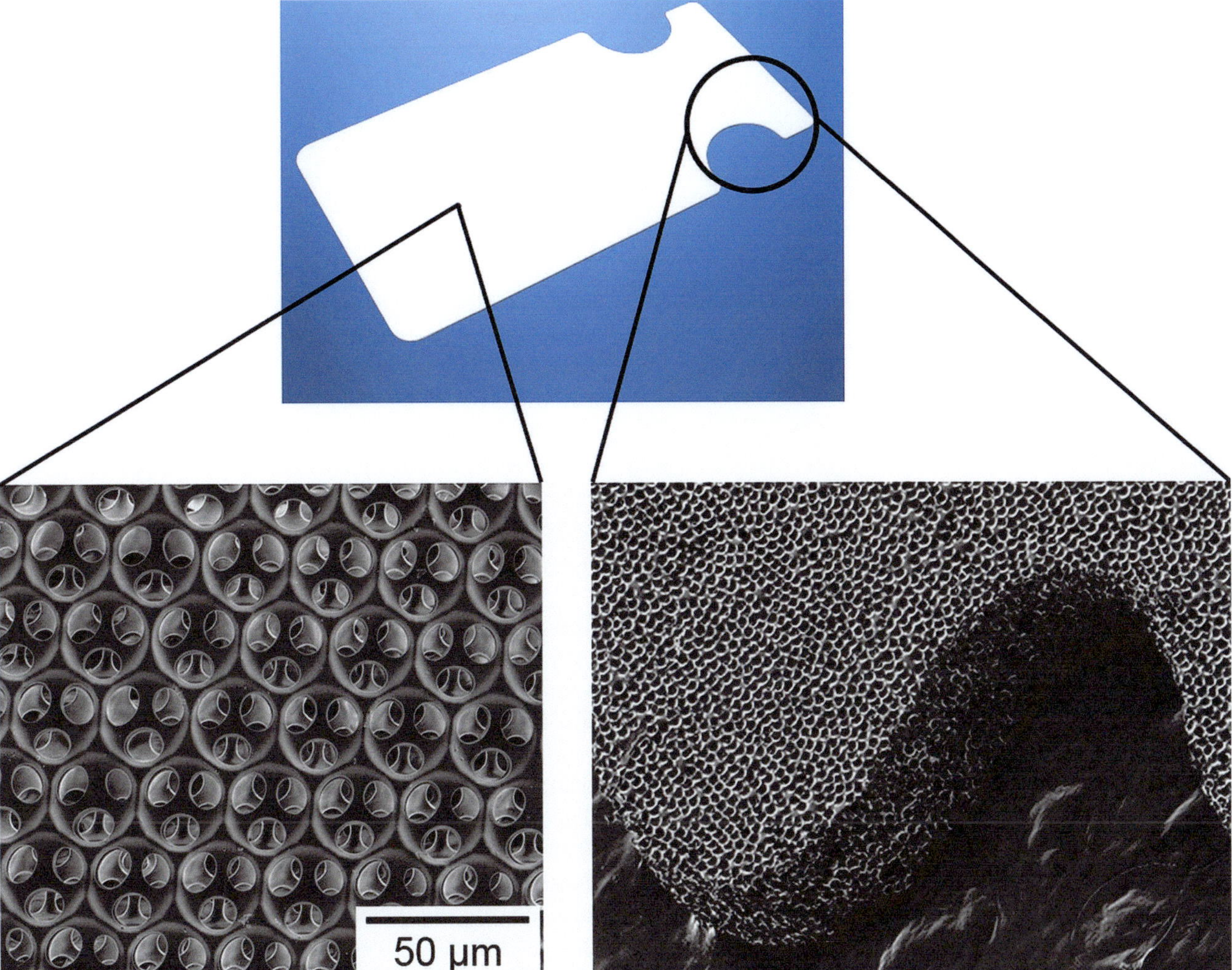



**Fig. 22.11** SEM of the STARflo device entirely made of STAR® Biomaterial

require the use of anti-fibrotic agents such as mitomycin C (MMC) or 5-fluorouracil (5-FU). The surgical implantation procedure recommended by iSTAR Medical is animated in Video 22.1, although the choice of anesthesia and method or technique to implant the drainage device is upon surgeon discretion.

A fornix-based conjunctival peritomy is first created, followed by a superficial, rectangular scleral flap (50 % thick, 8 mm wide, 3 mm long) as depicted in Fig. 22.13a. The second layer of sclera is then cautiously incised to reveal the choroid tissue, parallel to the limbus and leaving a scleral bridge of 1–2 mm (Fig. 22.13b). A 3-mm-wide incision is performed to reach the anterior chamber through the trabecular meshwork and allows STARflo head to be introduced (Fig. 22.13c). A subscleral pocket is then created by separating the sclera from the choroid using a blunt spatula. The posterior aspect of the implant is gently guided into the suprachoroidal space (Fig. 22.13d). One corner of the STARflo head is then inserted into the anterior chamber through the previously created entry

at the level of the scleral spur, followed by the other corner (Fig. 22.13e). When correctly placed, the implant neck is centered in the 3 mm incision and lays flat on the sclera without folds. The implant head is parallel to the iris to avoid incarceration or shunt-to-cornea touch and endothelial trauma. The scleral incision is then closed in a watertight fashion to avoid bleb formation. Finally, conjunctiva is sutured watertight. At all times, it is recommended to keep the implant moist using viscoelastic or sterile saline solution as a dry implant might compromise device performances. The use of non-toothed, blunt forceps is also recommended as well as avoidance of grasping the implant body.

## Technical Characteristics

STAR® Biomaterial has a controlled and predictable resistance to fluid flow. The measured flow resistivity of the 27-µm-pore-sized STAR material is 0.08 mmHg/(µl/min).

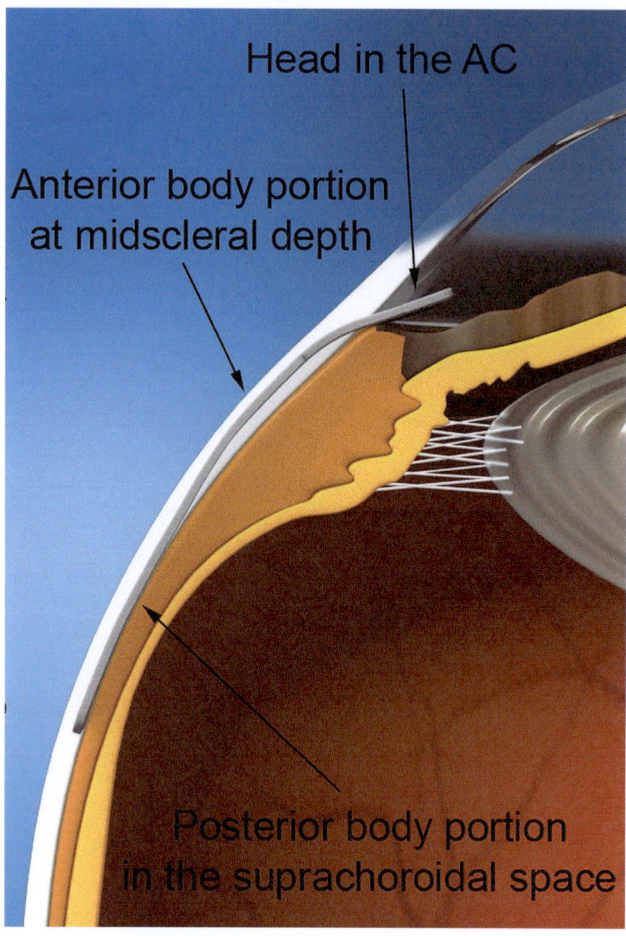



**Fig. 22.12** Illustration of the anatomical placement of the STARflo device. The head of the implant is inserted in the anterior chamber, the anterior portion of the body rests under a scleral flap, and the posterior portion of the body is placed within the suprachoroidal space

For the specific shape of the STARflo device, modeling provides an estimated in vitro flow resistance of 0.4 mmHg/(µl/min) for aqueous transfer into the head section, through the neck and then dispersion from the body. This value is comparable to in vitro values for the well-established devices with tube connection between the anterior chamber and subconjunctively located drainage plates. Under in vitro conditions, the device can convey 2.5 µl/min, equivalent to the normal aqueous inflow rate, with a pressure drop of 1 mmHg. In vivo, the natural differential in pressure between the anterior chamber and the suprachoroidal space permits the aqueous humor to drain through the STARflo device. STARflo does not rely on a subconjunctival bleb for IOP control, a well-known source of postoperative complications. However, formation of a small and transient bleb may be observed immediately after implantation, creating balancing back pressure to flow from the anterior chamber. Over time, as material integration with the choroid and sclera proceeds, it is hypothesized that

infiltration of the STARflo pores by capillaries from the choroidal vasculature network provides enhanced fluid contact for stable fluid absorption from the eye.

## Animal Study

Pre-market STARflo studies have been conducted on rabbits to assess safety in eye tissues and on dogs to assess performance in lowering IOP. At that time, implantation procedure recommended to create a full limbal-based scleral flap of the size of the implant body (8 mm in length by 6 mm in width) and to place the seton on the exposed choroid, followed by suturing the large scleral flap. Since then, STARflo surgery has evolved towards a trabeculectomy-like approach mainly to reduce risks of hyphema, choroidal prolapse, and choroidal hemorrhage.

## Rabbit Study

A sponsored 6-month preclinical study was conducted on rabbits by NAMSA (Northwood, USA) to evaluate the ocular irritation and toxicity potential of the STARflo. The protocol, entitled "Ocular Irritation Study of STARflo Glaucoma Implant Following Implantation in the Anterior Chamber of the Rabbit Eye," followed the US FDA Guidelines for Aqueous Shunts 510(k) clearance. This study closely duplicated the rabbit study performed with the CELLplant device but with the substitution of the STARflo device [30].

In total, 14 non-glaucomatous rabbits were implanted with the STARflo Glaucoma Implant in one eye. For ease of surgery, the body of the device was positioned mid-scleral depth. Based on the results of ocular examinations, no ocular irritation or toxicity was associated with the implantation of the STARflo device.

Histology images at both 12 and 26 weeks showed a progression in tissue integration along the length of the implant from the anterior chamber to the intrasclerally placed posterior portion. In Fig. 22.14, the extent of the STARflo device from the anterior chamber (on the left) into sclera (on the right) is clearly observed. In enlargement Fig. 22.14a, pores of the device in the anterior chamber are acellular and open to flow. In limbus area (enlargement Fig. 22.14b), STARflo integration with adjacent tissue is observed without the formation of a fibrous capsule. The pores appear to contain fibroblasts. In the anterior scleral area (enlargement Fig. 22.14c), further away from the anterior chamber, some vascularized capsule is formed and pores are highly vascularized; macrophages surrounding the capillary structures are shown in high magnification in Fig. 22.15 [31]. In the

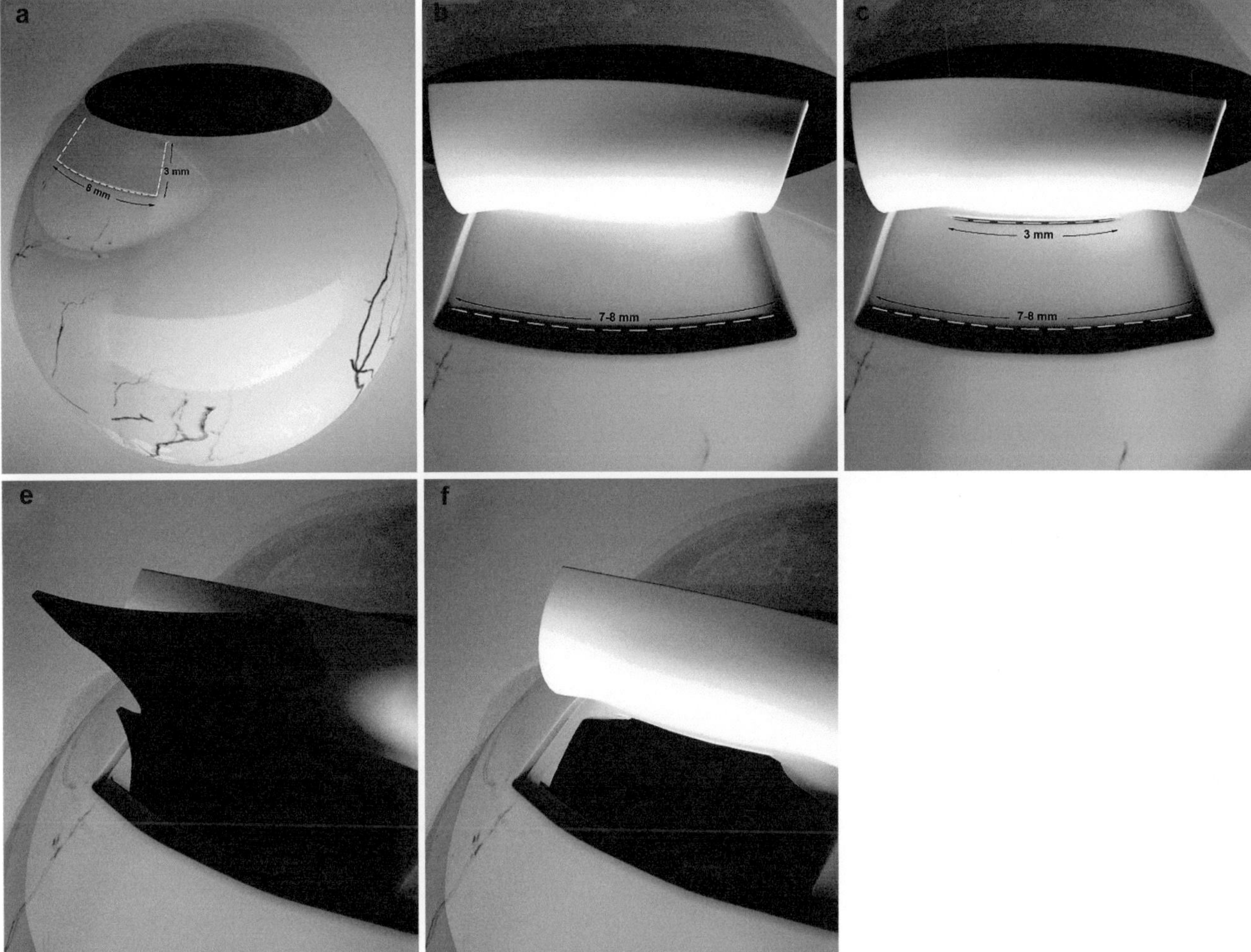

**Fig. 22.13** Key sequences of the STARflo surgical procedure recommended by iSTAR Medical SA. A half-thickness scleral flap (8 mm wide, 3 mm long) is performed (panel **a**) followed by a posterior full-thickness scleral incision (panel **b**). A 3-mm-wide entry is created into the anterior chamber (panel **c**). Body implant is guided into the suprachoroidal space (panel **d**) while the head of the implant is inserted into the anterior chamber (panel **e**)

posterior scleral area (enlargement Fig. 22.14d), pores are also highly vascularized and populated with macrophages.

Histology images at 6 months also showed that a robust capillary network persists within the pores long term. These capillaries within the pores and within the capsule tissue immediately adjacent to the implant appear to provide the transport surface area for drainage of the aqueous fluid.

Those observations are similar to previous results on the STAR® Biomaterial implanted in other tissue areas and demonstrate that the STARflo device exhibits excellent biointegration properties with minimal fibrotic tissue interface formation [27]. The device exerts minimal stress on surrounding tissue and conforms to the anatomic shape of the eye due to its spongy, flexible, and soft structure, hence removing potential irritation and promoting fast healing of the incisions with minimum foreign body reaction.

## Canine Study: The ClarifEYE

In collaboration with Dr. Craig Woods, CEO of TR BioSurgical, LLC (Chandler, Arizona), the STARflo device was initially introduced in 2008 for canine glaucoma veterinary use under the trade name ClarifEYE.

In a pilot study, glaucomatous dogs experiencing severe pain and unresponsive to maximum drug doses were implanted with ClarifEYE. Follow-up on two eyes over a 13-month period demonstrated that an IOP maintained between 10 and 20 mmHg after 1-year implantation (baseline IOP of 61.3 mmHg) and that needed medication could be decreased by 50 % [32]. The implant was observed to be well tolerated with minimal tissue reaction. To date, ClarifEYE has been implanted in more than 30 dogs of various breeds with glaucomatous eyes.

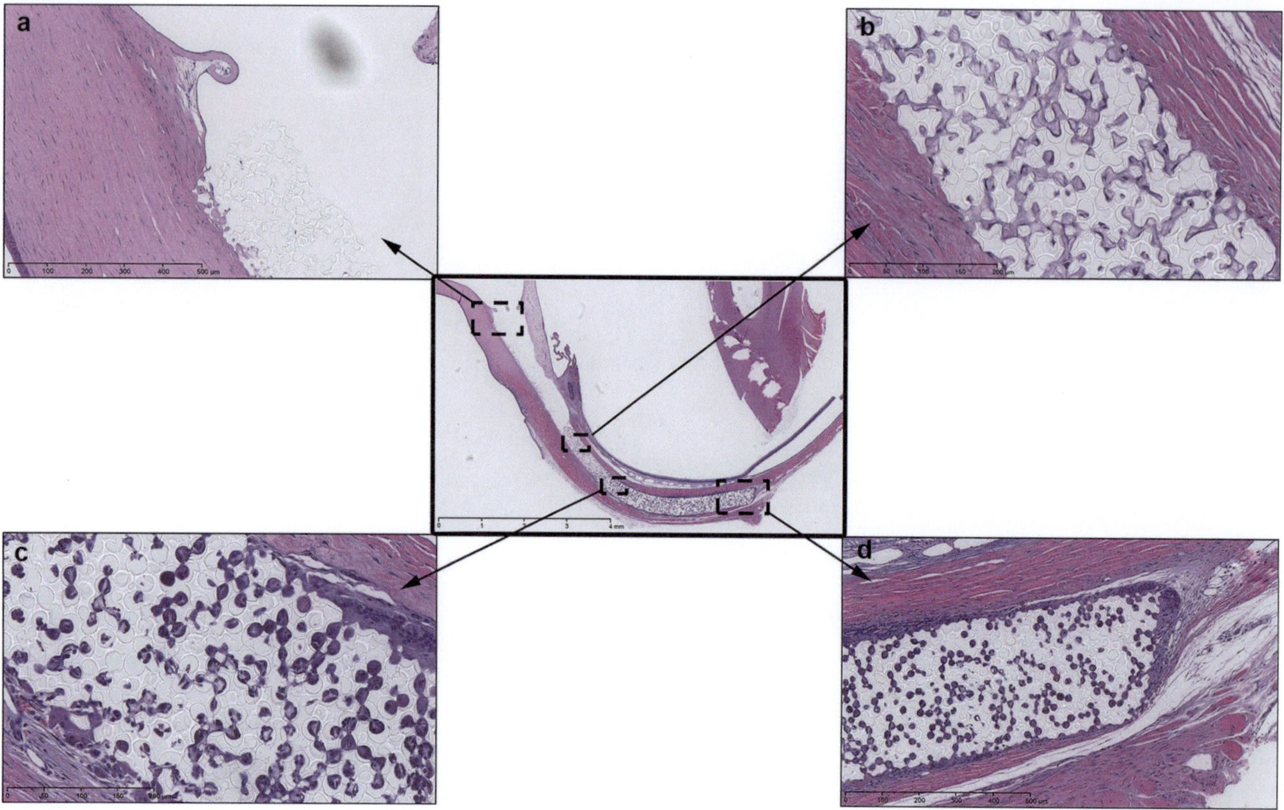

**Fig. 22.14** Histology image and its enlargements taken 12 weeks after STARflo implantation within the sclera, H&E stain. In the anterior chamber, pores are acellular and open to flow (panel **a**). In limbus area, STARflo integration with adjacent tissue is observed without the formation of fibrous capsule (panel **b**). In the anterior sceral area, pores are highly vascularized (panel **c**). In the posterior scleral area, pores are also highly vascularized and populated with macrophages (panel **d**)

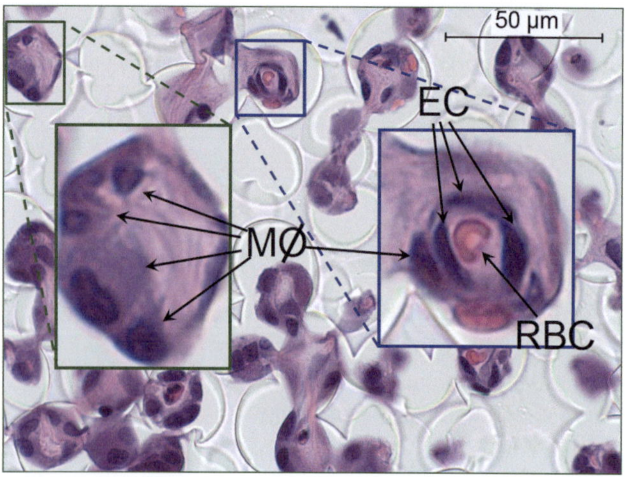


**Fig. 22.15** Capillary network in STAR pores at 6 months for intrascleral implant in rabbit, with vascular endothelial cells (*EC*) surrounding red blood cell (*RBC*) and macrophages (*MØ*) lining the pore walls; H&E stain [31]

## Human Clinical Study

A prospective, multicenter, feasibility trial was conducted to evaluate the safety and performance of the STARflo™ Glaucoma Implant in patients with open-angle glaucoma.

This study started in June 2011 and will close after 12-month follow-up. The study took place in three clinical sites in Belgium.

### Study Protocol

The aim of the study was to evaluate the safety of the STARflo Glaucoma Implant (i.e., implantation feasibility, incidence of device and procedure-related complications, and unanticipated adverse device effects) and its performance (i.e., reduction in IOP from preoperative baseline and reduction in number of glaucoma medications from preoperative baseline). The study protocol was approved by the respective ethics committees of the clinical sites. All patients signed an informed consent form to participate in the study.

The inclusion criteria for the clinical study were the following: (1) age of 18 years or older; (2) one or both eyes diagnosed with open-angle glaucoma or pseudoexfoliation glaucoma; (3) ability and willingness to return for up to 12 months of scheduled visits; (4) a documented IOP >21 mmHg in the study eye on medical therapy at two visits at least 48 h apart, within 2 months prior to study entry and at day of implantation; and (5) concurrent treatment with ocular hypotensive medications in the study eye or prescription of anti-inflammatory and acetazolamide approximately 3 weeks before the surgery till 2 days before the surgery.

The exclusion criteria were (1) diagnosis of traumatic, uveitic, or active neovascular glaucoma; (2) previous surgery with any aqueous shunt device in the same eye quadrant; (3) clinically significant corneal disease (e.g., corneal dystrophy); (4) any previous ophthalmic surgery in the same eye quadrant other than trabeculectomy, trabeculoplasty, and cataract surgery within 3 months prior to study entry; (5) anterior chamber anatomic configuration of high risk for development of angle-closure glaucoma; (6) laser trabeculoplasty within 3 months prior to study; (7) active proliferative/inflammatory retinopathy; (8) clinically significant intraocular inflammation or infection within 6 months prior to study; (9) uveitis within previous 6 months before the surgery; (10) evidence of crystalline lens subluxation or luxation; (11) evidence of vitreous loss in the anterior chamber; (12) uncontrolled systemic disease (e.g., diabetes, hypertension); (13) pregnancy; (14) participation in any study involving an investigational drug or device within the past 3 months; and (15) intolerance or hypersensitivity to topical anesthetics, mydriatics, or components of the device.

## Patient Follow-Up

Four patients (four eyes) with end-stage, medically uncontrolled IOP/refractory glaucoma were enrolled in this clinical study. Results for 6-month follow-up were collected to date.

### First Patient

In 2011, a 43-year-old male consulted because of severe pain in the almost nonfunctional right eye and headache since 3 months. The patient was known with high intraocular pressure in the right eye (48 mmHg) for which he was treated with Cosopt and Travatan since 3 years. He was using a combination therapy – paracetamol and codeine – for his headaches nearly twice a week. In 1978, he had a limbal perforation resulting in a low visual acuity (+1 LogMAR) probably due to irregular astigmatism, followed by cataract extraction in 1988. His IOP began to rise in 2005. His visual acuity in his right eye was very low (>+1 LogMAR). Biomicroscopy showed a Binkhorst pupillary fixated IOL with iridectomy at 11 o'clock without any signs of inflammation. Fundoscopy showed an optic disc excavation of 0.9 and normal maculae. On gonioscopy, the angle was wide open. Glaucoma in the right eye might be related to low-grade subclinical chronic inflammation. The left eye was normal with an IOP of 17 mmHg.

Patient was implanted with STARflo in his right eye under retrobulbar anesthesia. Intraocular pressure in the implanted eye and medications prescribed during the study follow-up are listed in Table 22.1. Postoperative observations during this period were the following:

**Table 22.1** IOP and medications for the first patient during the study follow-up

| Visit | IOP (mmHg) | Medications |
|---|---|---|
| Surgery | 48 | Atropine |
| | | Antibiotic and steroids |
| Day 1 | 2 | Topical combination therapy of antibiotics/steroids |
| Week 1 | 5 | Atropine |
| Month 1 | 29 | |
| Month 2 | 29 | |
| Month 3 | 38 | Atropine was stopped spontaneously 3 weeks before the visit |
| | | Antibiotics/steroids combination was continued |
| | | Cosopt was started |
| Month 4.5 | 42 | Cyclophotocoagulation (270°) → study discontinuation |

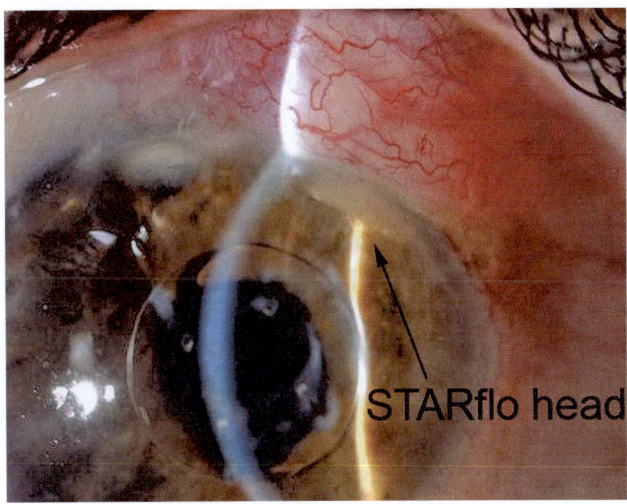


**Fig. 22.16** Slit lamp image of the first patient taken 1 month postoperatively. The head of the STARflo is visible in the anterior chamber at the 1 o'clock position, not touching the iris or cornea

- Severe eye/headache pain resolved on the first-week postoperative visit, but mild headache without eye pain started 3 months after the surgery.
- Mild inflammatory postoperative reaction in the anterior chamber resolved within 1 month.
- Moderate conjunctival vascularization at the implant site.
- Mild conjunctival edema resolved within 3 months.
- No changes in the fundus during the follow-up.
- No signs of choroidal hemorrhage or retinal detachment.
- Visual acuity remained unchanged from baseline.
- Small subconjunctival bleb started to encapsulate at the first-month postoperative examination (Fig. 22.16) but disappeared at the 3-month visit.

At the 4.5-month visit, the patient was suffering from mild headache and photophobia, probably not related to the STARflo device, but the IOP rise (42 mmHg on the right eye with Cosopt). The biomicroscopical scores remained unchanged. To reduce the IOP, a cyclophotocoagulation was performed (sparing the superonasal quadrant). At this point, the patient was discontinued from the study due to a lack of sufficient efficacy of the STARflo Glaucoma Device. After 10 days, a control visit showed an IOP of 10 mmHg in the right eye which slowly increased to 28 mmHg without pressure-lowering medication. Eleven months after the implantation, the STARflo device was removed because of persistent photophobia since the cyclodestruction, periocular pain, and conjunctival injection at the superonasal and inferior quadrants. The explant surgery went smoothly without any adverse event or complications. After a few days of hypotony, the IOP was again 24 mmHg 1 month after the explantation. Pain disappeared for a few months but relapsed afterwards. Photophobia was less, but not resolved. Six months after the removal of the implant, some anterior chamber inflammatory cells were seen for the first time, being a sign of chronic ocular inflammation. Probably a subclinical inflammation might have been the cause of the IOP rise from the start.

After this first implantation of STARflo in human, the surgical procedure was slightly adjusted based on surgeon's recommendation. The width of the superficial scleral flap and of the second layer of the sclera was assessed as too small (6 mm) for an easy implantation and for a watertight closure and was therefore increased to 7–8 mm for next surgeries.

## Second Patient

A 56-year-old male consulted in 2011 because of severe eye pain. Cataract surgery was performed 3 years ago. Patient was diagnosed with primary wide open-angle glaucoma in the left eye since 4 years and was treated with Cosopt and Travatan. His right eye was normal. The visual acuity of the left eye was only light perception, and the IOP was 32 mmHg. The biomicroscopy showed a moderate conjunctival redness, a severe corneal edema with no inflammatory reaction in the anterior chamber. Fundoscopy showed a severe excavated optic nerve in the left eye. The patient was implanted with STARflo under general anesthesia. Key sequences of the implantation are available on Video 22.2.

IOP in the implanted eye and medications prescribed during the study follow-up are listed in Table 22.2. Postoperative observations during this period were the following:

- Ocular pain and pain sensation around the eye globe disappeared within 1 month postoperatively.
- Some diffuse conjunctival fluid was observed the day after the surgery.
- Severe, preoperative corneal edema decreased progressively and resolved on the 6-month postoperative visit.
- Moderate cells and trace of flare in the anterior chamber without signs of inflammation resolved within 2 months.

**Table 22.2** IOP and medications for the second patient during the study follow-up

| Visit | IOP (mmHg) | Medications |
|---|---|---|
| Surgery | 32 | Paracetamol |
| | | Antibiotic |
| Day 1 | 2 | Nonsteroidal anti-inflammatory drug (NSAID) |
| | | Tropicamide |
| | | Combination drops of antibiotics/steroids |
| | | Antibiotic |
| Week 1 | 6 | Paracetamol |
| | | Tropicamide |
| | | Combination drops of antibiotics/steroids |
| | | NSAID |
| Week 2 | 26 | Acetazolamide 250 mg was added because of signs of topical drug toxicity |
| | | Antibiotic delivered in a single dose |
| | | Steroid delivered in a single dose |
| Month 1 | 22 | Steroid |
| | | Antibiotic |
| | | Acetazolamide 250 mg |
| Month 2 | 23 | Steroids |
| | | NSAID |
| | | Antibiotic |
| | | Acetazolamide 250 mg |
| Month 3 | 19 | Acetazolamide 250 mg |
| Month 6 | 20 | |

- Small choroidal detachment was observed superiorly in the fundus, probably related to the surgical procedure, and resolved within 2 weeks.
- Diffuse bleb resolved within the first month after surgery.
- Visual acuity remained light perception.
- Preoperative cystoid macula edema decreased from grade 3 (severe) to grade 1 (mild) 2 months after the surgery.

Six months after the surgery, the overall situation remained satisfactory.

## Third Patient

A 79-year-old female consulted in 2011 for an uncontrolled IOP in the left eye. The ophthalmological antecedents were congenital nystagmus and cataract surgery in both eyes. The patient was treated for primary open-angle glaucoma since 1994 in both eyes. Preoperatively, the eye pressure was 17 mmHg in the right eye and 29 mmHg in the left eye under Xalatan and Azopt. The visual acuity was only light perception in the left eye. Biomicroscopical exam revealed a mild corneal edema and a moderate corneal staining. The patient had abnormal macula and excavated optic nerve.

The patient underwent an operation with STARflo implant in 2011 in the left eye. The surgery was performed under general anesthesia. Intraocular pressure in the implanted eye and medications prescribed during the study follow-up are listed in Table 22.3. Postoperative observations during this period were the following:

**Table 22.3** IOP and medications for the third patient during the study follow-up

| Visit | IOP (mmHg) | Medications |
|---|---|---|
| Surgery | 29 | Antibiotic |
| | | Steroids |
| | | NSAID |
| Day 1 | 10 | NSAID |
| Week 1 | 6 | Cycloplegic drops |
| | | Acetazolamide 250 mg is added because of peripheral choroidal detachment. Because of the conjunctival redness, an oral treatment was preferred to antihypertensive drops |
| | | NSAID |
| Month 1 | 28 | Xalatan |
| | | Acetazolamide 250 mg (oral treatment) is preferred to eye drops because of the redness and conjunctival toxicity |
| | | Combination drops of antibiotics/steroids |
| Month 2 | 26 | Xalacom |
| | | Combination drops of antibiotics/steroids |
| Month 3 | 18 | Xalacom |
| Month 6 | 15 | |

**Table 22.4** IOP and medications for the fourth patient during the study follow-up

| Visit | IOP (mmHg) | Medications |
|---|---|---|
| Surgery | 39 | Steroid |
| Day 1 | 4 | Antibiotic |
| Week 1 | 6 | |
| Month 1 | 8 | Antibiotics were stopped |
| | | Steroids drops were continued because of the inflammatory reaction due to the exfoliative glaucoma and the combined procedure |
| Month 3.5 | NA | Steroid drops were spontaneously stopped by the patient |
| Month 4.5 | 40 | Cosopt was added |
| | | Intensive topical steroid was added to tamper the inflammation of the anterior chamber |
| Month 6 | 14 | Cosopt continued because of lack of persistency in medication use |
| | | Intensive topical steroid |

- Calm anterior chamber.
- Ocular pain and discomfort, probably due to the surgery, resolved in 2 weeks.
- Mild conjunctival edema resolved within 2 week.
- Moderate conjunctival redness resolved within 1 month.
- Small bleb resolved within 1 month.
- No differences in the fundus from baseline.
- Small choroidal detachment was observed superonasally in the left fundus, probably due to the surgical procedure, and resolved within the first month.
- Visual acuity remained light perception although hand movement perception was reported on 1-month visit.

Six months after the surgery, the overall situation remained satisfactory.

## Fourth Patient

A 83-year-old male patient from Morocco presented in 2011 because of progressive decrease of the vision especially in the left eye over 2 years. His ophthalmological history was blank. His visual acuity was +0.12 LogMAR in the right eye and nearly +2 LogMAR in the left eye with his hyperopic correction. Slit lamp examination showed cataract in both eyes. The anterior chambers were slightly smaller than normal. Signs of exfoliation syndrome were observed on both lenses. The IOPs were 24 mmHg in the right eye and 37 mmHg in the left eye. Gonioscopy examination showed in both eyes a narrow angle in all the quadrants with a marked Sampaolesi's line. There were no visible posterior synechia in dynamic gonioscopy. In fundi after dilatation, a normal optic disc was observed with an excavation of 0.3 and normal rim in the right eye and a total excavation of the left optic nerve, C/D 0.9+ with an overall loss of rim. A peripheral iridotomy (PI) was performed as first treatment, and prostaglandins (PG) were prescribed. The IOP remained high despite of PI and PG treatment. A combination therapy Cosopt was added to PG. In 2011, the IOP was 23.5 mmHg in the right eye and 39 mmHg in the left eye.

A combined operation, phacoemulsification cataract surgery first, followed by STARflo implantation, was performed on the left eye. Intraocular pressure in the implanted eye and medications prescribed during the study follow-up are listed in Table 22.4. Postoperative observations during this period were the following:

- Severe corneal edema and erosion, mainly caused by a complex cataract surgery, were resolved after 1 week.
- Small bleb resolved within 1 month.
- Merely due to the lack of compliance and the annulation of the third postoperative appointment by the patient, the following symptoms were observed 4.5 months after the surgery:
  - Signs of severe inflammatory reaction in the anterior chamber of the left eye resolved under intensive topical steroid drops.
  - Fibrin formation in front of the intraocular lens and on the STARflo head resolved on the 6-month postoperative visit.
  - Signs of synechia between the temporal angle of the STARflo head and the endothelium, still present on the 6-month visit but without disturbing the vision.
- Visual acuity slightly improved from +2.0 LogMAR to +1.2 LogMAR with postoperative correction.

On the 6-month postoperative control, the patient had neither complains nor pain even touching the site of operation.

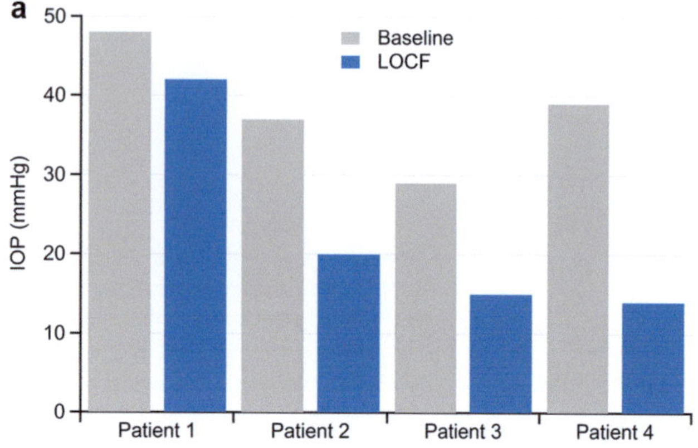


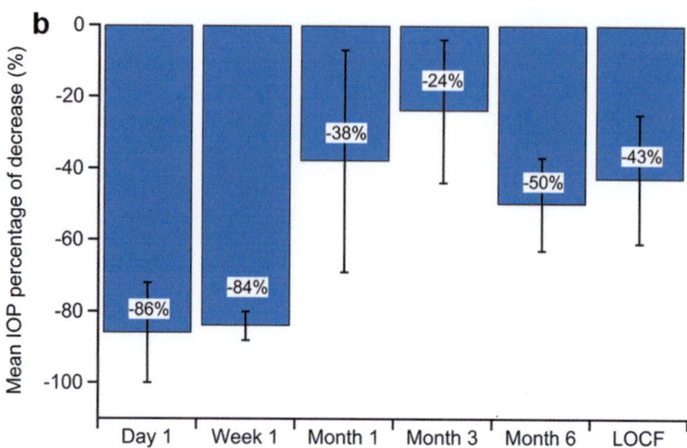


**Fig. 22.17** Comparison of IOP per patient at baseline and LOCF (panel **a**) and mean IOP percentage decrease at visit time (panel **b**). Patient 1 was discontinued after 4.5 months. *LOCF* last observation carried forward, e.g., at 4.5 months postoperatively for patient 1 and 6 months for patients 2, 3, and 4

**Fig. 22.18** Comparison of glaucoma medication per patient at baseline and LOCF (last observation carried forward, e.g., 4.5 months postoperatively for patient 1 and 6 months for patients 2, 3, and 4)

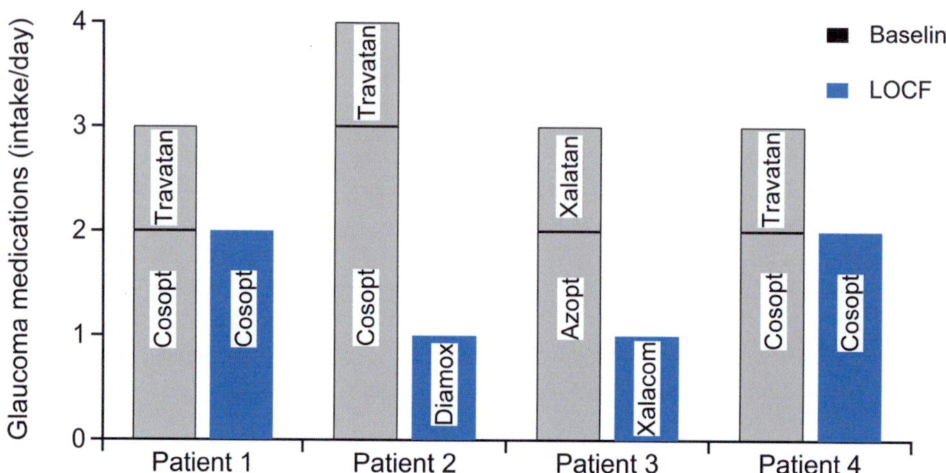


## Clinical Trial Summary

From a clinical perspective, the 6-month results of the STARflo clinical study showed that all the safety and the efficacy endpoints were achieved:

- For all patients, the STARflo implantation procedure was feasible without adverse events during or immediately after surgery.
- No device-related adverse events were reported.
- Transient choroidal detachment was encountered in two patients and probably procedure related, which resolved within the first month after surgery.
- Transient hypotony (IOP < 6 mmHg) resolved within 1 week in three patients and within 1 month in one patient.
- Postoperative bleb was seen in all four patients and disappeared between 1 week and 3 months.
- After 6-month follow-up (three cases), mean IOP percentage of decrease was 50 %, and an IOP < 21 mmHg was reported for all three patients still in study at that time (Fig. 22.17).
- After 6-month follow-up (three cases), the mean daily intake of glaucoma medication decreased by 60 % (Fig. 22.18).

However, despite the fact that a mean decrease in IOP and IOP-lowering medications was reported, no statistical significance between baseline and the last observations can be claimed due to the limited size of the studied cohort.

Concerning the first implanted patient whom been dropped out of the study, the scleral flap of 6 mm in width was too small to obtain watertight closure and was related to a more sustained filtering bleb (filtering up to 1 month, encapsulated bleb up to 3 months). Whether this might be related to an insufficient STARflo efficacy in lowering IOP remains an open question. STARflo devices placed in subsequent patients were inserted using a larger incision, and each exhibited a transient bleb and satisfactory IOP-lowering efficacy. On the other hand, this eye had probably a chronic low-grade inflammation which is a known risk factor for early fibrosis and failure in all filtering procedures.

## Conclusion

STARflo Glaucoma Implant is a new suprachoroidal drainage device that combines Nordquist's designs and the unique biointegration properties of the STAR® Biomaterials to enhance the natural uveoscleral outflow, hence reducing the intraocular pressure without the formation of a filtering bleb and its associated complication.

The STARflo device relies on extensive research and studies conducted for several years on the STAR® Biomaterial as implantable material and on STARflo predecessors in the ophthalmic field – the CELLplant and the ClarifEYE. In the ophthalmic field, the safety and the performances of the STARflo device were demonstrated on animals while early results on human shows encouraging results in the control of the IOP with a reduction of glaucoma medications. Although long-term success still has to be demonstrated, this newly CE-marked device exhibiting anti-fibrotic properties is promising as a novel, suprachoroidal implant for bleb-free, intraocular pressure reduction for patient suffering from refractory open-angle glaucoma. iSTAR Medical SA is currently running a controlled market rolled-out phase during which each new case is carefully followed.

**Acknowledgments** The authors express warm thanks to M. Maginness (PhD, Healionics Corporation), Dr. R.E. Norquist (PhD, Wound Healing Of Oklahoma, Inc.), and Dr. C. Woods (DVM, BioVeteria Life Sciences, LLC) for their contribution and inputs in this chapter.

# References


1. Bill A, Philips CI. Uveoscleral drainage of aqueous humor in human eye. Exp Eye Res. 1971;12(3):275–81.
2. Toris CB, Yablonski ME, Wang YL, Camras CB. Aqueous humor dynamics in the aging human eye. Am J Ophthalmol. 1999;127(4):407–12.
3. Weinreb RN. Uveoscleral outflow: the other outflow pathway. J Glaucoma. 2000;9(5):343–5.
4. Weinreb RN, Toris CB, Gabelt BT, Lindsey JD, Kaufman PL. Effects of prostaglandins on the aqueous humor outflow pathways. Surv Ophthalmol. 2002;47 Suppl 1:S53–64.
5. Mosaed S, Minckler DS. Aqueous shunt in the treatment of glaucoma. Expert Rev Med Devices. 2010;7(5):661–6.
6. Boyle JW, Netland PA. Incisional therapies: shunts and valved implants. In: Schacknow PN, Samples JR, editors. The glaucoma book – a practical, evidence-based approach to patient care. New York: Springer; 2010. p. 813–30.
7. Ratner BD, Marshall A, inventors; University of Washington, assignee. Porous biomaterials. United States patent US 7972628 B2, 5 July 2011.
8. Ratner BD, Marshall A, inventors; University of Washington, assignee. Crosslinked porous biomaterials. United States Patent US 8318193, 27 Nov 2012.
9. Ratner BD, Marshall A, inventors; University of Washington, assignee. Novel porous biomaterials that support vascular ingrowth. European Patent EP 1670385, 23 Jan 2013.
10. Nordquist RE, Li B, inventors; Wound Healing of Oklahoma, assignee. Method and apparatus for lowering the intraocular pressure of an eye. United States Patent US 5704907, 6 Jan 1998.
11. Nordquist RE, Li B, inventors; Premier Laser Systems Inc., assignee. Method and apparatus for lowering the intraocular pressure of an eye. United States Patent US 6102045, 15 Aug 2000.
12. Rollet M, Moreau M. Traitement de l'hypopyon par le drainage capillaire de la chambre antérieure. Rev Gen Ophthalmol (Paris). 1906;25:481–9. French.
13. Hong C-HH, Arosemena A, Zurakowski D, Ayyala RS. Glaucoma drainage devices: a systematic literature review and current controversies. Surv Ophthalmol. 2005;50(1):48–60.
14. Luntz MH, Harrison R. Alloplastic devices in glaucoma surgery: setons. In: Lim ASM, series editor. Glaucoma surgery. Singapore: World Scientific; 1994. p. 153–63.
15. Lisk JR, Memmen JE, Hampton SM, Nordquist RE, Robledo PV, Tai M-K, inventors; Medtronic-Xomed INc, assignee. Article and method for ocular aqueous drainage. United States Patent US 7160264 B2, 9 Jan 2007.
16. Lisk JR, Memmen JE, Hampton SM, Nordquist RE, Robledo PV, Tai M-K, inventors; Medtronic-Xomed Inc., assignee. Device for ocular aqueous drainage. European Patent EP 1578319B1, 23 Jan 2010.
17. Sabbagh L. Early results good with glaucoma seton. Ophthalmol Times. 1995;20(40):10–2.
18. Intraocular Implantation Study in the Rabbit. NAMSA study protocol and report # 02T0101300, 2002.
19. Martson M, Viljanto J, Hurme T, Laippala P, Saukko P. Is cellulose degradable or stable as implantation material? An in vivo subcutaneous study in the rat. Biomaterials. 1999;20(21):1989–95.
20. Marshall AJ, Ratner BD. Quantitative characterization of sphere-templated porous biomaterials. AIChE J. 2005;51(4):1221–32.
21. Marshall A. Hydrogels with well-defined pore structure for biomaterials applications. PhD dissertation, University of Washington; 2004: AAT 3151637.
22. Krombach F, Münzing S, Allmeling AM, Gerlach JT, Behr J, Dörger M. Cell size of alveolar macrophages: an interspecies comparison. Environ Health Perspect. 1997;105 Suppl 5:1261–3.
23. Brauker JH, Carr-Brendel VE, Martinson LA, Crudele J, Johnston WD, Johnson RC. Neovascularization of synthetic membranes directed by membrane microarchitecture. J Biomed Mater Res. 1995;29(12):1517–24.
24. Sharkaway AA, Klitzman B, Truskey GA, Reichert WM. Engineering the tissue which encapsulates subcutaneous implants. II. Plasma-tissue exchange properties. J Biomed Mater Res. 1998;40(4):586–97.
25. Bae HB, Kim CS, Ahn BH. A membranous drainage implant in glaucoma filtering surgery: animal trial. Korean J Opthalmol. 1988;2:49–56.
26. Terasaki D, Sobel M, Irvin C, Wijelath E, Ratner BD. Biomaterial-Induced Angiogenesis To Adress Peripheral Vascular Disease: The Application of Sphere Templated Hydrogels. In: Scholz C, Kressler J, editors. Tailored polymer architectures for pharmaceutical and biomedical applications. ACS Symp Ser 2013. p. 245–57.
27. Madden LR, Mortisen DJ, Sussman EM, Dupras SK, Fugate JA, Cuy JL, et al. Proangiogenic scaffolds as functional templates for cardiac tissue engineering. Proc Natl Acad Sci U S A. 2010;107(34):15211–6.
28. Marshall AJ, Alvarez M, Maginness M, inventors; Healionics Corporation, assignee. Implantable medical devices having microporous surface layers and method for reducing foreign body response to the same. United States Patent US 2011/0257623 A1, 20 Oct 2011.
29. Ayyala RS, Michelini-Norris B, Flores A, Haller E, Margo CE. Comparison of different biomaterials for glaucoma drainage devices: part 2. Arch Ophthalmol. 2000;118(18):1081–4.
30. Ocular Irritation Study of STARflo glaucoma implant following implantation in the anterior chamber of the rabbit eye. NAMSA study protocol and report # 10T5296802, 2010.
31. Biotechnol Bioeng. 2012;109(8):C1.
32. Roberts S, Woods C. Preliminary report: effect of a novel porous implant in refractory glaucomatous dogs. In: Veterinary ophthalmology. Abstracts: 39th annual meeting of the American College of Veterinary Ophthalmologists, Boston, 15–18 Oct 2008, p. 423.

# SOLX Suprachoroidal Shunt

Parul Ichhpujani and Marlene R. Moster

## Introduction

The nonphysiological nature of subconjunctival filtration, risk of hypotony and other complications, unpredictable wound healing, and flow control modulation led to the advent of newer glaucoma surgical approaches which enhance the physiologic mechanisms of aqueous outflow [1]. Ozdamar and colleagues introduced the first successful suprachoroidal drainage technique in which aqueous humor was diverted from the anterior chamber to suprachoroidal space by a modified Krupin eye valve [2].

This chapter addresses all aspects pertaining to glaucoma shunt draining in the suprachoroidal space.

## Suprachoroidal Space: Anatomical Considerations

The two physiologic outflow pathways in the normal human eye are the pressure-dependent, conventional pathway and the pressure-independent, uveoscleral outflow pathway. However, the pressure dependence or independence of these pathways is not absolute [3]. The conventional pathway consists of the trabecular meshwork, Schlemm's canal, and distal intrascleral and episcleral venous plexi. The uveoscleral outflow pathway consists of the interstitium of the ciliary body, the suprachoroidal space, and ultimately the scleral or choroidal vasculature [4].

P. Ichhpujani, MS, MD (✉)
Glaucoma Service, Department of Ophthalmology,
Level III, Block D, Government Medical College
and Hospital, Sector 32 A, Chandigarh 160031, India
e-mail: parul77@rediffmail.com

M.R. Moster, MD
Anne and William Goldberg Glaucoma Service,
Wills Eye Institute, Jefferson Medical College,
840 Walnut Street, Suite 1140, Philadelphia, PA 19107, USA
e-mail: marlenemoster@aol.com

The suprachoroid lies between the choroid and the sclera and is composed of closely packed layers of long pigmented processes derived from each tissue [5]. The suprachoroidal space is a potential space providing a pathway for uveoscleral outflow. Aqueous humor that flows into the suprachoroidal space leaves this space via the scleral channels [6] or via the choriocapillaris [7]. The outflow function of the choroid has been demonstrated by visualizing the suprachoroidal drainage following the implantation of a silicone cyclodialysis glaucoma implant, using MRI of the aqueous flow [8]. Furthermore, outflow capacity of the choroid from the suprachoroidal space has been demonstrated in other animal models [9, 10].

Aqueous inflow or outflow seems to be closely correlated with the hydrostatic pressure in the suprachoroidal space [11].The hydrostatic pressure difference between the anterior chamber and the suprachoroidal space is significantly correlated to the intraocular pressure. This hydrostatic pressure difference is mainly generated by the colloid osmotic absorption of the choroidal vessels and partly by the outflow of fluid across the sclera and emissaria. The pressure differential from the anterior chamber to the suprachoroidal space is the driving force for uveoscleral outflow [11].

In comparison to the subconjunctival space, the suprachoroidal space is attributed with less fibroblast colonization and activity.

## Suprachoroidal Drainage Shunt

### Concept

Two key observations were responsible for the inception of Gold Shunt. First, the investigation of uveoscleral outflow in monkeys revealed that intraocular pressure (IOP) in the suprachoroidal space is always negative when compared with the IOP in the anterior chamber [7]. Researchers at SOLX hypothesized that a device connecting these two areas might be able to take advantage of this negative gradient to lower IOP without creating a bleb. The second observation per-

J.R. Samples, I.I.K. Ahmed (eds.), *Surgical Innovations in Glaucoma*,
DOI 10.1007/978-1-4614-8348-9_23, © Springer Science+Business Media New York 2014

tained to a jeweler who had a piece of gold removed from his eye after 10 years. A laboratory analysis showed that the metal was completely free of proteins and cells. This discovery suggested that gold, if optimized, could provide a superior material base for a biocompatible device and minimize issues related to wound healing and the formation of scar tissue [12].

## Device

The Gold Shunt concept was developed based on a quote from Anders Bill in the book titled *Uveoscleral Outflow:*

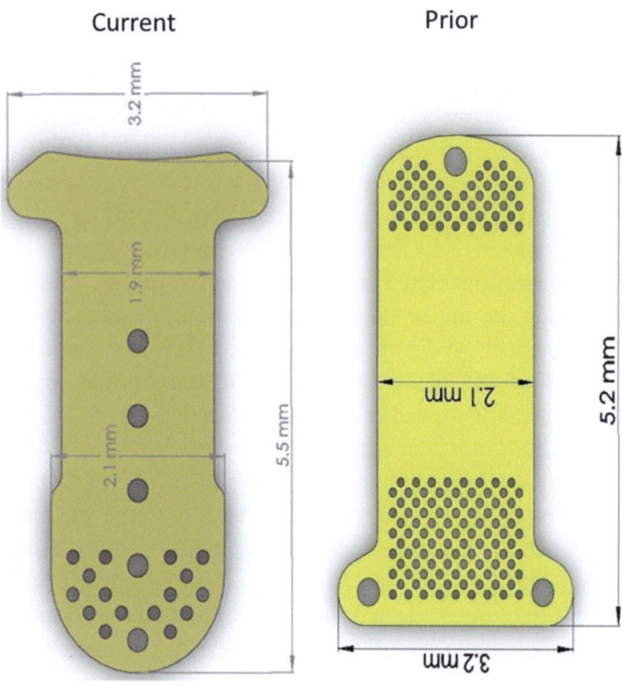


**Fig. 23.1** Current model of SOLX Shunt, GMS Plus, and the prior model GMS

*Biology and Clinical Aspects* (April 13, 1975). "More quantitatively controllable laser and/or surgical techniques to increase uveoscleral outflow should be developed." The Gold Shunt was a technology invented and developed by Gabriel Simon, MD, PhD. The Gold Shunt is cleared in Canada and has CE Mark in Europe. A pivotal trial is currently ongoing in the USA (Fig. 23.1).

The initial studies were done with the earlier model, Gold Micro Shunt, GMS, which was a non-valved flat-plate drainage device made from 24-karat medical-grade (99.95 %) gold. The shunt was 3.2 mm wide and 5.2 mm long and weighs 6.2 mg. It had a long rectangular shape, with rounded edges and finlike tabs on the distal end for anchoring the device in the suprachoroidal space. The aqueous entered the shunt at the proximal end, where 60 holes (100 mm in diameter) and one 300-mm through hole were present. The distal end provided drainage through the microchannels of the fluid from the AC into the suprachoroidal space. Nineteen channels were present, of which 10 were closed and 9 were open, with a lumen width of 24 μ and a height of 50 μ. The posterior end of the shunt contained a grid of 117 holes (110 mm in diameter) on each side of the implant to allow a free flow of the fluid from the device. The proximal and the distal ends also contained 12 and 10 additional 50-mm lateral channels, respectively, in order to increase flow [13].

The latest model, GMS Plus, is 3.2 mm wide and 5.5 mm long, weighs 9.2 mg, and has larger channels, which are essentially like posts and add to the tensile strength of the device. This model also has five central fixation holes for easier implantation (Fig. 23.2).

## Indications

- Refractory glaucoma
- Failure of a previous glaucoma surgical intervention

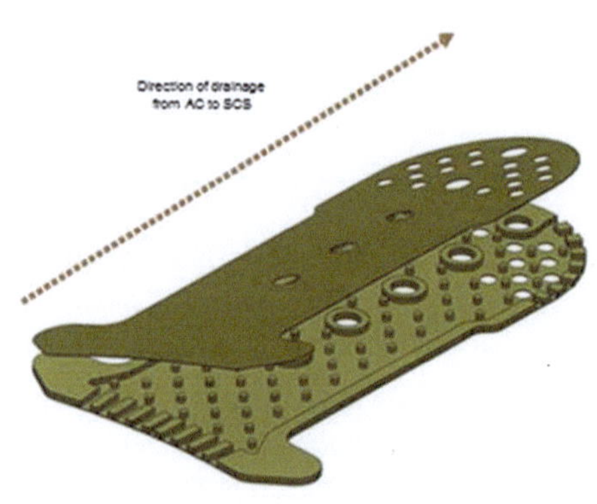


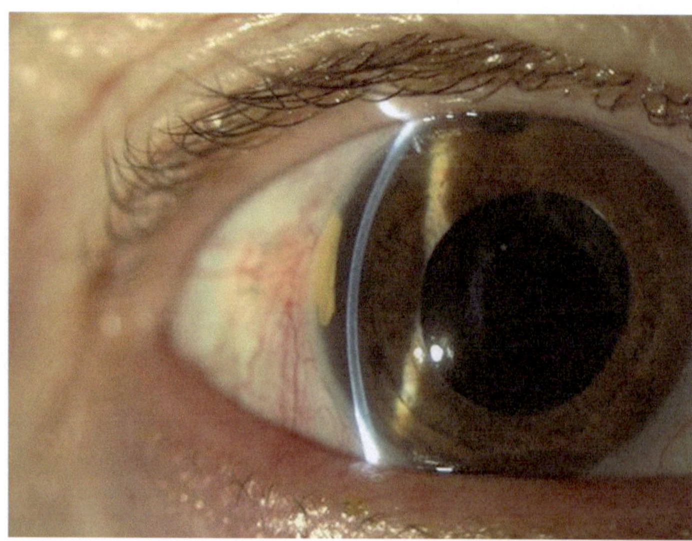

**Fig. 23.2** GMS Plus implanted in temporal quadrant of the eye

## Mechanism of Action

Enhancement of the aqueous filtration across the sclera may be one of the possible outflow pathways exploited by the shunt. The hypoechogenic space around the device detected by 20-MHz ultrasound and AS-OCT suggests increased flow through the supraciliary and suprachoroidal space [13]. From the suprachoroidal space, the aqueous humor can drain into the choroidal vascular system or permeate through the sclera.

## Surgical Technique

Patients can be operated on under local anesthesia using either a sub-Tenon or a peribulbar injection. A bridle suture is placed around the superior rectus muscle; alternatively, a corneal traction suture can be placed at 12 o'clock. The gold shunt can be implanted in any quadrant, but the scleral tissue in the area of surgery should be healthy. Temporal quadrant is the most suitable quadrant. Furthermore, the angle in the area of intended implantation should be open and free of any peripheral anterior synechia.

A fornix-based conjunctival flap is fashioned, followed by meticulous cautery of episcleral vessels. A 4 mm (wide) by 3.5 mm (long) scleral flap about 90 % in depth is created. Dissection is done up to clear cornea and scleral spur is identified. After measuring 1.5 mm posterior from scleral spur, a 3-mm-long mark at both scleral spur and 1.5-mm point is made. These steps should be performed with the eye pressurized to facilitate the scleral dissection.

A full-thickness incision 3 mm wide is made into the suprachoroidal space. A cyclodialysis spatula is used to ensure that wound is 100 % open end to end. This is followed by injection of a small amount of viscoelastic into the suprachoroidal space. Then a superficial ledge incision (approximately 50 µm) is created, and anterior chamber is entered with a 2.85-mm keratome, parallel to the iris.

The device is checked for mobility. Sclera is grasped with a .12 forceps just outside of the flap for countertraction.

The flared distal end of GMS Plus that is inserted into the AC allows for consistent fixation and more reproducible placement in the angle.

"Shoulders" of the device are passed through the incision site one at a time. Using either a cystotome needle or a Sinskey hook, the device is pushed forward out of the inserter using the positioning holes on the gold shunt. Once the tail of the device clears the suprachoroidal space incision site, the lower lip of the wound is grasped and lifted. Then the implant is pulled gently into the suprachoroidal space.

It is better to go hole by hole like climbing a ladder. The shoulders of the device will stop once they get to the angle. It is best to have the device as deep into the angle as possible. The scleral incision is closed with 10-0 nylon sutures and the conjunctiva is closed at the limbus. It is best to have no flow from flap; however, if there is a small amount of egress and a small bleb forms, realize it is only temporary and will resolve. If device is pushed out of the angle during suturing, simply insert a cyclodialysis spatula through the paracentesis port and push it back into the angle.

## Advantages

- Gold is known to be biocompatible, with no long-term toxicity in the human eye.
- No external filtering bleb.
- Chances of hypotony less.
- Reduced probability of developing endophthalmitis due to the exposure to the implant.
- Absence of conjunctival erosion.
- Absence of extraocular muscle imbalance.

## Disadvantages

- Presence of a permanent implant in the anterior chamber and suprachoroidal space

## Complications

The complications seen to date most commonly include hyphema and hypotony, which are minor and transient in nature and normally resolve by 1–2 weeks. Complications in the first published study of 38 patients included shunt exposure in 1 patient (3 %); synechiae formation, 1 patient (3 %); mild hyphema, 6 patients (16 %); moderate hyphema, 2 patients (5 %); and exudative inferior retinal detachment, 1 patient (3 %) [13]. Localized conjunctival congestion, mild hyphema, and mild cellular reaction generally resolve within a few days.

## Scientific Evidence So Far

Previous studies of GMS implantation into the rabbit eye confirmed that the device was safe and did not trigger any inflammatory response in adjacent tissues [14].

Melamed and colleagues reported outcome of 38 patients undergoing surgery with GMS in a prospective, noncomparative case series in 2009 [13]. In this study surgical success (defined as an IOP >5 and <22 mmHg with or without antiglaucoma medications in the last follow-up) was achieved in 30 patients (79 %). Complete success (defined as an IOP >5 and <22 mmHg without antiglaucoma medication in the last follow-up) was achieved in 5 patients (13.2 %). Two-thirds of the patients still used some form of antiglaucoma medication to achieve adequate IOP control. Despite the fact that more than 50 % of the eyes in this series had at least one failed trabeculectomy, glaucoma drainage device, or laser trabeculoplasty, patients with a GMS achieved a decrease in IOP of more than 30 %.

Mastropasqua et al. reported an observational case series of 14 glaucoma patients with a history of multiple prior failed incisional surgeries. The mean postoperative IOP percentage reduction at last follow-up visit was 22.6 % and was without relevant postoperative complications and the formation of filtering blebs [15].

Figus and colleagues evaluated the efficacy of GMS in 55 patients with refractory glaucoma. After 2 years of follow-up, qualified success was achieved in 37 eyes (67.3 %), and complete success was achieved in 3 eyes (5.5 %) [16]. Mild side effects occurred in 21 patients, with mild or moderate postoperative hyphema being the most frequent one. Development of a thin membrane, obstructing the anterior holes, was the most important factor affecting the efficacy of this device; it was found to be present in 12 patients from the failure group (66.7 % of failures).

Agnifili and colleagues studied the histological findings of five eyes of five glaucomatous patients with unsuccessful GMS implantation who underwent shunt removal [17]. Each device was sectioned into three portions: proximal or anterior chamber portion, middle or scleral portion, and distal or suprachoroidal portion. The main feature was the presence of a thick connective capsule-like reaction surrounding both the proximal and distal ends and invading the posterior and anterior grid holes, whereas a more loosely arranged connective tissue was observed within the inner channels. Signs of surface fibrosis of the middle-scleral portion and inflammatory cell infiltration of the device were not documented in any of the cases.

Harasymowycz recently presented a retrospective case series of 16 patients with glaucoma. The patients underwent deep sclerectomy with GMS implantation in the suprachoroidal space. The average IOP and IOP-lowering medication preoperatively were 33.6 mmHg and 3.0 medications, respectively. At 6 months, the average IOP was 16.3 on an average of 1.3 medications. No intra- or postoperative cases of choroidal detachment, hyphema, uveitis, or corneal edema or opacification were noted [18].

## References


1. Hong CH, Arosemena A, Zurakowski D, et al. Glaucoma drainage devices: a systematic literature review and current controversies. Surv Ophthalmol. 2005;40:48–60.
2. Ozdamar A, Aras C, Karacorlu M. Suprachoroidal seton implantation in refractory glaucoma: a novel surgical technique. J Glaucoma. 2003;12:354–9.
3. Becker B, Neufeld AH. Pressure dependence of uveoscleral outflow. J Glaucoma. 2002;11:545.
4. Bill A. Some aspects of aqueous humour drainage. Eye (Lond). 1993;7(Pt 1):14–9.
5. Hogan MJ, Alvarado JA, Weddell JE, editors. Choroid. In: Histology of the human eye. Philadelphia: W.B. Saunders; 1971. p. 320–92.
6. Bill A. The aqueous humor drainage mechanism in the cynomolgus monkey (Macaca irus) with evidence for unconventional routes. Invest Ophthalmol. 1965;4:911.
7. Pederson JE, Gaasterland DE, MacLellan HM. Uveoscleral aqueous outflow in the rhesus monkey: importance of uveal reabsorption. Invest Ophthalmol. 1977;16:1008.
8. Lee KY, Lashkari K, Kwong KK, et al. Magnetic resonance imaging of the aqueous flow in eyes implanted with the trabeculo-suprachoroidal glaucoma seton. Invest Ophthalmol Vis Sci. 1992;33:948.
9. Cole DF, Monro PA. The use of fluorescein-labelled dextrans in investigation of aqueous humour outflow in the rabbit. Exp Eye Res. 1976;23:571–85.
10. Krohn J, Bertelsen T. Corrosion casts of the suprachoroidal space and uveoscleral drainage routes in the pig eye. Acta Ophthalmol Scand. 1997;75:28–31.
11. Emi K, Pederson JE, Toris CB. Hydrostatic pressure of the suprachoroidal space. Invest Ophthalmol Vis Sci. 1989;30(2):233–8.
12. Sen SC, Ghosh A. Gold as an intraocular foreign body. Br J Ophthalmol. 1983;67(6):398–9.
13. Melamed S, Ben Simon GJ, Goldenfeld M, Simon G. Efficacy and safety of gold micro shunt implantation to the supraciliary space in patients with glaucoma: a pilot study. Arch Ophthalmol. 2009;127(3):264–9.
14. Orozco MA, Fernandez V, Acosta AC, et al. Biocompatibility of gold versus polydimethylsiloxane for glaucoma implants [ARVO abstract 988]. Invest Ophthalmol Vis Sci. 2004;45:B961.
15. Mastropasqua L, Agnifili L, Ciancaglini M, Nubile M, Carpineto P, Fasanella V, Figus M, Lazzeri S, Nardi M. In vivo analysis of conjunctiva in gold micro shunt implantation for glaucoma. Br J Ophthalmol. 2010;94(12):1592–6.
16. Figus M, Lazzeri S, Fogagnolo P, Iester M, Martinelli P, Nardi M. Supraciliary shunt in refractory glaucoma. Br J Ophthalmol. 2011;95(11):1537–41.
17. Agnifili L, Costagliola C, Figus M, Iezzi G, Piattelli A, Carpineto P, Mastropasqua R, Nardi M, Mastropasqua L. Histological findings of failed gold micro shunts in primary open-angle glaucoma. Graefes Arch Clin Exp Ophthalmol. 2012;250(1):143–9.
18. Harasymowycz P. Deep sclerectomy augmented with suprachoroidal gold micro shunt (GMS): 6 month results [P5.44, 10thEGS congress, 2012 abstract].

Steven L. Mansberger

Cataract surgery is the most common surgery performed in the United States according to the Agency for Health Care Research and Quality [1]. Many patients who are glaucoma suspects or have glaucoma have cataract surgery. The purpose of this chapter is to review the recent studies on the effect of cataract surgery on intraocular pressure (IOP), the mechanism of IOP lowering after cataract surgery, and how to decide between cataract surgery alone or cataract surgery combined with glaucoma surgery when operating on your glaucoma and glaucoma suspect patients.

## Recent Studies Examining the Effect of Cataract Surgery on Intraocular Pressure

Even as early as 1970 with intracapsular cataract surgery, Bigger and Becker suggested that cataract surgery lowered IOP [2]. Recent studies with modern clear cornea phacoemulsification cataract surgery suggest that cataract surgery lowers intraocular pressure in normal, glaucoma suspect, and glaucomatous eyes. One study by Shingleton [3] reported the long-term effect of cataract surgery in approximately 150 patients with a diagnosis of either glaucoma, glaucoma suspect, or cataract who underwent cataract surgery and were followed for at least 3 years. The study reported a mean decrease of approximately 1.5 mmHg in all three groups at 3 years. Many eyes were treated with ocular hypotensive medications both before and after surgery, and many did not have elevated IOP. The authors concluded that cataract surgery should not replace glaucoma surgery when significant IOP lowering is required, but it may be useful in patients with controlled early glaucoma who may want to continue glaucoma medication use.

S.L. Mansberger, MD, MPH
Devers Eye Institute at Legacy Health,
Portland, OR, USA
e-mail: smansberger@deverseye.org

Poley [4, 5] reported IOP changes after cataract surgery in patients who had a follow-up of 4 years or greater. They stratified the level of preoperative IOP and found it positively correlated with the amount of IOP lowering. In other words, their study documented that the higher the level of preoperative IOP, the greater the reduction in IOP after cataract surgery. For example, the IOP reduction was 6.5 mmHg in 19 eyes with preoperative IOP between 23 and 31 mmHg but only 1.6 mmHg in eyes with preoperative IOP in the 15–17 mmHg range.

A prospective study by Samuelson [6] reported the results of a regulatory trial including a "cataract surgery only" group. At 12 months, they found an IOP reduction of 8.5±4.3 mmHg with cataract surgery alone in a group of ocular hypertension and early glaucoma patients. This result is greater than Shingleton [3] and Poley [4, 5]. However, 35 % of these eyes were back on ocular hypotensive medications at 12 months.

These studies have suggested that the amount of IOP lowering is generally proportional to presurgical IOP. However, these previous studies used only a single preoperative intraocular pressure measurement, were retrospective, included a mixture of treated and untreated patients with ocular hypotensive medications, and were usually from a single-center. Finally, several of these previous studies included patients with multiple different diagnoses of glaucoma such as pigmentary dispersion, pseudoexfoliation, and primary open-angle glaucoma. While useful, these studies may be affected by regression of the mean or differential bias to the effect of cataract surgery on IOP lowering because ocular hypotensive medications were used preoperatively and postoperatively.

The Ocular Hypertension Treatment Study (OHTS) recently published a manuscript [7] regarding the change in IOP after cataract surgery. The OHTS is a multicenter, randomized clinical trial to determine the safety and efficacy of ocular hypotensive medications in delaying or preventing the onset of primary open-angle glaucoma in individuals with elevated intraocular pressure. The inclusion criteria for the study were those aged 40–80 years old, intraocular pres-

J.R. Samples, I.I.K. Ahmed (eds.), *Surgical Innovations in Glaucoma*,
DOI 10.1007/978-1-4614-8348-9_24, © Springer Science+Business Media New York 2014

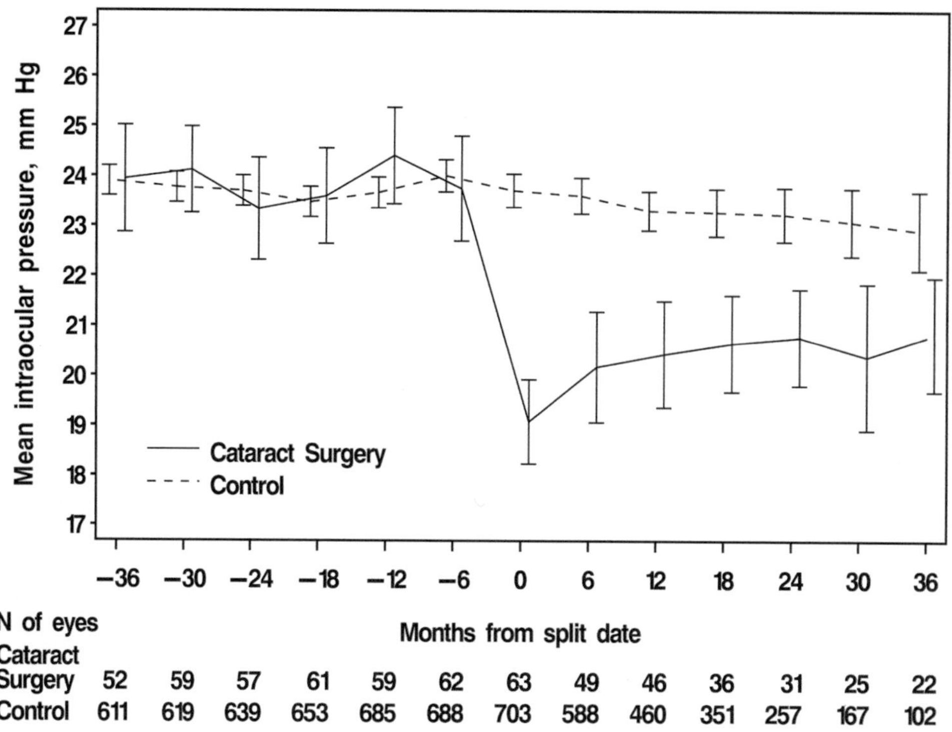



**Fig. 24.1** Intraocular pressure (IOP) before and after cataract surgery in the Ocular Hypertension Treatment Study. Month 0 is the *split date* or the study visit that the participant reported cataract surgery, or a randomly selected, corresponding date in the control group. Preoperative IOP was the mean IOP of up to three visits prior to the split date. Postoperative IOP was the mean IOP of up to three visits including the split date (0, 6, and 12 months). In the cataract surgery group, the mean postoperative IOP was lower than the mean preoperative IOP (23.9 ± 3.2 vs. 19.8 ± 3.2 mmHg, *p* < .0001, mixed model analysis of variance). In the control group, the mean IOP before and after the split date IOP were 23.8 ± 3.6 vs. 23.4 ± 3.9 mmHg, *p* < .002, respectively. Error bars are ± two standard errors of the mean

| N of eyes | | | | | | | | | | | | | |
|---|---|---|---|---|---|---|---|---|---|---|---|---|---|
| Cataract Surgery | 52 | 59 | 57 | 61 | 59 | 62 | 63 | 49 | 46 | 36 | 31 | 25 | 22 |
| Control | 611 | 619 | 639 | 653 | 685 | 688 | 703 | 588 | 460 | 351 | 257 | 167 | 102 |

sure between 24 and 32 mmHg in one eye and between 21 and 32 mmHg in the other eye, no evidence of glaucomatous structural or functional damage by standard clinical measures, and best-corrected visual acuity of at least 20/40 with no evidence of visually significant cataract. The study began recruitment in 1994 and continued for more than 10 years.

The study included 42 participants (63 eyes) who underwent cataract surgery in at least one eye and compared the results to a control group of 743 participants (743 eyes) who did not undergo cataract surgery. The study excluded participants if (1) they were ineligible for cataract surgery because of aphakia or pseudophakia at the enrollment visit, (2) they had a history of trabeculectomy surgery after enrollment, (3) they used topical ocular hypotensive medication use, and (4) they had less than 1 year of follow-up. The study also included up to three IOP measurements prior to cataract surgery and up to three visits subsequent to cataract surgery to determine postoperative intraocular pressure. The IOP data was censored after events that could alter the natural history of postoperative IOP. These included (1) laser iridotomy, (2) laser-assisted in situ keratomileusis (LASIK), and (3) initiation of topical ocular hypotensive medication.

Figure 24.1 shows that the mean postoperative IOP in the cataract surgery group was significantly lower compared to the mean preoperative IOP (19.8 ± 3.2 vs. 23.9 ± 3.2 mmHg). The estimated mean decrease in IOP postoperatively in the cataract surgery group was 4.0 mmHg. The overall average percent decrease from preoperative IOP was 16.5 % with 39.7 % of eyes having a postoperative IOP greater than 20 % below preoperative IOP. However, 11.1 % of participants had an increase in their postoperative IOP from the preoperative IOP. In these seven eyes, the percentage increase in IOP was between 0.7 and 18.3 %. The study also documented the long duration of IOP lowering after cataract surgery because postoperative IOP had not returned to the level of preoperative IOP by 36 months. However, the results do not last forever, with the figure showing an increasing IOP over time.

The OHTS study provided important new information regarding the effect of cataract surgery in a well-characterized group of patients with ocular hypertension. The study included multiple measurements of pre- and postoperative IOP to better characterize IOP. Another strength is that it only included eyes that were untreated, eliminating the effect of ocular hypotensive medications on both preoperative and postoperative IOP. Finally, it included a large diverse group of patients with multiple ethnicities and included multiple different clinical centers. This suggests that the results may be generalized to other ocular hypertensive patients.

However, one should avoid extrapolating the OHTS results to eyes with lower IOP, higher IOP, and to eyes with glaucoma. Similarly, the results may not be used to recommend a particular treatment (e.g., medications, laser, surgery) for ocular hypertension because the participants were not randomized to cataract surgery.

Overall, these recent studies examining the effect of cataract surgery on intraocular pressure are informative. They show that cataract surgery lowers IOP for a long period of time (at least 3 years). They show a moderate decrease in IOP of 1.5–8 mmHg with and without medications. However, a large proportion of glaucoma patients continue to require glaucoma medications after cataract surgery.

## Predicting the Response in IOP from Cataract Surgery

All of the previous studies show the wide variability in postoperative IOP after cataract surgery. In particular, the OHTS study [7] showed a 40 % *decrease* in IOP in some ocular hypertension participants, but other participants had an 18 % *increase* in IOP. For eye care providers performing cataract surgery and taking care of glaucoma and glaucoma suspect patients, the key questions are as follows: "*Who would have the most IOP lowering from cataract surgery?*" and "*Who may have minimal benefit from cataract surgery and require simultaneous or subsequent glaucoma surgery?*".

The OHTS study examined whether one could predict the IOP lowering after cataract surgery based on patient characteristics. Age, race, gender, and central corneal thickness were not predictive of subsequent IOP lowering. The only variable associated with postoperative IOP was preoperative IOP, which was similar to the results of Poley [4, 5] above. In other words, higher preoperative IOP was associated with a greater percentage drop in postoperative IOP. The mean change in IOP in those with a preoperative IOP below 22.3 mmHg was only −11.0 %. In those with a preoperative IOP between 22.3 and 25.0 mmHg, the mean percent change in postoperative IOP was −16.2 %. Finally, in the group with preoperative IOP greater than 25 mmHg, the mean change in postoperative IOP was −22.5 %.

The overall results of these studies suggest that preoperative IOP was the only consistent factor associated with the amount of postoperative lowering of intraocular pressure. This creates the classic dilemma of "risk versus benefits." Those glaucoma and glaucoma suspect patients with visually significant cataract and the highest IOP have the highest risk of worsening glaucoma but also may have the greatest response to cataract surgery. If cataract surgery does not lower IOP adequately, they are also most likely to require urgent glaucoma surgery. Overall, eye surgeons should counsel their patients regarding the wide differences in response to cataract surgery and the possibility of subsequent glaucoma surgery if their IOP is not controlled with topical ocular hypotensive medications.

In the future, other potential predictive factors for IOP lowering would be informative. These may include anterior chamber configuration [8] with the hypothesis that eyes with a more narrow anterior chamber angle experience a greater decrease in IOP after cataract surgery than eyes with open angles. Other factors may include the amount of pigmentation of the trabecular meshwork, the size of the intumescent cataract, the characteristics of the cataract surgery such as phacoemulsification time, the amount of postoperative inflammation and pigment release, and the characteristics of the intraocular lens on the lens capsule. Several of these factors have been previously associated with success of laser or glaucoma surgery for lowering intraocular pressure.

## What Is the Mechanism of IOP Lowering with Cataract Surgery?

The mechanisms for IOP lowering after cataract surgery could be separated into mechanical or biologic processes. The mechanical process suggests that cataract surgery exposes a larger area of the trabecular meshwork to aqueous humor. One can demonstrate this phenomenon by performing gonioscopy after unilateral cataract surgery. Gonioscopy in the pseudophakic eye commonly shows more angle structures than the contralateral phakic eye. This may occur because the iris moves posterior, exposing more angle structures to aqueous humor. Another explanation of the mechanical hypothesis is that the implanted intraocular lens creates zonular tension, which creates centripetal forces on the longitudinal tendon of the ciliary body. This subsequently pulls on the scleral spur, creating widening trabecular spaces and decreased outflow resistance. This mechanism of action is utilized by miotic medications such as pilocarpine. This mechanism was demonstrated in a postmortem study [9] in human eyes, which demonstrated an association between increased facility of outflow and tension on the lens zonule in eyes with open angles. Similarly to the latter study, Meyer [10] and Kee [11] demonstrated increased outflow facility by tonography after phacoemulsification in eyes without glaucoma.

The biologic process of how cataract surgery lowers intraocular pressure was studied by Wang in 2003 [12]. He showed that there was an increased amount of interleukin and tumor necrosis factor alpha (TNFα) released by trabecular meshwork cells after subjected to phacoemulsification. This may increase uveoscleral outflow. Whether it is a mechanical, biologic, or combination of processes, the exact mechanism of IOP lowering after cataract surgery is unknown.

## How to Decide Between Cataract Surgery Alone Versus Cataract Surgery Combined with a Glaucoma Procedure

One should recognize that cataract surgery frequently results in an increase in intraocular pressure within the first 12 h after cataract surgery. Ranier [13] documented the natural change in IOP after cataract surgery in normal patients and showed that 70 % of normal patients will have a spike in IOP to 30 mmHg or more. Krupin showed that 60 % of glaucoma patients will have a 10 mmHg rise in intraocular pressure after extracapsular cataract surgery (Krupin 1989, Ophthalmology). He also showed that combined cataract and glaucoma surgery (posterior lip sclerostomy) resulted in only 21 % having an IOP greater than 25 mmHg, but cataract surgery alone had a 77 % chance of IOP than 25 mmHg.

Therefore, the first question to ask yourself is *"Whether or not your patient can tolerate severely elevated intraocular pressure over the first 24 h after cataract surgery?"*. If they can't tolerate this elevation in their pressure, they should have a cataract combined with a glaucoma procedure. The second question is *"Whether or not the patient wants to stay on glaucoma medications?"*. Samuelson [6] showed that 35 % of patients with a diagnosis of glaucoma or glaucoma suspect required one or more glaucoma medications after cataract surgery. Therefore, if a patient wants to have the highest chance of eliminating a daily glaucoma ocular hypotensive treatment, they should choose a cataract combined with a glaucoma procedure.

The best candidates for cataract surgery alone are those with visually significant cataract and have well-controlled early glaucoma and/or those who are glaucoma suspects. No studies have examined clear lens extraction in glaucoma or glaucoma suspectsline, therefore, one should not perform cataract surgery in the open-angle glaucoma patient for IOP control unless they have a visually significant cataract.

### Conclusions

Cataract surgery is the most common surgery performed in the United States, and many patients with a diagnosis of glaucoma and glaucoma suspect require cataract surgery. Cataract surgery will lower IOP between 1.5 and 8.0 mmHg from preoperative IOP, and the IOP lowering will last a long time – at least 3 years on average. Those with the highest preoperative IOP will have the most IOP lowering but are at most risk of developing worsening glaucoma and subsequent glaucoma surgery. The best candidates for cataract surgery as a potential procedure to lower IOP are those with visually significant cataract and have well-controlled early glaucoma and/or those who are glaucoma suspects.

## References

1. Russo C, Owens P, Steiner C, Josephsen J. Ambulatory surgery in U.S. hospitals, 2003. 2007. http://archive.ahrq.gov/data/hcup/factbk9/. Accessed 1 May 2013.
2. Bigger JF, Becker B. Cataracts and primary open-angle glaucoma: the effect of uncomplicated cataract extraction on glaucoma control. Trans Am Acad Ophthalmol Otolaryngol. 1971;75(2):260–72.
3. Shingleton BJ, Pasternack JJ, Hung JW, O'Donoghue MW. Three and five year changes in intraocular pressures after clear corneal phacoemulsification in open angle glaucoma patients, glaucoma suspects, and normal patients. J Glaucoma. 2006;15(6):494–8.
4. Poley BJ, Lindstrom RL, Samuelson TW. Long-term effects of phacoemulsification with intraocular lens implantation in normotensive and ocular hypertensive eyes. J Cataract Refract Surg. 2008;34(5):735–42.
5. Poley BJ, Lindstrom RL, Samuelson TW, Schulze Jr R. Intraocular pressure reduction after phacoemulsification with intraocular lens implantation in glaucomatous and nonglaucomatous eyes: evaluation of a causal relationship between the natural lens and open-angle glaucoma. J Cataract Refract Surg. 2009;35(11):1946–55.
6. Samuelson TW, Katz LJ, Wells JM, Duh YJ, Giamporcaro JE. Randomized evaluation of the trabecular micro-bypass stent with phacoemulsification in patients with glaucoma and cataract. Ophthalmology. 2011;118(3):459–67.
7. Mansberger SL, Gordon MO, Jampel H, et al. Reduction in intraocular pressure after cataract extraction: the Ocular Hypertension Treatment Study. Ophthalmology. 2012;119(9):1826–31.
8. Shrivastava A, Singh K. The effect of cataract extraction on intraocular pressure. Curr Opin Ophthalmol. 2010;21(2):118–22.
9. Van Buskirk EM. Changes in the facility of aqueous outflow induced by lens depression and intraocular pressure in excised human eyes. Am J Ophthalmol. 1976;82(5):736–40.
10. Meyer MA, Savitt ML, Kopitas E. The effect of phacoemulsification on aqueous outflow facility. Ophthalmology. 1997;104(8):1221–7.
11. Kee C, Moon SH. Effect of cataract extraction and posterior chamber lens implantation on outflow facility and its response to pilocarpine in Korean subjects. Br J Ophthalmol. 2000;84(9):987–9.
12. Wang N, Chintala SK, Fini ME, Schuman JS. Ultrasound activates the TM ELAM-1/IL-1/NF-kappaB response: a potential mechanism for intraocular pressure reduction after phacoemulsification. Invest Ophthalmol Vis Sci. 2003;44(5):1977–81.
13. Rainer G, Menapace R, Schmid KE, et al. Natural course of intraocular pressure after cataract surgery with sodium chondroitin sulfate 4%-sodium hyaluronate 3% (Viscoat). Ophthalmology. 2005;112(10):1714–8.

Diamond Y. Tam

## Introduction and Classification

The incidence of angle-closure glaucoma (ACG) worldwide appears to be growing [1], and while it represents a lower proportion of all glaucomas in white [2–10] and black [11–13] ethnic populations, it has been and remains a significant problem in Inuit [14–16], Chinese [17–21], and other Asian [22–30] populations. Globally, it has been estimated that 0.7 % of people over the age of 40 years have angle-closure glaucoma and 21 million people are projected to have angle-closure glaucoma by the year 2020 [31]. In China alone, the approximately 91 % of bilateral blindness cases have been attributed to ACG, and 1.5 million individuals suffer from unilateral blindness (defined as visual acuity <3/60 or visual field ≤10°) from primary ACG [32]. It is imperative that proper understanding, diagnosis, and therapy of this potentially devastating disease is critical to the ophthalmologist both now and ever more so in the future.

The natural history of primary ACG typically begins with anatomical narrowing of the anterior chamber angle with a normal intraocular pressure (IOP) and visual fields and absence of peripheral anterior synechiae (PAS), also termed primary angle-closure suspect (PACS). In PACS patients, iridotrabecular contact (ITC) may be observed on non-compressive gonioscopy, with iris touching the posterior pigmented trabecular meshwork or more anterior structures. The next stage is by the closure of the angle or development of PAS accompanied by elevation of the IOP, termed primary angle closure (PAC) (Video 25.1). Finally, anatomical angle closure with the presence of glaucomatous optic neuropathy and an accompanying visual field defect is known as primary angle-closure glaucoma (PACG). PACG, while potentially sudden, painful, and with severe vision loss, well known to ophthalmologists as acute angle-closure glaucoma (AACG), is often

also asymptomatic and insidious. It is thus important to understand that ACG may present as acute, subacute or intermittent, and chronic. These variations may also be found in the same patient and even in the same eye, at different time points.

## Diagnosis and Mechanism of Disease

The proper timely diagnosis and treatment of angle closure is critical to the preservation of vision. The initial evaluation of the patient should begin with assessing the refractive status. Hyperopic eyes, especially in the elderly, commonly have narrower anterior chamber angles [33] and are also at increased risk of PAC [34]. Following this, attention should be given to the pupil. Reactivity, size, shape, and presence of a relative afferent pupillary defect should all be noted and may suggest chronic angle closure and optic nerve damage or herald an acute attack. IOP should be ascertained, and a careful slit lamp examination should follow, giving special attention to any corneal findings (edema, microcysts, pigmented deposits on the endothelium, endothelial cell loss), central and peripheral anterior chamber depth, iris abnormalities (posterior synechiae, irregular shape, poor reactivity, diffuse or focal atrophy), and finally lens changes (cataract, central lens rise or vault, glaukomflecken).

While all of examination is important, perhaps the most critical element is the gonioscopy. Both eyes should be carefully examined with regard to angle anatomy, any areas of ITC, and presence or absence of PAS. When performing gonioscopy, it is recommended that the light in the room as well as the slit lamp be made dim and care taken not to pass light into the pupil to create artificial widening of the angle through pupillary constriction (Fig. 25.1) [35]. When faced with the situation of determining the difference between an angle that

D.Y. Tam, MD
Department of Ophthalmology, University of Toronto,
340 College Street, Suite 400, Toronto, ON M5T 3A9, Canada
e-mail: diamondtam@gmail.com

**Electronic supplementary material** Supplementary material is available in the online version of this chapter at http://dx.doi.org/10.1007/978-1-4614-8348-9_25. Videos can also be accessed at http://www.springerimages.com/videos/978-1-4614-8347-2

J.R. Samples, I.I.K. Ahmed (eds.), *Surgical Innovations in Glaucoma*,
DOI 10.1007/978-1-4614-8348-9_25, © Springer Science+Business Media New York 2014

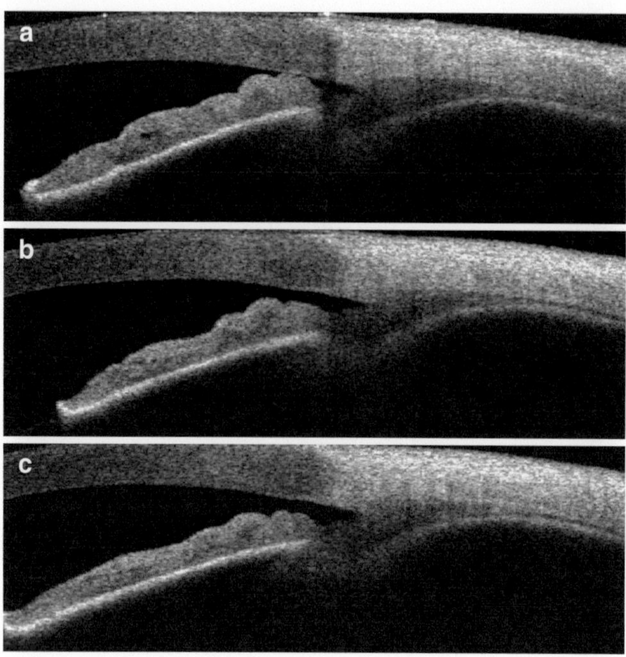

**Fig. 25.1** (**a**) Anterior segment OCT (AS-OCT) image of the angle in a patient in dark conditions. (**b**) Angle of the same patient with light shone onto the iris surface. (**c**) Angle of the same patient with light shone into the pupil. The angle can be seen to be closed with iridotrabecular contact in dark conditions, while this contact is relieved with light (Images courtesy of Ike K. Ahmed, MD)

is appositional and true synechiae, compression or indentation gonioscopy is a valuable tool. Mere ITC should be separable and the trabecular meshwork visualized, but PAS should remain on compression and no meshwork structures be visible. It should be noted that PAS can be broken on occasion with compression gonioscopy, and in fact AACG attacks may occasionally too be broken with compression techniques.

Finally, as an adjunct to the clinical examination, diagnostic imaging modalities may be extremely useful in angle closure. Anterior segment optical coherence tomography (AS-OCT), Scheimpflug imaging, and ultrasound biomicroscopy (UBM) may all be useful adjunctive modalities in the accurate diagnosis of the underlying factors resulting in angle closure.

When thinking about the proper approach to an angle-closure patient and the most appropriate therapeutic intervention, it is useful to first consider the predominant mechanism of the angle closure. While not independent of each other and commonly angle closure can be multifactorial, the main mechanisms to be considered should be pupillary block, lenticular causes, plateau iris, and retrolenticular.

## Treatment

Thought to be the most common form of angle closure, pupillary block refers to the phenomenon of aqueous humor build up in the posterior chamber space between the posterior iris and the anterior lens capsule. This may occur as a result of iris proximity to the anterior lens capsule or a forward position of the lens capsule resulting in apposition and trapping of aqueous humor in the posterior chamber. Without a conduit to allow for equalization of pressure between the posterior and anterior chamber, the mid-peripheral iris is pushed forward in a gradually increasing manner eventually causing iridotrabecular apposition in the "iris bombé" configuration. In order to alleviate the mechanism of pupillary block, relative or absolute, a pathway is required for fluid to exit the posterior chamber and enter into the anterior chamber, most commonly achieved via the creation of a peripheral iris opening to allow for equalization of fluid pressure, typically performed with a neodymium-doped yttrium aluminum garnet (Nd:YAG) laser. In cases where a peripheral iridotomy is not possible for reasons such as corneal edema and complete apposition of the peripheral iris to the cornea, pupillary block may also be relieved by using a needle to lift up the iris from the lens capsule, which can be performed at the slit lamp with the assistance of ophthalmic viscosurgical devices (OVD), providing a way for aqueous humor to exit the posterior chamber into the anterior chamber. Care must be taken not to injure the anterior lens capsule when performing this maneuver.

Although no conclusive clinical study has proven the benefit of laser iridotomy (LPI) for PACS, the relative ease and quickness of the procedure along with the relatively favorable safety profile of the minor procedure has given way to its more common and widespread use in attempts to prevent the more serious and grave consequences of AACG or PACG. Although LPI may be the first step in therapy, it is often insufficient in PAC or PACG to halt the disease process and does not address PAS or anatomical closure of the angle. It has been reported that nearly 1 out of 3 PAC eyes which received LPI continue to have significant ITC after treatment [36–38]. The term plateau iris configuration may be used to refer to eyes which appear to have a deep central anterior chamber with the peripheral iris continuing to appear in close apposition to the trabecular meshwork or have frank ITC. In cases of plateau iris configuration where IOP spikes occur following LPI, plateau iris syndrome may be diagnosed. Although the treatment of plateau iris is not the focus of this chapter and argon peripheral laser iridoplasty remains the standard treatment for plateau iris syndrome after LPI, surgical strategies to deal with plateau iris when combined with lensectomy will be discussed later on in this chapter.

Lenticular causes of angle closure can be a result of many different factors. Increase in lens thickness or lens vault, particularly in hyperopic eyes with smaller anterior segments, weakening of the zonular apparatus resulting in a forward position of the crystalline lens, and lens-induced pupillary block may all be implicated. It is well established that lensectomy widens the anterior chamber angle in ACG eyes as well as those with narrow, occludable angles [39–43]. Furthermore, in both prospective and retrospective studies comparing lens extraction with surgical iridectomy or trabeculectomy in acute and non-acute ACG, lensectomy patients were shown to have decreased postoperative medication requirements as well as a lower rate of complications [44–54].

In one study which randomized AACG patients to cataract surgery versus peripheral iridotomy alone, patients with an IOP >55 mmHg who underwent early lens extraction were found to be less likely to require IOP-lowering therapy [44]. In certain situations, lensectomy may be accompanied by other surgical procedures such as goniosynechialysis to release PAS, endocyclophotocoagulation, or filtration surgery. In one study randomizing 51 medically uncontrolled CACG eyes to cataract surgery alone versus combined phacotrabeculectomy, IOP was found to be lower in the combined surgery group as well as less postoperative dependence on topical medications, but the phacotrabeculectomy group had a significantly higher rate of complications, as well as progression of optic neuropathy [55]. In their study, 14.8 % of lensectomy-only eyes required subsequent filtration surgery.

The same group also performed the same randomized trial comparing phacoemulsification versus trabeculectomy head-to-head in 50 uncontrolled CACG eyes without cataractous lens opacities. No significant difference in IOP reduction between the two groups was found, but the trabeculectomy group required less postoperative medications. However, surgical complications were reported as 46 % in the trabeculectomy group as compared with only 4 % in the phacoemulsification-alone group ($P=0.001$) and one third of the trabeculectomy eyes demonstrated cataract development during the 24-month follow-up [56]. Finally, in patients with medically controlled CACG who were randomized to lensectomy alone versus phacotrabeculectomy, there was no statistically significant difference between IOP at 12- and 24-month follow-up and no difference in disease progression rates, and while the phacotrabeculectomy group was on a mean of 0.8 medications less than the lensectomy-alone group, the phacotrabeculectomy group suffered significantly more postoperative complications [57]. When faced with deciding which procedure to most appropriately perform in a patient with ACG, one should consider whether lens extraction is likely to relieve the pre-trabecular meshwork obstruction, allowing for control of the IOP and opening of the angle, with or without medications, before deciding to pursue filtration or combined phacoemulsification and filtration surgery, which, as these studies have shown, result in more postoperative and potential long-term complications for the patient. In certain cases, lensectomy without filtration surgery may be combined with other non-bleb-forming procedures, to be discussed later, which have a more favorable risk profile.

The final consideration in the patient with angle closure is that of retrolenticular causes. This includes situations such as choroidal expansion, malignant glaucoma, ciliary effusions, or any other posterior-pushing mechanism. Although not

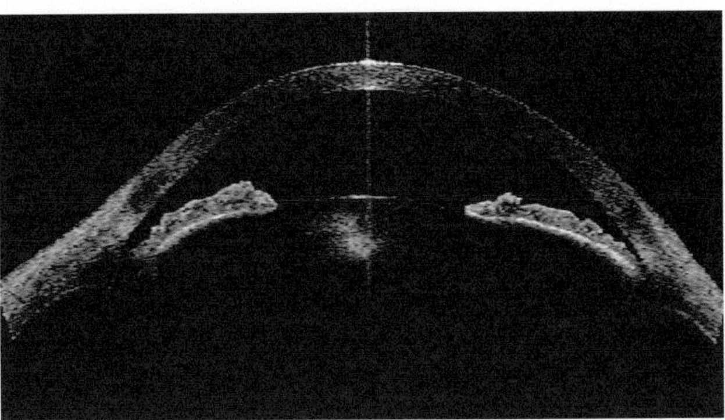

**Fig. 25.2** AS-OCT image of a patient with high lens vault and also relative pupillary block seen with a convex iris contour

classically considered in the category of primary angle closure and not within the scope of this chapter, a brief discussion on surgical considerations in malignant glaucoma will also be included in this chapter.

## Surgical Technique and Considerations

Lensectomy in the angle-closure eye may present many unique challenges to the surgeon. The difficulties may range from poor visibility due to an edematous cornea, flat anterior chamber, abnormal iris behavior, intumescent lens, and loose or missing zonules to predisposition to malignant glaucoma both intraoperatively and postoperatively.

The surgical approach to the angle-closure patient begins preoperatively. It is ideal if any AACG attack is broken prior to surgical intervention and, as well, the eye as quiet as possible from inflammation with the use of topical steroids or nonsteroidal anti-inflammatory medications. Topical, with or without, the use of systemic medications to obtain as normal an IOP as possible prior to surgery is also advisable. Specular microscopy with a corneal endothelial cell count may be helpful in determining the state of cornea. AS-OCT may provide information as to the amount of anterior chamber space one will have to work with intraoperatively (Fig. 25.2) as well as potentially suggest diagnostic etiologies related to poor zonular support such as ACG due to spherophakia (Fig. 25.3). Finally, UBM imaging may provide a view to the ciliary processes, with anteriorly positioned ciliary processes seen commonly in plateau iris syndrome (Fig. 25.4).

Intraoperatively, the first objective of surgery is to achieve an adequate view of the anterior segment to effectively and safely perform lens extraction. If the epithelium is edematous preventing an adequate view, topical glycerin may be used, or manual removal of the corneal epithelium is occasionally required. Once an adequate view has been achieved to proceed, the next objective is to protect the cornea, typically most effectively achieved by the use of a dispersive OVD injected into the anterior chamber via a paracentesis incision.

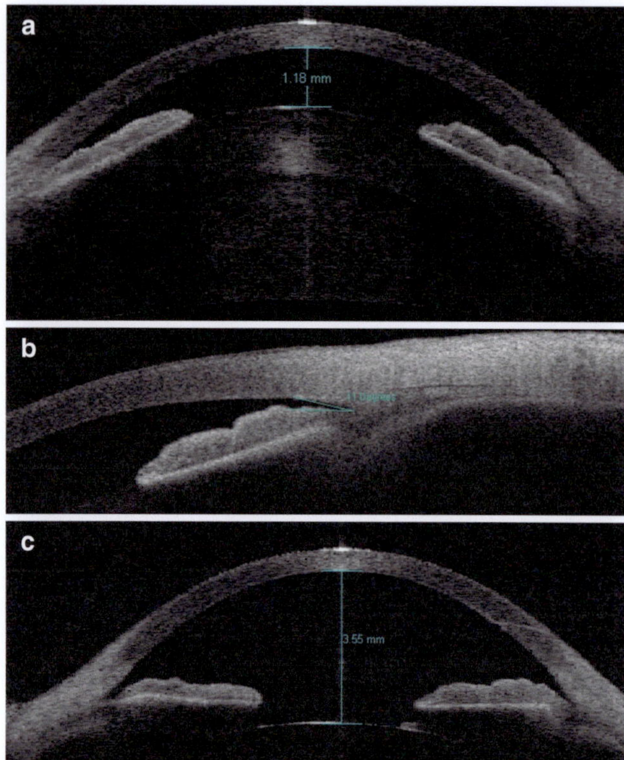

**Fig. 25.3** (**a**) Spherophakia lens-induced angle closure with anterior chamber depth of 1.18 mm as measured on AS-OCT. (**b**) Angle view of the same patient. (**c**) Postoperative imaging of the same patient after lens extraction and goniosynechialysis showing anterior chamber depth of 3.55 mm. (**d**) Postoperative angle image of same patient (Images courtesy of Ike K. Ahmed, MD)

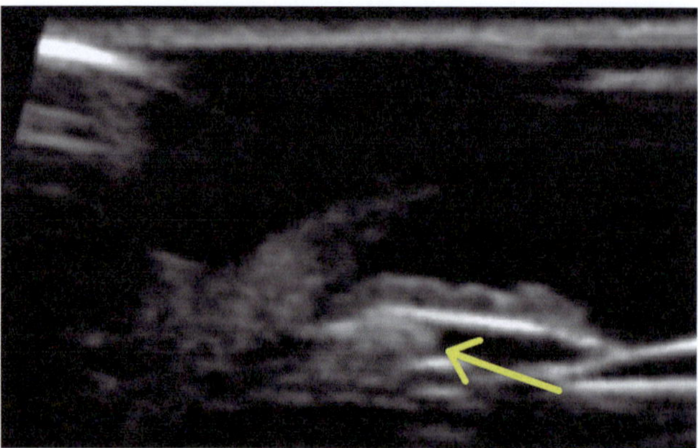

**Fig. 25.4** Ultrasound biomicroscopy image of a plateau iris patient showing anteriorly positioned ciliary processes (*arrow*) propping up the peripheral iris causing a narrow angle

Stabilization and deepening of the anterior chamber, often achieved with a cohesive OVD, should then be attained. In the occasional case, the anterior chamber cannot be deepened or formed with OVD, even with a high-viscosity agent such as Healon 5 (Abbott Medical Optics, Inc., Illinois, USA). In such cases, a pars plana tap to reduce posterior pressure can be an invaluable tool and technique in order to allow deepening of the anterior chamber for effective removal of the lens and as well providing a safe space for phacoemulsification and manipulations to occur away from the likely already-traumatized corneal endothelium [58].

The proper technique should involve a localized conjunctival peritomy and light cautery for hemostasis, followed by a careful measurement and marking with a caliper of 4 mm radially posterior to the limbus. A microvitreoretinal (MVR) blade is then used to enter the posterior segment with care taken to aim the blade posteriorly towards the optic nerve, to comfortably avoid the crystalline lens. Without the use of a separate infusion, the automated vitrectomy device is then placed into the posterior segment through the created incision, with care taken to point the guillotine and aspiration ostium posteriorly away from the lens. Vitrectomy with suction is then performed, and within a few seconds and with a very small volume of vitreous removed, sufficient decompression of the posterior segment will have occurred as to produce a dramatic and often surprising increase in the capacity to deepen the anterior chamber (Video 25.2).

Once the anterior chamber has been stabilized, the pupil may need to be addressed prior to lens extraction. Posterior synechiae from the iris to the lens capsule may need to be released, or pupil manipulation and expansion may be required. These maneuvers may be achieved using simple iris hook instruments such as the Kuglen or Lester hooks, pupil dilators such as the Beehler instrument, anterior segment microscissors to perform mini-sphincterotomies, or devices to maintain pupil dilation during surgery such as the Malyugin Ring or disposable iris retractors. Viscodilation with a visco-adaptive OVD is also often a useful adjunct in managing iris in these cases. In some cases, patients with atonic mid-dilated irides, or those with focal atrophy, may benefit from suture pupilloplasty to reduce photophobia and restore a more anatomically physiologic shape for both visual function and cosmesis. This is typically achieved using 10-0 polypropylene suture on a long curved needle to place either multiple interrupted sutures to close focal defects or occasionally a cerclage or partial cerclage suture to close circumferential or large clock-hour iris defects or areas of atonicity. Iris sutures may be tied using the McCannel [59], Siepser [60], any modification of the two, or intraocular microinstrument-mediated tying techniques (Videos 25.3 and 25.4).

In angle-closure eyes, creating a continuous curvilinear capsulorhexis (CCC) may be challenging, as these patients often have a lens or anterior capsule that is vaulted forward. As a result, an anterior CCC has the tendency to run out peripherally towards the lens equator. The use of high-viscosity OVD agents may be employed to flatten the anterior capsule, and as well, erring on the side of making the CCC slightly smaller may be useful strategies. If the lens cortex is hydrated, white, and intumescent, prior to commencing the CCC, a short hypodermic needle on a syringe half filled with balanced saline solution may be utilized to puncture the anterior capsule, immediately aspirating and decompressing the internal contents of the capsular bag to decrease the amount of forward pressure on the anterior capsule (Video 25.5). Should the CCC begin to stray peripherally during its creation, a tear-in technique is very useful to rescue the capsulorhexis (Video 25.6) [61]. If zonular issues are present in an angle-closure patient undergoing cataract extraction, a CCC is critical to permit the use of capsular tension devices. Without an intact CCC, capsular tension support devices are very challenging to use and may in fact be detrimental [62, 63].

Zonular weakness is frequently encountered in angle-closure eyes, from mild laxity allowing or causing the lens to vault forward into a configuration causing pupillary block or simply an overall forward position of the lens-iris apparatus with a crowded anterior segment. Occasionally the zonular laxity can present in the extreme and severe forms such as in microspherophakia as the cause of angle closure. While zonular weakness may occasionally be elucidated at the preoperative examination, this may be very subtle or difficult to observe in the angle-closure eye, especially after an AACG attack. Furthermore, patients with frank phacodonesis and lens movement typically will have enough space, even if only intermittent between saccades, between the iris and lens capsule to allow aqueous humor to pass from the posterior to the anterior chamber.

Intraoperatively, several signs may suggest moderate or severe zonulopathy: capsular wrinkling when attempting to puncture the anterior capsule, difficulty puncturing the anterior capsule, ovalization of the CCC, movement of the entire lens during creation of the CCC, or tilting or lens movement during phacoemulsification [64]. In angle-closure patients, capsular tension devices may serve to stabilize weak zonules or support an area of focalized weakened zonules, distribute forces along the capsular bag circumference evenly, expand the equator of the capsule, recenter a mildly subluxed capsular bag, and keep the capsular bag in an anatomically acceptable position. Although a small series, one study has shown with UBM postoperative imaging that implantation of a CTR placed the bag equator and CTR in an anatomically favorable position between the IOL haptics and the ciliary body without posterior iris touch [65]. Other studies have also suggested similar findings [66].

When confronted with weak zonules, the first decision to be made is whether a mere capsular tension ring will be sufficient to support the capsular bag. A CTR is suitable for use in cases where mild generalized zonular weakness or a localized focal zonulolysis area of less than four clock hours is sus-

pected. As well, where no overt or gross lens subluxation is present, even in cases of suspected progressive zonulopathies, a CTR may be sufficient [67].

If the zonular weakness is in excess of these criteria, it is likely that more than a CTR alone will be required to stabilize the capsular bag. If more extensive support is required, one can select a Cionni-modified CTR (M-CTR) which consists of a CTR with one or two eyelets for suturing positioned 0.25 mm anterior to the equatorial ring or an Ahmed capsular tension segment (CTS). While the M-CTR encompasses the entire circumference, it is not injectable and must be manually inserted into the capsular bag.

This may be quite challenging especially in cases where the assistance of the device is required before the capsular bag contents are removed and may in fact damage zonules further. Also, it is ideal to position the eyelet for suturing into the area of greatest zonular weakness or absence, something which may require even further manual manipulation and rotation once the device is in the capsular bag. In these cases, an Ahmed CTS may be used, which is composed of a 120° arc length PMMA ring segment with a 5 mm radius of curvature. Like the M-CTR, it has an anterior positioned eyelet for suturing to the sclera. The CTS is more relatively easily maneuvered in the eye and into the capsular bag, without the need for rotational movements, which may further damage existing zonules. Further, because it is designed to slide into the capsular bag, it is more readily placed into the particular quadrant or zone where it is most needed and, with caution, can be used in cases of a discontinuous CCC or a posterior capsular tear.

The main body of the device is designed to sit in the capsular equator with the central eyelet remaining anterior to the anterior capsule. It can easily be placed prior to cataract extraction and may be supported intraoperatively with an inverted iris retractor through a paracentesis incision and sutured later on after the cataract has been removed. While the CTS provides focal support transversely to the scleral wall, it may be used in conjunction with a CTR to provide circumferential support and distribution of zonular tension. Finally, multiple CTS may be used if the zonular weakness or absence is profound. These may be sutured to the sclera through an ab externo technique using a 9-0 polypropylene suture or larger-caliber suture such as GORE-TEX expanded polytetrafluoroethylene (ePTFE) material (W.L. Gore & Associates, Inc., USA) for greater longevity and reduced suture breakage risk (Video 25.7) [67].

Once the decision has been made to employ the use of a CTR in surgery, the decision must be made whether to place it in the capsular bag prior to or after phacoemulsification. There are advantages and disadvantages to each approach. If there is suspicion of significant zonular weakness from either preoperative evaluation, intraoperative signs, or a concern for the capsular equator collapsing centrally, then consideration should be given to placing the CTR early on, prior to lens removal. The technique to achieve this involves careful and thorough viscodissection creating a plane between the capsular bag and the cortical material. A diligent viscodissection will prevent any cortical lens material entrapment by the CTR when placed prior to phacoemulsification. If moderate or severe zonular weakness is encountered, iris retractors may be used and placed gently on the CCC to stabilize the capsular bag while viscodissection and CTR injection is performed (Video 25.8). The CTR may be injected also after a CTS has been placed if this was required (Video 25.9).

After successful insertion of the CTR, hydrodissection and hydrodelineation may proceed as per the surgeon's usual technique. The main advantage of early placement includes expansion of the capsular equator alleviating the concern of equatorial collapse and inadvertent bag injury during phacoemulsification. As well, the expanded capsular equator may serve in certain cases to barricade any vitreous that would otherwise be able to prolapse forward in an area of zonular dehiscence. In some cases, without early capsular tension device placement, phacoemulsification would be very challenging to achieve uneventfully in a very mobile lens and capsular bag complex.

While advantageous in early stabilization of the zonules, some disadvantages of early placement include the potential to injure or dehisce more zonules because of rotational forces transmitted to the zonular apparatus during CTR insertion. The potential for injury to the capsular bag itself during insertion, the potential entrapment of cortical material if viscodissection is not done properly making for challenging cortical removal, and the possibility of posterior dislocation of the CTR into the posterior segment should a posterior capsular tear occur during subsequent phacoemulsification. Finally, as the CTR expands the capsular equator and places tension on the posterior capsule, a taut capsule may be more easily torn or appear to move the posterior capsule into a more forward configuration during the latter stages of phacoemulsification and irrigation/aspiration.

Injection of a CTR late after the contents of the capsular bag have been removed can be advantageous in ease of insertion, but in cases where zonulopathy is moderate or severe, the capsular bag equator may collapse increasing the risk of inadvertent injury potentially eliminating the possibility that a CTR can even be considered.

It is worth noting that in angle-closure eyes, and eyes with suspected zonulopathy, direct chopping lens disassembly techniques such as phaco chop have some advantages over techniques such as divide and conquer. Phaco chop has been shown to dissipate significantly less phaco power and time into the eye [68, 69], being advantageous to the corneal endothelium [70] and other anterior segment structures such as the trabecular meshwork, which both may be already compromised in angle closure. Further, in the divide and conquer technique, a downward pressure is transmitted onto the zonular apparatus during sculpting maneuvers, which may further injure or break already-weakened zonules.

Vector forces in phaco chop techniques, when performed properly, are transmitted endocapsularly with shearing or cracking of the lens material and minimal tension placed on zonules.

Once the crystalline lens material is removed and all required capsular tension devices have been placed properly, an intraocular lens (IOL) can be inserted, preferably into the capsular bag if sufficiently intact. Although different IOL models and designs may be used, it is the author's experience that a soft foldable acrylic one-piece IOL unfolds slowly and gently in a manner which is gentle on the zonules and is the easiest to control in terms of endocapsular placement, rotation, and manipulations.

In the case of a non-intact posterior capsule, a three-piece IOL with thin polymethyl methacrylate, polypropylene, or polyimide haptics may be placed in the ciliary sulcus with posterior optic capture through an intact CCC for added stability. Although certainly possible to perform successfully, caution is advised when placing IOLs in the ciliary sulcus of eyes with crowded anterior segments. The bulky acrylic haptics such as those found on the one-piece acrylic IOL platforms should never be placed in the ciliary sulcus as they will chafe the posterior iris surface resulting in complications such as uveitis-glaucoma-hyphema syndrome. Finally, if capsular support is absent and not viable for IOL support, the iris claw IOL (Ophtec BV, Netherlands) may be used if the anterior chamber depth has been sufficiently improved after lens extraction and in the presence of a healthy corneal endothelium [71–73]. Should corneal or anterior chamber depth criteria not be met, a three-piece IOL may be fixated to the posterior chamber using the scleral-glued technique [74].

## Combined Surgery

In certain clinical situations, the decision may be made to combine lens extraction with adjunctive glaucoma procedures including endocyclophotocoagulation (ECP) and goniosynechialysis (GSL), or even in cases with advanced disease where it is felt that lens extraction alone with adjunctive medications may not achieve the target IOP, filtration surgery including trabeculectomy, Ex-PRESS mini shunt, and long tube shunt implantation may be considered concurrently. Although filtration and tube shunt surgery are covered elsewhere in this book, a brief discussion of ECP and GSL will be included.

Although lens extraction may alone be completely therapeutic in angle closure due solely to lens vault, phacomorphic ACG, or lens-induced pupillary block, the angle may remain narrow after lens extraction alone, this being particularly so in cases of plateau iris [75]. In cases of angle closure undergoing cataract surgery where the primary cause is thought to be plateau iris configuration or where a mixed

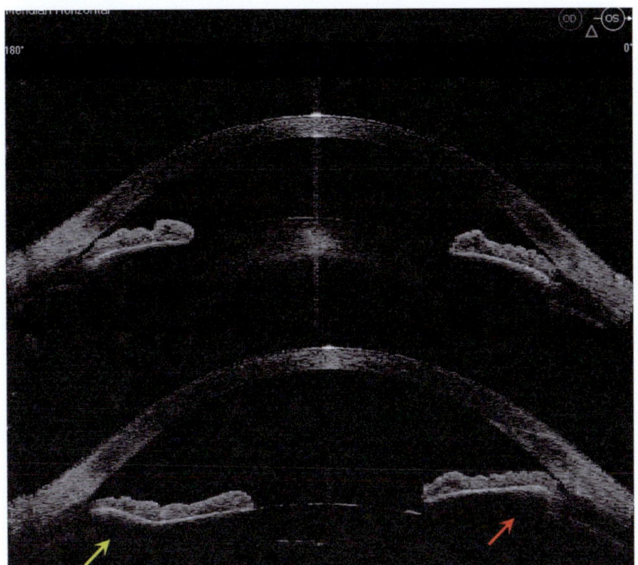

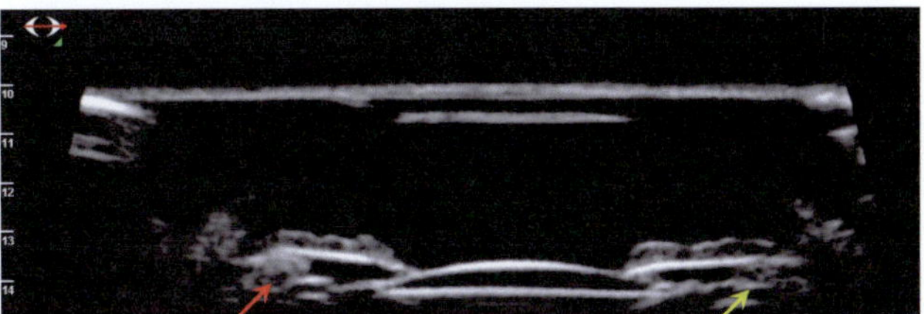

**Fig. 25.6** Ultrasound biomicroscopy of the same patient as seen in Fig. 25.5 showing again the temporal ciliary processes (*red arrow*) and the shrunken nasal ciliary processes (*yellow arrow*)

**Fig. 25.5** Noncontact AS-OCT image of anterior chamber in an eye after lens extraction and endocycloplasty (ECPL). Because of the 270° treatment performed during surgery, the temporal angle (*red arrow*) remains narrow with the peripheral iris propped up by the anteriorly positioned ciliary processes, while the nasal angle (*yellow arrow*) is dramatically opened with the peripheral iris able to fall back from the angle and trabecular meshwork with the ciliary processes shrunken posteriorly from the treatment (Image courtesy of Ike K. Ahmed, MD)

mechanism of lens-related causes and plateau iris is felt to be contributory, ECP may be considered as a way to widen the angle and increase the separation between the peripheral iris and the trabecular meshwork. While traditional ECP techniques have been reported as a treatment for refractory open-angle glaucoma, ECP may be a very effective tool in angle-closure glaucoma as well. In a technique that has been termed "endocycloplasty" [76], the diode laser beam and energy are directed and applied to the posterior aspect of the ciliary processes, pulling the entire ciliary process posteriorly away from the posterior iris surface. This allows the peripheral iris to fall back posteriorly away from the trabecular meshwork and angle.

This treatment is typically performed for 270° arc length via the same incision by which the phacoemulsification or lens extraction was performed. It is important to note that in this technique, the location of the laser application on the tail of the ciliary process is critical to its success. Treatment at the posterior tail of the process directs the entire ciliary process including the anterior head to shrink posteriorly.

The treatment should shrink and whiten the ciliary process, but care be taken to attempt to avoid "popping" as this may lead to increased postoperative inflammation and breakdown of the blood-aqueous barrier (Video 25.10). Although further study is required, the early results of this technique have appeared very promising in improving angle configuration (Figs. 25.5 and 25.6 – Visante post-ECPL, UBM post-ECPL).

While lensectomy and even ECPL may deepen the anterior chamber, if peripheral anterior synechiae are present, more may need to be done for the control of IOP in synechial angle-closure patients. Goniosynechialysis has been reported to be effective and safe in the reduction of IOP [77] and even more so when combined with lens extraction [78–81]. UBM imaging has also shown the restoration of an open anterior chamber angle after GSL [82]. Although controversial, the success of GSL may be dependent on the duration of the presence of PAS. Existing data from studies which showed efficacy of GSL suggested that it is best performed in cases where PAS has been present for 6 months or less, although when presented with an ACG, it may be difficult to know how long PAS have been present and no data currently exists directly comparing the efficacy of GSL when performed at varying time points of PAS presence. However, given the relatively favorable safety profile of GSL, it may be beneficial to consider performing GSL prior to making the decision to proceed with more invasive and higher-risk filtration surgery, even if it is suspected that the PAS have been present for greater than 6 months.

GSL may be performed with varying techniques, but the author's preferred technique is under gonioscopic visualization with the use of anterior segment microinstrumentation to precisely grasp the peripheral iris tissue and view the angle structures as the PAS are released (Video 25.11). In cases where the cornea does not permit an adequate view of the angle via a gonio mirror, endoscopic visualization may be utilized to assist in performance of GSL (Video 25.12) [83]. It should be noted that it is common for lens extraction to be performed in conjunction with both ECPL and GSL, as a very useful technique to release PAS, maximize angle space, and minimize risk of PAS recurrences.

## Additional Considerations: Malignant Glaucoma

Although the mechanism by which the challenging entity of malignant glaucoma remains a subject of debate [84, 85], it is generally agreed that eyes with crowded anterior segments and angle closure are more prone to it [86], with a recent study suggesting that plateau iris configuration could be an additional risk factor [87]. Although malignant glaucoma is traditionally thought of as occurring after filtration surgery, it has been reported after laser iridotomy [88] and routine cataract surgery [89] as well.

Various different treatments have been proposed for the effective treatment of this difficult entity, including first medical therapy with cycloplegic agents, IOP-reducing agents, and osmotic agents [90–92]; laser therapy to disrupt the anterior hyaloid face [93–95]; transscleral cyclodiode laser [89, 96, 97]; and pars plana vitrectomy [98, 99], but perhaps the most important and key concept in successfully treating malignant glaucoma is the concept of creating a "unicameral" eye where there is a free and unimpeded communication between the posterior segment and the anterior chamber. This has been described as being created with a pars plana anterior vitrectomy, hyaloido-zonulectomy, and iridectomy [100], or by the term vitrectomy-hyaloidotomy-iridectomy (VHI) [101].

Creation of the VHI can be performed from either an anterior chamber or a pars plana approach with the use of an automated vitrectomy instrument to cut through the iris, zonules, and vitreous. If malignant glaucoma or excessive posterior positive pressure occurs intraoperatively during phacoemulsification or other anterior segment surgery, even in an eye where a pars plana tap has already been performed, a VHI can be performed concurrently to definitively deepen the anterior chamber. Care should be taken in a phakic patient, or when performed with concurrent phacoemulsification, to avoid injuring the capsule by placing the vitrector as peripheral as possible to clear the lens equator (Video 25.13). Once malignant glaucoma has been encountered, careful consideration should be given to performing a prophylactic VHI as part of the surgical management in the fellow eye if still phakic and planning for lens extraction and the eye exhibits signs of being at potential risk for malignant glaucoma.

Finally, careful selection of postoperative topical therapy can be very influential to the postoperative success of surgery. In cases of malignant glaucoma, it is the author's opinion that maintaining cycloplegia postoperatively to stretch zonules posteriorizes the ciliary processes and the IOL-capsular bag complex, is of paramount importance in stabilizing the eye. Conversely, miotics anteriorize the ciliary processes as well as the IOL-capsular bag complex and may even, in some cases, precipitate or aggravate malignant glaucoma. It is best to avoid the use of miotics in malignant glaucoma postoperatively but, on the other hand, may be beneficial in angle closure due to plateau iris. In postoperative lens extraction with or without ECP and GSL for plateau iris, miotics act to contract and pull iris tissue away from the angle potentially aiding in the prevention of postoperative PAS reformation in cases where GSL or combined ECP/GSL have been performed. Once the postoperative inflammation has improved or resolved, the miotic may be observantly discontinued monitoring closely for reformation of PAS. Choosing carefully between postoperative miotic or cycloplegic agents should be individualized to the mechanism believed to be the main cause of angle closure but may be very important to the ultimate success in the overall management of the condition.

## Conclusions

Although angle closure may be a challenging entity to manage successfully, careful preoperative examination with the use of adjunctive imaging and a resultant understanding of the predominant cause of the angle closure in each individual case is of paramount importance. Unique challenges may be encountered during lens extraction relating to the cornea, adequate anterior chamber space, iris distortion, lens capsule, and zonules, requiring a systematic and expectant approach to each obstacle. In certain cases, adjunctive surgical procedures may be performed with lens extraction, such as ECP, GSL, more invasive filtration or tube shunt surgery, and, in some cases, a VHI for malignant glaucoma cases. With careful surgical planning, lens extraction, with or without adjunctive procedures, is a pivotal and indispensable management tool and can be the definitive therapy in angle closure, especially in recalcitrant and stubborn cases.

## References


1. Foster PJ. The epidemiology of primary angle closure and associated glaucomatous optic neuropathy. Semin Ophthalmol. 2002;17:50–8.
2. Bonomi L, Marchini G, Marraffa M, et al. Prevalence of glaucoma and intraocular pressure distribution in a defined population. The Egna-Neumarkt Study. Ophthalmology. 1998;105:209–15.
3. Mitchell P, Smith W, Attebo K, Healey PR. Prevalence of open-angle glaucoma in Australia. The Blue Mountains Eye Study. Ophthalmology. 1996;103:1661–9.
4. Bankes JL, Perkins ES, Tsolakis S, Wright JE. Bedford glaucoma survey. Br Med J. 1968;1:791–6.
5. Coffey M, Reidy A, Wormald R, et al. Prevalence of glaucoma in the west of Ireland. Br J Ophthalmol. 1993;77:17–21.
6. Hollows FC, Graham PA. Intra-ocular pressure, glaucoma, and glaucoma suspects in a defined population. Br J Ophthalmol. 1966;50:570–86.
7. Wensor MD, McCarty CA, Stanislavsky YL, et al. The prevalence of glaucoma in the Melbourne Visual Impairment Project. Ophthalmology. 1998;105:733–9.
8. Klein BE, Klein R, Sponsel WE, et al. Prevalence of glaucoma. The Beaver Dam Eye Study. Ophthalmology. 1992;99:1499–504.
9. Dielemans I, Vingerling JR, Wolfs RC, et al. The prevalence of primary open-angle glaucoma in a population-based study in The Netherlands. The Rotterdam Study. Ophthalmology. 1994;101:1851–5.
10. Bengtsson B. The prevalence of glaucoma. Br J Ophthalmol. 1981;65:46–9.
11. Tielsch JM, Katz J, Singh K, et al. A population-based evaluation of glaucoma screening: the Baltimore Eye Survey. Am J Epidemiol. 1991;134:1102–10.

12. Buhrmann RR, Quigley HA, Barron Y, et al. Prevalence of glaucoma in a rural East African population. Invest Ophthalmol Vis Sci. 2000;41:40–8.

13. Rotchford AP, Kirwan JF, Muller MA, et al. Temba glaucoma study: a population-based cross-sectional survey in urban South Africa. Ophthalmology. 2003;110:376–82.

14. Van Rens GH, Arkell SM, Charlton W, Doesburg W. Primary angle-closure glaucoma among Alaskan Eskimos. Doc Ophthalmol. 1988;70:265–76.

15. Arkell SM, Lightman DA, Sommer A, et al. The prevalence of glaucoma among Eskimos of northwest Alaska. Arch Ophthalmol. 1987;105:482–5.

16. Bourne RR, Sorensen KE, Klauber A, et al. Glaucoma in East Greenlandic Inuit – a population survey in Ittoqqortoormiit (Scoresbysund). Acta Ophthalmol Scand. 2001;79:462–7.

17. Congdon NG, Quigley HA, Hung PT, et al. Screening techniques for angle-closure glaucoma in rural Taiwan. Acta Ophthalmol Scand. 1996;74:113–9.

18. He M, Foster PJ, Ge J, et al. Prevalence and clinical characteristics of glaucoma in adult Chinese: a population-based study in Liwan District, Guangzhou. Invest Ophthalmol Vis Sci. 2006;47:2782–8.

19. Foster PJ, Baasanhu J, Alsbirk PH, et al. Glaucoma in Mongolia. A population-based survey in Hovsgol province, northern Mongolia. Arch Ophthalmol. 1996;114:1235–41.

20. Xu L, Zhang L, Xia CR, et al. The prevalence and its effective factors of primary angle-closure glaucoma in defined populations of rural and urban in Beijing [in Chinese]. Zhonghua Yan Ke Za Zhi. 2005;41:8–14.

21. Foster PJ, Oen FT, Machin D, et al. The prevalence of glaucoma in Chinese residents of Singapore: a cross-sectional population survey of the Tanjong Pagar district. Arch Ophthalmol. 2000;118:1105–11.

22. Casson RJ, Newland HS, Muecke J, et al. Prevalence of glaucoma in rural Myanmar: the Meiktila Eye Study. Br J Ophthalmol. 2007;91:710–4.

23. Salmon JF, Mermoud A, Ivey A, et al. The prevalence of primary angle closure glaucoma and open angle glaucoma in Mamre, Western Cape, South Africa. Arch Ophthalmol. 1993;111:1263–9.

24. Dandona L, Dandona R, Mandal P, et al. Angle-closure glaucoma in an urban population in southern India. The Andhra Pradesh eye disease study. Ophthalmology. 2000;107:1710–6.

25. Bourne RR, Sukudom P, Foster PJ, et al. Prevalence of glaucoma in Thailand: a population based survey in Rom Klao District, Bangkok. Br J Ophthalmol. 2003;87:1069–74.

26. Vijaya L, George R, Arvind H, et al. Prevalence of angle-closure disease in a rural southern Indian population. Arch Ophthalmol. 2006;124:403–9.

27. Ramakrishnan R, Nirmalan PK, Krishnadas R, et al. Glaucoma in a rural population of southern India: the Aravind comprehensive eye survey. Ophthalmology. 2003;110:1484–90.

28. Rahman MM, Rahman N, Foster PJ, et al. The prevalence of glaucoma in Bangladesh: a population based survey in Dhaka division. Br J Ophthalmol. 2004;88:1493–7.

29. Shiose Y, Kitazawa Y, Tsukahara S, et al. Epidemiology of glaucoma in Japan – a nationwide glaucoma survey. Jpn J Ophthalmol. 1991;35:133–55.

30. Yamamoto T, Iwase A, Araie M, et al. The Tajimi Study report 2: prevalence of primary angle closure and secondary glaucoma in a Japanese population. Ophthalmology. 2005;112:1661–9.

31. Quigley HA. Number of people with glaucoma worldwide in 2010 and 2020. Br J Ophthalmol. 2006;90:262–7.

32. Foster PJ, Johnson GJ. Glaucoma in China: how big is the problem? Br J Ophthalmol. 2001;85:1277–82.

33. Van Herick W, Shaffer RN, Schwartz A. Estimation of width of angle of anterior chamber. Incidence and significance of the narrow angle. Am J Ophthalmol. 1969;68:626–9.

34. Lowe RF. Aetiology of the anatomical basis for primary angle-closure glaucoma. Biometrical comparisons between normal eyes and eyes with primary angle-closure glaucoma. Br J Ophthalmol. 1970;54:161–9.

35. Gazzard G, Foster PJ, Friedman DS, et al. Light to dark physiological variation in iridotrabecular angle width. Br J Ophthalmol. 2004. Available at: http://bjo.bmj.com/cgi/content/full/88/11/DC1/1. Accessed 20 Apr 2013.

36. Quigley HA. Long-term follow-up of laser iridotomy. Ophthalmology. 1981;88:218–24.

37. He M, Friedman DS, Ge J, et al. Laser peripheral iridotomy in primary angle-closure suspects: biometric and gonioscopic outcomes: the Liwan Eye Study. Ophthalmology. 2007;114:494–500.

38. He M, Friedman DS, Ge J, et al. Laser peripheral iridotomy in eyes with narrow drainage angles: ultrasound biomicroscopy outcomes. The Liwan Eye Study. Ophthalmology. 2007;114:1513–9.

39. Greve EL. Primary angle closure glaucoma: extracapsular cataract extraction or filtering procedure? Int Ophthalmol. 1988;12:157–62.

40. Steuhl KP, Marahrens P, Frohn C, Frohn A. Intraocular pressure and anterior chamber depth before and after extracapsular cataract extraction with posterior chamber lens implantation. Ophthalmic Surg. 1992;23:233–7.

41. Yang CH, Hung PT. Intraocular lens position and anterior chamber angle changes after cataract extraction in eyes with primary angle-closure glaucoma. J Cataract Refract Surg. 1997;23:1109–13.

42. Hayashi K, Hayashi H, Nakao F, Hayashi F. Changes in anterior chamber angle width and depth after intraocular lens implantation in eyes with glaucoma. Ophthalmology. 2000;107:698–703.

43. Tham CC, Lai JS, Lam DS. Changes in AC angle width and depth after IOL implantation in eyes with glaucoma. Ophthalmology. 2001;108:428–9.

44. Lam DS, Leung DY, Tham CC, et al. Randomized trial of early phacoemulsification versus peripheral iridotomy to prevent intraocular pressure rise after acute primary angle closure. Ophthalmology. 2008;115:1134–40.

45. Wishart PK, Atkinson PL. Extracapsular cataract extraction and posterior chamber lens implantation in patients with primary chronic angle-closure glaucoma: effect on intraocular pressure control. Eye (Lond). 1989;3(Pt 6):706–12.

46. Gunning FP, Greve EL. Uncontrolled primary angle closure glaucoma: results of early intercapsular cataract extraction and posterior chamber lens implantation. Int Ophthalmol. 1991;15:237–47.

47. Acton J, Salmon JF, Scholtz R. Extracapsular cataract extraction with posterior chamber lens implantation in primary angle-closure glaucoma. J Cataract Refract Surg. 1997;23:930–4.

48. Gunning FP, Greve EL. Lens extraction for uncontrolled angle-closure glaucoma: long-term follow-up. J Cataract Refract Surg. 1998;24:1347–56.

49. Roberts TV, Francis IC, Lertusumitkul S, et al. Primary phacoemulsification for uncontrolled angle-closure glaucoma. J Cataract Refract Surg. 2000;26:1012–6.

50. Hayashi K, Hayashi H, Nakao F, Hayashi F. Effect of cataract surgery on intraocular pressure control in glaucoma patients. J Cataract Refract Surg. 2001;27:1779–86.

51. Jacobi PC, Dietlein TS, Luke C, et al. Primary phacoemulsification and intraocular lens implantation for acute angle-closure glaucoma. Ophthalmology. 2002;109:1597–603.

52. Khokar K, Pangtey M. Phacoemulsification in filtered chronic angle closure glaucoma eyes. Clin Experiment Ophthalmol. 2002;30:256–60.

53. Ming Zhi Z, Lim AS, Yin Wong T. A pilot study of lens extraction in the management of acute primary angle-closure glaucoma. Am J Ophthalmol. 2003;135:534–6.

54. Kubota T, Toguri I, Onizuka N, Matsuura T. Phacoemulsification and intraocular lens implantation for angle closure glaucoma after the relief of pupillary block. Ophthalmologica. 2003;217:325–8.

55. Tham CC, Kwong YY, Leung DY, et al. Phacoemulsification versus combined phacotrabeculectomy in medically uncontrolled chronic angle closure glaucoma with cataract. Ophthalmology. 2009;116:725–31.

56. Tham CC, Kwong YY, Baig N, et al. Phacoemulsification versus trabeculectomy in medically uncontrolled chronic angle closure glaucoma without cataract. Ophthalmology. 2013;120:62–7.

57. Tham CC, Kwong YY, Leung DY, et al. Phacoemulsification versus combined phacotrabeculectomy in medically controlled chronic angle closure glaucoma with cataract. Ophthalmology. 2008;115:2167–73.

58. Chang DF. Pars plana vitreous tap for phacoemulsification in the crowded eye. J Cataract Refract Surg. 2001;27(12):1911–4.

59. McCannel MA. A retrievable suture idea for anterior uveal problems. Ophthalmic Surg. 1976;7:98–103.

60. Siepser SB. The closer chamber slipping suture technique for iris repair. Ann Ophthalmol. 1994;26:71–2.

61. Little BC, Smith JH, Packer M. Little capsulorhexis tear-out rescue. J Cataract Refract Surg. 2006;32(9):1420–2.

62. Bopp S, Lucke K. Chronic cystoid macular edema in an eye with a capsule defect and posteriorly dislocated capsular tension ring. J Cataract Refract Surg. 2003;29:603–8.

63. Bhattacharjee H, Bhattacharjee K, Das A, et al. Management of a posteriorly dislocated endocapsular tension ring and a foldable acrylic intraocular lens. J Cataract Refract Surg. 2004;30:243–6.

64. Hasanee K, Ahmed IK. Capsular tension rings: update on endocapsular support devices. Ophthalmol Clin North Am. 2006;19:507–19.

65. Boomer JA, Jackson DW. Anatomic evaluation of the Morcher capsular tension ring by ultrasound biomicroscopy. J Cataract Refract Surg. 2006;32(5):846–8.

66. Tribus C, Alge CS, Haritoglou C, et al. Indications and clinical outcome of capsular tension ring (CTR) implantation: a review of 9528 cataract surgeries. Clin Ophthalmol. 2007;1:65–9.

67. Hasanee K, Butler M, Ahmed IK. Capsular tension rings and related devices: current concepts. Curr Opin Ophthalmol. 2006;17:31–41.

68. DeBry P, Olson RJ, Crandall AS. Comparison of energy required for phaco-chop and divide and conquer phacoemulsification. J Cataract Refract Surg. 1998;24:689–92.

69. Wong T, Hingorani M, Lee V. Phacoemulsification time and power requirements in phaco chop and divide and conquer nucleofractis techniques. J Cataract Refract Surg. 2000;26:1374–8.

70. Pirazzoli G, D'Eliseo D, Ziosi M, Acciarri R. Effects of phacoemulsification time on the corneal endothelium using phacofracture and phaco chop techniques. J Cataract Refract Surg. 1996;22:967–9.

71. Guell JL, Velasco F, Malecaze F, et al. Secondary Artisan-Verisyse aphakic lens implantation. J Cataract Refract Surg. 2005;31:2266–71.

72. Tahzib NG, Nuijts RM, Wu WY. Long-term study of Artisan phakic intraocular lens implantation for the correction of moderate to high myopia. Ophthalmology. 2007;114:1133–42.

73. Saxena R, Boekhoorn SS, Mulder PG, et al. Long-term follow-up of endothelial cell change after Artisan phakic intraocular lens implantation. Ophthalmology. 2008;115:608–13.

74. Agarwal A, Jacob S, Kumar DA, et al. Handshake technique for glued intrascleral haptic fixation of a posterior chamber intraocular lens. J Cataract Refract Surg. 2013;39:317–22.

75. Tran HV, Liebmann JM, Ritch R. Iridociliary apposition in plateau iris persists after cataract extraction. Am J Ophthalmol. 2003;135:40–3.

76. Podbielski DW, Varma DK, Tam DY, Ahmed IIK. Endocycloplasty: a new technique for managing angle-closure glaucoma secondary to plateau iris syndrome. Glaucoma Today. Oct 2010.

77. Shingleton BJ, Chang MA, Bellows AR, Thomas JV. Surgical goniosynechialysis for angle-closure glaucoma. Ophthalmology. 1990;97:551–6.

78. Tanihara H, Nishiwaki K, Nagata M. Surgical results and complications of goniosynechialysis. Graefes Arch Clin Exp Ophthalmol. 1992;230:309–13.

79. Teekhasaenee C, Ritch R. Combined phacoemulsification and goniosynechialysis for uncontrolled chronic angle-closure glaucoma after acute angle-closure glaucoma. Ophthalmology. 1999;106:669–74.

80. Harasymowycz PJ, Papamatheakis DG, Ahmed I, et al. Phacoemulsification and goniosynechialysis in the management of unresponsive primary angle closure. J Glaucoma. 2005;14:186–9.

81. Fakhrale G, Vahedian Z, Moghimi S, et al. Phacoemulsification and goniosynechialysis for the management of refractory acute angle closure. Eur J Ophthalmol. 2012;22:714–8.

82. Canlas OA, Ishikawa H, Liebmann JM, et al. Ultrasound biomicroscopy before and after goniosynechialysis. Am J Ophthalmol. 2001;132:570–1.

83. Fang AW, Yang XJ, Nie L, Qu J. Endoscopically controlled goniosynechialysis in managing synechial angle-closure glaucoma. J Glaucoma. 2010;19:19–23.

84. Luntz MH, Rosenblatt M. Malignant glaucoma. Surv Ophthalmol. 1987;32:73–93.

85. Quigley HA, Friedman DS, Congdon NG. Possible mechanisms of primary angle-closure and malignant glaucoma. J Glaucoma. 2003;12:167–80.

86. Razeghinejad MR, Amini H, Esfandiari H. Lesser anterior chamber dimensions in women may be predisposing factor for malignant glaucoma. Med Hypotheses. 2005;64:572–4.

87. Prata TS, Dorairaj S, De Moraes CG, et al. Is pre-operative ciliary body and iris anatomical configuration a predictor of malignant glaucoma development? Clin Experiment Ophthalmol. 2013;41:541–5.

88. Cashwell LF, Martin TJ. Malignant glaucoma after laser iridotomy. Ophthalmology. 1992;99:651–8.

89. Muqit MM, Menage MJ. Malignant glaucoma after phacoemulsification: treatment with diode laser cyclophotocoagulation. J Cataract Refract Surg. 2007;33:130–2.

90. Simmons RJ. Malignant glaucoma. Br J Ophthalmol. 1972;56:263–72.

91. Chander PA, Grant WM. Mydriatic-cycloplegic treatment in malignant glaucoma. Arch Ophthalmol. 1962;68:353–9.

92. Weiss DI, Shaffer RN, Harrington DO. Treatment of malignant glaucoma with intravenous mannitol infusion. Medical reformation of the anterior chamber by means of an osmotic agent: a preliminary report. Arch Ophthalmol. 1963;69:154–8.

93. Little BC. Treatment of aphakic malignant glaucoma using Nd:YAG laser posterior capsulotomy. Br J Ophthalmol. 1994;78:499–501.

94. Brown RH, Lynch MG, Tearse JE, Nunn RD. Neodymium-YAG vitreous surgery for phakic and pseudophakic malignant glaucoma. Arch Ophthalmol. 1986;104:1464–6.

95. Epstein DL, Steinert RF, Puliafito CA. Neodymium-YAG laser therapy to the anterior hyaloid in aphakic malignant (ciliovitreal block) glaucoma. Am J Ophthalmol. 1984;98:137–43.

96. Carassa RG, Bettin P, Fiori M, Brancato R. Treatment of malignant glaucoma with contact transscleral cyclophotocoagulation. Arch Ophthalmol. 1999;117:688–90.

97. Stumpf TH, Austin M, Bloom PA, et al. Transscleral cyclodiode laser photocoagulation in the treatment of aqueous misdirection syndrome. Ophthalmology. 2008;115:2058–61.

98. Sharma A, Sii F, Shah P, Kirkby GR. Vitrectomy-phacoemulsification-vitrectomy for the management of aqueous misdirection syndromes in phakic eyes. Ophthalmology. 2006;113:1968–73.

99. Harbour JW, Rubsamen PE, Palmberg P. Pars plana vitrectomy in the treatment of phakic and pseudophakic malignant glaucoma. Arch Ophthalmol. 1996;114:1073–8.

100. Bitrian E, Caprioli J. Pars plana anterior vitrectomy, hyaloido-zonulectomy, and iridectomy for aqueous humor misdirection. Am J Ophthalmol. 2010;150:82–7.

101. Dave P, Senthil S, Rao HL, Garudadri CS. Treatment outcomes in malignant glaucoma. Ophtholmology. 2013;120:984–90.

**Part VIII**

**Future Developments**

# Adopting New Surgical Methods: How I Do It and How I Choose: Going with the Flow

E. Randy Craven

## Historical Background and Identifying the Need for "New Procedures"

Are you a cowboy or conservative? For years glaucoma surgeons have desired a less invasive surgical option to lower the intraocular pressure (IOP). If you, the surgeon, are looking for something better and try it early in its development, does that make you a cowboy? The search for this "better glaucoma surgery" revolves around avoiding blebs and taping into the natural outflow system of the eye. Blebs come from transscleral filtration caused by a hole or stent/tube running into the subconjunctival space. Surgeons looking at new procedures could be considered a "cowboy"—but I might argue that they may be conservative. They want to get away from blebs and the problems they bring to the table. The options available fall into new/old, high risk/low risk, and bleb/no bleb. All these procedures arise out of a need.

Today we see great interest in "new" glaucoma procedures designed to avoid a bleb; these procedures are done with a small instrument and usually are done ab interno. The goal is to try to avoid a bleb and tap into the trabecular outflow and Schlemm's canal system [1, 2] or get into the uveoscleral system and create a controlled cyclodialysis cleft [3]. Unfortunately, our understanding of the outflow system is not perfect, so what we think we may be achieving with the procedure may not, in fact, be the case [4, 5]. The story of glaucoma procedures evolving seems to have some recurrent themes when you look at the past glaucoma surgical procedures and changes thereunto. The continued search for a "procedure that makes sense" and has lower risk has led to the micro-invasive glaucoma surgical (MIGS) procedures [6]. Our hopes with MIGS are fewer hassles in performing the procedure and less postoperative complications. The evolution to MIGS procedures has been a long-time coming. We have continued to struggle with controlling outflow through our full-thickness holes or were trying to get more safety through partial-thickness procedures [7]. All these efforts were "new," and the struggle for the surgeon was how to move from a successful procedure, the trabeculectomy, to something with better safety but perhaps not the long-term success with intraocular pressure (IOP) control [8–10].

Before we focus on how to incorporate new surgical options, let us look at the evolution of former glaucoma procedures and see if that might lead us to a better ability to predict what to expect with regard to success or failure seen with "new" glaucoma surgeries. Take the trabeculectomy. Cairns' original description of the trabeculectomy was in a sense a minimal incision procedure and was an attempt to just remove the area of suspected blockage, the meshwork. There was minimal or no opening into the sub-Tenon's space [11, 12]. The more formal sclerokeratectomy (what most call a trabeculectomy) had issues associated with the incision size and location, leading to modifications designed to avoid complications and hoping to improve surgical success [13]. Adjusting flow seemed to hold promise: we cut sutures and vented or obturated tubes [14, 15]. With every new modification of the incisional procedures came hope for less flat anterior chambers and better IOP control. The location, size, and tightness of the conjunctival or scleral incision only went so far in helping to achieve success with glaucoma surgery [16–18]. Later we mostly focused on wound healing by modifying the Tenon's and subconjunctival fibrosis. Steroids were showed to increase success and then antimetabolites [19–22]. Not too long ago, "new adopters" were those using antimetabolites for the trabeculectomy, which was an option evolving to solve the issue of wound healing, but with that came unforeseen issues related to blebs. Debates broke out discussing the "cowboys" using high-dose antimetabolites and causing ischemic blebs. Through the search for a better outcome, we ended up with a better success rate with "new" complications such as a higher incidence of hypotony and bleb-related issues [23].

E.R. Craven, MD
Division of Glaucoma, Department of Ophthalmology,
Wilmer Eye Institute at Johns Hopkins University,
King Khaled Eye Specialist Hospital, 600 N. Wolfe St, Room 110,
Baltimore, MD 21287, USA
e-mail: ecraven1@jhmi.edu; ercraven@yahoo.com

J.R. Samples, I.I.K. Ahmed (eds.), *Surgical Innovations in Glaucoma*,
DOI 10.1007/978-1-4614-8348-9_26, © Springer Science+Business Media New York 2014

When considering the significance and degree of the risks associated with a given glaucoma surgery, the amount of IOP reduction or likelihood of the surgery achieving non-progressing glaucoma is our main fulcrum. So, if we do a procedure with less IOP reduction and then supplement with medications to get to the IOP goal, is that acceptable? Should we do a more aggressive procedure because we need a lower IOP? Evidence-based medicine has shown us the importance of IOP reduction in stabilizing glaucoma. Glaucoma surgery can lead to significant IOP reduction [24–28]. Reaching a desired IOP target for patients with open-angle glaucoma has led some surgeons to consider surgery as an earlier treatment option. The procedures we see today may open the surgical door for options. Many would argue that because of compliance concerns and since no patient is perfect with adherence, we want as good of IOP reduction as possible for the patient undergoing surgery. A patient with a significant glaucomatous hemifield defect most likely needs a lower IOP compared to a patient with healthy optic nerves and no field loss. If we find a low-risk procedure that does not harm the patient and keeps them seeing, that is our main goal.

Herein we see the struggle for the surgeon when considering glaucoma surgery: "when is the risk to the patient small enough that I cross the surgical threshold and recommend the surgery?" If a patient has definite risk for losing field and progressing due to inadequate IOP reduction, surgery seems reasonable to consider. However, this has not been the case. For many surgeons and patients, the problems associated with trabeculectomy may lead us to say "let's wait for significant field loss or nerve atrophy before we do that!"

Several years ago the English evaluated the option of using trabeculectomy early on for patients with open-angle glaucoma. Their experience in treating newly diagnosed glaucoma with trabeculectomy originally began with the hope that a full-thickness glaucoma procedure (with expected superior IOP lowering to medications) would help to prevent glaucoma progression and save money [10, 29, 30]. Despite fairly good evidence that trabeculectomy did achieve a lower pressure, the eye care community continued to search for the Holy Grail of glaucoma surgical procedures: what procedure would provide great IOP reduction but not harm the patient? "New procedures" arise from surgeons considering the anatomy and physiology of the glaucoma outflow system and looking for a better option less influenced by wound healing.

Looking back to the 1970s, we see that John Edward Cairns wanted to avoid flat chambers by adjusting the flow through the fistula created from sclerostomies [11, 12, 31]. All of the ab externo incisional procedures, including the trabeculectomy, are influenced by wound healing [32]. Cairns' modification of the original scleral incision moved to a clear corneal incision with the hopes of avoiding a bleb and reestablishing physiologic outflow. At the same time Cairns searched for achieving outflow through the trabecular meshwork (and subsequently Schlemm's canal and the collector channels), we see various "new" procedures appear designed to establish the flow of aqueous through the physiologic outflow pathway. These are the "nonpenetrating" procedures. They are a group of surgical procedures that hopefully leave a layer of tissue intact (Descemet's membrane) to resist outflow and help avoid overfiltration some. It may be that it is only a "window" of tissue, but it provides some resistance to outflow. Aqueous will take more of the natural outflow route rather than go transscleral like what we see with the high-flow trabeculectomy.

Some nonpenetrating procedures glaucoma surgical procedure developed:

- Krasnov by Sinusotomy (1968) [33]
- Zimmerman: "Nonpenetrating Trabeculectomy" (1984) [34]
- Fyodorov: "Deep Sclerectomy" (1989) [35]
- Kozlov: "Nonpenetrating deep sclerectomy with collagen" (1989) [36]
- Stegmann: "Viscocanalostomy" (1999) [7]
- Lewis: "Canaloplasty" (2007) [37]

On this list is the canaloplasty (see Chap. 14). Many consider the canaloplasty to be a "new procedure" and are trying it for the first time today. Most likely the surgical success of the canaloplasty is based on where we see the aqueous is going—transscleral outflow versus the suture enhancing the natural outflow system or both [9, 38]. Some disagreement exists if the procedure (or any nonpenetrating glaucoma procedure for that matter) is really a guarded filtration procedure leading to a bleb, or is really taping into the trabecular outflow system and the success is not based on a bleb. Our understanding of how we achieve the success in the nonpenetrating procedures has led to a lot of confusion as to how they work. Some say the canaloplasty is a "bleb-less" procedure, while others say it does develop a bleb and has transscleral outflow. Some say the canaloplasty is a canal-based procedure and others not. There does seem to be fairly good evidence that when transscleral outflow is present, then we probably achieve a better IOP reduction [39, 40]. This means wound healing is a significant part of the success for nonpenetrating procedures. Therefore, antimetabolites may help them work better. In the late 1980s, the experience with delaying conjunctival healing showed us that if we wanted to have transscleral flow, we would have to deal with fibrosis and healing. This led to the era of antimetabolites and the collateral issues of hypotony, dysesthesia from blebs, and higher risk of endophthalmitis. Some surgeons do use antimetabolites with the nonpenetrating procedures because of this belief. Others do not. Surgeons are using lasers and differently shaped and sized collagen implants as "new options" for a better and safer result [41].

The micro-invasive glaucoma surgeries (MIGS) family of procedures is surgical options that we use to move toward small incision surgery with fewer problems associated with wound healing and to better avoid hypotony. The evolution of nonpenetrating procedures has some parallels to the evolution of MIGS: more control over unwanted postoperative events. The trabecular bypass stent (iStent, see Chap. 13) may be without the risk of problems from blebs but may not always give us as low of an IOP that we want. Some surgeons may take a less invasive trabecular bypass stent and use a medication to achieve a goal, versus a more aggressive trabeculectomy that others might choose hoping to get the patient off of medications. Even with MIGS, we are still in search of the "perfect" procedure. The MIGS procedures give the patients and the surgeon options to try if the surgeon or the patients are concerned about specific risks, for example, bleb issues. When considering these new procedures, the balance is as follows: what does the surgeon have comfort with and will the patient be willing to accept tradeoffs for achieving safety or a lower IOP?

## Time to Decide: New or Old Procedures? What Fits for Your Patient? When Is It Time to Adopt a New Technique or Go with an Old One?

As the surgeon sits with the patient, there are past experiences for the surgeon and evidence from the literature that start to shape the surgeon's choice for a procedure. The patient's choice for a procedure, however, may be coming from a totally different set of concerns. Sometimes the surgeon wants safety and sometimes he or she wants significant IOP reduction. This is where the discussion about the risk-to-benefit ratio of a specific procedure is appropriate for the patient. If the patient has a significant risk of nerve damage and subsequent vision loss, IOP reduction is most likely paramount.

Let's say you do want to use a new procedure, which one might be best? Often open-angle glaucoma is treated different than a closed-angle because the angle has not been scarred down too much. Usually the choice for a given surgery is influenced by the following:

1. The surgeon has experience and success with certain procedures and techniques that lead to safety and success.
2. The disease state of the patient is such that the optic nerve damage is substantial and the risk of more nerve damage is significant; with that comes the potential to lose vision.
3. The patient's prior experiences and trust in the surgeon influence their comfort with choice of which procedure and the risks associated with a procedure and the risk of loss of vision.
4. Where the procedure is done: office or operating room (OR) can lead to the patient's comfort or concern.

As we look at a given patient, the anatomy of the eye lends itself to some procedures being a better option than

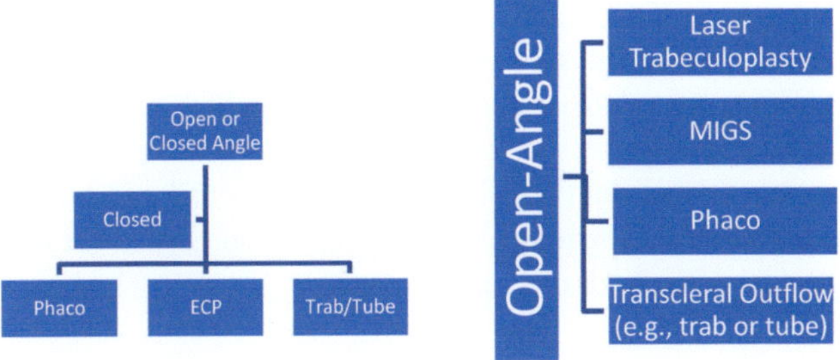



**Fig. 26.1**  Open- or closed-angle options

others, so *in looking at the anatomy, consider the angle type when making your choice for surgery.*

If the patient has a closed angle, really the options are limited (Fig. 26.1). Removing the lens can help to open the angle and hopefully prevent chronic IOP elevation that develops with chronic closure; for chronic angle-closure glaucoma (CACG), a trabeculectomy might be one of our few choices to achieve better IOP control [42–45]. Some have advocated ECP and others goniosynechialysis for angle closure with cataract surgery [46]. These especially might be an option with the earlier phase of angle closure and not with the long-standing CACG. One might argue that for ACG or CACG, the "new procedure" is considering a phaco to open the angle. Suprachoroidal stents may offer a possibility here but have no studies to support from the literature to show that is an option at present.

For open-angle glaucoma, there are many more "new-technique" options. In the open-angle glaucoma patient, consider the level of the disease (based on optic nerve and visual field damage) when picking the surgery. The amount of optic nerve damage correlates with how much IOP reduction you want. The amount of glaucomatous damage shown on the visual field usually parallels the nerve considerations. Patients with advance loss usually require a lower IOP. So, step one for the open-angle patient is how low you do want the IOP to be.

## IOP Goals

### Lowest IOP Range (Often Looking for Near Single-Digit IOP Here)

Usually the procedures that achieve the lowest IOP are tubes, deep sclerectomy (with enhancements to achieve more transscleral flow—like using mitomycin), sclerostomy, sclerectomy, or trabeculectomy (filtering procedures). Antimetabolites or other medications designed to inhibit wound healing usually lead to the lowest IOP. Using IOP-lowering medications after these procedures can help to achieve a lower IOP. There are patients whose prior experience with a filtering procedure was not optimal. Perhaps it led to poor IOP control, or perhaps there were postoperative issues making the surgeon or patient reluctant to wanting a filtering procedure. A good example is the high myope who experiences decreased vision due to macular folds and may have a double-digit IOP. Patients who never had a history of a high IOP may require a more significant surgery to get IOP reduction to the desired target range.

## Patient Has Glaucoma That Can Probably Tolerate Mid-Teens

This opens the MIGS door. Patients who tolerate IOP in the 17–20 range may be a great MIGS candidate. Laser trabeculoplasty (LT) might be a first consideration in this group of patients. Patients with an IOP goal of 13 might be able to get to this goal with an MIGS and medications. These patients should be the ones who can tolerate some glaucoma medication usage. Glaucoma suspects or early open-angle glaucoma patients that you do not feel will rapidly progress but who also have a cataract can be considered for phaco alone or phaco plus an MIGS. If I have a patient with a mild cataract and who will accept an MIGS option, sometimes we go straight to the surgery (depending on the visual disability), and sometimes a laser trabeculoplasty delays the need for further intervention.

## Patient Can Tolerate an IOP of 20 or More

Here considering a phaco with or without LT and/or medications may be a very logical choice. Certainly if the patient wants the option of long-term IOP control or the hope of no medications in the future, MIGS or incisional surgery might be a consideration.

Another IOP consideration is the highest IOP on record. It seems that patients with very high IOP, such as 40 or 50, may best be served by an incisional surgery since it seems to have lower risk of postoperative spikes (which the MIGS can have). Also, if the nerve cannot tolerate an IOP spike, considering an incisional surgery is reasonable. I have had patients with significant IOP spikes on record, who are monocular with significant glaucoma that repeatedly refuses incisional surgery and who will consider an MIGS. For this group, I do see them on the same day of the surgery if possible, leave them on their medications, and, if possible, use an anterior chamber maintainer instead of viscoelastic for maintaining the anterior chamber during surgery. This seems to give a lower risk of IOP spikes but they do not go away.

Patients with specific ocular situations that would be problematic with a bleb are sometimes appropriate to consider for an MIGS procedure. Examples that might fall into this group are patients with significantly scarred conjunctiva or who have ocular cicatricial pemphigoid. So a patient who had a scleral buckle is a reasonable patient to consider here. Patients with significant proptosis from, for example, Graves' orbitopathy, may be MIGS candidates. If a patient has had bleb revisions in the other eye, history of endophthalmitis from a bleb in the other eye, then, again, MIGS may be a great option for this group.

Sometimes I shy away from MIGS. Patients with neovascularization are not good MIGS candidates. Increased episcleral venous pressure (ESVP) also may limit the MIGS procedures from success. The high-ESVP patients are ones we want to avoid over filtration. When considering alternative surgical options for high-ESVP patients, my choice was to try a canaloplasty for many of such patients. This was based on significant choroidal effusions and bleeding associated with trabeculectomy and valves, so this option evolved out of exploring safe options for patients. Surprisingly, I have had good success with this surgical option in this select group. Considering new techniques as an attempt to avoid a known problem is what led to this choice. If the patient had a prior angle surgery, they may not be the best candidate for MIGS. So a patient with a prior Trabectome would not be a good trabecular bypass candidate, but they may be a good Trabectome candidate if they have had a prior trabecular bypass (anatomy dictating this exclusion; if the TM is cut out, you cannot put a stent into it). Thus, we might end up with sequential glaucoma (excluding phaco here) events that look something like this:

1. Laser trabeculoplasty (Table 26.1)
2. Trabecular bypass (Table 26.2)
3. Suprachoroidal bypass (Table 26.2)
4. Trabectome or canaloplasty (Tables 26.2 and 26.3)
5. If canaloplasty, conversion to a full-thickness procedure with YAG to the Descemet's window; if it is a Trabectome, then a deep sclerectomy or sclerokeratectomy/trabeculectomy (Tables 26.3 and 26.4)
6. Trabeculectomy or valve (Table 26.4)
7. Cyclodestruction (put at the end for purposes of illustration but could some at any point based on the patient's diagnosis—I tend to avoid cyclodestruction until the last step if possible) (Table 26.1)

Of course, changing the order or combination of options would be dictated by the patient or surgeon's special circumstances.

The next consideration are specific anatomic and past surgical procedures that dictate consideration of specific and possibly MIGS surgical options for a given eye and patient. For example, a patient with the history of a prior scleral buckle in the eye needing a glaucoma surgery may be a better MIGS candidate than those without that history. High myopia is also a circumstance where the patient may

**Table 26.1** Office-based and no-incision procedures that do not create a bleb

| No incision<br>No bleb | Most likely<br>mechanism of action | Angle type | IOP range | Downside | Upside | Ref # |
|---|---|---|---|---|---|---|
| Laser trabeculoplasty | Conventional outflow | OAG | 14–20 | 25 % nonresponder rate; 2- to 5-year life | No bleb, minimal post-op | [47–52] |
| Laser iridotomy/iridoplasty | Relieve ACG | ACG | N/A | IOP rise after PI and not enough to reduce ACG; may not affect IOP | Potential immediate reversal | [53, 54] |
| Pneumatic trabeculoplasty | Conventional outflow | OAG | N/A | Efficacy not clear | Inexpensive; minimal equipment | [55] |
| Transscleral cyclophotocoagulation | Decreased aqueous production | ACG/OAG | 0–50 | Fix loss, CME, iritis, hypotony, phthisis, less predictable IOP reduction | Can be successful when filtration procedures haven't worked. No incision for vascular eyes | [56, 57] |

**Table 26.2** OR-based procedures with no incision into the conjunctiva and no bleb created

| No incision into the conjunctiva<br>No bleb | Most likely<br>mechanism of action | Angle type | Low IOP range | Downside | Upside | Ref # |
|---|---|---|---|---|---|---|
| Suprachoroidal bypass (ab interno CyPass and iStent Supra) | Uveoscleral outflow | OAG (no data on ACG) | 13–18 | Hyphema | May work if SLT or meds fail. Repeatable | [58] |
| Goniotomy (ab interno) | Conventional outflow | OAG (developmental) | 17–25 | Hyphema Little adult data | Opens access to canal system | [59–61] |
| Trabectome with or without endoscope (ab interno) | Conventional outflow | OAG | 16–25 | Efficacy; limited open publications | Controls bleeding | [62–64] |
| Trabecular bypass (iStent, ab interno) | Conventional outflow | OAG | 16–19 | Efficacy; placement to achieve IOP reduction | Little bleeding; leaves TM intact | [1, 2, 4, 65–67] |
| Sclerothalomotomy | Conventional outflow | OAG | 12–17 | Little published data, scleral shrinkage | IOP control | [68] |
| Trabecular bypass with canal dilation (Hydrus, ab interno) | Conventional outflow | OAG | 12–17 | Little published data | A trabecular bypass and dilates canal | [69] |
| Endoscopic cyclophotocoagulation | Cyclodestructive with decreased aqueous production | OAG/ACG | 17–20s | Poor response with exfoliation, IOP spike; can help open angle | No bleeding | [56, 70, 71] |
| Excimer trabeculostomy | Conventional outflow | OAG | 18 | Little published data | No bleeding | [72–74] |
| Phaco alone | Conventional outflow (prob.) | OAG/ACG | 18 | IOP spike, no effect on IOP for some | Low risk for most patients | [1, 2, 75–78] |
| Goniosynechialysis | Opens angle | ACG | N/A | Opening angle | Can restore out trabecular flow | [79] |

be at a risk of suffering a loss of best corrected vision due to hypotony or macular folds. For patients who are allergic to many or most glaucoma medications, they may need procedures likely to achieve a lower IOP without them; if an MIGS is picked as a surgical option, considering a second one may be a possibility for that patient if further IOP reduction is required after the first MIGS.

## Where the Procedure Should Be Done, in the Office or Operating Room?

There are procedures that are office based and use primarily laser and the result is to increase the conventional trabecular outflow (Table 26.1). Bridging between office type of procedures and OR procedures are the no-conjunctival-incision

**Table 26.3** Conjunctival incision to allow a scleral incision in order to enter the canal space—but not for the intent of creating a bleb or creating transscleral filtration

| Conjunctiva incision and scleral incision but no purposeful fistula creation | Most likely mechanism of action | Angle type | Low IOP range | Downside | Upside | Ref # |
|---|---|---|---|---|---|---|
| Trabeculotomy | Conventional outflow | OAG and congenital | 14–25 | May have bleb | Less concerns with fibrosis stopping transscleral flow | [59, 80] |
| Deep sclerectomy with or without collagen implant | Conventional outflow | OAG | 10–20 | May need conversion to transscleral filtering procedure with YAG—goniopuncture. May have bleb | Less formal bleb; less likely to get hypotony | [9, 35, 36, 41, 58, 81–88] |
| Viscocanalostomy | Conventional outflow | OAG | 16–18 | May have bleb | Less formal bleb; less likely to get hypotony | [7, 89–92] |
| Canaloplasty | Conventional outflow | OAG | 15–19 | May have bleb; difficulty with learning; bleeding | Less formal bleb; less likely to get hypotony | [37, 38, 40, 61, 92–96] |

**Table 26.4** The bleb-creating procedures. Two types: no conjunctival incision or a conjunctival incision with either incision type leading to a full-thickness hole or a stent/shunt with an end result of bleb creation

| *No incision into the conjunctiva with full-thickness ocular penetration* | Most likely mechanism of action | Angle type | Low IOP range | Downside | Upside | Ref # |
|---|---|---|---|---|---|---|
| Ab interno sclerostomy with collagen wick to control flow through fistula (AquaSys with Implant) | Full-thickness ostomy with bleb creation | OAG (?ACG) | 14–16 | Bleb | No incision into conjunctiva | [97, 98] |
| Sclerectomy (or ostomy) ab interno (including laser and trephine) | Full-thickness ostomy with bleb creation | OAG/ACG | 8 | Bleb; profound hypotony immediate post-op at times; bleeding | Access 360 of angle for bleb creation (inferonasal bleb creation) | [99–103] |
| *Conjunctival incision w/o ocular penetration* | Most likely mechanism of action | Type | Low IOP range | Downside | Upside | Ref # |
| Express Mini-Shunt | Bleb formation | OAG | 12 | Bleb | Fibrosis, stent erosion | [104, 105] |
| Suprachoroidal bypass ab externo (Gold Shunt) | Uveoscleral outflow | OAG | 17–25 | Corneal edema, erosion, bleeding, late closure | Usually no bleb; potentially titratable | [58, 106] |
| Trabeculectomy and sclerokeratectomy | Bleb | OAG/ACG | 6–18 | Hypotony, bleeding, fibrosis, and need for antimetabolite | IOP control | [9, 14, 19–22, 92, 107–113] |
| Sclerectomy ab externo (including cautery and trephine) | Bleb | OAG/ACG | 8 | Hypotony can be profound | Low IOP | [99–103] |
| Tube shunts | Bleb | OAG/ACG | 11 | Tube erosion, corneal edema, hypotony | Can very control IOP post-op | [111, 114–116] |

(i.e., clear corneal incision) procedures. These are ab interno techniques to access the outflow system or open the angle (Table 26.2). Someday these may be done in the office. The doctor or the patient may have specific reasons for wanting an office-based procedure, and someday we may see injectable drug delivery systems that would allow even more procedures possible in the office. The real strengths of office procedures are the ability to schedule it easily, the perception by the patient that it is avoiding the operating room, and cost savings. When starting out with new surgical options, certainly having the comfort of surgical suites may lead to using the OR as the choice for the surgeon with new procedures.

I believe we will continue to see an evolution in glaucoma surgery until the day we have a no-risk great IOP control procedure. As we keep refining our surgical options, patients will benefit, and doctor's satisfaction with these new glaucoma procedures will grow as we find which patients are best served by a given procedure. To shake off the past beliefs that you have to get profound IOP reduction from a procedure may be difficult. Many surgeons will be reluctant to try MIGS as a result of this. However, as more surgeons expand into the arena of MIGS, we should see better what the true place of the "newer" procedures will be. My guess for now, we will see a similar evolution as to what happened with the trabeculectomy and deep sclerectomy—continued refinements. There will be surgeons who believe in some procedures strongly and others will not. Keeping an open mind can be difficult when you try new things. If the first "new" procedure you do doesn't appear to work, was it because you were expecting it to be a trabeculectomy result? Were you disappointed because it took months to see the benefit (such as SLT or trabecular bypass), or was it because the procedure required a different surgical skill set than you had experienced before? Whatever the reasons for liking or not liking MIGS or newer procedures are, the test of time will reveal the true place these options will have for us and our patients.

## References


1. Samuelson TW, Katz LJ, Wells JM, Duh YJ, Giamporcaro JE, iStent Study Group. Randomized evaluation of the trabecular micro-bypass stent with phacoemulsification in patients with glaucoma and cataract. Ophthalmology. 2011;118(3):459–67. PubMed PMID: 20828829.
2. Craven ER, Katz LJ, Wells JM, Giamporcaro JE, iStent Study Group. Cataract surgery with trabecular micro-bypass stent implantation in patients with mild-to-moderate open-angle glaucoma and cataract: two-year follow-up. J Cataract Refract Surg. 2012;38(8):1339–45. PubMed PMID: 22814041.
3. Ozdamar A, Aras C, Karacorlu M. Suprachoroidal seton implantation in refractory glaucoma: a novel surgical technique. J Glaucoma. 2003;12(4):354–9.
4. Johnson DH. Trabecular meshwork and uveoscleral outflow models. J Glaucoma. 2005;14(4):308–10.
5. Johnstone MA. The aqueous outflow system as a mechanical pump: evidence from examination of tissue and aqueous movement in human and non-human primates. J Glaucoma. 2004;13(5):421–38.
6. Saheb H, Ahmed II. Micro-invasive glaucoma surgery: current perspectives and future directions. Curr Opin Ophthalmol. 2012;23(2):96–104. PubMed PMID: 22249233.
7. Stegmann R, Pienaar A, Miller D. Viscocanalostomy for open-angle glaucoma in black African patients. J Cataract Refract Surg. 1999;25(3):316–22.
8. Folgar FA, De Moraes CG, Teng CC, Tello C, Ritch R, Liebmann JM. Effect of successful and partly successful filtering surgery on the velocity of glaucomatous visual field progression. J Glaucoma. 2012;21(9):615–8. PubMed PMID: 21623221.
9. Razeghinejad MR, Fudemberg SJ, Spaeth GL. The changing conceptual basis of trabeculectomy: a review of past and current surgical techniques. Surv Ophthalmol. 2012;57(1):1–25. PubMed PMID: 22137574.
10. Landers J, Martin K, Sarkies N, Bourne R, Watson P. A twenty-year follow-up study of trabeculectomy: risk factors and outcomes. Ophthalmology. 2012;119(4):694–702. PubMed PMID: 22196977.
11. Cairns JE. Trabeculectomy. Preliminary report of a new method. Am J Ophthalmol. 1968;66:673–9.
12. Cairns JE. Trabeculectomy. Sub-title: "a surgical method of reducing intra-ocular pressure in chronic simple glaucoma without sub-conjunctival drainage of aqueous humour". Trans Ophthalmol Soc U K. 1969;88:231–3.
13. Watson PG, Barnett F. Effectiveness of trabeculectomy in glaucoma. Am J Ophthalmol. 1975;79:831–45.
14. Savage JA, Condon GP, Lytle RA, Simmons RJ. Laser suture lysis after trabeculectomy. Ophthalmology. 1988;95:1631–8.
15. Broadway DC, Chang LP. Trabeculectomy, risk factors for failure and the preoperative state of the conjunctiva. J Glaucoma. 2001;10(3):237–49.
16. Birchall W, Wakely L, Wells AP. The influence of scleral flap position and dimensions on intraocular pressure control in experimental trabeculectomy. J Glaucoma. 2006;15(4):286–90. doi:10.1097/01.ijg.0000212241.18842.83.
17. Ralli M, Nouri-Mahdavi K, Caprioli J. Outcomes of laser suture lysis after initial trabeculectomy with adjunctive mitomycin C. J Glaucoma. 2006;15(1):60–7.
18. Aykan U, Bilge AH, Akin T, Certel I, Bayer A. Laser suture lysis or releasable sutures after trabeculectomy. J Glaucoma. 2007;16(2):240–5. doi:10.1097/IJG.0b013e31802d6ded.
19. Starita RJ, Fellman RL, Spaeth GL, Poryzees EM, Greenidge KC, Traverso CE. Short- and long-term effects of postoperative corticosteroids on trabeculectomy. Ophthalmology. 1985;92:938–46.
20. Araujo SV, Spaeth GL, Roth SM, Starita RJ. A ten-year follow-up on a prospective, randomized trial of postoperative corticosteroids after trabeculectomy. Ophthalmology. 1995;102(12):1753–9.
21. Singh KMK, Shaikh NM, Tsai JC, Moster MR, Budenz DL, Greenfield DS, Chen PP, Cohen JS, Baerveldt GS, Shaikh S. Trabeculectomy with intraoperative mitomycin C versus 5-fluorouracil: prospective randomized clinical trial. Ophthalmology. 2000;107(12):2305–9.
22. Goldenfeld MKT, Ruderman JM, Wong PC, Rosenberg LF, Ritch R, Liebmann JM, Gieser DK. 5-Fluorouracil in initial trabeculectomy. A prospective, randomized, multicenter study. Ophthalmology. 1994;101:1024–9.
23. Solus JF, Jampel HD, Tracey PA, Gilbert DL, Loyd TL, Jefferys JL, Quigley HA. Comparison of limbus-based and fornix-based trabeculectomy: success, bleb-related complications, and bleb morphology. Ophthalmology. 2012;119(4):703–11. PubMed PMID: 22226886.
24. Lichter PR. Expectations from clinical trials: results of the early manifest glaucoma trial. Arch Ophthalmol. 2002;120(10):1371–2.
25. Musch DC, Gillespie BW, Niziol LM, Cashwell LF, Lichter PR, Collaborative Initial Glaucoma Treatment Study Group. Factors associated with intraocular pressure before and during 9 years of treatment in the Collaborative Initial Glaucoma Treatment Study. Ophthalmology. 2008;115(6):927–33.
26. De Moraes CV, Juthani VJ, Liebmann JM, Teng CC, Tello C, Susanna R, Ritch R. Risk factors for visual field progression in treated glaucoma. Arch Ophthalmol. 2010;129(5):562–8.
27. Kim JDL, Ederer F, Gaasterland DE, VanVeldhuisen PC, Blackwell B, Sullivan EK, Prum B, Shafranov G, Beck A, Spaeth GL, Agis Investigators Group. The Advanced Glaucoma Intervention Study (AGIS): 14. Distinguishing progression of glaucoma from visual field fluctuations. Ophthalmology. 2004;111(11):2109–16.
28. Leske MC, Heijl A, Hussein M, Bengtsson B, Hyman L, Komaroff E, The Early Manifest Study Group. Factors for glaucoma progression and the effect of treatment: the early manifest glaucoma trial. Arch Ophthalmol. 2003;121(1):48–56.
29. Migdal C, Gregory W, Hitchings R. Long-term functional outcome after early surgery compared with laser and medicine in open-angle glaucoma. Ophthalmology. 1994;101:1651–6.
30. Edmunds B, Bunce CV, Thompson JR, Salmon JF, Wormald RP. Factors associated with success in first-time trabeculectomy for patients at low risk of failure with chronic open-angle glaucoma. Ophthalmology. 2004;111(1):97–103. PubMed PMID: 14711719.

31. Phillips CI. Trabeculectomy "ab externo". Trans Ophthalmol Soc U K. 1969;88:681–91.

32. Jampel HD, Friedman DS, Lubomski LH, Kempen JH, Quigley HA, Congdon N, Levkovitch-Verbin H, Robinson KA, Bass EB. Effect of technique on intraocular pressure after combined cataract and glaucoma surgery: an evidence-based review. Ophthalmology. 2002;109(12):2215–24.

33. Krasnov MM. Sinusotomy in glaucoma. Vestn Oftalmol. 1964;77: 37–41.

34. Zimmerman TJ, Kooner KS, Ford VJ. Trabeculectomy vs nonpenetrating trabeculectomy: a retrospective study of two procedures in phakic patients with glaucoma. Ophthalmic Surg. 1984;15:734–40.

35. Fyodorov SN, Kozlov VI, Timoshkina NT, et al. Non-penetrating deep sclerectomy in open angle glaucoma. IRTC Eye Microsurgery Moscow: RSFSR Ministry of Public Health. 1989:52–5.

36. Kozlov VI, Bagrov SN, Anisimova SY, et al. Non-penetrating deep sclerectomy with collagen. IRTC Eye Microsurgery Moscow: RSFSR Ministry of Public Health. 1989:44–6.

37. Lewis RA, von Wolf K, Tetz M, Korber N, Kearney JR, Shingleton B, Samuelson TW. Canaloplasty: circumferential viscodilation and tensioning of Schlemm's canal using a flexible microcatheter for the treatment of open-angle glaucoma in adults: interim clinical study analysis. J Cataract Refract Surg. 2007;33(7):1217–26. PubMed PMID: 17586378.

38. Ayyala RS, Chaudhry AL, Okogbaa CB, Zurakowski D. Comparison of surgical outcomes between canaloplasty and trabeculectomy at 12 months' follow-up. Ophthalmology. 2011;118(12):2427–33. PubMed PMID: 21856008.

39. O'Brart DPS, Rowlands E, Islam N, Noury AMS. A randomised, prospective study comparing trabeculectomy augmented with antimetabolites with a viscocanalostomy technique for the management of open angle glaucoma uncontrolled by medical therapy. Br J Ophthalmol. 2002;86(7):748–54.

40. Klink T, Panidou E, Kanzow-Terai B, Klink J, Schlunck G, Grehn FJ. Are there filtering blebs after canaloplasty? J Glaucoma. 2012;21(2):89–94. PubMed PMID: 21278586.

41. Muñoz G. Nonstitch suprachoroidal technique for T-flux implantation in deep sclerectomy. J Glaucoma. 2009;18(3):262–4. doi:10.1097/IJG.0b013e3181812812.

42. Tarongoy P, Ho CL, Walton DS. Angle-closure glaucoma: the role of the lens in the pathogenesis, prevention, and treatment. Surv Ophthalmol. 2009;54(2):211–25. PubMed PMID: 19298900.

43. Husain R, Gazzard G, Aung T, Chen Y, Padmanabhan V, Oen F, et al. Initial management of acute primary angle closure: a randomized trial comparing phacoemulsification with laser peripheral iridotomy. Ophthalmology. 2012;119(11):2274–81. PubMed PMID: 22885123.

44. Tham CC, Kwong YY, Leung DY, Lam SW, Li FC, Chiu TY, et al. Phacoemulsification versus combined phacotrabeculectomy in medically uncontrolled chronic angle closure glaucoma with cataracts. Ophthalmology. 2009;116(4):725–31, 31.e1–3. PubMed PMID: 19243831.

45. Tham CC, Kwong YY, Baig N, Leung DY, Li FC, Lam DS. Phacoemulsification versus trabeculectomy in medically uncontrolled chronic angle-closure glaucoma without cataract. Ophthalmology. 2013;120(1):62–7. PubMed PMID: 22986111.

46. Teekhasaenee C. Combined phacoemulsification and goniosynechialysis for uncontrolled chronic angle-closure glaucoma after acute angle-closure glaucoma. Ophthalmology. 1999;106(4): 669–75.

47. Hodge WG, Damji KF, Rock W, Buhrmann R, Bovell AM, Pan Y. Baseline IOP predicts selective laser trabeculoplasty success at 1 year post-treatment: results from a randomised clinical trial. Br J Ophthalmol. 2005;89(9):1157–60. PubMed PMID: 16113372. Pubmed Central PMCID: 1772832.

48. Pham H, Mansberger S, Brandt JD, Damji K, Ramulu PY, Parrish RK. Argon laser trabeculoplasty versus selective laser trabeculoplasty. Surv Ophthalmol. 2008;53(6):641–6. PubMed PMID: 19026324.

49. Ramulu PY, Parrish III RK. Asking the right question in laser trabeculoplasty: "which patient", not "which laser"? Surv Ophthalmol. 2008;53(6):652–4.

50. Alvarado JA, Shifera AS. Progress towards understanding the functioning of the trabecular meshwork based on lessons from studies of laser trabeculoplasty. Br J Ophthalmol. 2010;94:1417–8. PubMed PMID: 20962351.

51. Koucheki B, Hashemi H. Selective laser trabeculoplasty in the treatment of open-angle glaucoma. J Glaucoma. 2012;21(1):65–70. PubMed PMID: 21278588.

52. Prasad N, Murthy S, Dagianis JJ, Latina MA. A comparison of the intervisit intraocular pressure fluctuation after 180 and 360 degrees of selective laser trabeculoplasty (SLT) as a primary therapy in primary open angle glaucoma and ocular hypertension. J Glaucoma. 2009;18(2):157–60. doi:10.1097/IJG.0b013e3181752c97.

53. Jiang Y, Chang DS, Foster PJ, He M, Huang S, Aung T, et al. Immediate changes in intraocular pressure after laser peripheral iridotomy in primary angle-closure suspects. Ophthalmology. 2012;119(2):283–8. PubMed PMID: 22036632.

54. Quigley HA. Long-term follow-up of laser iridotomy. Ophthalmology. 1981;88(3):218–24.

55. Eldaly MA. Pneumatic trabecular bypass (PTB): pilot study. J Glaucoma. 2010;19(1):31–4. PubMed PMID: 19373109.

56. Lin SC. Endoscopic and transscleral cyclophotocoagulation for the treatment of refractory glaucoma. J Glaucoma. 2008;17(3): 238–47. doi:10.1097/IJG.0b013e31815f2539.

57. Ramli N, Htoon HM, Ho CL, Aung T, Perera S. Risk factors for hypotony after transscleral diode cyclophotocoagulation. J Glaucoma. 2012;21(3):169–73. PubMed PMID: 21336153.

58. Figus M, Bartolomei MP, Lazzeri S, Nardi M. Very deep sclerectomy. J Glaucoma. 2011;20(1):67. doi:10.1097/IJG.0b013e3182073e5d.

59. Iwao K, Inatani M, Tanihara H, Japanese Steroid-Induced Glaucoma Multicenter Study Group. Success rates of trabeculotomy for steroid-induced glaucoma: a comparative, multicenter, retrospective cohort study. Am J Ophthalmol. 2011;151(6):1047–56.e1. PubMed PMID: 21396622.

60. Francis BA, Minckler D, Dustin L, Kawji S, Yeh J, Sit A, et al. Combined cataract extraction and trabeculotomy by the internal approach for coexisting cataract and open-angle glaucoma: initial results. J Cataract Refract Surg. 2008;34(7):1096–103. PubMed PMID: 18571075.

61. Grieshaber MC, Fraenkl S, Schoetzau A, Flammer J, Orgul S. Circumferential viscocanalostomy and suture canal distension (canaloplasty) for whites with open-angle glaucoma. J Glaucoma. 2011;20(5):298–302. PubMed PMID: 20577106.

62. Francis BA, See RF, Rao NA, Minckler DS, Baerveldt G. Ab interno trabeculectomy: development of a novel device (trabectome(TM)) and surgery for open-angle glaucoma. J Glaucoma. 2006; 15(1):68–73.

63. Ferrari E, Ortolani F, Petrelli L, Contin M, Pognuz DR, Marchini M, et al. Ab interno trabeculectomy: ultrastructural evidence and early tissue response in a human eye. J Cataract Refract Surg. 2007;33(10):1750–3. PubMed PMID: 17889771.

64. Ting JL, Damji KF, Stiles MC, Trabectome Study Group. Ab interno trabeculectomy: outcomes in exfoliation versus primary open-angle glaucoma. J Cataract Refract Surg. 2012;38(2):315–23. PubMed PMID: 22322166.

65. Zhou J, Smedley GT. A trabecular bypass flow hypothesis. J Glaucoma. 2005;14(1):74–83.

66. Belovay GW, Naqi A, Chan BJ, Rateb M, Ahmed II. Using multiple trabecular micro-bypass stents in cataract patients to treat open-angle glaucoma. J Cataract Refract Surg. 2012;38(11): 1911–7. PubMed PMID: 22980724.

67. Bahler CK, Smedley GT, Zhou J, Johnson DH. Trabecular bypass stents decrease intraocular pressure in cultured human anterior segments. Am J Ophthalmol. 2004;138(6):988–94. PubMed PMID: 15629290.

68. Pajic B, Pajic-Eggspuehler B, Haefliger I. New minimally invasive, deep sclerotomy ab interno surgical procedure for glaucoma, six years of follow-up. J Glaucoma. 2011;20(2):109–14. PubMed PMID: 20520572.

69. Lorens K, Norbert P, Ramirez M, Scharioth G, Tets M; Vass C, Grisanti S, Samuelson T. 6 month results from a prospective, multicenter study of a nickel-titanium Schlemm's canal scaffold for IOP reduction in open angle glaucoma. New York: American Glaucoma Society; 2012.

70. Netland PA, Mansberger SL, Lin S. Uncontrolled intraocular pressure after endoscopic cyclophotocoagulation. J Glaucoma. 2007; 16(2):265–7. doi:10.1097/01.ijg.0000243475.36213.41.

71. Lima FE, Magacho L, Carvalho DM, Susanna RJ, Ávila MP. A prospective, comparative study between endoscopic cyclophotocoagulation and the Ahmed drainage implant in refractory glaucoma. J Glaucoma. 2004;13(3):233–7.

72. Francis BA, Singh K, Lin SC, Hodapp E, Jampel HD, Samples JR, et al. Novel glaucoma procedures: a report by the American Academy of Ophthalmology. Ophthalmology. 2011;118(7): 1466–80. PubMed PMID: 21724045.

73. Wilmsmeyer S, Philippin H, Funk J. Excimer laser trabeculotomy: a new, minimally invasive procedure for patients with glaucoma. Graefes Arch Clin Exp Ophthalmol. 2006;244:670–6.

74. Babighian S, Rapizzi E, Galan A. Efficacy and safety of ab interno excimer laser trabeculotomy in primary open-angle glaucoma: two years of follow-up. Ophthalmologica. 2006;220(5):285–90. PubMed PMID: 16954703. Epub 2006/09/07. eng.

75. Poley BJ, Lindstrom RL, Samuelson TW. Long-term effects of phacoemulsification with intraocular lens implantation in normotensive and ocular hypertensive eyes. J Cataract Refract Surg. 2008;34(5):735–42. PubMed PMID: 18471626.

76. Hudovernik M, Pahor D. Intraocular pressure after phacoemulsification with posterior chamber lens implantation in open-angle glaucoma. Klin Monatsbl Augenheilkd. 2003;220: 835–9.

77. Shingleton BJ, Pasternack JJ, Hung JW, O'Donoghue MW. Three and five year changes in intraocular pressures after clear corneal phacoemulsification in open angle glaucoma patients, glaucoma suspects, and normal patients. J Glaucoma. 2006;15(6):494–8. doi:10.1097/01.ijg.0000212294.31411.92.

78. Mochizuki H, Takenaka J, Sugimoto Y, Takamatsu M, Kiuchi Y. Cataract surgery in primary angle closure: can it replace iridotomy? J Glaucoma. 2012;21(4):274–5. doi:10.1097/ IJG.0b013e31824c7859.

79. Fang AW, Yang XJ, Nie L, Qu J. Endoscopically controlled goniosynechialysis in managing synechial angle-closure glaucoma. J Glaucoma. 2010;19(1):19–23. PubMed PMID: 20075673.

80. Tanito M, Park M, Nishikawa M, Ohira A, Chihara E. Comparison of surgical outcomes of combined viscocanalostomy and cataract surgery with combined trabeculotomy and cataract surgery. Am J Ophthalmol. 2002;134(4):513–20.

81. Mansouri K, Tran VH, Ravinet E, Mermoud A. Comparing deep sclerectomy with collagen implant with the new method of very deep sclerectomy with collagen implant: a single-masked randomized controlled trial. J Glaucoma. 2011;20(1):67–8. doi:10.1097/ IJG.0b013e3182073e84.

82. Mendrinos E, Mermoud A, Shaarawy T. Nonpenetrating glaucoma surgery. Surv Ophthalmol. 2008;53(6):592–630. PubMed PMID: 19026321.

83. Anand N, Kumar A, Gupta A. Primary phakic deep sclerectomy augmented with mitomycin C: long-term outcomes. J Glaucoma. 2011;20(1):21–7. PubMed PMID: 20179623.

84. Bissig A, Rivier D, Zaninetti M, Shaarawy T, Mermoud A, Roy S. Ten years follow-up after deep sclerectomy with collagen implant. J Glaucoma. 2008;17(8):680–6. doi:10.1097/IJG.0b013e318182ed9e.

85. Mermoud A, Schnyder CC, Sickenberg M, Chiou AGY, Hédiguer SEA, Faggioni R. Comparison of deep sclerectomy with collagen implant and trabeculectomy in open-angle glaucoma. J Cataract Refract Surg. 1999;25(3):323–31.

86. Ambresin A, Shaarawy T, Mermoud A. Deep sclerectomy with collagen implant in one eye compared with trabeculectomy in the other eye of the same patient. J Glaucoma. 2002;11(3):214–20.

87. Galassi F, Giambene B. Deep sclerectomy with SkGel implant: 5-year results. J Glaucoma. 2008;17(1):52–6. doi:10.1097/ IJG.0b013e3180d0a885.

88. Goldsmith JA, Ahmed IK, Crandall AS. Nonpenetrating glaucoma surgery. Ophthalmol Clin North Am. 2005;18(3):443–60, vii. PubMed PMID: 16055001.

89. Lüke C, Dietlein TS, Jacobi PC, Konen W, Krieglstein GK. A prospective randomized trial of viscocanalostomy versus trabeculectomy in open-angle glaucoma: a 1-year follow-up study. J Glaucoma. 2002;11(4):294–9.

90. Yalvac IS, Sahin M, Eksioglu U, Midillioglu IK, Aslan BS, Duman S. Primary viscocanalostomy versus trabeculectomy for primary open-angle glaucoma: three-year prospective randomized clinical trial. J Cataract Refract Surg. 2004;30(10):2050–7. PubMed PMID: 15474813.

91. Carassa RG, Bettin P, Fiori M, Brancato R. Viscocanalostomy versus trabeculectomy in white adults affected by open-angle glaucoma. Ophthalmology. 2003;110(5):882–7.

92. Chai C, Loon SC. Meta-analysis of viscocanalostomy versus trabeculectomy in uncontrolled glaucoma. J Glaucoma. 2010;19(8): 519–27. PubMed PMID: 20179632.

93. Lewis RA, von Wolff K, Tetz M, Koerber N, Kearney JR, Shingleton BJ, et al. Canaloplasty: circumferential viscodilation and tensioning of Schlemm canal using a flexible microcatheter for the treatment of open-angle glaucoma in adults: two-year interim clinical study results. J Cataract Refract Surg. 2009;35(5): 814–24. PubMed PMID: 19393879.

94. Lewis RA, von Wolff K, Tetz M, Koerber N, Kearney JR, Shingleton BJ, et al. Canaloplasty: three-year results of circumferential viscodilation and tensioning of Schlemm canal using a microcatheter to treat open-angle glaucoma. J Cataract Refract Surg. 2011;37(4):682–90. PubMed PMID: 21420593.

95. Grieshaber MC, Pienaar A, Olivier J, Stegmann R. Canaloplasty for primary open-angle glaucoma: long-term outcome. Br J Ophthalmol. 2010;94(11):1478–82. PubMed PMID: 20962352.

96. Godfrey DG, Fellman RL, Neelakantan A. Canal surgery in adult glaucomas. Curr Opin Ophthalmol. 2009;20(2):116–21. PubMed PMID: 19240543.

97. Varma R. Devices in development: AqueSys implant. Glaucoma Today. 2012;10(6):44–5.

98. Palmberg P. Conjunctival sparing surgery: breakthrough or fad? In: 6th international congress on glaucoma surgery. Edinburgh; 2012. p. 19.

99. Brown RH, Lynch MG, Denham DB, Parel JM, Palmberg P, Brown DD. Internal sclerectomy with an automated trephine for advanced glaucoma. Ophthalmology. 1988;95(6):728–34. PubMed PMID: 3211473. Epub 1988/06/01. eng.

100. Higginbotham EJ, Kao G, Peyman G. Internal sclerostomy with the Nd: YAG contact laser versus thermal sclerostomy in rabbits. Ophthalmology. 1988;95(3):385–90.

101. Iwach AG, Hoskins HD. Laser sclerostomy for the management of glaucoma. Curr Opin Ophthalmol. 1993;4:85–92.

102. Latina MA, Melamed S, March WF, Kass MA, Kolker AE. Gonioscopic ab interno laser sclerostomy. A pilot study in glaucoma patients. Ophthalmology. 1992;99:1736–44.

103. Lin P, Wollstein G, Glavas IP, Schuman JS. Contact transscleral neodymium:yttrium-aluminum-garnet laser cyclophotocoagulation

long-term outcome. Ophthalmology. 2004;111(11):2137–43. PubMed PMID: 15522383. Pubmed Central PMCID: 1950289.

104. Seider MI, Rofagha S, Lin SC, Stamper RL. Resident-performed Ex-PRESS shunt implantation versus trabeculectomy. J Glaucoma. 2012;21(7):469–74. PubMed PMID: 21522022.

105. Patel HY, Wagschal LD, Trope GE, Buys YM. Economic analysis of the Ex-PRESS miniature glaucoma device versus trabeculectomy. J Glaucoma. 2012. doi:10.1097/IJG.0b013e31827a06f4. [Epub ahead of print].

106. Melamed S, Ben Simon GJ, Goldenfeld M, Simon G. Efficacy and safety of gold micro shunt implantation to the supraciliary space in patients with glaucoma: a pilot study. Arch Ophthalmol. 2009;127(3):264–9.

107. Radhakrishnan S, Quigley HA, Jampel HD, Friedman DS, Ahmad SI, Congdon NG, et al. Outcomes of surgical bleb revision for complications of trabeculectomy. Ophthalmology. 2009;116(9):1713–8. PubMed PMID: 19643490.

108. AGIS(Advanced Glaucoma Intervention Study) Investigators. The advanced glaucoma intervention study: 8. Risk of cataract formation after trabeculectomy. Arch Ophthalmol. 2001;119:1771–9. PubMed PMID: 11735786.

109. Gedde SJ, Herndon LW, Brandt JD, Budenz DL, Feuer WJ, Schiffman JC, et al. Postoperative complications in the Tube Versus Trabeculectomy (TVT) study during five years of follow-up. Am J Ophthalmol. 2012;153(5):804–14.e1. PubMed PMID: 22244522.

110. Radcliffe NM, Musch DC, Niziol LM, Liebmann JM, Ritch R, Collaborative Initial Glaucoma Treatment Study Group. The effect of trabeculectomy on intraocular pressure of the untreated fellow eye in the collaborative initial glaucoma treatment study. Ophthalmology. 2010;117(11):2055–60. PubMed PMID: 20570363. Pubmed Central PMCID: 3334525.

111. Gedde SJ, Schiffman JC, Feuer WJ, Herndon LW, Brandt JD, Budenz DL. Treatment outcomes in the tube versus trabeculectomy study after one year of follow-up. Am J Ophthalmol. 2007;143(1):9–22. PubMed PMID: 17083910.

112. Law SK, Shih K, Tran DH, Coleman AL, Caprioli J. Long-term outcomes of repeat vs initial trabeculectomy in open-angle glaucoma. Am J Ophthalmol. 2009;148(5):685–95.e1. PubMed PMID: 19596220.

113. Anand N, Khan A. Long-term outcomes of needle revision of trabeculectomy blebs with mitomycin C and 5-fluorouracil: a comparative safety and efficacy report. J Glaucoma. 2009;18(7):513–20. PubMed PMID: 19223788.

114. Gedde SJ, Schiffman JC, Feuer WJ, Herndon LW, Brandt JD, Budenz DL, et al. Three-year follow-up of the tube versus trabeculectomy study. Am J Ophthalmol. 2009;148(5):670–84. PubMed PMID: 19674729.

115. Gedde SJ, Schiffman JC, Feuer WJ, Herndon LW, Brandt JD, Budenz DL, et al. Treatment outcomes in the Tube Versus Trabeculectomy (TVT) study after five years of follow-up. Am J Ophthalmol. 2012;153(5):789–803.e2. PubMed PMID: 22245458.

116. Prata TS, Mehta A, De Moraes CG, Tello C, Liebmann J, Ritch R. Baerveldt glaucoma implant in the ciliary sulcus: midterm follow-up. J Glaucoma. 2010;19(1):15–8. PubMed PMID: 19373099.

Paul A. Knepper, Algis Grybauskas, Paulius V. Kuprys, Kevin Skuran, and John R. Samples

Primary open-angle glaucoma (POAG) is a chronic, degenerative optic neuropathy characterized by concurrent loss of retinal ganglion cells and their axons resulting in optic nerve cupping and visual field loss [1]. POAG is the most common type of glaucoma, the second leading cause of blindness worldwide, and the leading cause of blindness in African-Americans [1]. Increased intraocular pressure (IOP) is common in POAG; some patients have IOP in the normal range and are classified as "normal-tension glaucoma." Results of the 2010 ocular hypertension treatment study [2] provided strong evidence that increased intraocular pressure (IOP) is associated with the progression of ocular hypertension to POAG. Other risk factors are greater cup-to-disc ratio, lesser central corneal thickness, and age. If all these factors are present, an individual's risk for POAG is greater than 33 % in 5 years [3]. For every 1-mmHg increase in IOP,

P.A. Knepper, MD, PhD (✉)
Department of Ophthalmology and Visual Sciences,
University of Illinois at Chicago, 150 East Huron,
Suite 1000, Chicago, IL 60611, USA

Department of Ophthalmology, Northwestern
University Medical School, Chicago, IL USA
e-mail: pknepper@northwestern.edu

A. Grybauskas • P.V. Kuprys
Department of Ophthalmology and Visual Sciences,
University of Illinois at Chicago,
1855 West Taylor Street Building 902 Room B1,
Chicago, IL 60612, USA
e-mail: agrybaus11@gmail.com; paulkuprys@gmail.com

K. Skuran
Department of Ophthalmology and Visual Sciences,
University of Illinois, 1855 West Taylor Street
Building 902 Room B1, Chicago, IL 60612, USA
e-mail: kskuran@gmail.com

J.R. Samples, MD
Department of Surgery, Rocky Vista University, Parker, CO, USA

Western Glaucoma Foundation, Portland, OR, USA

Cornea Consultants of Colorado, Littleton, CO, USA

The Eye Clinic, Portland, OR, USA

there was a 10 % increase in relative risk of POAG [4]. The most predictive factor of visual field loss, however, is the presence of an optic nerve head hemorrhage [5].

POAG is associated with genetic mutations at several loci [6, 7], but the vast majority of POAG patients do not have known genetic mutations. How each of the known genetic mutation leads to POAG is not exactly understood. Therefore, it remains a primary neuronal disease [8] without a definable cause. Surgical intervention is required if the IOP is not under control or the patient continues to have progressive visual field loss. Nonetheless, surgical intervention is not always successful. Classically, a set of defined events occur during and after surgery: hemostasis, inflammatory reaction, angiogenesis, and cellular remodeling. We have examined known biomarkers of POAG in human studies and have excluded physiologic or imaging technologies in order to search for predictive biomarkers of surgical success. In principle, a biomarker is an indicator of a biochemical feature or facet that can be used to diagnose or monitor the progress of a disease [9]. Signature biomarkers of diseases such as cardiovascular [10] and Alzheimer's disease [11, 12] are nearly impossible due to the multifactorial etiologies, but recent progress in biomarkers has facilitated the diagnosis and risk management of these diseases.

We have cataloged all known biomarkers in the aqueous humor, trabecular meshwork (TM), optic nerve, and blood serum/plasma in patients with POAG. To facilitate comparisons and to offer mechanistic clues, biochemical changes such as up- or downregulation of biomarkers that have been reported in POAG are organized into four categories; namely, ECM, cell signaling molecules, aging/stress, and immunity-related changes are listed, respectively, in Tables 27.1 [13–28], 27.2 [29–41], 27.3 [42–58], and 27.4 [59–78]. Notably, POAG has multiple systemic

**Electronic supplementary material** Supplementary material is available in the online version of this chapter at http://dx.doi.org/10.1007/978-1-4614-8348-9_27. Videos can also be accessed at http://www.springerimages.com/videos/978-1-4614-8347-2

**Table 27.1** Extracellular matrix (ECM) changes in POAG

| | Aqueous humor | Trabecular meshwork | Optic nerve | Systemic (serum/plasma) |
|---|---|---|---|---|
| ECM elements | | | | |
| CD44 | | ↓ [13] | | |
| Cochlin | | ↑ [14] | | |
| Chondroitin sulfate | | ↑ [15] | | |
| Collagen type IV | | nc [16] | | |
| Elastin | | ↑ [17] | ↑ [18] | |
| Fibronectin | nc [19] | nc [16] | | |
| Hyaluronic acid | ↓↓ [20] | ↓↓↓↓ [15] | ↓ [21] | |
| GAGase-resistant material | | ↑↑↑↑ [15] | | |
| Tenascin | | | ↑ [22] | |
| Thrombospondin-1 | | ↑ [23] | | |
| ECM remodeling enzymes and inhibitors | | | | |
| MMP-1 | | ↑ [24] | ↑ [25] | |
| MMP-3 | nc [26] | ↑ [24] | ↑ [25] | |
| MT1-MMP | | | | ↑ [27] |
| TIMP-1 | nc [26] | ↑ [24] | | |
| TIMP-2 | ↑ [28] | | | |

*GAGase* glycosaminoglycan-degrading enzyme, *MMP* matrix metalloproteinase, *MT1* membrane type 1, *TIMP* tissue inhibitor for MMP
A statistically significant difference in the changes comparing POAG and control patients is indicated by ↑ or ↓
If two arrows are shown, this indicates a twofold change, three arrows indicate a threefold change, four arrows indicate a fourfold change, and nc indicates that there is no change between POAG and controls

**Table 27.2** Cell signaling changes in POAG

| | Aqueous humor | Trabecular meshwork | Optic nerve | Systemic (serum/plasma) |
|---|---|---|---|---|
| Angiopoietin-like 7 | ↑↑↑ [29] | | | |
| Aquaporin-9 | | | ↓ [30] | |
| Erythropoietin | ↑ [31] | | | |
| Endothelin-1 | ↑ [32] | | | ↑ [32, 33] |
| Hepatocyte growth factor | ↑ [34] | | | |
| Phospholipase A2 | ↑ [35] | | | |
| Plasminogen activator inhibitor-1 | ↑↑↑ [36] | | | |
| Soluble CD44 | ↑↑ [37, 38] | | | |
| Thymulin | | | | ↑↑↑ [39] |
| Vascular endothelial growth factor | ↑ [40] | | | ↑ [41] |

A statistically significant difference in the changes comparing POAG and control patients is indicated by ↑ or ↓
If two arrows are shown, this indicates a twofold change, and three arrows indicate a threefold change

features which may serve as a platform for evaluating and predicting surgical success in POAG.

## ECM Changes in POAG

The ECM and TM endothelium are essential for maintenance of the normal aqueous humor outflow [79]. In the TM of POAG eyes, excessive, abnormal accumulations as well as decreases of other ECM materials (Table 27.1) have been documented [80, 81]. The ECM produced by the cells is composed of multidomain macromolecules such as collagens, cell-binding glycoproteins, and proteoglycans that link together to form a structurally stable composite. It is now well documented that ECM is a dynamic entity determining and controlling the behavior and biologic characteristics of the cells [82].

One key component of the ECM in the TM is proteoglycans which are macromolecules consisting of a core protein to which glycosaminoglycan side chains are covalently attached. This class of molecules has been implicated in the maintenance of resistance to aqueous humor outflow. In the TM tissue, proteoglycans form gel-like networks that may function as a gel filtration system. The major types identified include chondroitin, dermatan, and heparan sulfate proteoglycans that may represent decorin, biglycan, versican, perlecan, and syndecan [82, 83].

The relative amounts of each type of glycosaminoglycan in the TM tissue have been determined [15, 80]. Hyaluronic acid

**Table 27.3** Oxidative stress and senescence changes in POAG

| | Aqueous humor | Trabecular meshwork | Optic nerve/retina | Systemic (serum/plasma/red blood cells) |
|---|---|---|---|---|
| Acetylcholinesterase | | | | ↑ [42] |
| Asymmetric dimethylarginine | | | | ↑ [43] |
| 3-α-Hydroxysteroid dehydrogenase | | | | ↓ [44, 45] |
| Ascorbic acid | ↑ ↑ ↑ [46] | | | |
| Citrate | | | | ↓ [47] |
| Cortisol | | | | ↑ [48] |
| Diadenosine tetraphosphate | | | | ↑ [44] |
| Dimethylarginine | | | | ↑ [43] |
| ELAM-1 | | ↑ [49] | | |
| Fatty acid | | | | |
| Eicosapentaenoic | | | | ↓ [50] |
| Choline plasmalogens | | | | ↓ [51] |
| Docosahexaenoic | | | | ↓ [51] |
| Ω-3 | | | | ↓ [51] |
| Glutathione | ↑ ↑ ↑ [52] | | | ↓ [53] |
| Nitric oxide | ↑ [54] | | | |
| Nitric oxide synthase | | | | ↑ [55] |
| NF-κB | | ↑ [56] | | |
| HIF-1α | | | ↑ [57] | |
| Senescence-associated β-galactosidase | | ↑ [58] | | |

*ELAM* endothelial cell leukocyte adhesion molecule, *NF* nuclear factor, *HIF* hypoxia-inducible factor
A statistically significant difference in the changes comparing POAG and control patients is indicated by ↑ or ↓
If two arrows are shown, this indicates a twofold change, and three arrows indicate a threefold change

and chondroitin–dermatan sulfates are the major constituents, with heparan sulfate and keratan sulfate present in smaller amounts. A depletion in hyaluronic acid and an accumulation of chondroitin sulfates and undigestible glycosaminoglycan material have been associated with POAG conditions [15]. Both chondroitin sulfate and hyaluronic acid have been shown to contribute to flow resistance and influence flow rate in vitro [80]. The flow rate was decreased when hyaluronic acid and chondroitin sulfate were used at POAG concentrations. If glycosaminoglycan chain biosynthesis is distributed by sodium chlorate or β-xyloside, outflow facility increases in perfusion cultures [81]. Of note, the level of an ectodomain fragment of hyaluronic acid receptor CD44 (sCD44) was found to be elevated (Table 27.2) in the aqueous humor of POAG patients [37], and the concentration was highly correlated with the clinical visual field loss which characterizes POAG. sCD44 is internalized in TM cells and localizes in part to mitochondria [84]. sCD44 is cytotoxic to TM cells [85].

Fibronectin, laminin, vitronectin, and matricellular proteins that include tenascin and thrombospondin-1 have been localized in the TM [82]. These glycoproteins are crucial in biologic processes such as cell attachment, spreading, and cell differentiation [82]. Overexpression of fibronectin, laminin, and collagen type IV results in a decrease in the TM cell monolayer permeability [86, 87]. In addition, the expression of thrombospondin-1 has been shown to be increased [23] in the TM of POAG eyes (Table 27.1).

Elastin is localized to the central core of sheath-derived plaques or elastic-like fibers in the TM [86]. Fibrillin-1, a component of microfibrils, is found in both the core and the surrounding sheath of the elastic-like fibers. Fibrillin-1 and collagen type VI are also constituents of long-spacing collagens in the TM [86, 87]. In trabecular lamellae and in juxtacanalicular tissue, accumulation of long-spacing collagens and sheath-derived plaques has been documented in POAG and aged eyes [86, 88]. The cochlin deposits in the glaucomatous TM (Table 27.1) appear to increase with age and are associated with proteoglycans. Such deposits have been proposed to contribute to the increase of ECM resistance to outflow and the POAG pathology [12].

The ECM is constantly modified by the surrounding cells through enzymes such as matrix metalloproteinase (MMP) family member and inhibitors such as tissue inhibitors of matrix metalloproteinase (TIMPs) found in the TM [83]. Ongoing ECM turnover, initiated by MMPs, appears to be essential for maintenance of the aqueous outflow homeostasis. MMP-3, and possibly also MMP-9, may be responsible for the efficacy of laser trabeculoplasty, a clinically useful alternative treatment to reduce IOP in patients with glaucoma [83, 86]. Addition or induction of MMP-3 in perfused human anterior segment organ cultures increases, whereas blocking the endogenous activity of the MMPs in the TM reduces, the aqueous humor outflow facility [83].

**Table 27.4** Innate and adaptive immunity changes in POAG

| | Aqueous humor | Trabecular meshwork | Optic nerve/retina | Systemic (serum/plasma) |
|---|---|---|---|---|
| Innate immunity | | | | |
| Receptors | | | | |
| TLR 2 | | | ↑ ↑ [59] | |
| TLR 4 | | | ↑ ↑ ↑ [59] | |
| TLR 7 | | | ↑ [59] | |
| TLR 8 | | | ↑ [59] | |
| Associated proteins | | | | |
| MyD88 | | | ↑ [59] | |
| CD44 | | ↑ [13] | | |
| Ligands (pathogen-associated molecular patterns) | | | | |
| Hsp 60 (bacterial) | | | | ↑ [60, 61, 63] |
| *H. pylori* | ↑ ↑ ↑ [62] | | | |
| Heat shock proteins | | | | |
| Hsp 27 | | | ↑ ↑ ↑ ↑ [64] | ↑ [65] |
| αB-crystallin | | | ↑ ↑ ↑ [59, 61] | ↑ [65] |
| Hsp 60 | | | ↑ ↑ ↑ ↑ [59] | ↑ [65] |
| Hsp 70 | | | ↑ ↑ ↑ ↑ [59] | ↑ [65] |
| Serum amyloid A | | ↑ ↑ [66] | | |
| Adaptive immunity | | | | |
| Cytokines | | | | |
| IL-2 | | | | ↑ [67] |
| IL-4 | | | | ↑ ↑ [68] |
| IL-8 | | | | ↑ ↑ [68–70] |
| IL-12 | | | | ↑ ↑ [68] |
| TGF-β2 | ↑ [71, 72] | | | |
| TNF α | nc [73] | | ↑ [25] | ↓ [68] |
| Autoantibodies | | | | |
| Anti-phosphatidylserine | | | | ↑ [74] |
| Fodrin | | | | ↑ [75] |
| Glial fibrillary acidic protein | | | | ↓ [74] |
| Glutathione S-transferase | | | | ↑ [76] |
| Myelin basic protein | | | | ↑ [74] |
| Neuron-specific enolase | | | | ↑ [77] |
| Retinaldehyde-binding protein | | | | ↑ [74] |
| Retinal S-antigen | | | | ↑ [78] |
| Vimentin | | | | ↑ [65] |
| γ-Enolase | | | | ↑ [74] |
| 14-3-3 | | | | ↓ [74] |
| Monoclonal gammopathy | | | | ↑ [76] |

*TLR* Toll-like receptor, *MyD88* myeloid differential primary response gene 88, *IL* interleukin, *TGF* transforming growth factor, *TNF* tumor necrosis factor

A statistically significant difference in the changes comparing POAG and control patients is indicated by ↑ or ↓

If two arrows are shown, this indicates a twofold change, three arrows indicate a threefold change, four arrows indicate a fourfold change, and nc indicates that there is no change between POAG and controls

The ECM in the TM may also be remodeled in response to exogenous stimuli such as glucocorticoids and oxidative stress [82, 86]. Mechanical stretch caused an increase in MMP-1 and MMP-3 activities and alteration of ECM molecules including proteoglycans and matricellular proteins [89]. The ECM is modulated by cytokines. The most studied cytokine in the TM is transforming growth factor-beta (TGF-β). A higher than normal level [73] of TGF-β2 was found in the aqueous humor of patients with POAG (Table 27.4). In TGF-β2-perfused organ cultures, focal accumulation of fine fibrillar extracellular material was observed in TM tissues. Furthermore, TGF-β2 perfusion reduced outflow facility and elevated IOP [90], and adenoviral gene transfer of active TGF-β2 elevated IOP and reduced outflow facility in rodent eyes [91]. These results suggest that the increased TGF-β2 level in the aqueous humor may be related to the pathogenesis of glaucoma. Other cytokines such as tumor necrosis factor-α (TNF-α) that is increased in the optic nerve head of POAG (Table 27.4) also modulate the ECM, probably via regulation of MMP and TIMP expressions [82, 92].

## Signaling Molecules in POAG

The TM and optic nerve utilize local and probably systemic cell signaling pathways to maintain cell viability. Locally in the TM, the Rho family of small guanosine triphosphatases (GTPase) has been shown to be of vital importance in the outflow system [93–95]. Sphingosine-1-phosphate and endothelin-1 activate Rho/Rho kinase signaling pathway decrease the aqueous humor outflow facility [93–95]. Endothelin-1 has been reported to be increased in the aqueous humor [32] and blood [33] of POAG patients (Table 27.2).

The aqueous humor also modulates TM cell signaling. It contains albumin as a major constituent. Other components encompass hydrogen peroxide ($H_2O_2$), ascorbic acid, cytokines such as TGF-β, hepatocyte growth factor and vascular endothelial growth factor (VEGF), and molecules including MMPs, proteinase inhibitors, sCD44, and hyaluronic acid [82]. In both POAG aqueous humor and Alzheimer's cerebrospinal fluid [96], hepatocyte growth factor [34] and VEGF [40] increase, indicating modulation of these fluids in the disease process. Increased levels of angiopoietin-like 7, aquaporin-9, erythropoietin, plasminogen activator inhibitor-1, sCD44, interleukin-2, phospholipase A2, thymulin (Table 27.2), glutathione, ascorbic acid (Table 27.3), and TGF-β2 (Table 27.4) but, significantly, a decreased level of hyaluronic acid (Table 27.1) have been reported in the aqueous humor of POAG eyes. Of note, the decrease in aqueous hyaluronic acid concentration parallels that in the TM, and the increase in sCD44 (the ectodomain portion of the CD44 receptor) also parallels the CD44 receptor increase in the TM (Table 27.1). Only sCD44 has been tested in rodents; adenoviral gene transfer of sCD44 resulted in a sustained increase in IOP in mice [97]. The sCD44 found in the POAG aqueous humor is hypophosphorylated [98]. The hypophosphorylated form has high cytotoxicity and low hyaluronic acid-binding affinity and is suggested to represent a pathophysiologic feature of the disease process [98].

## Stress and Aging in POAG

TM cellularity is reduced with aging [99, 100]. Morphologic studies have also revealed thickened basement membranes and accumulation of sheath-derived plaques and long-spacing collagens in the TM of aged eyes [90]. The number of senescent cells which stain positive for senescence-associated β-galactosidase is increased (Table 27.3) in the

TM of POAG eyes [56], supporting further that POAG is an age-related disease [82, 101]. Oxidative damage and stress (Table 27.3) have also been implicated to contribute to the morphologic and physiologic alterations in the aqueous outflow pathway in aging and glaucoma [102]. The TM is subjected to chronic oxidative stress [86]. Superoxide dismutase, an enzyme involved in the protection against oxidative damage, has been shown to decline with age in human TM tissues [101]. TM cells also synthesized a specific set of proteins, such as αB-crystallin, that may act as molecular chaperones to prevent oxidative or heat shock protein damage [41]. Markers of oxidative damage [102, 103], abnormalities in mitochondrial DNA [104], and diminished blood levels of oxidant scavenger glutathione [52] are found in POAG patients. It appears that oxidative stress that exceeds the capacity of TM cells for detoxification is involved in damaging the cells and alteration of the aqueous humor outflow, leading to increased IOP. Moreover, stress-/aging-related changes also occur in the red blood cell phospholipid composition which may alter red blood cell flexibility in POAG [51], causing reduced ocular blood flow and optic nerve axon loss. Linear regression analysis suggests that a decrease in phosphatidylcholine-carrying docosahexaenoic acid (DHA, an omega-3 fatty acid) occurs years before the onset of POAG. This underscores the notion that aging, and specifically membrane lipid composition, is a risk factor in POAG [51]. In a longitudinal study, a decrease in phospholipid composition correlates with the development of Alzheimer's disease [105]. There is, however, a possible correction for the change in lipid composition of membranes. One effect of dietary omega-3 is downregulation of Toll-4 innate immune receptors [106], whereas supplement-free fatty acids upregulate Toll-4 [107].

## Innate and Adaptive Immunity in POAG

The immune system is actively involved in the POAG disease process. Innate immunity is the first line of defense and is rapidly activated by surgery (see Fig. 27.1), leading to NF-kB activation responsive genes [108]. Toll-4 receptor recognizes low molecular weight hyaluronic acid fragments and many others [108]. Significantly, a number of Toll-like receptors are increased in the retina of POAG patients (Table 27.4). Upregulation of acute stress response protein amyloid in TM of POAG patients [66] further supports the notion that POAG has ocular altered protein expression. Treatment of cultured human TM cells with recombinant serum amyloid A affects gene expression, including a 22-fold upregulation of interleukin-8 [66]. Toll-like receptors are expressed on monocytes, dendritic cells, neutrophils, mucosal epithelial cells, and endothelial cells [109]. Notably, low molecular weight hyaluronic acid activates monocyte

                                                                                                                    

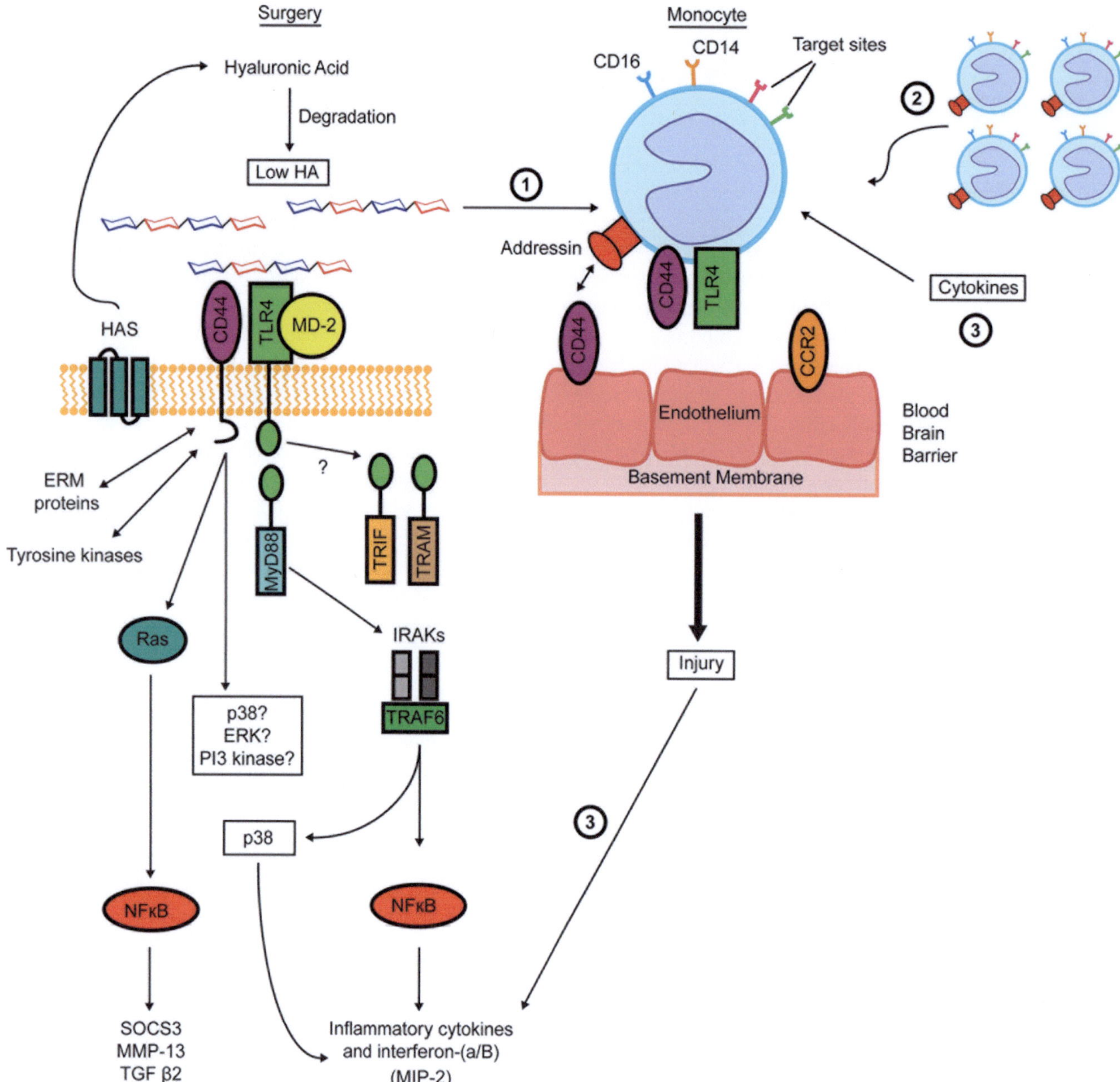


**Fig. 27.1** (**a**) Putative activation of Toll-4-like receptors occurs by breakdown of hyaluronic acid into hyaluronic acid oligosaccharides depicted as red-blue saccharides and are released from the ECM as a result of surgery. These oligosaccharides bind to Toll-4 receptor (*TLR4*) along with co-accessory molecules lymphocyte antigen 96 (*MD-2*) and the CD44 receptor. This receptor complex utilizes ERM proteins (ezrin, radixin, moesin) and myeloid differentiation primary response gene 88 (*MyD88*). Rat sarcoma g proteins (*Ras*) and nuclear factor kappa light chain enhancer of activated β-cells (*NF-κB*) are upregulated, leading to downstream effectors including matrix metalloproteinase (*MMP-13*), transforming growth factor-beta 2 (*TGF-β2*.), suppressor of cytokine signaling 3 (*SOCS3*), and inflammatory cytokines. Ligand binding to TLR4 activates certain factors (IRAK, interleukin-1 receptor kinase and TRAFs, tumor necrosis factor receptor-associated kinases) that amplify the signal leading to the inflammatory response and its modulation of the ECM, cell signaling molecules, stress response, and immunity-related changes. The pathway includes TIR-domain-containing adaptor-inducing interferon-B (*TRIF*), TRIF-related adaptor molecule (*TRAM*), extracellular-signal-regulated kinase (*ERK*), and macrophage inflammatory protein 2 (*MIP-2*). (**b**) Theoretical monocyte activation and recruitment involvement in site-specific injury. Approximately 48 h after sustaining injury, monocytes are recruited from the bone marrow to an injured area by C-C chemokine receptor (*CCR-2*). Three pathways are shown for monocyte activation: (1) low molecular weight hyaluronic acid, (2) recruitment of additional monocytes, and (3) inflammatory cytokines and chemokines. During the initial inflammatory cascade, cells synthesize hyaluronic acid by hyaluronan synthases (*HAS*). HA binds to CD44 on monocytes and endothelium, leading to extravasation of monocytes from the blood vessel into the surgical site. The activation of the NF-κB pathway upregulates both CD44 and HAS. Addressins are a family of cell identity makers, putative target sites for monocyte surveillance

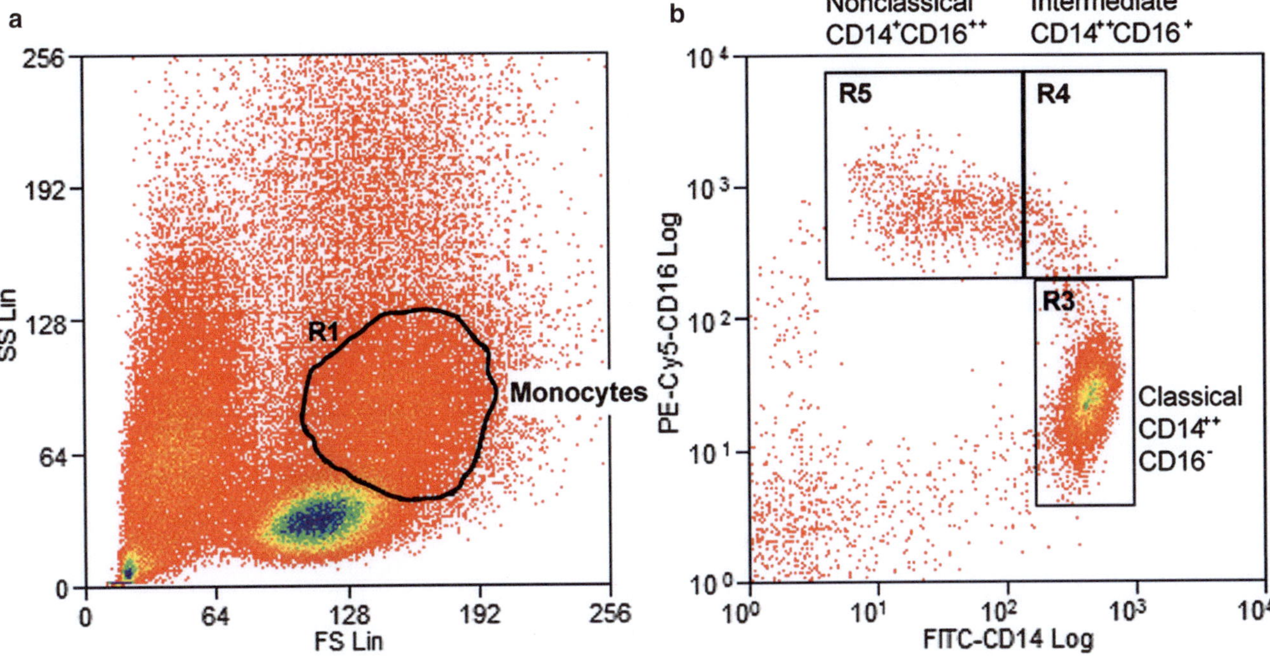

**Fig. 27.2** Flow cytometry of monocyte subtypes. (**a**) Monocyte population was identified by forward scatter (*FS*) and side scatter (SS), enclosed in R1. (**b**) Events within R1 were plotted against CD14 and CD16 fluorochromes and subsequently divided into the three monocyte subtypes: CD14++CD16−, classical monocyte (*R3*); CD14++CD16+, intermediate (*R4*); and CD14+ CD16++, nonclassical (*R5*)

expression. Monocytes from the blood extravasate through the blood vessel walls using the multifaceted CD44, the homing receptor for leucocytes. Once monocytes arrive in the wound site, monocytes differentiate into macrophages. Upon activation, the macrophages induce new ECM and stimulate the local cells to re-epithelize the wound. Figure 27.1 depicts three pathways in which monocytes are activated: (1) low molecular weight hyaluronic acid, (2) cytokines and chemokines, and (3) recruitment of other monocytes. The monocyte activation creates positive feedback loop leading to extensive scar tissue and aberrant wound healing. See Fig. 27.1. One idea that we are exploring is that the expression of CD44 message and its numerous variants are changed in POAG. Although CD44 expression on keloid cells is similar to normal dermal cells [110], keloid tissue exhibits a different miRNA profile [111, 112] and increased hyaluronic acid [110]. The 3′ untranslated region of CD44 is very active in miRNA binding and influences disease progression [113]. The overexpression of sCD44 in the aqueous of African-Americans with POAG [37] is important since CD44 contributes to inflammation and fibrosis in response to injury. CD44 promotes the activation of TGF-β via an MMP-dependent mechanism leading to fibroblast migration and recruitment [114]. We have used flow cytometry to characterize monocyte activation. See Fig. 27.2. Recently, three monocyte subset populations were identified as classical (CD14++CD16−), intermediate (CD14++CD16+), and nonclassical (CD14+ CD16++) [115]. In healthy individuals the

classical monocytes represent ~90 % of monocytes, while the intermediate and nonclassical comprise the other 10 [116]. The relative concentrations of intermediate and nonclassical monocytes have been implicated in a number of diseases, such as HIV-1 infection [117], cancer [118], and stroke [119]. Notably, monocyte profile predicts the clinical course and prognosis human stroke [119]. Monocyte subtypes have already been identified in Eales disease [120], but to our knowledge have not been examined in POAG. If monocyte subtypes are different in POAG from normal patients, monocyte subtypes may provide a reliable biomarker of the disease as well as information about patient's status after glaucoma-associated surgery. Interestingly, a recent paper identified that radiation treatment has been found to prevent glaucoma in a mouse model by disrupting monocyte migration [121]. One particular element that was disrupted was L-selectin, which, when activated, aids in trans-endothelial cell migration. The intermediate monocytes (CD14++CD16+) overexpress L-SELECTIN, which might implicate this monocyte subtype as a prime facilitator of glaucoma [122]. If these results are supported, patients undergoing surgery might benefit from having their monocyte subtypes examined using flow cytometry.

The adaptive immune system is also a defense and relies on antigen-presenting cells required for lymphocyte activation and effector cells that eliminate antigens [109]. Cytokines are secreted by the cells of innate and adaptive immunity system in response to a variety of inflammatory and antigenic stimuli [123]. Excessive amounts or actions of cytokines can lead to pathological consequences. In both POAG aqueous humor [69, 70] and Alzheimer's cerebrospinal fluid [124], interleukin-8 is increased. See Table 27.4 for changes in cytokines in the aqueous humor, optic nerve, and blood in POAG patients. It is of note that Alvarado et al. have shown that conditioned media obtained from irradiated TM and cytokines modulated aqueous outflow in vitro [125, 126]. In addition, autoantibodies also are present in the blood of POAG patients (Table 27.4).

The exact role of each biomarker is sketchy at present and a direct link to POAG remains to be established. One important key in successful surgery is wound healing. Although there are numerous factors, the innate immunity is the first line of defense. Monocytes, for example, typically appear on day 2 of injury to promote wound healing. A second line in defense is the vascularization of the wound. Park et al. observed nail bed hemorrhages in 20 % of POAG patients [127]. The use of nail fold capillaroscopy to describe and detect various connective tissue diseases has been well established. Nail fold capillaroscopy demonstrates morphologic changes in the nail fold capillaries of systemic sclerosis patients and can establish the progression of the disease [128]. Capillary changes have been determined in other autoimmune disorders such as systemic lupus erythematosus and Sjogren's syndrome [129, 130]. Of note, hemorrhages were found to be prevalent in the nail fold capillaries of Sjogren's syndrome patients [130]. The discovery of microhemorrhages in the nail fold capillaries of POAG patients indicates possible systemic manifestations which are characteristic of connective tissue diseases.

Recently we used nail bed capillaroscopy to observe hemorrhages in POAG. See Video 27.1. Nail fold hemorrhages were observed in all low-tension POAG patients ($n=7$). If nail fold hemorrhages occur before the onset of the clinical manifestations of POAG or are more abundant in the progression of the disease process, close monitoring of nail bed hemorrhage may prove to be useful in the diagnosis and management of POAG. The direct cause of the nail fold microhemorrhages remains undetermined. Microhemorrhages in the nail folds may correlate to optic disc hemorrhages and may assist surgeons in deciding when surgery is needed and what type of surgical intervention is appropriate and minimizing surgical failures.

We cataloged all known ocular biomarkers in the aqueous humor, trabecular meshwork, optic nerve, as well as systemic biomarkers in blood serum. We present a theoretical model to show possible signaling pathways of the ECM, cell signaling, and innate immune response through activation of Toll-4 receptor and monocyte activation which may impact the success of glaucoma surgery. The innate immune system is driven by the danger signal, a low molecular weight hyaluronic acid, and the activation of monocytes. Subtyping monocytes to characterize the innate immunity and documenting nail fold hemorrhages may prove useful in predicting the success of glaucoma surgery. For example, preoperative evaluation of a POAG patient who has marked monocyte activation and extensive nail fold hemorrhages may indicate a high-risk surgery patient. The surgeon may decide that surgical intervention may be necessary sooner rather than later or may even influence the type of surgery that is performed. In addition, the Toll-4 and monocyte activation could be countered by adjunct therapy since it well recognized that naloxone is a Toll-4 antagonist [131, 132]. Thus, the future direction of POAG surgical success may be influenced by the modulation of the innate immune system.

## References


1. Kwon YH, Fingert JH, Kuehn MH, Alward WLM. Primary open-angle glaucoma. N Engl J Med. 2009;360(11):1113–24.
2. Kass MA, Gordon MO, Gao F, Heuer DK, Higginbotham EJ, Johnson CA, et al. Delaying treatment of ocular hypertension: the ocular hypertension treatment study. Arch Ophthalmol. 2010;128(3):276–87.
3. Gordon MO, Torri V, Miglior S, Beiser JA, Floriani I, Miller JP, et al., Ocular Hypertension Treatment Study Group, European Glaucoma Prevention Study Group. Validated prediction model for the development of primary open-angle glaucoma in individuals with ocular hypertension. Ophthalmology. 2007;114(1):10–9.
4. Weinreb RN. IOP and the risk of progression to glaucoma. Graefes Arch Clin Exp Ophthalmol. 2005;243(6):511–2.
5. De Moraes CG, Liebmann JM, Park SC, Teng CC, Nemiroff J, Tello C, Ritch R. Optic disc progression and rates of visual field change in treated glaucoma. Acta Ophthalmol. 2013;91(2):e86–91.
6. Allingham RR, Liu Y, Rhee DJ. The genetics of primary open-angle glaucoma: a review. Exp Eye Res. 2009;88(4):837–44.
7. Bhattacharya SK, Lee RK, Grus FH, Seventh ARVO/Pfizer Ophthalmics Research Institute Conference Working Group. Molecular biomarkers in glaucoma. Invest Ophthalmol Vis Sci. 2013;54(1):121–31.
8. Caprioli J. Glaucoma is a neuronal disease. Eye. 2007;21:S6–10.
9. Ross JS, Symmans WF, Pusztai L, Hortobagyi GN. Pharmacogenomics and clinical biomarkers in drug discovery and development. Am J Clin Pathol. 2005;124 Suppl 1:S29–41.
10. de Lemos JA, Lloyd-Jones DM. Multiple biomarker panels for cardiovascular risk assessment. N Eng J Med. 2008;358(20):2172–4.
11. Ray S, Britschgi M, Herbert C, Takeda-Uchimura Y, Boxer A, Blennow K, et al. Classification and prediction of clinical Alzheimer's diagnosis based on plasma signaling proteins. Nat Med. 2007;13(11):1359–62.
12. Simonsen AH, McGuire J, Hansson O, Zetterberg H, Podust VN, Davies HA, et al. Novel panel of cerebrospinal fluid biomarkers for the prediction of progression to Alzheimer dementia in patients with mild cognitive impairment. Arch Neurol. 2007;64(3):366–70.
13. Knepper PA, Goossens W, Mayanil CS. CD44H localization in primary open-angle glaucoma. Invest Ophthalmol Vis Sci. 1998;39(5):673–80.
14. Picciani R, Desai K, Guduric-Fuchs J, Cogliati T, Morton CC, Bhattacharya SK. Cochlin in the eye. Prog Retin Eye Res. 2007;26(5):453–69.
15. Knepper PA, Goossens W, Hvizd M, Palmberg PF. Glycosaminoglycans of the human trabecular meshwork in primary open-angle glaucoma. Invest Ophthalmol Vis Sci. 1996;37(7):1360–7.

16. Hann CR, Springett MJ, Wang X, Johnson DH. Ultrastructural localization of collagen IV, fibronectin, and laminin in the trabecular meshwork of normal and glaucomatous eyes. Ophthalmic Res. 2001;33(6):314–24.

17. Umihira J, Nagata S, Nohara M, Hanai T, Usuda N, Segawa K. Localization of elastin in the normal and glaucomatous human trabecular meshwork. Invest Ophthalmol Vis Sci. 1994;35(2):486–94.

18. Pena JD, Netland PA, Vidal I, Dorr DA, Rasky A, Hernandez MR. Elastosis of the lamina cribrosa in glaucomatous optic neuropathy. Exp Eye Res. 1998;67(5):517–24.

19. Vesaluoma M, Mertaniemi P, Mannonen S, Lehto I, Uusitalo R, Sarna S, et al. Cellular and plasma fibronectin in the aqueous humour of primary open-angle glaucoma, exfoliative glaucoma and cataract patients. Eye. 1998;12(5):886–90.

20. Navajas EV, Martins JR, Melo Jr LA, Saraiva VS, Dietrich CP, Nader HB, et al. Concentration of hyaluronic acid in primary open-angle glaucoma aqueous humor. Exp Eye Res. 2005;80(6):853–7.

21. Gong H, Ye W, Freddo TF, Hernandez MR. Hyaluronic acid in the normal and glaucomatous optic nerve. Exp Eye Res. 1997;4(4):587–95.

22. Pena JD, Varela HJ, Ricard CS, Hernandez MR. Enhanced tenascin expression associated with reactive astrocytes in human optic nerve heads with primary open angle glaucoma. Exp Eye Res. 1999;68(1):29–40.

23. Flugel-Koch C, Ohlmann A, Fuchshofer R, Weige-Lussen U, Tamm ER. Thrombospondin-1 in the trabecular meshwork: localization in normal and glaucomatous eyes, and induction by TGF-β1 and dexamethasone in vitro. Exp Eye Res. 2004;79(5):649–63.

24. Ronkko S, Rekonen P, Kaarniranta K, Prustjarvi T, Terasvirta M, Uusitaol H. Matrix metalloproteinases and their inhibitors in the chamber angle of normal eyes and patients with primary open-angle glaucoma and exfoliation glaucoma. Graefes Arch Clin Exp Ophthalmol. 2007;245(5):697–704.

25. Yan X, Tezel G, Wax MB, Edward DP. Matrix metalloproteinases and tumor necrosis factor-α in glaucomatous optic nerve head. Arch Ophthalmol. 2000;118(5):666–73.

26. Schlotzer-Schrehardt U, Lommatzsch J, Kuchle M, Konstas AG, Naumann GO. Matrix metalloproteinases and their inhibitors in aqueous humor of patients with pseudoexfoliation syndrome/glaucoma and primary open-angle glaucoma. Invest Ophthalmol Vis Sci. 2003;44(3):1117–25.

27. Golubnitschaja O, Yeghiazaryan K, Liu R, Mönkemann H, Leppert D, Schild H, et al. Increased expression of matrix metalloproteinases in mononuclear blood cells of normal-tension glaucoma patients. J Glaucoma. 2004;13(1):66–72.

28. Maatta M, Tervahartiala T, Harju M, Airaksinen J, Autio-Harmainen H, Sorsa T. Matrix metalloproteinases and their tissue inhibitors in aqueous humor of patients with primary open-angle glaucoma, exfoliation syndrome, and exfoliation glaucoma. J Glaucoma. 2005;14(1):64–9.

29. Kuchtey J, Källberg ME, Gelatt KN, Rinkoski T, Komàromy AM, Kuchtey RW. Angiopoietin-like 7 secretion is induced by glaucoma stimuli and its concentration is elevated in glaucomatous aqueous humor. Invest Ophthalmol Vis Sci. 2008;49(8):3438–48.

30. Mizokami J, Kanamori A, Negi A, Nakamura M. A preliminary study of reduced expression of aquaporin-9 in the optic nerve of primate and human eyes with glaucoma. Curr Eye Res. 2011;36(11):1064–7.

31. Cumurcu T, Bulut Y, Demir HD, Yenisehirli G. Aqueous humor erythropoietin levels in patients with primary open-angle glaucoma. J Glaucoma. 2007;16(8):645–8.

32. Tezel G, Kass MA, Kolker AE, Becker B, Wax MB. Plasma and aqueous humor endothelin levels in primary open-angle glaucoma. J Glaucoma. 1997;6(2):83–9.

33. Emre M, Orgul S, Haufschild T, Shaw SG, Flammer J. Increased plasma endothelin-1 levels in patients with progressive open angle glaucoma. Br J Ophthalmol. 2005;89(1):60–3.

34. Hu DN, Ritch R. Hepatocyte growth factor is increased in the aqueous humor of glaucomatous eyes. J Glaucoma. 2001;10(3):152–7.

35. Ronkko S, Rekonen P, Kaarniranta K, Puustjarvi T, Terasvirta M, Uuusitiao H. Phospholipase A2 in chamber angle of normal eyes and patients with primary open angle glaucoma and exfoliation glaucoma. Mol Vis. 2007;13:408–17.

36. Dan J, Belyea D, Gertner G, Leshem I, Lusky M, Miskin R. Plasminogen activator inhibitor-1 in the aqueous humor of patients with and without glaucoma. Arch Ophthalmol. 2005;123(2):220–4.

37. Nolan MJ, Giovingo MC, Miller AM, Wertz RD, Ritch R, Liebmann JM, et al. Aqueous humor sCD44 concentration and visual field loss in primary open-angle glaucoma. J Glaucoma. 2007;16(5):419–29.

38. Budak YU, Akdogan M, Huysal K. Aqueous humor level of sCD44 in patients with degenerative myopia and primary open-angle glaucoma. BMC Res Notes. 2009;8(2):224.

39. Noureddin BN, Al-Haddad CE, Bashshur Z, Safieh-Garabedian B. Plasma thymulin and nerve growth factor levels in patients with primary open angle glaucoma and elevated intraocular pressure. Graefes Arch Clin Exp Ophthalmol. 2006;244(6):750–2.

40. Hu DN, Ritch R, Liebmann J, Liu Y, Cheng B, Hu MS. Vascular endothelial growth factor is increased in aqueous humor of glaucomatous eyes. J Glaucoma. 2002;11(5):406–10.

41. Lip PL, Felmeden DC, Blann AD, Matheou N, Thakur S, Cunliffe IA, et al. Plasma vascular endothelial growth factor, soluble VEGF receptor FLT-1, and von Willebrand factor in glaucoma. Br J Ophthalmol. 2002;86(11):1299–302.

42. Zabala L, Saldanha C, Martins e Silva J, Souza-Ramalho P. Red blood cell membrane integrity in primary open angle glaucoma: ex vivo and in vitro studies. Eye. 1999;13(1):101–3.

43. Javadiyan S, Burdon KP, Whiting MJ, Abhary S, Straga T, Hewitt AW, et al. Elevation of serum asymmetrical and symmetrical dimethylarginine in patients with advanced glaucoma. Invest Ophthalmol Vis Sci. 2012;53(4):1923–7.

44. Kokotas H, Kroupis C, Chiras D, Grigoriadou M, Lamnissou K, Petersen MB, Kitsos G. Biomarkers in primary open angle glaucoma. Clin Chem Lab Med. 2012;50(12):2107–19.

45. Weinstein BI, Iyer RB, Binstock JM, Hamby CV, Schwartz IS, Moy FH, et al. Decreased 3α-hydroxysteroid dehydrogenase activity in peripheral blood lymphocytes from patients with primary open angle glaucoma. Exp Eye Res. 1996;62(1):39–45.

46. Lee P, Lam KW, Lai M. Aqueous humor ascorbate concentration and open-angle glaucoma. Arch Ophthalmol. 1977;95(2):308–10.

47. Fraenkl SA, Muser J, Groell R, Reinhard G, Orgul S, Flammer J, Goldblum D. Plasma citrate levels as potential biomarker for glaucoma. J Ocul Pharmacol Ther. 2011;27(6):577–80.

48. McCarty GR, Schwartz B. Reduced plasma cortisol binding to albumin in ocular hypertension and primary open-angle glaucoma. Curr Eye Res. 1999;18(6):467–76.

49. Wang N, Chintala SK, Fini ME, Schuman JS. Ultrasound activates the TM ELAM-1/IL-1/NF-kappaB response: a potential mechanism for intraocular pressure reduction after phacoemulsification. Invest Ophthalmol Vis Sci. 2003;44(5):1977–81.

50. Ren H, Magulike N, Ghebremeskel K, Crawford M. Primary open-angle glaucoma patients have reduced levels of blood docosahexaenoic and eicosapentaenoic acids. Prostaglandins Leukot Essent Fatty Acids. 2006;74(3):157–63.

51. Acar N, Berdeaux O, Juaneda P, Grégoire S, Cabaret S, Joffre C, et al. Red blood cell plasmalogens and docosahexaenoic acid are independently reduced in primary open-angle glaucoma. Exp Eye Res. 2009;89(6):840–53.

52. Ferreira SM, Lerner SF, Brunzini R, Evelson PA, Llesuy SF. Oxidative stress markers in aqueous humor of glaucoma patients. Am J Ophthalmol. 2004;137(1):62–9.

53. Gherghel D, Griffiths HR, Hilton EJ, Cunliffe IA, Hosking SL. Systemic reduction in glutathione levels occurs in patients with primary open-angle glaucoma. Invest Ophthalmol Vis Sci. 2005; 46(3):877–83.

54. Tsai DC, Hsu WM, Chou CK, Chen SJ, Peng CH, Chi CW, et al. Significant variation of the elevated nitric oxide levels in aqueous humor from patients with different types of glaucoma. Ophthalmologica. 2002;216(5):346–50.

55. Fernández-Durango R, Fernández-Martínez A, García-Feijoo J, Castillo A, de la Casa JM, García-Bueno B, et al. Expression of nitrotyrosine and oxidative consequences in the trabecular meshwork of patients with primary open-angle glaucoma. Invest Ophthalmol Vis Sci. 2008;49(6):2506–11.

56. Wang N, Chintala SK, Fini ME, Schuman JS. Activation of a tissue-specific stress response in the aqueous outflow pathway of the eye defines the glaucoma disease phenotype. Nat Med. 2001;7(3):304–9.

57. Tezel G, Wax MB. Hypoxia-inducible factor-1α in the glaucomatous retina and optic nerve head. Arch Ophthalmol. 2004;122(9): 1348–56.

58. Liton PB, Challa P, Stinnett S, Luna C, Epstein DL, Gonzalez P. Cellular senescence in the glaucomatous outflow pathway. Exp Gerontol. 2005;40(8–9):745–8.

59. Luo C, Yang X, Kain A, Powell D, Kuehn MH, Tezel G. Glaucomatous tissue stress and the regulation of immune response through the glial Toll-like receptor signaling. Invest Ophthalmol Vis Sci. 2010;51(11):5697–707.

60. Cancino-Diaz ME, Sanchez-Becerra M, Elizondo-Olascoaga C, Rodrguez-Martínez S, Cancino-Diaz JC. Amino acid regions 357–368 and 418–427 of Streptococcus pyogenes 60kDa heat shock protein are recognized by antibodies from glaucomatous patient sera. Microb Pathog. 2010;48(6):239–44.

61. Wax MB, Tezel G, Kawase K, Kitazawa Y. Serum autoantibodies to heat shock proteins in glaucoma patients from Japan and the United States. Ophthalmology. 2001;108(2):296–302.

62. Kountouras J, Mylopoulos N, Konstas AG, Zavos C, Chatzopoulos D, Boukla A. Increased levels of Helicobacter pylori IgG antibodies in aqueous humor of patients with primary open-angle and exfoliation glaucoma. Graefes Arch Clin Exp Ophthalmol. 2003; 241(11):884–90.

63. Deshpande N, Lalitha P, Krishna das SR, Jethani J, Pillai RM, Robin A, Karthik. Helicobacter pylori IgG antibodies in aqueous humor and serum of subjects with primary open angle and pseudo-exfoliation glaucoma in a South Indian population. J Glaucoma. 2008;17(8):605–10.

64. Tezel G, Seigel GM, Wax MB. Autoantibodies to small heat shock proteins in glaucoma. Invest Ophthalmol Vis Sci. 1998;39(12): 2277–87.

65. Joachim SC, Bruns K, Lackner KJ, Pfeiffer N, Grus FH. Antibodies to αB-crystallin, vimentin, and heat shock protein 70 in aqueous humor of patients with normal tension glaucoma and IgG antibody patterns against retinal antigen in aqueous humor. Curr Eye Res. 2007;32(6):501–9.

66. Wang WH, McNatt LG, Pang IH, Hellberg PE, Fingert JH, McCartney MD, et al. Increased expression of serum amyloid A in glaucoma and its effect on intraocular pressure. Invest Ophthalmol Vis Sci. 2008;49(5):1916–23.

67. Yang J, Patil RV, Yu H, Gordon M, Wax MB. T cell subsets and sIL-2R/IL-2 levels in patients with glaucoma. Am J Ophthalmol. 2001;31(4):421–6.

68. Huang P, Zhang SS, Zhang C. Erratum: the two sides of cytokine signaling and glaucomatous optic neuropathy. J Ocul Biol Dis Infor. 2009;2(3):98–103.

69. Kuchtey J, Rezaei KA, Jaru-Ampornpan P, Sternberg PJ, Kuchtey RW. Multiplex cytokine analysis reveals elevated concentration of interleukin-8 in glaucomatous aqueous humor. Invest Ophthalmol Vis Sci. 2010;51(12):6441–7.

70. Janciauskiene S, Westin K, Grip O, Krakau T. Detection of Alzheimer peptides and chemokines in the aqueous humor. Eur J Ophthalmol. 2011;21(1):104–11.

71. Picht G, Welge-Luessen U, Grehn F, Lutjen-Drecoll E. Transforming growth factor β2 levels in the aqueous humor in different types of glaucoma and the relation to filtering bleb development. Graefes Arch Clin Exp Ophthalmol. 2001;239(3):199–207.

72. Ochiai Y, Ochiai H. Higher concentration of transforming growth factor-beta in aqueous humor of glaucomatous eyes and diabetic eyes. Jpn J Ophthalmol. 2002;46(3):249–53.

73. Sawada H, Fukuchi T, Tanaka T, Abe H. Tumor necrosis factor-alpha concentrations in the aqueous humor of patients with glaucoma. Invest Ophthalmol Vis Sci. 2010;51(2):903–6.

74. Gramlich OW, Bell K, von Thun Und Hohenstein-Blaul N, Wilding C, Beck S, Pfeiffer N, et al. Autoimmune biomarkers in glaucoma patients. Curr Opin Pharmacol. 2013;13(1):90–7.

75. Grus FH, Joachim SC, Bruns K, Lackner KJ, Pfeiffer N, Wax MB. Serum autoantibodies to alpha-fodrin are present in glaucoma patients from Germany and the United States. Invest Ophthalmol Vis Sci. 2006;47(3):968–76.

76. Tezel G, Yang J, Wax MB. Heat shock proteins, immunity and glaucoma. Brain Res Bull. 2004;62(6):473–80.

77. Maruyama I, Ikeda Y, Nakazawa M, Ohguro H. Clinical roles of serum autoantibody against neuron-specific enolase in glaucoma patients. Tohoku J Exp Med. 2002;197(3):125–32.

78. Reichelt J, Joachim SC, Pfeiffer N, Grus FH. Analysis of autoantibodies against human retinal antigens in sera of patients with glaucoma and ocular hypertension. Curr Eye Res. 2008;33(3):253–61.

79. Barany EH. The effect of different kinds of hyaluronidase on the resistance to flow through the angle of the anterior chamber. Acta Ophthalmol. 1956;34(5):397–403.

80. Knepper PA, Fadel JR, Miller AM, Goossens W, Choi J, Nolan MJ, et al. Reconstitution of trabecular meshwork GAGs: influence of hyaluronic acid and chondroitin sulfate on flow rates. J Glaucoma. 2005;14(3):230–8.

81. Keller KE, Bradley JM, Kelley MJ, Acott TS. Effects of modifiers of glycosaminoglycan biosynthesis on outflow facility in perfusion culture. Invest Ophthalmol Vis Sci. 2008;49(6):2495–505.

82. Knepper PA, Yue BYJT. Abnormal trabecular meshwork outflow pathway. In: Levin LA, Albert DM, editors. Ocular disease: mechanisms and management. London: Elsevier; 2010. p. 171–7.

83. Acott TS, Kelley MJ. Extracellular matrix in the trabecular meshwork. Exp Eye Res. 2008;86(4):543–61.

84. Nolan M, Koga T, Walker L, McCarty R, Grybauskas A, Giovingo M, et al. sCD44 internalization in human trabecular meshwork cells. Invest Ophthalmol Vis Sci. 2013;54(1):592–601.

85. Choi J, Miller AM, Nolan MJ, Yue BY, Thotz ST, Clark AF, et al. Soluble CD44 is cytotoxic to trabecular meshwork and retinal ganglion cells in vitro. Invest Ophthalmol Vis Sci. 2006;46(1):214–22.

86. Yue BYJT. Cellular mechanisms in the trabecular meshwork affecting the aqueous humor outflow pathway. In: Albert DM, Miller JW, editors. Albert and Jakobiec's principles and practice of ophthalmology. 3rd ed. Oxford: Elsevier; 2007. p. 2457–74.

87. Tane N, Dhar S, Roy S, Pinheiro A, Shira A, Roy S. Effect of excess synthesis of extracellular matrix components by trabecular meshwork cells: possible consequence on aqueous outflow. Exp Eye Res. 2007;84(5):832–42.

88. Lutjen-Drecoll E, Rohen JW. Morphology of aqueous outflow pathways in normal and glaucomatous eyes. In: Ritch R, Shields MB, Krupin T, editors. The glaucomas. St. Louis: CV Mosby; 1996. p. 89–123.

89. Vittal V, Rose A, Gregory KE, Kelley MJ, Acott TS. Changes in gene expression by trabecular meshwork cells in response to mechanical stretching. Invest Ophthalmol Vis Sci. 2005;46(8): 2857–68.

90. Gottanka J, Chan D, Eichhorn M, Lutjen-Drecoll E, Ethier CR. Effects of TGF-β2 in perfused human eyes. Invest Ophthalmol Vis Sci. 2004;45(1):153–8.

91. Shepard AR, Millar JC, Pang IH, Jacobson N, Wang WH, Clark AF. Adenoviral gene transfer of active human transforming growth factor-{beta}2 elevates intraocular pressure and reduces outflow facility in rodent eyes. Invest Ophthalmol Vis Sci. 2010; 51(4):2067–76.

92. Kelley MJ, Rose AY, Song K, Chen Y, Bradley JM, Rookhuizen D, et al. Synergism of TNF and IL-1 in the induction of matrix metalloproteinases-3 in the trabecular meshwork. Invest Ophthalmol Vis Sci. 2007;48(6):2634–43.

93. Tan JCH, Peters DM, Kaufman PL. Recent developments in understanding the pathophysiology of elevated intraocular pressure. Curr Opin Ophthalmol. 2006;17(2):168–74.

94. Tian B, Geiger B, Epstein DL, Kaufman PL. Cytoskeletal involvement in the regulation of aqueous humor outflow. Invest Ophthalmol Vis Sci. 2000;41(3):619–23.

95. Rao PV, Epstein DL. Rho GTPase/Rho kinase inhibition as a novel target for the treatment of glaucoma. BioDrugs. 2007;21(3):167–77.

96. Olson L, Humpel C. Growth factors and cytokines/chemokines as surrogate biomarkers in cerebrospinal fluid and blood for diagnosing Alzheimer's disease and mild cognitive impairment. Exp Gerontol. 2010;45(1):41–6.

97. Giovingo M, Nolan M, McCarty R, Pang I-H, Clark AF, Beverley RM, et al. sCD44 overexpression increases intraocular pressure and aqueous outflow resistance. Molecular Vision. 2013;19:2151–64.

98. Knepper PA, Miller AM, Wertz CJ, Choi J, Nolan MJ, Goossens W, et al. Hypophosphorylation of aqueous humor sCD44 and primary open angle glaucoma. Invest Ophthalmol Vis Sci. 2005;46(8):2829–37.

99. Alvarado JA, Murphy CG, Polansky JR, Juster R. Age-related changes in trabecular meshwork cellularity. Invest Ophthalmol Vis Sci. 1981;21(5):714–27.

100. Alvarado J, Murphy C, Juster R. Trabecular meshwork cellularity in primary open-angle glaucoma and non-glaucomatous normals. Ophthalmology. 1984;91(6):564–79.

101. Sacca SC, Izzotti A, Rossi P, Traverso C. Glaucomatous outflow pathway and oxidative stress. Exp Eye Res. 2007;84(3):389–99.

102. De La Paz MA, Epstein DL. Effect of age on superoxide dismutase activity of human trabecular meshwork. Invest Ophthalmol Vis Sci. 1996;37(9):1849–53.

103. Abu-Amero KK, Morales J, Bosley TM. Mitochondrial abnormalities in patients with primary open-angle glaucoma. Invest Ophthalmol Vis Sci. 2006;47(6):2533–41.

104. Izotti A, Saccà SC, Longobardi M, Cartiglia C. Mitochondrial damage in the trabecular meshwork of patients with glaucoma. Arch Ophthalmol. 2010;128(6):724–30.

105. Schaefer EJ, Bongard V, Beiser AS, Lamon-Fava S, Robins SJ, Au R, et al. Plasma phosphatidylcholine docosahexaenoic acid content and risk of dementia and Alzheimer disease: the Framingham Heart Study. Arch Neurol. 2006;63(11):1545–50.

106. Lee JY, Plakidas A, Lee WH, Heikkinen A, Chanmugam P, Bray G, et al. Differential modulation of Toll-like receptors by fatty acids: preferential inhibition by n-3 polyunsaturated fatty acids. J Lipid Res. 2003;44(3):479–86.

107. Chapkin RS, Kim W, Lupton JR, McMurray DN. Dietary docosahexaenoic and eicosapentaenoic acid: emerging mediators of inflammation. Prostaglandins Leukot Essent Fatty Acids. 2009;81(2–3):187–91.

108. Taylor KR, Yamasaki K, Radek KA, Di Nardo A, Goodarzi H, Golenbock D, et al. Recognition of hyaluronan released in sterile injury involves a unique receptor complex dependent on Toll-like receptor 4, CD44, and MD-2. J Biol Chem. 2007;282(25):18265–75.

109. Beutler BA. TLRs and innate immunity. Blood. 2009;113(7): 1399–407.

110. Alaish SM, Yager DR, Diegelmann RF, Cohen IK. Hyaluronic acid metabolism in keloid fibroblasts. J Pediatr Surg. 1995;30: 949–52.

111. Kasiyama K, Mitsutake N, Matsuse M, Ogi T, Saenko VA, Ujifuku A, Hirano A, Yamashita S. miR-196a downregulation increases the expression of Type I and III collagens in keloid fibroblasts. J Invest Dermatol. 2012;132(6):1597–604.

112. Liu Y, Yang D, Xiao Z, Zhang M. miRNA expression profiles in keloid tissue and corresponding normal skin tissue. Aesthetic Plast Surg. 2012;36(1):193–201.

113. Jeyapalan Z, Deng Z, Shatseva T, Fang L, He C, Yang BB. Expression of CD44 3′-untranslated region regulates endogenous microRNA functions in tumorigenesis and angiogenesis. Nucleic Acids Res. 2009;39:3026–41.

114. Acharya PS, Majumdar S, Jacob M, Hayden J, Mrass P, Weninger W, et al. Fibroblast migration is mediated by CD44-dependent TGFβ activation. J Cell Sci. 2008;121:1393–402.

115. Ziegler-Heitbrock L, Ancuta P, Crowe S, Dalod M, Grau V, Hart DN, et al. Nomenclature of monocytes and dendritic cells in blood. Blood. 2010;116(16):e74–80.

116. Ziegler-Heitbrock HW. Heterogeneity of human blood monocytes: the CD14+ CD16+ subpopulation. Immunol Today. 1996;17(9): 424–8.

117. Ellery PJ, Tippett E, Chiu YL, Paukovics G, Cameron PU, Solomon A, et al. The CD16+ monocyte subset is more permissive to infection and preferentially harbors HIV-1 in vivo. J Immunol. 2007;178(10):6581–9.

118. Feng AL, Zhu JK, Sun JT, Yang MX, Neckenig MR, Wang XW, et al. CD16+ monocytes in breast cancer patients: expanded by monocyte chemoattractant protein-1 and may be useful for early diagnosis. Clin Exp Immunol. 2011;164:57–65.

119. Urra X, Villamor N, Amaro S, Gómez-Choco M, Obach V, Oleaga L, et al. Monocyte subtypes predict clinical course and prognosis in human stroke. J Cereb Blood Flow Metab. 2009;29(5): 994–1002.

120. Sen A, Chowdhury IH, Mukhopadhyay D, Paine SK, Mukherjee A, Mondal LK, et al. Increased toll-like receptor-2 expression on nonclassic CD16+ monocytes from patients with inflammatory stage of Eales' disease. Invest Ophthalmol Vis Sci. 2011;52: 6940–8.

121. Howell GR, Soto I, Zhu X, Ryan M, Macalinao DG, Sousa GL, et al. Radiation treatment inhibits monocyte entry into the optic nerve head and prevents neuronal damage in a mouse model of glaucoma. J Clin Invest. 2012;122(4):1246–61.

122. Eshkar Sebban L, Ronen D, Levartovsky D, Elkayam O, Caspi D, Aamar S, et al. The involvement of CD44 and its novel ligand galectin-8 in apoptotic regulation of autoimmune inflammation. J Immunol. 2007;179(2):1225–35.

123. Balistreri CR, Colonna-Romano G, Lio D, Candore G, Caruso C. TLR4 polymorphisms and ageing: implications for the pathophysiology of age-related diseases. J Clin Immunol. 2009;29(4):406–15.

124. Zhang J, Sokal I, Peskind ER, Quinn JF, Jankovic J, Kenney C, et al. CSF multianalyte profile distinguishes Alzheimer and Parkinson diseases. Am J Clin Pathol. 2008;129(4):526–9.

125. Alvarado JA, Alvarado RG, Yeh RF, Franse-Carman L, Marcellino GR, Brownstein MJ. A new insight into the cellular regulation of aqueous outflow: how trabecular meshwork endothelial cells drive a mechanism that regulates the permeability of Schlemm's canal endothelial cells. Br J Ophthalmol. 2005;89(11): 1500–5.

126. Alvarado JA, Katz LJ, Trivedi S, Shifera AS. Monocyte modulation of aqueous outflow and recruitment to the trabecular meshwork

following selective laser trabeculoplasty. Arch Ophthalmol. 2010;128(6):731–7.

127. Park H, Park S, Oh Y, Park C. Nail bed hemorrhage: a clinical marker of optic disc hemorrhage in patients with glaucoma. Arch Ophthalmol. 2011;129(10):1299–304.

128. Cutolo M, Sulli A, Pizzorni C, Accardo S. Nailfold videocapillaroscopy assessment of microvascular damage in systemic sclerosis. J Rheumatol. 2000;27(1):155–60.

129. Redisch W, Messina EJ, Hughes G, McEwen C. Capillaroscopic observations in rheumatic diseases. Ann Rheum Dis. 1970;29: 244–53.

130. Tektonidou M, Kaskani E, Skopouli FN, Moutsopoulos HM. Microvascular abnormalities in Sjogren's syndrome: nailfold capillaroscopy. Rheumatology. 1999;38:826–30.

131. Stevens CW, Aravind S, Das S, Davis RL. Pharmacological characterization of LPS and opioid interactions at the toll-like receptor 4. Br J Pharmacol. 2013;168(6):1421–9.

132. Wagner EL, Grybauskas A, Burdi RA, Walker L, Yue B, Samples JR, Knepper PA. Naloxone as a neuroprotectant in glaucoma: its role in the TLR4 pathway and innate immunity. ARVO meeting E-Abstract: 3474, May 2012; Fort Lauderdale, FL.

# Index




J.R. Samples, I.I.K. Ahmed (eds.), *Surgical Innovations in Glaucoma*,
DOI 10.1007/978-1-4614-8348-9, © Springer Science+Business Media New York 2014